Applications of Nanomaterials in Agriculture, Food Science, and Medicine

Mohd Amin Bhat
Higher Education Department, Government of Jammu and Kashmir, India

Irshad Ahmad Wani
Government Degree College for Boys, Anantnag, India

Shah Ashraf
National Institute of Technology Srinagar (NIT Srinagar), India

IGI Global
PUBLISHER of TIMELY KNOWLEDGE

A volume in the Advances in Chemical and Materials Engineering (ACME) Book Series

Published in the United States of America by
IGI Global
Engineering Science Reference (an imprint of IGI Global)
701 E. Chocolate Avenue
Hershey PA, USA 17033
Tel: 717-533-8845
Fax: 717-533-8661
E-mail: cust@igi-global.com
Web site: http://www.igi-global.com

Library of Congress Cataloging-in-Publication Data

Names: Bhat, Mohd Amin, 1979- editor. | Wani, Irshad Ahmad, 1983- editor. | Shah, Mohammad Ashraf, 1968- editor.
Title: Applications of nanomaterials in agriculture, food science, and medicine / Mohd Amin Bhat, Irshad Ahmad Wani, and Mohammad Ashraf Shah, editors.
Description: Hershey, PA : Engineering Science Reference, an imprint of IGI Global, [2021] | Includes bibliographical references and index. | Summary: "This book examines applications of nanomaterials in agriculture, food science, and medicine"-- Provided by publisher.
Identifiers: LCCN 2020009639 (print) | LCCN 2020009640 (ebook) | ISBN 9781799855637 (hardcover) | ISBN 9781799855644 (paperback) | ISBN 9781799855651 (ebook)
Subjects: LCSH: Nanostructured materials--Industrial applications.
Classification: LCC TA418.9.N35 A6667 2021 (print) | LCC TA418.9.N35 (ebook) | DDC 620.1/15--dc23
LC record available at https://lccn.loc.gov/2020009639
LC ebook record available at https://lccn.loc.gov/2020009640

This book is published in the IGI Global book series Advances in Chemical and Materials Engineering (ACME) (ISSN: 2327-5448; eISSN: 2327-5456)

British Cataloguing in Publication Data
A Cataloguing in Publication record for this book is available from the British Library.

For electronic access to this publication, please contact: eresources@igi-global.com.

Advances in Chemical and Materials Engineering (ACME) Book Series

J. Paulo Davim
University of Aveiro, Portugal

ISSN:2327-5448
EISSN:2327-5456

MISSION

The cross disciplinary approach of chemical and materials engineering is rapidly growing as it applies to the study of educational, scientific and industrial research activities by solving complex chemical problems using computational techniques and statistical methods.

The **Advances in Chemical and Materials Engineering (ACME) Book Series** provides research on the recent advances throughout computational and statistical methods of analysis and modeling. This series brings together collaboration between chemists, engineers, statisticians, and computer scientists and offers a wealth of knowledge and useful tools to academics, practitioners, and professionals through high quality publications.

COVERAGE

- Ceramics and glasses
- Metallic Alloys
- Polymers Engineering
- Heat Treatments
- Coatings and surface treatments
- Multifuncional and Smart Materials
- Computational methods
- Biomaterials
- Toxicity of Materials
- Electrochemical and Corrosion

IGI Global is currently accepting manuscripts for publication within this series. To submit a proposal for a volume in this series, please contact our Acquisition Editors at Acquisitions@igi-global.com or visit: http://www.igi-global.com/publish/.

The Advances in Chemical and Materials Engineering (ACME) Book Series (ISSN 2327-5448) is published by IGI Global, 701 E. Chocolate Avenue, Hershey, PA 17033-1240, USA, www.igi-global.com. This series is composed of titles available for purchase individually; each title is edited to be contextually exclusive from any other title within the series. For pricing and ordering information please visit http://www.igi-global.com/book-series/advances-chemical-materials-engineering/73687. Postmaster: Send all address changes to above address.

Titles in this Series

For a list of additional titles in this series, please visit: http://www.igi-global.com/book-series/advances-chemical-materials-engineering/73687

Technology Development for Adsorptive Heat Energy Converters Emerging Research and Opportnities
Kostyantyn M. Sukhyy (Ukrainian State University of Chemical Engineering, Ukraine) Elena A. Belyanovskaya (Ukrainian State University of Chemical Engineering, Ukraine) and Mikhailo P. Sukhyy (Ukrainian State University of Chemical Engineering, Ukraine)
Engineering Science Reference • © 2021 • 305pp • H/C (ISBN: 9781799844327) • US $195.00

Nanotechnologies and Clusters in the Spaces of Higher Dimension Emerging Research and Opportunities
Gennadiy Vladimirovich Zhizhin (Independent Researcher, Russia)
Engineering Science Reference • © 2021 • 286pp • H/C (ISBN: 9781799837848) • US $195.00

Advanced Surface Coating Techniques for Modern Industrial Applications
Supriyo Roy (Haldia Institute of Technology, India) and Goutam Kumar Bose (Haldia Institute of Technology, India)
Engineering Science Reference • © 2021 • 342pp • H/C (ISBN: 9781799848707) • US $215.00

Handbook of Research on Advancements in Supercritical Fluids Applications for Sustainable Energy Systems
Lin Chen (Institute of Engineering Thermophysics, Chinese Academy of Sciences, China & University of Chinese Academy of Sciences, China)
Engineering Science Reference • © 2021 • 821pp • H/C (ISBN: 9781799857969) • US $415.00

Inspiration and Design for Bio-Inspired Surfaces in Tribology Emerging Research and Opportunities
Hisham Abdel-Aal (Drexel University, USA)
Engineering Science Reference • © 2021 • 367pp • H/C (ISBN: 9781799816478) • US $195.00

Advanced Applications of 2D Nanostructures
Subhash Singh (National Institute of Technology Jamshedpur, India) and Kartikey Verma (Indian Institute of Technology, Kanpur, India)
Engineering Science Reference • © 2020 • 300pp • H/C (ISBN: 9781799829911) • US $225.00

Innovative Applications of Layered Materials and Structures
Sarmila Sahoo (Heritage Institute of Technology, Kolkata, India)
Engineering Science Reference • © 2020 • 300pp • H/C (ISBN: 9781799835875) • US $225.00

IGI Global
PUBLISHER of TIMELY KNOWLEDGE

701 East Chocolate Avenue, Hershey, PA 17033, USA
Tel: 717-533-8845 x100 • Fax: 717-533-8661
E-Mail: cust@igi-global.com • www.igi-global.com

Table of Contents

Detailed Table of Contents

In modern research, nanotechnology is a very attractive technology and helps to reduce infectious diseases. Nanoparticles have gained significantly more important than the bulk counterparts due to their unique properties. This chapter gives knowledge about the general introduction of nanoparticles with classification and also discussed the effect of nanoparticles impact on public health. Nanotechnology is most widely used to reduced different types of infectious diseases such as bacterial, viral, parasitic diseases, etc. Nanotechnology is applied to detect different types of diseases such as cancer, diabetes, and other diseases. Nanotechnology is a useful technique to develop novel drug delivery systems due to their high specificity, high drug-carrying capacity, and high stability. Nanotechnology can be able to improve human health but on the other hand, we have seen a negative impact on human health and environmental health. The solubility and toxicity of nanoparticles is a major issue worldwide.

Nanotechnology has emerged as one of the most promising tools for the present revolution in the field of agri-food sector. Engineered nano materials (ENMs) are a part of nanotechnology which has led to the invention of smart and active materials such as nanosensors, nanofertilizers, nanopesticides, etc. Bioinspired and biosynthesis approach for the synthesis of nanomaterials using various eco-friendly green chemistry methods has overcome the various problem associated with the use of toxic chemicals and harsh reaction conditions. Thus, use of these nanomaterial in this sector has tremendously increased the crop yield and quality thereby reducing the use of toxic crop protecting agents.

Bacterial contamination is an unusual menace for human well-being. Nanotechnology proposes diverse techniques to nurture new inorganic antibacterial agents. Nano-inorganic metal oxides possess an auspicious potential to diminish bacterial effluence. Magnesium oxide (MgO) is a significant inorganic oxide and has been widely employed in numerous arenas such as catalysis, ceramics, toxic waste remediation, antibacterial activity, and as an additive in paint and superconductor products by virtue of its distinctive properties. Numerous studies have shown that magnesium oxide nanostructures possess remarkable antibacterial activity. Therefore, in this direction, few synthesis methods such as hydrothermal method, sol-gel method, etc., antibacterial activity, and antibacterial mechanisms of magnesium oxide nanostructures have been incorporated in this chapter.

Nanotechnology as an emerging scientific field has enabled humanity to manipulate the environment at molecular and atomic level and has touched and even revolutionized all scientific fields due to its characteristic features. Medicine is one of the important fields that witnessed a nanotechnological revolution that guided medical scientists to device new approaches to study pathologies and explore genuine therapeutic tricks by exploring nanotechnology to operate on more specific molecular targets and to reduce the adverse risks and side effects imposed by the conventional approaches. By manipulating drugs and other materials, the fundamental properties and bioactivity of the materials can be altered at the nano scale. These tools can led to the different characteristics of drugs or agents such as a) modulation in solubility and blood pool retention time, b) controlled release over short or long durations, c) environmentally triggered controlled release or highly specific site-targeted deliver.

Nanotechnology offers multiple benefits. Nanomedicine and nanodelivery systems are relatively new areas in nanotechnology. There are number of outstanding applications of the nanomedicine in diagnosing diseases, delivering drugs to its target location, and thus treating human diseases. Here materials in the nanoscale range are employed to serve as means of diagnostic tools and also to deliver precise medicines to specific targeted sites in a controlled manner. Also, metal nanoparticles offer great interest in modern chemistry and materials research because of their applications in diverse fields such as photochemistry, nanoelectronics, optics, and catalysis. Chemistry provides various nanostructured materials either synthetic or isolated from natural sources offers opportunities and challenges in drug delivery and their applications including biomedical imaging, biosensing, diagnostic, and therapy. Thymoquinone, a bioactive compound in Nigella sativa, after encapsulation in lipid nanocarrier, has been found to show six-fold increase in bioavailability in comparison to free thymoquinone. In addition to this, organic nanomaterials have recently become of great interest for photovoltaic applications also.

Among various nanoparticles (NPs), gold nanoparticles (GNPs) gained valuable attention in the field of medicine because of some unique properties like small size and high surface area-to-volume ratio, inert nature, stability, high dispersity, non-cytotoxicity, and biocompatibility. These NPs are evolving as promising agents especially in drug carriers, cancer therapy, and constantly being exploring as photothermal agents, contrast agents, and radiosensitisers. Besides, GNPs interact with thiols that provides an effective and selective means of controlled intracellular release. At the present, cancer patients are increasing rapidly at national and international levels. In this chapter, efforts have taken to highlight the importance of GNPs, their critical mediation in drug delivery, as sensors for probing and imaging tumors and anti-angiogenesis. More importantly, this short piece of analysis highlights the photothermal effect of GNPs in therapy and as radiosensitizers. Finally, the current challenges and future perspectives of GNP's in cancer management are also discussed.

Metamaterials are novel artificial materials with periodic arrangement of structural meta-atoms which exhibit unique properties. Field localization and enhancement at the surface of the meta-atoms allow the structure to be an effective tool for sensing applications. This chapter discusses the emerging field of nanostructured electromagnetic metamaterials in sensing applications. The first section introduces nanostructured metamaterials based on their structures, properties, and fabrication techniques. The following section encompasses the applications of metamaterial-based nano-sensors in medicine and food science. For biomedical sensing, the applications of metamaterial-based nano biosensors in medical field are highlighted. For food science sensing, the applications of nano metamaterials in food contamination detection and food quality control are discussed. The last section discusses the future trends of nanostructured metamaterials in shifting towards reconfigurable, controllable, and multi-functional meta-devices.

As the energy demand is rapidly increasing worldwide, one of the main challenges of this century is to fulfill the energy needs for the sustenance of life. There is clearly an urgent need to develop alternative renewable energy harvesting technologies. This chapter emphasizes nano-structured materials which hold the key to fundamental advances in energy storage and conversion. Nano-structured materials offer unique properties as electrodes and electrolytes in a range of energy devices. Among the fundamental technologies in energy storage and conversion influenced by nanostructured materials, photovoltaic cells, lithium ion batteries, supercapacitors, and electro catalysts for fuel cells are highlighted in this chapter. The principles involved for hydrogen generation and nanostructured materials used for photocatalytic hydrogen generation are also discussed.

The possibility of both energy and environmental crisis that may arise due to use of fossil fuels has resulted in intense research activities in the past decade on the development of technologies for harvesting and storage of energy from renewable sources. In order to meet the energy requirements for an ever-increasing population, there is a need for high performance electrochemical energy harvesting as well as storage devices. Nanomaterials and nanocomposites with diverse composition, structure, and morphologies have been applied in various energy related applications ranging from photocatalytic hydrogen generation, solar electricity generation, electric energy storage by lithium ion batteries and supercapacitors, hydrogen storage systems, etc. The aim of this chapter is to provide an overview of the recent developments in the technological advancements brought about by the use of nanotechnology in energy harvesting and storage appliances with specific focus on dye sensitized solar cells for electricity generation, lithium ion batteries, and supercapacitors for energy storage.

Renewable energy resources have been investigated as alternatives to fossil fuels. Though the energy density of these renewable sources is not comparable to the fossil fuels, their abundance make them highly interesting. There are three main steps in the renewable energy utilization: harvesting, conversion, and storage. Thus, after harvesting renewable energy, storing this energy is an important aspect for its large-scale end use. Considering the fact that the energy is a basic need for life on earth, there has been a strong scientific temperament towards the renewable energy utilization. The electrical energy storage maintains the key to promote the use of renewable energy. Among the storage devices, the rechargeable lithium ion batteries (LIBs) are the most promising energy storage devices. Among various cathodes proposed for LIBs, the most promising one is the spinel lithium manganese oxide (LiMn2O4). Its non-toxicity, low cost, abundance, and ease of synthesis, besides being environmentally friendly, make it suitable for next generation green LIBs.

The 21st century has seen a massive spring up in the applications of nanobiotechnology. Incorporation of functionalized and modified nanostructures in various biomedical applications has generated significant research interests such as implant and tissue engineering, diagnosis, and therapy, thereby aiding in improvement of human health. The unique properties of nanoparticles including non-toxicity and biocompatibility with a large surface area make it possible to modify their surface with different chemicals including different polymers, antibodies, and drug molecules. Therefore, they are utilized for targeted drug delivery in order to carry drugs and selectively release them in desired tissues which reduces destructive effects on healthy cells. This chapter mainly covers the basic properties of nanoparticles including nanomedicine, their preparation and focuses on their diagnosis, and therapeutic applications in disease including cancer and other challenging ailments.

Nano particles (NPs) have superior properties and hence can be used for various applications. The cold storage is most widely used in the preservation of agricultural and horticultural products. The cold storage maybe operated by vapour compression or vapour absorption cooling system. The operating cost of this system can be reduced by using renewable energy systems and thermal energy storage systems. The NPs are used to increase the performance of renewable energy and thermal storage systems. In recent years, phase change materials are used to increase heat transfer rate in solar cold storage units. The NPs can be used to absorb the ethylene gas produced during storage of fruits, so that the shelf life, freshness, firmness, and texture of the fruits can be maintained for longer storage duration. The NPs coatings also increases the shelf life and freshness of the fruits. This chapter discusses NPs, types of NPs, basics of cold storage systems, use of NPs in solar integrated cold storage, and effect of NPs coatings on fruits stored in cold storage.

Preface

The first was the industrial revolution in late 18th and early 19th century, when man learned to harness matter at the millimeter scale (thousandth of a meter) with the invention like steam engine. The second technological revolution occurred in the mid twentieth century with the microelectronics, when man harnessed matter at the micrometer scale (millionth of a meter). The twentieth century has witnessed revolution in science and technology. The invention of lasers, computers and transistors has resulted in new technologies that have transformed our society, which we are witnessing. Discoveries have spanned the entire universe, from the world of very small to the world of very large and very complex. Quantum theory, relativity, new dimensions in time and space and expanding universe are examples that have transformed human thought and are the basis for the new quests for new frontiers.

The third technological revolution has already been taking place in the twenty first century with the rise of nanotechnology, which will enable man to control matter at the atomic scale that at billionth of a meter. In the twenty first century, new discoveries are being made at a dazzling speed and these discoveries are finding way in our day to day life. It has affected the society in every respect--- human health (medicine), human information (internet), human existence (environment) and human survival. Globalization drives the integration of human resources, capital and technology, making it impossible for any nation to influence the global economy in the significant way without a strong science base. The nano era may remove the barrier further and life may acquire a seamless link with nature. It will offer better built, longer lasting, cleaner, safer and smarter products for home, for communication, for medicine, for transportation, for agriculture and for industry in general. Such potential strides explain why nanotechnology is viewed as key to future economic growth and why technologically advanced countries and developing countries are earnestly pursuing its development.

In recent past, nanotechnology has gained good momentum in agriculture by providing new agrochemical agents and promises to reduce pesticide applications. In order to improve the crop production, it has also provided new delivery systems. In order to improve crop production and quality, Nanotechnology is working to provide nano formulations of agrochemicals, nanodevices for plant genetic engineering and plant disease diagnostics. Precision farming is being introduced using nanotechnology to improve the crop yields with no damage done to soil and water. This can also preserve the soil microorganisms and reduce the nitrogen loss due to leaching. Nanotechnology is also applied in agriculture to minimize the spraying of plant protection agents. The rising concerns about the quality and health benefits of food have compelled the research community to find the ways to improve both the quality and nutritional values of the food. In this regard, nanotechnology has come to the rescue and has revolutionized the food sector over the past few decades in terms of quality and nutritional value.

Nanoparticle based food products have been incorporated in the market which contains essential ingredients. Such nano based food products have been found to be stable at higher temperatures. Nanotechnology has offer complete solution from food manufacturing, food processing to packaging. Many nanotechnology research organizations are coming up with novel techniques that have not only enhanced the quality and safety of food products and there health benefits. Despite promising developments in food technology, there are still many issues which need to be addressed like devising tools to analyze the safety of nanoparticles in consumer food products.

Nanotechnology has its applications in medical sector. Nanomaterials have been used in medical sector for various applications like bio-tagging or labeling, drug delivery etc, since size of nanoparticles lies in the size domain as that of most biomolecules such as proteins and DNA. Mostly biological or molecular coatings such as antibodies, biopolymers are used on the surface of nanoparticles as interfaces for interaction with the biological targets. Due to the unique optical properties of nanoparticles they are also used in optical detection techniques in biological research to visualize some specific type of infected or target cells. The various physicochemical properties of nanomaterials can affect their interaction with the biological systems such as cells, other animals, humans and environment and may exert adverse effects on human health and the environment, which needs to be evaluated at greater details.

These fields are strongly interlinked with the nano-world. It is necessary to make our studies more interdisciplinary in order to enable us to understand the world of nano-science. A basic understanding of these diverse disciplines through nanotechnologies will help the researchers to develop and potentially change the way of living in near future by an appreciation of the wider aspects of sciences and technologies involved in it. The book will provide an opportunity to the researchers and experts of same and other fields to acquire an over view of principles and utilities of nanotechnologies in agriculture and health sectors. This book covers a wide range of topics such as "Synthesis and Characterization of Nanomaterials", "Nanomaterials in Health and Medicine", "Nanostructured Materials for Sensing Applications", "Nanomaterials for Efficient Energy Harvesting, Conversion and Storage" "Nanomaterials in Cold Storage" "Nanomaterials for Food Packaging and Agriculture", "Applications of Nanomaterials for Environmental Remediation".

The various topics given in this book are detailed enough to accumulate and capture the interest of curious readers and at the same time to motivate them further exploration of the subjects in future. A brief summary of each chapter in the book is presented here.

Chapter 1, "Molecularly Imprinted Nanomaterial-Based Surface Plasmon Resonance Biosensors in Molecular Diagnosis," describes the development of new generation analytical techniques in the diagnosis. In contrast, biosensors are performed quick and selective detection of various markers. This chapter primarily focuses on the status and applications of nano-MIP based SPR biosensors for the molecular diagnosis.

Chapter 2, "Nanotechnology and Its Applications in Environmental Remediation," explains the efficacy of nanotechnology in environmental remediation. The use of nanotechnology to enhance the performance of remediation processes has developed research interest in modern day due to the high reactivity and environmental friendliness associated with nanoparticles. This book chapter explores the science behind the application of nanotechnology in environmental remediation, the processes used in decontaminating environmental media and the various categories of nanomaterials. Various examples based on literature are used to enhance insight on the subject.

Chapter 3, "Nanostructured Electromagnetic Metamaterials for Sensing Applications," focused on how Metamaterials are novel artificial materials with periodic arrangement of structural meta-atoms which exhibit unique properties, could be an effective tool for sensing applications. The first section introduces nanostructured metamaterials based on their structures, properties and fabrication techniques. The following section encompasses the applications of metamaterial-based nano-sensors in medicine and food science. For biomedical sensing, the applications of metamaterial-based nano biosensors in medical field are highlighted. For food science sensing, the applications of nano metamaterials in food contamination detection and food quality control are discussed. The last section discusses the future trends of nanostructured metamaterials in shifting towards reconfigurable, controllable and multi-functional meta-devices.

Chapter 4, "Nanomaterials for Food and Agriculture," briefly explains how nanotechnology has emerged as one of the most promising tools for the present revolution in the field of agri-food sector. Engineered Nano Materials (ENMs) are a part of nanotechnology which has led to the invention of smart and active materials such as nano-sensors, nanofertilizers, nanopesticides etc. Bio-inspired and biosynthesis approach for the synthesis of nanomaterials using various Eco-friendly green chemistry methods has overcome the various problems associated with the use of toxic chemicals and harsh reaction conditions. Thus, use of these nanomaterials in this sector has tremendously increased the crop yield and quality thereby reducing the use of toxic crop protecting agents.

Chapter 5, "Magnesium Oxide (MgO): A Viable Agent for Antimicrobial Activity," deals with the various strategies related to new inorganic antibacterial agents. Nano-inorganic metal oxides possess an auspicious potential to diminish bacterial effluence. Magnesium oxide (MgO) is a significant inorganic oxide and has been widely employed in numerous arenas such as catalysis, ceramics, toxic waste remediation, antibacterial activity and as an additive in paint and superconductor products by virtue of its distinctive properties. Numerous studies have shown that magnesium oxide nanostructures possess remarkable antibacterial activity. Therefore, in this direction, few synthesis methods such as hydrothermal method, sol-gel method, etc., antibacterial activity and antibacterial mechanisms of magnesium oxide nanostructures have been incorporated in this chapter.

Chapter 6, "Nanotechnology as an Emerging Field in the Arena of Medicine," explains efficacy of nanotechnology as an emerging scientific field has enabled humanity to manipulate the environment at molecular and atomic level and has touched and even revolutionized all scientific fields due to its characteristic features. Medicine is one of the important fields that witnessed a nanotechnological revolution that guided medical scientists to manipulate drugs and other materials, the fundamental properties and bioactivity of the materials can be altered at the nano scale. This chapter briefly explains how the tools can led to the different characteristics of drugs or agents such as: a) modulation in solubility and blood pool retention time, b) controlled release over short or long durations, c) environmentally triggered controlled release or highly specific site-targeted deliver.

Chapter 7, "Applications of Organic Chemistry in Nano-Medicine: Current and Future Prospects," focuses how organic chemistry provides various nanostructured materials either synthetic or isolated from natural sources offers opportunities and challenges in drug delivery and their applications including biomedical imaging, biosensing, diagnostic and therapy. The organic chemistry molecule "Thymoquinone" a bioactive compound in extracted *from Nigella sativa*, after encapsulation in lipid nano-carrier has been found to show six-fold increase in bioavailability in comparison to free thymoquinone. In addition to this organic nanomaterials have recently become of great interest for photovoltaic applications also.

Chapter 8, "Role of Gold Nanoparticles in Drug Delivery and Cancer Therapy," focuses on recent advances and current challenges of gold nanoparticles (GNP's) which gained valuable attention in the field of medicine because of some unique properties like small size and high surface area-to-volume ratio, inert nature, stability, high dispersity, non-cytotoxicity and biocompatibility. These NP's are evolving as promising agents especially in drug carriers, cancer therapy and constantly being exploring as photo thermal agents, contrast agents and radio-sensitizers. In this book chapter efforts have taken to highlight the importance of GNP's, their critical mediation in drug delivery, as sensors for probing and imaging tumors and anti-angiogenesis. More importantly, this short piece of analysis highlight the photo thermal effect of GNP's in therapy and as radio sensitizers. Finally, the current challenges and future perspectives of GNP's in cancer management are also discussed.

Chapter 9, "Nanomaterials Useful in Health and Medicine to Improve Public Health," describes the development of modern research in nanotechnology which is a very attractive technology and helps to reduce infectious diseases. Nanoparticles have gained significantly more important than bulk counterparts due to their unique properties. This chapter gives knowledge about the general introduction of nanoparticles with classification and also discussed the effect of nanoparticles impact on public health. Nanotechnology is applied to detect different types of diseases such as cancer, diabetes and other diseases. Nanotechnology is a useful technique to develop novel drug delivery systems due to their high specificity, high drug-carrying capacity, and high stability.

Chapter 10, "Nano-Structured Materials for Efficient Energy Storage and Conversion," is a resurgence of interest in food science due to high energy demand worldwide, which could be fulfilled by developing alternative renewable energy harvesting technologies. This chapter emphasizes nano-structured materials which hold the key to fundamental advances in energy storage and conversion. As nano-structured materials offer unique properties as electrodes and electrolytes in a range of energy devices. Among the fundamental technologies in energy storage and conversion influenced by nanostructured materials, photovoltaic cells, lithium ion batteries, super capacitors and electro catalysts for fuel cells are highlighted in this chapter. The principles involved for hydrogen generation and nanostructured materials used for photo catalytic hydrogen generation are also discussed.

Chapter 11, "Nanomaterials for Energy Harvesting and Storage: An overview," focuses how both energy and environmental crisis that may arise due to use of fossil fuels has resulted in intense research activities in the past decade on the development of technologies for harvesting and storage of energy from renewable sources. The aim of this chapter is to provide an overview of the recent developments in the technological advancements brought about by the use of nanotechnology in energy harvesting and storage appliances with specific focus on dye sensitized solar cells for electricity generation, lithium ion batteries and super capacitors for energy storage.

Chapter 12, "Application of $LiMn_2O_4$ Nanostructures as Efficient Cathodes for Energy Storage Devices," focused on how renewable energy resources could be used as alternatives energy for fossil fuels. Considering the fact that the energy is a basic need for life on earth, there has been a strong scientific temperament towards the renewable energy utilization. The electrical energy storage maintains the key to promote the use of renewable energy. Among the storage devices, the rechargeable lithium ion batteries (LIBs) are the most promising energy storage devices. Among various cathodes proposed for LIBs, the most promising one is the spinel lithium manganese oxide (LiMn2O4). Its non-toxicity, low cost, abundance and ease of synthesis, besides being environmental friendly makes it suitable for next generation green LIBs.

Chapter 13, "Nanomaterials Clinical and Therapeutical Approaches in Drug Delivery System," focuses on the applications of nanobiotechnology Nanotechnology is a branch of science which deals with the engineering of functional systems at the molecular level and there target at diverse fields along with broad range of applicability i.e. surface science, organic chemistry, molecular engineering, nano-medicine, bio-materials and many more. Medical science has latterly advanced to the point where diagnosis and therapeutics can be carried out with high precision, even at the molecular level and there use clinical approaches and also explore role of nanomaterials in drug delivery.

Chapter 14, "Applications of Nanomaterials in Cold Storage," explains the efficacy of nano particles (NPs) could be used in preservation of agricultural and horticultural products in cold storage. This book chapter discusses NPs, types of NPs, basics of cold storage systems, use of NPs in solar integrated cold storage and effect of NPs coatings on fruits stored in cold storage.

Chapter15, "Nanomaterials in Food Packaging," is capable itself to solve the complex set of engineering and scientific challenges in food industry due to their size-dependent properties, high surface area, longer retention, easy absorption, and unique optical properties. The role of nanomaterials have been extended for increasing the stability and bioavailability of nutrients, encapsulation of flavors, bioactive, enhancing the physical and mechanical properties of food packaging (nanocomposites), pesticide and growth hormone delivery, antimicrobial agents to boost preservation of foodstuffs, detection of food borne pathogens, biodegradable nano-sensors for monitoring of temperature and moisture, etc. There are various types of nanomaterials like nanoparticles, nano-emulsions, and nano-clays which are synthesized by several methods to be used in the food industry. However, there is some food safety concerns associated with these nanomaterials when used in food systems. It is, therefore, very necessary to formulate and develop some method for the detection of nanomaterials, in particular when used in-vivo which are briefly discussed in this chapter.

Chapter 16, "Routes of Synthesis and Characterizations of Nanoparticles," explains briefly various synthesis procedures of nanomaterials across a range of sizes, shapes and chemical compositions. This chapter will concentrate on the different methods such as electron irradiation, laser ablation, and chemical reduction, biological methods, photochemical methods; microwave processing, Chemical Vapour Condensation (CVC), arc discharge, hydrogen plasma-metal reaction, and laser pyrolysis in the vapour phase. This chapter will also elaborate briefly regarding various characterization techniques for the conformation of nanomaterials such as UV-visible spectroscopy, X-ray diffraction, and electron microscopy (e.g. Transmission Electron Microscopy [TEM], Scanning Electron Microscopy [SEM], and Atomic Force Microscopy [AFM]).

Chapter 17, "Role of Nanostructured Materials in Health and Medicine," refers applications of nanotechnology in many devices which are devised at a lightning speed, which were earlier impossible to imagine. Nanotechnology offers multiple benefits in treating chronic human diseases by cite specific and target oriented delivery of precise medicines. This chapter describes the importance of nanoparticle based devices like nano-tubes, quantum dots, carbon nano-tubes, dendrimers etc and their applications for the treatment of several diseases. Applications of nanoparticles in drug delivery, tuberculosis treatment and cancer therapy are also explained in this chapter. Nanomedicines can also be used to detect diseases at much earlier stages.

Chapter 18 , "Implication of Nanoparticles in Drosophila Toxicology Research," focuses on how wide variety of nano particles and their impact on Drosophila melanogastsr's development, longevity, and characteristics of reproduction has been studied could be useful in the future research in modern scientific world.

Mohd Amin Bhat
Higher Education Department, Government of Jammu and Kashmir, India

Irshad Ahmad Wani
Government Degree College for Boys, Anantnag, India

Shah Ashraf
National Institute of Technology Srinagar (NIT Srinagar), India

Chapter 1
Molecularly-Imprinted Nanomaterial-Based Surface Plasmon Resonance Biosensors in Molecular Diagnosis

Emir Alper Türkoğlu
https://orcid.org/0000-0001-7850-6456
University of Health Sciences Turkey, Turkey

ABSTRACT

Molecular diagnosis is based on target detection associated with many diseases and abnormalities. Common analytical techniques have disadvantages in the diagnosis. In contrast, biosensors are performed quick and selective detection of various markers. Surface plasmon resonance (SPR) biosensor allows qualitative and quantitative measurements without labelling and frequently used in medical applications. Recent developments in various emerging disciplines have allowed the design of novel bioreceptors for SPR biosensors. In recent years, the use of bioreceptors combined with nanotechnology and molecular imprinting technologies has increased in SPR instruments. Molecularly imprinted polymers (MIPs) are synthetic polymeric materials and provide specific and selective recognition sites for the target of interest. MIPs as bioreceptor show unique features compared to natural receptors. Therefore, MIP-based bioreceptors in SPR sensors have gained more attention recently. This chapter primarily focuses on the status and applications of nano-MIP-based SPR biosensors for the molecular diagnosis.

INTRODUCTION

The talk of Richard Feynman titled 'There's plenty of room at the bottom' has induced to open a new era known as nanotechnology. Feynman never used the term 'nanotechnology' in his speech, but what Feynman meant by 'plenty of room' was the possible predictions of what we want to happen in the future when we exceed our molecular limits (Toumey, 2009). The term of nano originates from the Greek word of 'nanos' which means 'dwarf' (Dagar & Bagchi, 2020). Nanotechnology is the synthesis, design,

DOI: 10.4018/978-1-7998-5563-7.ch001

production and characterization of material, device and system with at least one dimension is on one nano nanometer equal to one billionth of a meter (Sahoo, Parveen, & Panda, 2007). Nanotechnology have applications in the areas of environment, agriculture, engineering, food science, security, space and medicine (Bhattacharyya, Singh, & Satnalika, 2009). Nanotechnology based therapies and diagnostics are two major application areas of this discipline for medical sciences (Saxena, Nyodu, Kumar, & Maurya, 2020).

Molecular diagnosis is based on bio-interactions between molecular targets and specific receptors. The selectivity in these interactions is important for the effectiveness of diagnosis. Effective selectivity enables the desired reliable measurement, quantification and validation in molecular diagnosis (Johnson, Zhukovsky, Cass, & Nagy, 2008). Nanotechnology-based disciplines and rapid advances in these disciplines have led to significant advances in diagnostic techniques. Nanomaterial-based molecular detection systems increase the speed, sensitivity, reliability, flexibility and reusability of diagnosis (Syedmoradi et al., 2017). Nanotechnology based diagnostic systems have detected biological targets which cannot be detected by some conventional techniques and provided more effective decision-making in the disease process, reduced treatment costs and effective treatment in early diagnosis. In addition, a cost-effective analysis process is carried out by working with small sample volumes with the use of nanomaterials as ligand. Although genomics, proteomic and microarray-based detection systems have been widely used, these techniques have some limitations in use. However, nanotechnology based biosensing systems have been the most outstanding candidates in molecular diagnosis (Jain, 2005).

BIOSENSORS

In recent decades, all human beings need certain early detection systems for the quality of their life due to the dramatic incidence of some metabolic diseases, cancer and exposed toxic substances with the rapidly growing world population (Ruzzin, 2012; Van Gosen, Blitz, Plumlee, Meeker, & Pierson, 2013; Wolf et al., 2010). There are several established techniques available for diagnosis of diseases such as biopsies, immunohistochemistry, fluorescent in situ hybridization analysis, ELISA, PCR and positron emission tomography. These techniques have the advantage of performing in low detection limits (Tsé, Gauchez, Jacot, & Lamy, 2012). However, these techniques have some drawbacks due to the need for trained personnel for the operation, the high cost of analysis, time-consuming procedures and lack of site-specific detection (Malhotra, Kumar, & Pandey, 2016). In order to overcome these problems, intensive efforts are being performed on the design of new types of analytical devices for rapid diagnosis of disease, helping better health care solutions and reducing stressful patient waiting time of clinical results dissemination with a special interest on biosensor platforms (Freitas, Nouws, & Delerue-Matos, 2018; Tothill, 2009). In recent years, great interests have been shown for biosensors by the scientific community and society due to their use in many fields such as food science, environmental interest, clinical diagnosis (da Silva et al., 2017; Mehrotra, 2016) and security (Conroy, Millner, Stewart, & Pollmann, 2010). Biosensors are analytical devices that mimic the structural, compositional and functional features of nature. The biological components react with the target analyte to produce data which is readily converted to an electrical signal by a chemical transducer (Guo, 2012). Biosensors offer practical solutions due to the advantages of their user friendly, cost-effective, rapid and multi analyte detection capabilities (Dincer et al., 2019). There are several cornerstones for medical perspective in the development of biosensor technology. The first biosensor was proposed for measuring glucose levels in 1962 by Clark and Lyons (Clark &

Lyons, 1962). Yellow Spring Instruments launched the first biosensor device in 1975 to detect blood glucose level. Suzuki et al. developed the first microbe-based biosensor in 1976 (Borgmann, Schulte, Neugebauer, & Schuhmann, 2012). Fibre-optic biosensor and first mediated amperometric biosensor to detect glucose were demonstrated by Schultz and Cass et al., respectively (Cass et al., 1984; Mansouri & Schultz, 1984). Some biosensor companies started to launch their commercial devices in 1987 and following years. Launches of MediSense ExacTech blood glucose sensor in 1987, i-STAT blood analyzer in 1992, in vivo glucose sensor by MiniMed in 1999 and wearable non-invasive biosensor for glucose monitoring by GlucoWatch were announced. In the following years, other types of biosensors have been designed to detect diseases, drugs, pollutants, pathogen bacteria and biomarkers from body fluids such as blood, urine, saliva and sweat. A typical biosensor consists of;

1. Analyte: Substance of interest to be determined.
2. Bioreceptor: Molecule and/or interface that recognize the analyte.
3. Transducer: Turns biointeraction into a measurable signal.
4. Electronics: It consists of electronic circuits. It is the part that processes the converted signal and prepares it before display.
5. Display: This section displays the data in a usable way with a combination of hardware and software (Metkar & Girigoswami, 2019).

Biosensors are classified according to their recognition elements and transducers. Receptors in biosensors are integrated to different signal transducers. Transducers convert molecular signals into an electrical or digital signal that can be quantified, viewed, or analyzed. Biosensors are mainly categorized in terms of their transducers as calorimetric, mass based, electrochemical and optical biosensors.

Electrochemical Biosensors

Electrochemical biosensors are widely used due to their low costs, portability, fast response time, high selectivity, ease of use and operation. In recent studies, electrochemical sensors are frequently designed for point-of-care analysis and can be operated even in doctor offices and/or clinics. There are two common electrochemical sensors: amperometric and potentiometric. In near future, electrochemical sensors, notably essential for personalized medicine and early diagnosis, can be integrated into small devices such as mobile phones with the effect of micro and nano fabrication processes, and they will be performed to analyze without the need for any special training (da Silva et al., 2017; Freitas et al., 2018).

Mass-Sensitive Biosensors

Piezoelectric and acoustic biosensors are two types of mass-sensitive biosensors. Piezoelectric biosensors are devices that measure mass change on the quarz crystal when potential energy is applied. The change in mass creates a frequency that is converted into a signal later. There are many investigations on the detection of cancer biomarkers by piezoelectric biosensors (Patel & Patel, 2017). In recent years, the use of new generation microcantilever based sensors has increased in cancer diagnosis. The operational principle of this sensor is based on the detection of changes in the resonant frequencies as a result of the affinity interactions of the biomolecule on the cantilever surface and the target molecule (Hansen & Thundat, 2005).

Calorimetric Biosensors

Calorimetric biosensors measure exothermic reactions. Many enzymatic processes generate heat, and heat changes are utilized to determine the target molecule concentration. Calorimetric biosensors are preferred less than other biosensor types especially in medical diagnostics. However, interest for calorimetric biosensors has been increased with the contribution of emerging technologies (Bohunicky & Mousa, 2011). It has been reported that cancerous cells have been detected by aptamer-based calorimetric biosensor (Medley et al., 2008).

Optical Biosensors

Optical biosensors are analytical sensing devices that contain optical converters using light absorption, fluorescence, luminescence, total internal reflection or surface plasmon resonance (Jerónimo, Araújo, & Conceição, 2007). In general, an optical sensor consists of a light source, a sensing platform, light waveguides, a light detector and a data processor. The working mechanism of optical sensors is based on the measuring the change of light before and after receptor interacts with the desired analyte. Changes in wavelength are converted with optical transducers and monitored as digital data and/or images as a result of analyte interaction. More effective and powerful optical sensors can be designed with the use of nano-sized receptors in the fields of environmental application, healthcare, biotechnology industry and disease diagnosis etc. (Ng, 2019). There are some types of biosensors that use optical principles (Martins et al., 2013) and surface plasmon resonance biosensors are one of optical biosensors that uses electromagnetic waves to monitor bio-interactions between the analyte and the immobilized receptor on sensor surface (Monošík, Streďanský, & Šturdík, 2012).

SURFACE PLASMON RESONANCE

A comprehensive survey of biosensor literature reveals that SPR biosensors are used in many fields from biological applications to clinical diagnosis. The basis of this success lies in the role of surface sciences in SPR sensors. At the beginning of the 20th century, the first studies on surface plasmon were carried out. Surface plasmon resonance was firstly observed by Wood in 1901 (Wood, 1902). Surface plasmon resonance phenomenon was explained by Rayleigh in 1907. Otto and Kretschmann demonstrated optical excitation of surface plasmons with the method of attenuated total reflection in 1968 (Couture, Zhao, & Masson, 2013). These marvelous investigations about the excitation of surface plasmons of Otto and Kretschmann with the studies of Raether composed a functional method in optics (Homola, 2008). In the early 1980s, Nylander *et al.* and Liedberg *et al.* used SPR sensors in gas detection and biosensing (Liedberg, Nylander, & Lunström, 1983; Nylander, Liedberg, & Lind, 1982).

The term SPR is used for the excitation and propagation of electromagnetic waves in a layer between the metal surface and the analyte. Stimulation of plasmons requires a prism for attenuated total reflection coated with a metal layer approximately 50 nm thick. Gold and silver surfaces are generally used as SPR biosensor surface (Steiner, 2004). When polarized light above a critical angle enters an environment with a higher refractive index (glass prism), it undergoes total internal reflection. In this case, the light, called self-damping wave, penetrates into the metal film. At a given refraction angle, this wave causes free electrons on the metal surface to form surface plasmon. Thus, the intensity of the reflected light decreases. This phenomenon is called surface plasmon resonance and is observed only at a certain angle called the resonance angle. The angle of resonance changes by adding analyte to the surface. This change can be made selective by modifying the surface relative to the target molecule. These processes form the basis of SPR biosensors (Situ, Mooney, Elliott, & Buijs, 2010).

Surface plasmon resonance theory is based on the principle of energy-carrying light photon coupling with electron of metal or energy transfer. The angle of light at which the energy transfer takes place varies with the features of the metal surface. Energy transfer occurs when a match and/or resonance is captured between light photons and electrons on the metal surface. This energy transfer is determined by measuring the amount of light reflected from the bottom surface of the metal film. Every light is reflected at many angles, however some of the light can be absorbed at the resonance angle. While s-polarized light cannot cause surface plasmons, only p-polarized light forms surface plasmon on metal surface (Szentirmay, 1992; Welford, 1991). Several metal surfaces can produce surface plasmon. However, it should contain suitable chemical properties for modifications required in detection purposes besides having suitable conductivity properties of metal. Gold is one of the rare metals with these two properties (Yuan et al., 2006).

SPR Biosensors

SPR biosensors have been used for real-time analysis of bio-interactions with rapid, sensitive, label free (Mittal, Kaur, Gautam, & Mantha, 2017) and low volume operation manner (Saylan, Akgönüllü, et al., 2017) in biotechnology, environmental and food monitoring (Nakamura, Hasegawa, Nakamura, & Miyake, 2003; Taylor et al., 2006; Uzun, Say, Ünal, & Denizli, 2009). Notably, the last four decades have witnessed countless efforts in the SPR biosensor technology and their applications in the fields of health-related disciplines (Ladd et al., 2004; Stigter, De Jong, & Van Bennekom, 2005). SPR based biosensors are versatile sensing platforms including the biointeractions of DNA/DNA, protein/DNA (Majka & Speck, 2006; Ritzefeld & Sewald, 2012), protein/RNA (Katsamba, Park, & Laird-Offringa, 2002), protein/protein (Karlssonz & Fält, 1997; Nikolovska-Coleska, 2015; Wegner, Lee, Marriott, & Corn, 2003), protein/carbohydrate (Duverger, Frison, Roche, & Monsigny, 2003; Linman, Taylor, Yu, Chen, & Cheng, 2008), protein/receptor (Mitchell & Wu, 2010), DNA/small molecule (Lin et al., 2005; Tsai & Hsu, 2012), biomolecule/artificial cell (Osman, Uzun, Beşirli, & Denizli, 2013; Sari, Üzek, Duman, & Denizli, 2016), ligand/artificial cell (Sari, Üzek, Duman, & Denizli, 2018; Yılmaz et al., 2017), whole cell/artificial cell (Idil, Hedström, Denizli, & Mattiasson, 2017; Yilmaz, Majidi, Ozgur, & Denizli, 2015).

Four assay approaches have been carried out in SPR biosensor according to size of analyte: (i) direct assay, (ii) sandwich assay, (iii) inhibition assay and (iv) competitive assay. In direct assay, receptors or recognition elements are immobilized to the surface and analytes interact with immobilized ligands. This assay is used for medium or large molecular weight (>10 kDa) targets (Homola et al., 2002). Other assay formats have been mainly performed to determine low molecular weight targets. In sandwich assay, a secondary recognition element is used to detect the target molecule captured by the receptor immobilized to the SPR sensor surface. The secondary recognition element is useful for improving the detection limit and verifying the captured target molecule. A molecule is attached on the surface of SPR sensor in inhibition assay format. The analyzed sample is preincubated with constant concentration of antibodies for target molecule and directed to the SPR sensor. The binding of the unreacted antibody to the molecule is determined. There is an inverse proportion between the concentration of the target molecule in the incubation solution and the sensor response. In competitive format, two samples compete to interact with the receptors immobilized to the SPR surface (Abdulhalim, Zourob, & Lakhtakia, 2008).

RECOGNITION ELEMENTS

Recognition elements are at the basis of biosensor platforms. At first, recognition elements were obtained from living organisms. However, they have been purified from living beings and also synthetically manufactured in laboratory (Chambers, Arulanandam, Matta, Weis, & Valdes, 2008). Natural recognition elements based on biomolecules such as enzymes, antibodies, nucleic acids and whole cell establish naturally evolved molecular interactions with the target molecule. These bioreceptors are classified as catalytic and affinity-based receptors according to their biological working mechanisms. While catalytic-based bioreceptors integrate with enzymes, tissues, and whole-cells, affinity-based bioreceptors interact specifically with the analyte using biomolecules such as antibodies, lectins, nucleic acids, and/ or aptamers. Interests have recently focused on affinity-based bioreceptors due to their simplicity, fast and selective detection characteristics (Farzin & Shamsipur, 2018). Although affinity-based bioreceptors possess high selectivity and specificity, they show some limitations due to their poor chemical and physical stability and low long-term stability, batch-to-batch variability, high cost and need of skilled staff (Haupt & Mosbach, 2000; Sapsford, Bradburne, Delehanty, & Medintz, 2008). In order to eliminate these limitations, efforts have focused on the design of new generation recognition elements. Imprinted polymers as synthetic receptors have become reasonable candidates to compete effectively with natural receptors. In recent studies, IgG imprinted polymer has demonstrated a binding affinity equivalent to protein A in terms of interaction with IgG (Moczko et al., 2019). Synthetic receptors interact with analyte by mimicking natural interactions. Pseudo-natural recognition elements, which are integrated with natural and artificial recognition elements, are receptors that provide recognition with a natural and synthetic approach (Morales & Halpern, 2018).

Molecular Recognition

The secret of life is hidden in molecular recognition according to Nobel winner scientist L. C. Pauling (Dabrowski, Lach, Cieplak, & Kutner, 2018). Molecular recognition is a basic biomechanism in nature (Marty & Mauzac, 2005) and has showed an important role in antibody/antigen interaction in the immune system, enzymatic processes, signal transduction in organisms and nucleic acid-based processes such as replication, transcription and translation. This unique recognition is largely run by non-covalent forces such as ionic interactions, hydrogen bonds, pi interactions, hydrophobic interactions and van der Walls forces (Chen, Piletsky, & Turner, 2002). Molecular recognition is based on the complex association between receptor and substrate exactly like the lock-and-key model first proposed by Emil Fischer. The formation between these pairs is the result of interactions between functional groups on the receptor and the substrate (analyte) (Jozefowicz & Jozefonvicz, 1997).

There have been much interests to synthesize structures that mimic or inspire molecular recognition processes in nature. Small ring systems and cage molecules including crown ethers, cryptates, cyclophanes and cyclodextrins were among the earliest studies. However, these structures have some disadvantages in preparation processes, usage and cost.

Antibodies, enzymes and receptors have been utilized in many disciplines such as affinity chromatography, immunoassay and biosensors for the detection, diagnosis and quantification of a target molecule. However, the utilization of biomolecules as recognition elements has some limitations in practice. For this reason, studies focused on new generation-materials that are more cost effective, stable, user friendly and other unique features (Table 1) (Marty & Mauzac, 2005).

Table 1. Comparison of MIPs with natural recognition elements

	MIP	Natural Recognition Element
Preparation	Easy to prepare	Time-consuming
Cost	Cost-effective	Expensive
Stability	High physicochemical stability	Low or limited stability
Storage	Long-term storage	Days at 25°C
Sensor integration	Full compatibility with several platforms	Poor compatible
Infrastructure required	Label free detection without any training	Need expensive analytical tools and trained staff

Source: (Ahmad, Bedwell, Esen, Garcia-Cruz, & Piletsky, 2019; Dabrowski et al., 2018; Kryscio & Peppas, 2012; Soper et al., 2006)

Molecular Imprinting

Molecular imprinting is an emerging discipline of creating and designing artificial recognition sites in a polymer matrix (Ahmad et al., 2019). Firstly, functional monomers are positioned to form a complex with the template in the presence of crosslinkers. Secondly, the complex is polymerized to fix the positions of functional groups. Finally, artificial recognition sites in terms of size, shape and chemical properties as well as template (analyte) are obtained by removing the template, and these sites in polymer matrix reversibly bind the analyte because of complementary and selective characteristics (Verheyen et al., 2011). Schematic representation of molecular imprinting process is given in Fig. 1.

Figure 1. Schematic illustration of molecular imprinting process

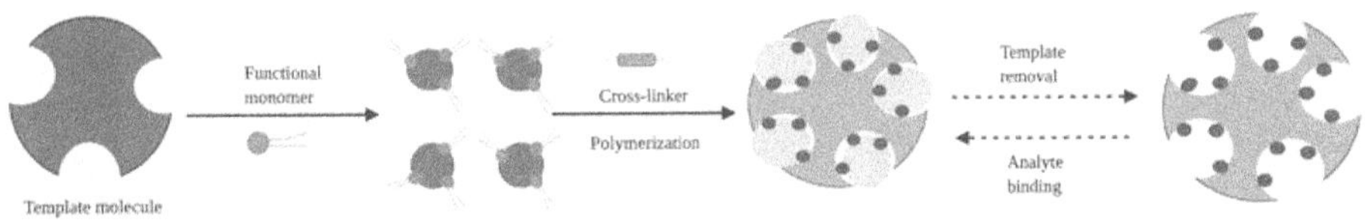

Molecular imprinting method is basically classified in three ways according to interactions between the functional monomer and the template. Complex in covalent imprinting is formed in the presence covalent interactions (Wulff, 1995). Functional monomers establish non-covalent interactions, i.e. hydrogen bonds, electrostatic interactions, hydrophobic interactions and Van der Waals forces, with the template in complexation (Ersöz, Denizli, Özcan, & Say, 2005). In the metal chelating one, the interaction between functional monomer and the template occur on the functional groups on the protein surface and the metal chelating functional monomers (Say, Ersöz, Türk, & Denizli, 2004).

Template

Template perform an active role in the arrangement of functional groups on functional monomers. Proper molecular architecture of the template provides the formation of successful recognition zones. A preferred template should possess some characteristic as (i) not containing functional groups preventing polymerization, (ii) stable and available functional groups of template molecule in polymerization process and (iii) easy bind formation with functional monomers (Pandey, Khare, Singh, & Singh, 2020). Amino acids, carbohydrates, peptides/proteins, nucleotides, hormones, cells, ions, drugs and pesticides can be used as template (Cormack & Mosbach, 1999).

Functional Monomers

Functional monomers serve the interactions to form a complex with the template. Optimization of template and functional monomer molar ratios is an important step for the effectiveness of imprinting (Pandey et al., 2020). Figure 2 illustrates the common functional monomers used in molecular imprinting approaches.

Figure 2. Structures of widely used monomers

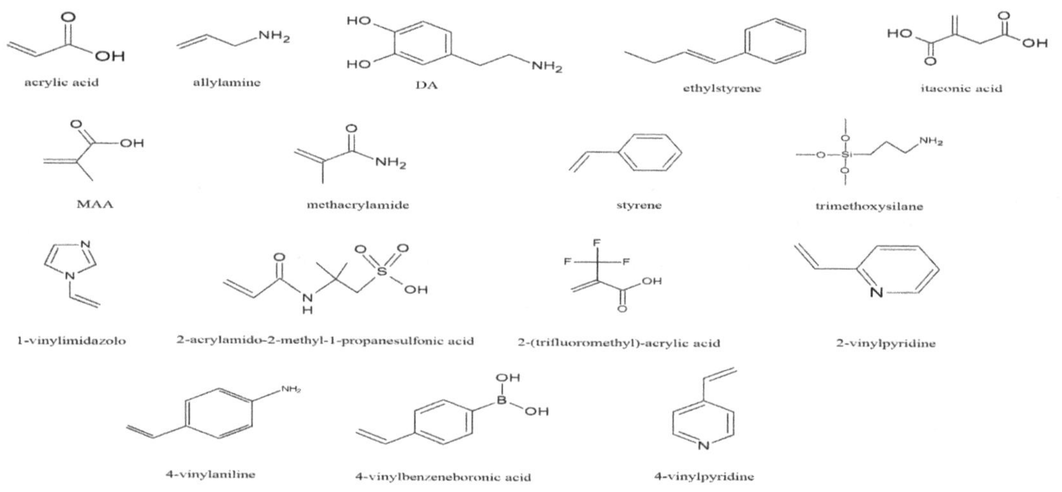

Cross-Linkers

Crosslinkers are used for the physicochemical stability of polymer. Crosslinkers interact with one or more functional monomers, therefore it is essential that they must establish non-spesific binds to the target. Water soluble or organic solvent soluble cross-linkers are successfully used in the preparation of protein imprinted polymers. Ethylene bis acrylamide (EBA) and methylene bis acrylamide (MBA) as water-soluble crosslinkers have been particularly used to design successful protein imprinting approaches (Yang, Zhang, Liang, & Zhang, 2012). The efficiency of imprinted polymers depends on the type and ratio of crosslinkers used in polymerization. It has been stated that the ratio of crosslinker and monomer should be 4:1 in the molecular imprinting process (Muhammad, Nur, Piletska, Yimit, & Piletsky, 2012). Some common cross-linkers are shown in Fig. 3.

Figure 3. Structures of common cross-linkers

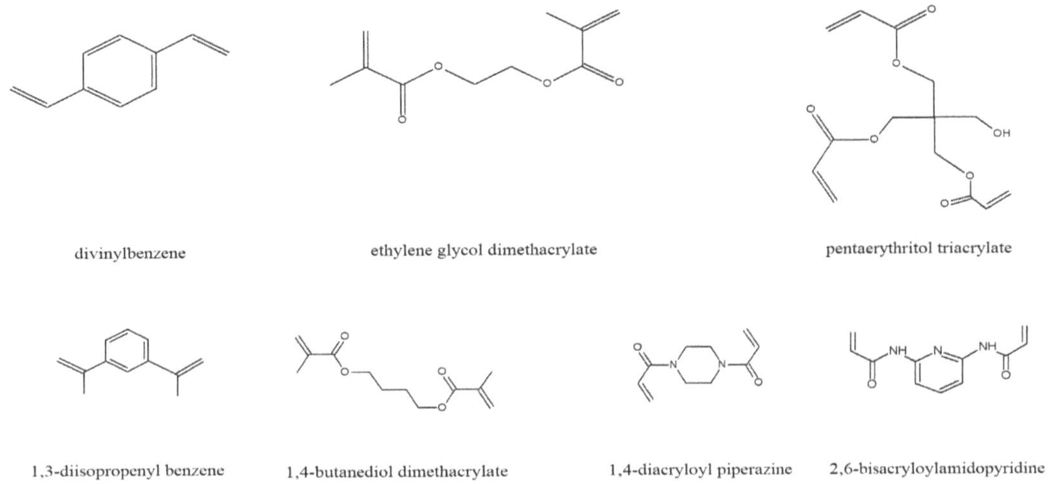

Initiators

Chemicals with certain properties are acted as initiators in free radical polymerization. The effectiveness of these chemicals depends on light, heat, chemical and/or electrochemical properties. The aim of initiator is to promote polymerization in the presence of template. The presence of oxygen is not preferred in free radical polymerization. For this reason, oxygen should be removed from the medium by ultra-sonication or an inert gas such as argon and nitrogen which pass through the medium (Pandey et al., 2020). Different initiators used in the literature are shown in Fig. 4.

Figure 4. Structure of various initiators types

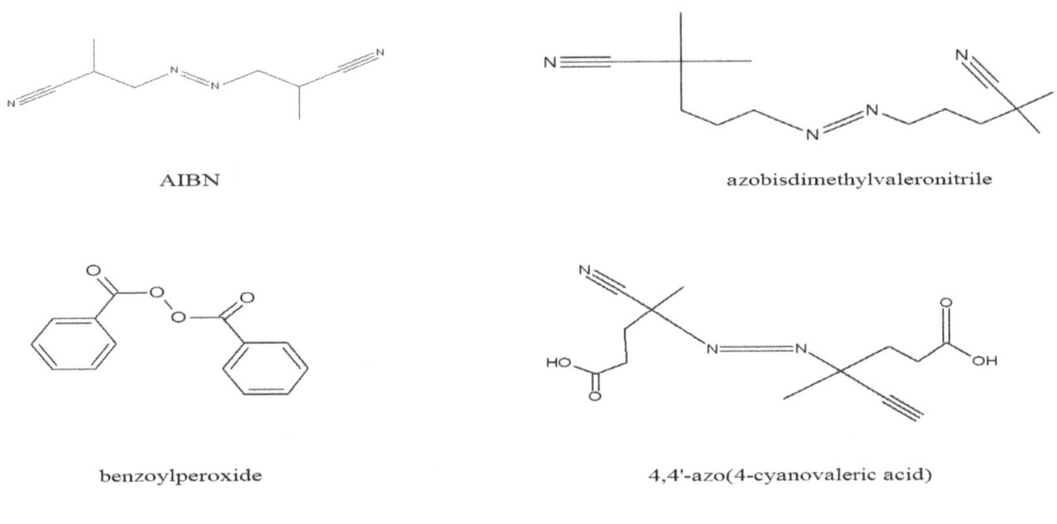

Solvents (Porogens)

Solvents are added to all polymerization media, i.e., template, functional monomer, cross-linker and initiator to bring all components into one phase. And they play significant role in the fabrication of macroporous polymers. Type and amount of porogen are important to manipulate morphology and total pore volume of macroporous polymers. While a thermodynamically good solvent contributes to the formation of polymers with well-developed pore structures and a high specific surface area, a weak solvent causes undesirable polymeric properties for the purpose. Besides these two properties, the choice of solvent should be considered in terms of bonding intensity between template and functional monomer. Toluene (Cormack & Elorza, 2004), acetonitrile, chloroform and tetrahydrofuran have been utilized for the efficiency of imprinting process (Yan & Row, 2006).

Molecularly Imprinted Polymers

Molecular imprinting of polymers is the most common, versatile, scalable and cost-effective option to use in the design of artificial molecular receptors (Ahmad et al., 2019). The imprinted molecular memory on a sensor surface provides a highly selective interaction for the target (analyte) (Selvolini & Marrazza, 2017). MIPs are more stable, cost-effective, easier to prepare and miniaturized than natural receptors. Lotierzo et al. reported that the proposed MIP system showed better performance than monoclonal antibodies with the detection feature and long-term stabilization under the same conditions (Lotierzo et al., 2004).

Applications of SPR Based MIP Nanobiosensor

There are two major fields in SPR applications: (i) identification and detection of biological targets (analytes) and (ii) biophysical analysis of biomolecular interactions (Rich & Myszka, 2002). First SPR biosensor application was performed in 1983 (Liedberg et al., 1983) and then several research group have focused on the interest on SPR biosensing. The study of kinetic and thermodynamic constants of biomolecular interactions were especially developed with real-time analysis of biointeractions in 1994. Earlier investigations of SPR biosensors focused on antigen-antibody interactions, reaction of biotin-streptavidin, IgG analysis, configuration of new SPR platforms for that period and design of surface chemistry (Homola et al., 1999). The use of MIP based SPR biosensor has increased rapidly especially in recent years. In addition, nano-MIPs platforms for SPR system have gained popularity in medical applications such as the detections of protein, antibody, hormone, microorganism, viruses and the monitoring of pharmaceuticals.

Detection of Proteins and Antibodies

Lysozyme is an enzyme that breaks the glycosidic bond between N-acetyl muramic acid and N-acetyl glucose amine in the peptidoglycan layer found in the cell wall of gram-positive bacteria. The enzyme is found in serum, urine, saliva and tears. The increased concentration of lysozyme in blood and urine is related to leukemia, renal and gastrointestinal diseases. Therefore, rapid and effective detection of lysozyme is vital for the diagnosis of these diseases. MIPs as artificial recognition elements for SPR platforms provide promising characteristics in lysozyme detection (Vasilescu et al., 2017). Şener et al. aimed to prepare a molecular imprinted biorecognition element for SPR biosensor to detect lysozyme.

In the study, lysozyme imprinted poly(ethylene glycol dimethacrylate-*N*-methacryloyl-l-histidine methylester) nanoparticles were synthesized by two-phase mini-emulsion polymerization approach and SEM and zetasizer were applied to determine the size and structure of nanoparticles. TEM results indicated that nanoparticles have ~50 nm size and spherical shape. According to zetasizer results, average size of prepared nanoparticles is 64.9 nm. Then imprinted nanoparticles were immobilized on the gold SPR sensor surface. Surface and structure analysis were characterized by FTIR, atomic force microscopy (AFM) and ellipsometry. Surface depth of the lysozyme imprinted SPR biosensor is 60.4 nm. This data confirmed both the results of TEM and zetasizer and the monolayer nanoparticle attachment was accomplished. Imprinted SPR nanosensor possessed the detection features from aqueous lysozyme solution and chicken egg white as natural source and limit of detection (LOD) of the biosensor was calculated as 84 pM. The SPR nanobiosensor was performed with albumin and cytochrome *c* to determine the selectivity of the sensor. After the selectivity studies, it was clear that imprinted SPR nanobiosensor specifically perform in the detection of lysozyme in both aqueous solution and chicken egg white. In this study, nanotechnology and molecular imprinting technology served promising solutions for lysozyme detection. Lysozyme imprinted SPR nanosensor showed the abilities to detect lysozyme from experimental and natural sources with high specificity, sensitivity and reusability (Sener, Uzun, Say, & Denizli, 2011). To compare this study with another study by the same group, Saylan and colleagues prepared hydrophobic nanoparticles as receptors in SPR biosensors to detect lysozyme. The detection limit of the biosensor was determined as 66 nM for lysozyme (Saylan, Yılmaz, Derazshamshir, Yılmaz, & Denizli, 2017). The comparison of two studies indicate that MIPs have a great advantage in the detection limit in nanoparticle-based platforms.

There are many studies in which MIPs (known as antibody mimics) could detect antibody and/or antigen molecules in the clinics. Ertürk et al. prepared F_{ab} fragment imprinted SPR biosensor for real time detection of IgG. Papain digestion procedure was carried out to obtain F_{ab} fragments from IgG and the collection of F_{ab} was performed by fast protein liquid chromatography (FPLC). Then F_{ab}-imprinted nanofilm were attached on SPR sensor surface. Chip surface was characterized by AFM, FTIR and contact angle measurement. According to characterization studies of AFM, surface deepness of the nanofilm was determined 30,00 nm. Proposed MIP-based SPR nanobiosensor detected IgG from both aqueous and natural sources with the detection limit of 56 ng/mL (Ertürk, Uzun, Tümer, Say, & Denizli, 2011). Türkoğlu and collaborators were also designed poly(2-hydroxyethyl methacrylate)/3-(2-imidazoline-1-yl) propyl(triethoxysilane) (PHEMA/IMEO) nanoparticles and attached the nanoparticles on the gold surface of SPR sensor for real-time detection of IgG. It was clear that it could not obtain a lower meaningful detection limit less than 0.05 mg/mL obtained within the kinetic study of the biosensor (Türkoğlu, Yavuz, Uzun, Akgöl, & Denizli, 2013). These two studies conducted by the same group are important in terms of revealing the superior feature of MIPs for sensor sensitivity.

Uzun et al. used hepatitis B surface antibody (HBsAb) as a template molecule for SPR biosensor studies. HBsAb-imprinted film for SPR sensor was formed to detect HBsAb from human serum. Surface depth of the SPR biosensor was determined as 15.6 nm by AFM. And the biosensor was performed in the kinetic studies with different concentrations of HBsAb positive human serums. According to result LOD was found as 208.2 mIU/mL. And control investigation were carried out to show that the HBsAb-imprinted sensor did not give a significant response to negative samples of HBsAb (Uzun et al., 2009).

Myoglobin is one of the biochemical cardiac biomarkers. Osman et al. used microcontact imprinting as another imprinting approach to detect myoglobin. The myoglobin imprinted poly(hydroxyethyl methacrylate-N-methacryloyl-L-tryptophan methyl ester) [poly(HEMA-MATrp)] nanofilms on the gold surface of SPR sensor was designed and performed in both aqueous and natural sources. The detection limit of the SPR based MIP sensor was determined as 87.6 ng/mL. According to result, this modified biosensor demonstrated high sensitivity and selectivity for the target molecule (Osman et al., 2013).

Prostate-specific antigen (PSA) is a protein which is produced in high levels during the malignant transformation of prostate gland cells. Diagnosis of PSA by biosensors in the men with prostate cancer is reliable and the quantitative results obtained with biosensors are more acceptable than the results from rectal examination or transrectal ultrasonography. 4.0 ng mL^{-1} PSA level in patient blood is a possible indication of prostate cancer. In recent studies, prostate cancer cases have been announced at below this level (Karami et al., 2019). Ertürk et al. developed imprinted SPR sensor for ultrasensitive and real-time detection of PSA. Microcontact imprinting method was applied to design PSA detection sites on the thin polymeric film. The thickness of the thin film was achieved as 125±1.54 nm by ellipsometric analysis, and the surface deepness of the polymeric layer was determined as 164±1.53 nm by AFM measurement. PSA-imprinted SPR nanobiosensor was run under the optimum conditions in the range of 0.1–50 ng mL^{-1} with the LOD of 91 pg mL^{-1}. The biosensor was performed with human serum albumin and lysozyme for selectivity studies. The performance of the biosensor was evaluated with 10 clinical samples and it was determined that imprinted biosensor showed 98% consistency between the results of ELISA measurements (Ertürk, Özen, Tümer, Mattiasson, & Denizli, 2016).

Detection of Microorganisms and Viruses

Microorganisms are one of the vital threats for public health in terms of emergence of antibiotic resistance, waterborne pathogens and food borne microorganism responsible for many diseases in the world. Microbial contamination affects all hygiene related issues in health sciences, and the rapid and reliable detection of these organisms is important for the prevention of many diseases. Several biochemical and analytical techniques are performed to identify and monitor microorganisms. Lab-based biochemical applications are based on conventional microbiology analysis. In addition to this, analytical methods have included nucleic acid and antibody-based applications to determine certain sequence of any organism's genome and fragment of surface of microorganisms. These approaches have possessed some drawbacks including trained staff, difficult preparation processes and need for labelling. The use of such devices and methods are also time-consuming to gain results in the laboratory and technical personnel can be exposed to more microbial contamination during the analysis. Therefore, novel, fast and reliable platforms are needed in the detection of microorganisms. As a result, MIP based biosensors have been one of the most important candidates to detect microorganism. Whole cell and/or a part of cell imprinted artificial receptors have gained much popularity recently (Jia et al., 2018).

The most common bacterial infections are painful and costly urinary tract infections (UTIs) that generally affect women due to their anatomical differences. The most common microorganism related to UTIs acquired in the community is uropathogenic *E. coli* (UPEC), which is responsible for about 85% of these infections. After the epithelial cells of the urinary system are invaded by this type of bacteria, UPEC can remain in dormant state. This bacterial settlement in the cells allows them to gain resistance to commonly used antibiotics. Early diagnosis of UPEC is required to minimize recurrence risk and mortality before effective treatment of UTIs. For this aim, surface imprinted Au nanoparticle based SPR biosensor was designed to detect *E. coli* to diagnose UTIs. *E. coli* imprinted SPR biosensor was characterized by AFM, SEM, contact angle measurement and ellipsometry. Au nanoparticle size was determined as ~15 nm by SEM. The thickness of *E. coli* imprinted SPR chip surface was 32.8±7.1 nm and 30 nm according to ellipsometer and AFM measurements, respectively. *E. coli* solutions with the concentration range of 1×10^3–0.5×10^1 CFU/mL were injected in SPR system for real time detection of the bacteria. *Pseudomonas aeruginosa, Klebsiella pneumoniae* and *Staphylococcus aureus* were carried out for selectivity and specificity studies of *E. coli* imprinted SPR nanobiosensor. According to result, surface imprinted SPR nanobiosensor has showed high selectivity efficiency for *E. coli*. The limit of detection for *E. coli* was achieved as 1 CFU/mL in the study. And *E. coli* detection were also achieved with artificial urine samples (Gür, Bakhshpour, & Denizli, 2019).

Microcontact *E. coli* imprinted artificial recognition sites for SPR biosensor were manufactured for real-time detection of *E. coli* from aqueous and urine mimicking solution. Ag nanoparticles were used in the polymerization process of *E. coli* imprinted polymer to enhance LOD of the biosensor. Contact angle measurement, ellipsometry, AFM and SEM were utilized to characterize the SPR sensor surface. The size of Au nanoparticles was determined as 31.55 nm. The thickness of imprinted sensor surface was found as 50.0±11.7 nm. *Staphylococcus* sp. and *Salmonella* sp. were chosen to investigate shape recognition and memory abilities of imprinted biosensor for selectivity studies. The lower limit of detection for *E. coli* was achieved as 0.57 CFU/mL in the study compared to previous study. Also imprinted SPR nanobiosensor can diagnose UTIs in urine mimicking solution with short analysis time and lower limit of detection (Özgür, Topçu, Yılmaz, & Denizli, 2020).

Poor water quality is important for public health notably in developing countries and there are still some problems on the access of clean drinking water. The drinking water used by about two million people has been contaminated by feces according to the data of World Health Organization. Fecal contamination in water is an important issue for the contamination of pathogenic microorganisms and several model microorganisms have been analyzed to monitor fecal pollution in water resources used for cooking, drinking, bathing and irrigation purposes. Enterococci are one of the indicator microorganisms for fecal pollution in water bodies due to their presences in intestinal flora of human and animal at high concentrations. And *Enterococcus faecalis* is one of the common species in human feces than other species of *Enterococcus*. *E. faecalis*-imprinted SPR sensor was developed for label-free detection of *E. fecalis* from artificial and natural water resources. After the polymerization of *E. faecalis*-imprinted nanoparticles, particle size of the nanoparticles was determined ~43 nm with the polydispersity index of 0.134 by zeta-size analysis. The thickness of *E. faecalis*-imprinted SPR biosensor was obtained as 70.8±6.0 nm by ellipsometer measurement. The imprinted SPR nanobiosensor was evaluated the range of 2×10^4–$1\text{x}10^8$ CFU/mL with the LOD of 1.05×10^2 CFU/mL. *E. coli*, *B. subtilis* and *S. aureus* are applied to SPR system due to selectivity analyses of *E. faecalis*-imprinted SPR nanobiosensor. According to selectivity studies, imprinted recognition sites on nanosensor selectively recognize *E. faecalis* than other species. Besides detecting of *E. faecalis* from water bodies, this proposed nanoplatform could find several applications from microbiome characterization to forensics (Erdem, Saylan, Cihangir, & Denizli, 2019).

Viruses are small in size, covered with a protective protein coat and have no metabolism. Since the inactivation of viruses are challenging in water sources, an intense interest is shown in this area. Enterically-transmitted viruses are one of the main sources of waterborne diseases for human beings. This kind of viruses remain stable in the environment for long periods of time and is infectious even at very low doses. Altintas et al. have reported molecularly imprinting approach for specific and sensitive adenovirus detection. MIP based nanoparticles were synthesized with the use of a novel solid phase approach to detect adenovirus. After the immobilization of MIP based recognition part on the sensor surface, SPR biosensor was tested in different concentration ranges (0.01–20 pM). And LOD of the biosensor was obtained as 0.02 pM. It was suggested that the proposed biosensor could be used for effective virus detection according to results of the study (Altintas, Pocock, Thompson, & Tothill, 2015).

Hormone Detection

Diagnosis of endocrine diseases is challenging, and these diseases can be determined by measuring the hormone levels in the blood directly or indirect measurement such as blood glucose measurement for diabetes mellitus. In clinical studies, SPR biosensors are suggested for hormone detection and effective solutions can be provided with this technology (Mariani & Minunni, 2014).

Cenci et al. created artificial recognition sites of N-terminus of the hormone hepcidin-25 by molecular imprinting approach. They exploited precipitation polymerization to synthesized MIP-nanoparticles (MIP-NPs) to detect hepcidin-25. The serum level of hepcidin-25 is associated with iron dis-metabolisms and doping. SEM and AFM measurements were applied to determine physical characterization of MIP-NPs. Morphological studies indicated that the size of MIP-NPs was in the range of 20-50 nm. Then modified MIP-NPs were immobilized onto the SPR biosensor surface. Hepcidin-25 concentration was observed in the range of 7.2–720 pM and LOD of the biosensor was calculated as 5 pM. Results of the study showed that the proposed imprinted SPR biosensor was achieved the detection sensitivity for Hepcidin-25 in picomolar range with the role of nanomaterials (Cenci et al., 2015).

Zhang et al. have designed a molecularly imprinted polymer film by photo copolymerization of methacrylic acid and 2-hydroxyethyl methacrylate as monomers, ethylene glycol dimethacrylate as cross-linker, polystyrene nanoparticles and testosterone as a template. The thickness of MIP film was measured as 177 nm by surface profiler. MIP based SPR nanobiosensor detected testosterone from aqueous solution and artificial urine sample with the LOD of 10^{-15} g/mL. The MIP based SPR biosensor showed about 84% affinity 10^{-15} g/mL target molecule after 8-month storage period (Zhang et al., 2014).

Progesterone is one of the main hormones for maintenance of human health and undesired secretion of the hormone has negative effects on biological activities in human body. Yu et al. prepared MIP based SPR biosensor to detect progesterone from some water bodies and human urine. MIP based recognition element was characterized by SEM. According to measurement results, the film whose thickness was ~100 nm possessed rough surface and there were many nano-sized recognition sites (cavities). The SEM images proved that MIP nanofilm was successfully immobilized on the SPR sensor surface. Sensing detection limit of the biosensor was achieved as 1×10^{-16} mol/L in aqueous solution. Imprinted SPR biosensor was applied to detect progesterone in human urine with the LOD of 3.94×10^{-13} (Yu, Jiao, Nawaz, Wang, & Wei, 2019).

Monitoring of Pharmaceuticals

Pharmaceuticals show huge benefits in many areas such as diagnosis, disease prevention, treatment including anti-inflammatory drugs, beta-blockers, antibiotics and analgesics. Pharmaceuticals are found in high levels in aquatic environments and/or foods. They cause tolerance in animals and humans and the development of resistance in microorganisms. (Altintas, Guerreiro, Piletsky, & Tothill, 2015). Therefore, this issue is an emerging concern for human and wildlife health. A study has revealed that erythromycin and its residues can directly affect public health. To date, many approaches and techniques have been developed to determine erythromycin and its residues. Analytical instruments have been successful, but some of them provide expensive, complicated, laborious and time-consuming procedures. Some electrochemical and UV based methods are simple but cannot provide satisfactory specifications. On the other hand, MIP based system show great benefit with operating-friendly biosensing structure. Sari et al. manufactured erythromycin imprinted nanoparticles for rapid and selective determination of erythromycin. Imprinted nanoparticles were characterized by SEM, FTIR and zetasizer. After the characterization studies of nanoparticles, they were immobilized on the gold sensor surface of SPR. The contact angle measurement was applied to the hydrophilic/hydrophobic features of modified MIP surface. According to SEM images, nanoparticles were around 40 nm, spherical and almost monosize. Zetasizer results also coincide with SEM result. The LOD of SPR nanobiosensor was determined as 0.29 ppm. Three chemical and structural analogs of erytromycin (kanamycin sulfate, neomycin sulfate and spiramycin) were injected to the SPR system as competitor agents for selectivity studies of SPR nanosensor. Erytromycin imprinted SPR nanosensor response showed highest selectivity for erythromycin than other three competitors (Sari et al., 2016).

Diclofenac is one of the important pharmaceuticals which widely used in the treatment of analgesic conditions and inflammation. The level of pharmaceuticals that contaminate aquatic environments ranges from ng mL^{-1} to g mL^{-1}. For this reason, effective detection systems have been developed to prevent the possible harm of pharmaceuticals. Although many analytical techniques are used in the detection of pharmaceuticals, these techniques are expensive, time-consuming and need trained personnel, laborious and not available for on-site detection. Altintas et al. proposed a new MIP based nanoparticle receptors which combined with SPR biosensor. Diclofenac imprinted nanoparticles were prepared using solid-phase synthesis with the use of photopolymerization. Nanoparticle size were determined $\sim 132.3 \pm 3.2$ nm and then particles were immobilized on the SPR sensor surface. The target molecule, diclofenac, was monitored in the range of 1.24–80 ng mL^{-1}. Affinity of nano recognition surfaces to diclofenac was confirmed using a solid phase – nanoMIP columns (SPE) and LC–MS. Uniformity, size and quality of MIP was tested during 12-month period for shelf-life analysis. According to results, it was determined that the particles demonstrated high affinity and stability during this period (Altintas, Guerreiro, et al., 2015).

Since the invention of penicillin, antibiotics have been used for the sustainability of living being's health. However, some concerns have arisen in terms of environment and human health after using antibiotics. These antibiotics are usually excreted from the body with urine and feces and a significant part of these ones have active metabolite forms. These antibiotics contaminate the environment without getting rid of household and pharmaceutical wastewater and hospital effluents (ul Ain et al., 2018).

Amikacin (AMIK) is a water-soluble, semi-synthetic antibiotic used in the treatment of gram-negative infections. AMIK provides a very narrow therapeutic range and can show undesirable side effects such as ototoxicity and nephrotoxicity. Therefore, it is important to monitor AMIK in patient metabolism. Although many analytical techniques have been used to detect amikacin, the use of SPR nanosensors has been reported in recent years for simple, selective and effective determination. Yola et al. fabricated a sensor to determine the AMIK from human blood. In this study, AMIK-imprinted poly(2-hydroxyethyl methacrylate-methacryloylamidoaspartic acid) [p(HEMA–MAAsp)] nanofilm was immobilized on the allyl mercaptane modified gold sensor surface. Contact angle measurements, AFM in tapping mode and FTIR measurements were performed to characterize the modified sensor surface. The recognition surface depth of AMIK-imprinted [p(HEMA–MAAsp)] SPR sensor was 20.24 ± 1.51 nm according to AFM measurements and the LOD of the sensor was determined as 0.0025 μg/mL. It was suggested that this study might contribute the designs of fast, simple and selective nanosensors to be fabricated for antibiotic detection in the future (Yola, Atar, & Eren, 2014).

Amoxicillin is a penicillin group antibiotic and widely used in bacterial infections, veterinary purposes, chemotherapeutic, prophylactic and growth promotion agents (Yola, Eren, & Atar, 2014). It is also considered to play a role in plant growth and be the most used antibiotic in the world. The European Union has determined the maximum limit of this antibiotic in animal tissues as 50 μg kg^{-1} and 4.0 μg

kg^{-1} in milk. To date, many analytical techniques such as some spectrophotometric and chromatography techniques have been used to detect amoxicillin. However, these techniques provide expensive, poor sensitivity and complex instrumentation processes. On the other hand, nanotechnology provides new generation recognition elements for high selectivity and sensitivity (ul Ain et al., 2018). Yola et al. developed a nanosensor that can detect amoxicillin in human plasma and chicken eggs. Amoxicillin-imprinted poly(2-hydroxyethyl methacrylate–methacryloylamidoglutamic acid) [p(HEMAGA)] nanofilm was immobilized on gold sensor surface. After the modified nanosensor surface was characterized by ellipsometry, FTIR and contact angle measurements. According to ellipsometry results, homogeneous and monolayer film formation was accomplished and the thickness of the nanosensor was determined as 15.23±0.082 nm. The detection limit of amoxicillin imprinted nanosensor was 0.022 ng/mL. Amoxicillin was also determined with LC-MS/MS in addition to SPR analysis. According to results, there were no important difference between the result of SPR and LC-MS/MS (Yola, Eren, et al., 2014).

Ayankoyo et al. developed a hybrid organic/inorganic MIP based SPR nanosensor to detect amoxicillin from aqueous solution. The surface thickness of amoxicillin imprinted nanofilm was characterized by ellipsometry and determined as 65 nm. The imprinted SPR biosensor could detect amoxicillin with limit of detection down 73 pM. The modified imprinted nanofilm achieved good reproducibility and can be stored at 25°C for a long time without losing stability (Ayankojo, Reut, Öpik, Furchner, & Syritski, 2018).

Kanamycin is an aminoglycoside antibiotic that is extensively used for the treatment of infectious diseases caused by gram-positive and gram-negative bacteria. This antibiotic is considered a comparatively narrow therapeutic index and the monitoring of kanamycin should be essential due to its accumulation in the bodies of human beings and notable adverse effects as nephrotoxicity and ototoxicity. To date, several approaches have been developed because of the detection importance of kanamycin. SPR biosensors with integrated MIP based artificial cells have emerged in the detection of kanamycin in recent years. A kanamycin imprinted SPR nanosensor was designed to detect kanamycin. 4-vinylbenzeneboronic acid, polyethylene glycol acrylate and 2,2′-azo isobutyl amidine hydrochloride were carried out in the polymerization of biosensor receptor as functional monomer, crosslinker and initiator, respectively. The surface morphology and thickness of kanamycin imprinted SPR biosensor were characterized by atomic force microscopy and MIP film thickness was estimated as 4.3 nm. The LOD of kanamycin imprinted SPR nanosensor was achieved as 4.33×10^{-8} mol/L and 1.20×10^{-8} mol/L for milk powder and honey, respectively (Zhang et al., 2018).

A MIP based SPR biosensor was prepared for selective detection of ciprofloxacin (CIP). Molecularly imprinted nanofilm was synthesized with in-situ photo-initiated polymerization method. The thickness of MIP nanofilm was determined as 54.0±11 nm under 50 s polymerization time. According to results, CIP imprinted-SPR nanobiosensor showed relatively lower LOD and wider detection range compared with SPE-LC–MS/MS and UHPLC–MS/MS. It was concluded that prepared MIP based SPR nanosensor presented good stability and repeatability (Luo, Yu, Shi, Wang, & Wu, 2016).

Ractopamine (RAC) is a food additive for animals and has been banned in certain countries due to the increasing behavior of its illegal adding to animal feeds. SPR based biosensors have been utilized for analyte detection in veterinary medicine and banned additives. Yao et al. developed a nano-hybrid film to function as receptor for RAC in SPR biosensor. For this purpose, a hybrid system was designed by covering MIPs with gold nanoparticles (GNPs) and reduced graphene oxides (rGO). Precipitation polymerization was performed to synthesize MIPs. After the preparation of GNPs/rGO composite system, MIP/GNPs/rGO hybrid film was attached on the sensor surface. The thickness of nano-hybrid receptor was 148.9–177.8 nm across the sensor surface with little variations. The detection limit of imprinted hybrid sensor was demonstrated as 5 ng/mL and designed nano-hybrid SPR biosensor was accomplished rapid detection and screening of RAC (Yao et al., 2016).

Detection of Other Important Molecules for Molecular Diagnosis

Uric acid (UA, urate, 2,6,8-trihydroxypurine) is an essential antioxidant to regulate antioxidant stress and blood pressure. UA levels are clinically important for healthy human body functions because changes in UA levels are associated with cardiovascular diseases, pneumonia, hypertension and Parkinson's disease. Many detection techniques are used to detect UA level in blood, saliva, urine, tear and nail (Wang, Wen, & Kong, 2019). Compared to these techniques, biosensors provide great advantages for fast, selective and desired operation procedures with low sample volume and short response time in UA detection. Göçenoğlu Sarıkaya et al. prepared SPR biosensor for the detection of uric acid. UA-imprinted nanoparticles were synthesized as recognition element for SPR biosensor. TEM analysis showed that UA-imprinted nanoparticle is around 100 nm with spherical structure. The average diameter of imprinted nanoparticles was found as 117.8 nm (polydispersity index: 0.223) by zeta size analysis. After the characterization studies, different UA concentrations in the range of 0.5-40 mg/L were applied to investigate the sensing abilities of UA imprinted SPR biosensor. The LOD for UA-imprinted biosensor was determined as 0.247 mg/L in aqueous solution. Imprinted SPR nanobiosensor also performed in urine. Prepared SPR nanobiosensor showed high sensitivity, selectivity and reusability in the detection of UA according to results (Göçenoğlu Sarıkaya, Osman, Çam, & Denizli, 2017).

Creatinine is the final product in the metabolism of creatinine, and the changes of this molecule level in the urine and blood cause some disorders such as muscular dystrophy, renal diseases, urinary tract obstruction. Therefore, creatinine is an important biomarker in the diagnosis of these diseases. Biosensors and integrated MIPs as bioreceptor can perform fast, cost effective, selective and sensitive analysis of biological fluids in clinical diagnosis. Topçu et al. designed creatinine recognition sites on the SPR gold surface. Before the kinetic studies, imprinted sensor surface was characterized by ellipsometry. This analysis showed that the thickness of creatinine imprinted SPR biosensor was 96±3 nm. Imprinted nanobiosensor performed analysis of creatinine in the range of 1-100 mM. The LOD of the biosensor was determined as 57 μM. Proposed nanobiosensor can selectively detect creatinine from aqueous and urine mimic solutions. And it was suggested that this biosensor platform could be alternative tool to measure creatinine levels for clinical purposes (Topçu, Özgür, Yılmaz, Bereli, & Denizli, 2019).

CONCLUSION

There have been great comforts among scientists, doctors, patients and industry with the development of biodiagnostic tests in medical industry. While laboratory-based diagnostic systems have achieved reliable and good results, the need for fast, on-site and cost-effective systems has increased in recent years. Biosensors are the most outstanding candidates to fill this need in medical applications with their unique instrumental characteristics. SPR biosensors have offered unique refinements and improvements in molecular diagnosis and biorecognition elements play an essential role to obtain effective results for SPR biosensor platforms. Combining MIPs with nanomaterials as bioreceptor is one of the solutions to overcome some common drawbacks and provides unique bioanalytical performance to the biosensors. Nano-sized materials have superior molecular, chemical and physical properties compared to their macro-sized counterparts such as increased surface to volume ration and binding sites, unique optical features, desired nanoparticle monodispersity and binding site homogeneity. Nano-sized MIP systems have at least 3 times more detection limits and sensitivity than macroMIPs. Integrating MIPs with nanoparticles and/or nanofilms is anticipated to achieve strategic results for effective real-time detection (Cenci et al., 2015). Nano-MIP based recognition elements are one of the options that will greatly increase the commercial success of biosensors. Therefore, it can be considered that SPR biosensors based the new generation nano-MIP for lab-on-chip, on-site and point-of-care (POC) platforms will show significant advances in the future.

REFERENCES

Abdulhalim, I., Zourob, M., & Lakhtakia, A. (2008). Surface plasmon resonance for biosensing: A mini-review. *Electromagnetics*, *28*(3), 214–242. doi:10.1080/02726340801921650

Ahmad, O. S., Bedwell, T. S., Esen, C., Garcia-Cruz, A., & Piletsky, S. A. (2019). Molecularly imprinted polymers in electrochemical and optical sensors. *Trends in Biotechnology*, *37*(3), 294–309. doi:10.1016/j.tibtech.2018.08.009 PMID:30241923

Altintas, Z., Guerreiro, A., Piletsky, S. A., & Tothill, I. E. (2015). NanoMIP based optical sensor for pharmaceuticals monitoring. *Sensors and Actuators. B, Chemical*, *213*, 305–313. doi:10.1016/j.snb.2015.02.043

Altintas, Z., Pocock, J., Thompson, K. A., & Tothill, I. E. (2015). Comparative investigations for adenovirus recognition and quantification: Plastic or natural antibodies? *Biosensors & Bioelectronics*, *74*, 996–1004. doi:10.1016/j.bios.2015.07.076 PMID:26264266

Ayankojo, A. G., Reut, J., Öpik, A., Furchner, A., & Syritski, V. (2018). Hybrid molecularly imprinted polymer for amoxicillin detection. *Biosensors & Bioelectronics*, *118*, 102–107. doi:10.1016/j.bios.2018.07.042 PMID:30056300

Bhattacharyya, D., Singh, S., Satnalika, N., Khandelwal, A., & Jeon, S.-H. (2009). Nanotechnology, big things from a tiny world : A review. *Science and Technology*, *2*(3), 29–38.

Bohunicky, B., & Mousa, S. A. (2011). Biosensors: The new wave in cancer diagnosis. *Nanotechnology, Science and Applications*, *4*, 1–10. doi:10.2147/NSA.S13465 PMID:24198482

Borgmann, S., Schulte, A., Neugebauer, S., & Schuhmann, W. (2012). Amperometric biosensors. In R. C. Alkire, D. M. Kolb, & J. Lipkowski (Eds.), *Bioelectrochemistry: Fundamentals, applications and recent developments* (Vol. 13, pp. 1–83)., doi:10.1002/9783527644117.ch1

Cass, A. E. G., Davis, G., Francis, G. D., Allen, H., Hill, H. A. O., Aston, W. J., ... Turner, A. P. F. (1984). Ferrocene-mediated enzyme electrode for amperometric determination of glucose. *Analytical Chemistry*, *56*(4), 667–671. doi:10.1021/ac00268a018 PMID:6721151

Cenci, L., Andreetto, E., Vestri, A., Bovi, M., Barozzi, M., Iacob, E., Busato, M., Castagna, A., Girelli, D., & Bossi, A. M. (2015). Surface plasmon resonance based on molecularly imprinted nanoparticles for the picomolar detection of the iron regulating hormone Hepcidin-25. *Journal of Nanobiotechnology*, *13*(1), 51. doi:10.118612951-015-0115-3 PMID:26311037

Chambers, J. P., Arulanandam, B. P., Matta, L. L., Weis, A., & Valdes, J. J. (2008). Biosensor recognition elements. *Current Issues in Molecular Biology*, *10*, 1–12. doi:10.21775/cimb.010.001 PMID:18525101

Chen, B., Piletsky, S., & Turner, A. P. F. (2002). Molecular recognition: Design of "keys.". *Combinatorial Chemistry & High Throughput Screening*, *5*(6), 409–427. doi:10.2174/1386207023330129 PMID:12470272

Clark, L. C. Jr, & Lyons, C. (1962). Electrode systems for continuous monitoring in cardiovascular surgery. *Annals of the New York Academy of Sciences*, *102*(1), 29–45. doi:10.1111/j.1749-6632.1962.tb13623.x PMID:14021529

Conroy, D. J. R., Millner, P. A., Stewart, D. I., & Pollmann, K. (2010). Biosensing for the environment and defence: Aqueous uranyl detection using bacterial surface layer proteins. *Sensors (Basel)*, *10*(5), 4739–4755. doi:10.3390100504739 PMID:22399904

Cormack, P. A. G., & Elorza, A. Z. (2004). Molecularly imprinted polymers: Synthesis and characterisation. *Journal of Chromatography. B, Analytical Technologies in the Biomedical and Life Sciences*, *804*(1), 173–182. doi:10.1016/j.jchromb.2004.02.013 PMID:15093171

Cormack, P. A. G., & Mosbach, K. (1999). Molecular imprinting: Recent developments and the road ahead. *Reactive & Functional Polymers*, *41*(1-3), 115–124. doi:10.1016/S1381-5148(99)00024-3

Couture, M., Zhao, S. S., & Masson, J. F. (2013). Modern surface plasmon resonance for bioanalytics and biophysics. *Physical Chemistry Chemical Physics*, *15*(27), 11190–11216. doi:10.1039/c3cp50281c PMID:23748491

da Silva, E. T. S. G., Souto, D. E. P., & Barragan, J. T. C., de F. Giarola, J., de Moraes, A. C. M., & Kubota, L. T. (. (2017). Electrochemical biosensors in point-of-care devices: Recent advances and future trends. *ChemElectroChem*, *4*(4), 778–794. doi:10.1002/celc.201600758

Dabrowski, M., Lach, P., Cieplak, M., & Kutner, W. (2018). Nanostructured molecularly imprinted polymers for protein chemosensing. *Biosensors & Bioelectronics*, *102*, 17–26. doi:10.1016/j.bios.2017.10.045 PMID:29101784

Dagar, G., & Bagchi, G. (2020). Nanoparticles as potential endocrine disruptive chemicals. In S. K. Saxena & S. M. P. Khurana (Eds.), *NanoBioMedicine* (pp. 411–429). Springer., doi:10.1007/978-981-32-9898-9_17

Dincer, C., Bruch, R., Costa-Rama, E., Fernández-Abedul, M. T., Merkoçi, A., Manz, A., Urban, G. A., & Güder, F. (2019). Disposable sensors in diagnostics, food, and environmental monitoring. *Advanced Materials*, *31*(30), 1806739. doi:10.1002/adma.201806739 PMID:31094032

Duverger, E., Frison, N., Roche, A. C., & Monsigny, M. (2003). Carbohydrate-lectin interactions assessed by surface plasmon resonance. *Biochimie*, *85*(1-2), 167–179. doi:10.1016/S0300-9084(03)00060-9 PMID:12765786

Erdem, Ö., Saylan, Y., Cihangir, N., & Denizli, A. (2019). Molecularly imprinted nanoparticles based plasmonic sensors for real-time Enterococcus faecalis detection. *Biosensors & Bioelectronics*, *126*, 608–614. doi:10.1016/j.bios.2018.11.030 PMID:30502683

Ersöz, A., Denizli, A., Özcan, A., & Say, R. (2005). Molecularly imprinted ligand-exchange recognition assay of glucose by quartz crystal microbalance. *Biosensors & Bioelectronics*, *20*(11), 2197–2202. doi:10.1016/j.bios.2004.07.030 PMID:15797316

Ertürk, G., Özen, H., Tümer, M. A., Mattiasson, B., & Denizli, A. (2016). Microcontact imprinting based surface plasmon resonance (SPR) biosensor for real-time and ultrasensitive detection of prostate specific antigen (PSA) from clinical samples. *Sensors and Actuators. B, Chemical*, *224*, 823–832. doi:10.1016/j.snb.2015.10.093

Ertürk, G., Uzun, L., Tümer, M. A., Say, R., & Denizli, A. (2011). Fab fragments imprinted SPR biosensor for real-time human immunoglobulin G detection. *Biosensors & Bioelectronics*, *28*(1), 97–104. doi:10.1016/j.bios.2011.07.004 PMID:21802938

Farzin, L., & Shamsipur, M. (2018). Recent advances in design of electrochemical affinity biosensors for low level detection of cancer protein biomarkers using nanomaterial-assisted signal enhancement strategies. *Journal of Pharmaceutical and Biomedical Analysis*, *147*, 185–210. doi:10.1016/j.jpba.2017.07.042 PMID:28869052

Freitas, M., Nouws, H. P. A., & Delerue-Matos, C. (2018). Electrochemical biosensing in cancer diagnostics and follow-up. *Electroanalysis*, *30*(8), 1584–1603. doi:10.1002/elan.201800193

Göçenoğlu Sarıkaya, A., Osman, B., Çam, T., & Denizli, A. (2017). Molecularly imprinted surface plasmon resonance (SPR) sensor for uric acid determination. *Sensors and Actuators. B, Chemical*, *251*, 763–772. doi:10.1016/j.snb.2017.05.079

Guo, X. (2012). Surface plasmon resonance based biosensor technique: A review. *Journal of Biophotonics*, *5*(7), 483–501. doi:10.1002/jbio.201200015 PMID:22467335

Gür, S. D., Bakhshpour, M., & Denizli, A. (2019). Selective detection of Escherichia coli caused UTIs with surface imprinted plasmonic nanoscale sensor. *Materials Science and Engineering C*, *104*, 109869. doi:10.1016/j.msec.2019.109869 PMID:31500013

Hansen, K. M., & Thundat, T. (2005). Microcantilever biosensors. *Methods (San Diego, Calif.)*, *37*(1), 57–64. doi:10.1016/j.ymeth.2005.05.011 PMID:16199177

Haupt, K., & Mosbach, K. (2000). Molecularly imprinted polymers and their use in biomimetic sensors. *Chemical Reviews*, *100*(7), 2495–2504. doi:10.1021/cr990099w PMID:11749293

Homola, J. (2008). Surface plasmon resonance sensors for detection of chemical and biological species. *Chemical Reviews*, *108*(2), 462–493. doi:10.1021/cr068107d PMID:18229953

Homola, J., Dostálek, J., Chen, S., Rasooly, A., Jiang, S., & Yee, S. S. (2002). Spectral surface plasmon resonance biosensor for detection of staphylococcal enterotoxin B in milk. *International Journal of Food Microbiology*, *75*(1-2), 61–69. doi:10.1016/S0168-1605(02)00010-7 PMID:11999118

Homola, J., Yee, S. S., & Gauglitz, G. (1999). Surface plasmon resonance sensors [Review]. *Sensors and Actuators. B, Chemical*, *54*(1-2), 3–15. doi:10.1016/S0925-4005(98)00321-9

Idil, N., Hedström, M., Denizli, A., & Mattiasson, B. (2017). Whole cell based microcontact imprinted capacitive biosensor for the detection of Escherichia coli. *Biosensors & Bioelectronics*, *87*, 807–815. doi:10.1016/j.bios.2016.08.096 PMID:27657842

Jain, K. K. (2005). Nanotechnology in clinical laboratory diagnostics. *Clinica Chimica Acta*, *358*(1-2), 37–54. doi:10.1016/j.cccn.2005.03.014 PMID:15890325

Jerónimo, P. C. A., Araújo, A. N., & Conceição, M. (2007). Optical sensors and biosensors based on sol-gel films. *Talanta*, *72*(1), 13–27. doi:10.1016/j.talanta.2006.09.029 PMID:19071577

Jia, M., Zhang, Z., Li, J., Ma, X., Chen, L., & Yang, X. (2018). Molecular imprinting technology for microorganism analysis. *Trends in Analytical Chemistry*, *106*, 190–201. doi:10.1016/j.trac.2018.07.011

Johnson, C. J., Zhukovsky, N., Cass, A. E. G., & Nagy, J. M. (2008). Proteomics, nanotechnology and molecular diagnostics. *Proteomics*, *8*(4), 715–730. doi:10.1002/pmic.200700665 PMID:18297650

Jozefowicz, M., & Jozefonvicz, J. (1997). Randomness and biospecificity: Random copolymers are capable of biospecific molecular recognition in living systems. *Biomaterials*, *18*(24), 1633–1644. doi:10.1016/S0142-9612(97)00145-2 PMID:9613811

Karami, P., Bagheri, H., Johari-Ahar, M., Khoshsafar, H., Arduini, F., & Afkhami, A. (2019). Dual-modality impedimetric immunosensor for early detection of prostate-specific antigen and myoglobin markers based on antibody-molecularly imprinted polymer. *Talanta*, *202*, 111–122. doi:10.1016/j.talanta.2019.04.061 PMID:31171159

Karlssonz, R., & Fält, A. (1997). Experimental design for kinetic analysis of protein-protein interactions with surface plasmon resonance biosensors. *Journal of Immunological Methods*, *200*(1-2), 121–133. doi:10.1016/S0022-1759(96)00195-0 PMID:9005951

Katsamba, P. S., Park, S., & Laird-Offringa, I. A. (2002). Kinetic studies of RNA-protein interactions using surface plasmon resonance. *Methods (San Diego, Calif.)*, *26*(2), 95–104. doi:10.1016/S1046-2023(02)00012-9 PMID:12054886

Kryscio, D. R., & Peppas, N. A. (2012). Critical review and perspective of macromolecularly imprinted polymers. *Acta Biomaterialia*, *8*(2), 461–473. doi:10.1016/j.actbio.2011.11.005 PMID:22100344

Ladd, J., Boozer, C., Yu, Q., Chen, S., Homola, J., & Jiang, S. (2004). DNA-directed protein immobilization on mixed self-assembled monolayers via a streptavidin bridge. *Langmuir*, *20*(19), 8090–8095. doi:10.1021/la049867r PMID:15350077

Liedberg, B., Nylander, C., & Lunström, I. (1983). Surface plasmon resonance for gas detection and biosensing. *Sensors and Actuators*, *4*, 299–304. doi:10.1016/0250-6874(83)85036-7

Lin, L. P., Huang, L. S., Lin, C. W., Lee, C. K., Chen, J. L., Hsu, S. M., & Lin, S. (2005). Determination of binding constant of DNA-binding drug to target DNA by surface plasmon resonance biosensor technology. *Current Drug Targets. Immune, Endocrine and Metabolic Disorders*, *5*(1), 61–72. doi:10.2174/1568008053174697 PMID:15777205

Linman, M. J., Taylor, J. D., Yu, H., Chen, X., & Cheng, Q. (2008). Surface plasmon resonance study of protein-carbohydrate interactions using biotinylated sialosides. *Analytical Chemistry*, *80*(11), 4007–4013. doi:10.1021/ac702566e PMID:18461973

Lotierzo, M., Henry, O. Y. F., Piletsky, S., Tothill, I., Cullen, D., Kania, M., Hock, B., & Turner, A. P. F. (2004). Surface plasmon resonance sensor for domoic acid based on grafted imprinted polymer. *Biosensors & Bioelectronics*, *20*(2), 145–152. doi:10.1016/j.bios.2004.01.032 PMID:15308215

Luo, Q., Yu, N., Shi, C., Wang, X., & Wu, J. (2016). Surface plasmon resonance sensor for antibiotics detection based on photo-initiated polymerization molecularly imprinted array. *Talanta*, *161*, 797–803. doi:10.1016/j.talanta.2016.09.049 PMID:27769483

Majka, J., & Speck, C. (2006). Analysis of protein-DNA interactions using surface plasmon resonance. In H. Seitz (Ed.), *Analytics of protein–DNA interactions. Advances in biochemical engineering/biotechnology* (Vol. 104, pp. 13–36). Springer., doi:10.1007/10_026

Malhotra, B. D., Kumar, S., & Pandey, C. M. (2016). Nanomaterials based biosensors for cancer biomarker detection. *Journal of Physics: Conference Series*, *704*(1), 012011. doi:10.1088/1742-6596/704/1/012011

Mansouri, S., & Schultz, J. S. (1984). A miniature optical glucose sensor based on affinity binding. *Nature Biotechnology*, *2*(10), 885–890. doi:10.1038/nbt1084-885

Mariani, S., & Minunni, M. (2014). Surface plasmon resonance applications in clinical analysis. *Analytical and Bioanalytical Chemistry*, *406*(9-10), 2303–2323. doi:10.100700216-014-7647-5 PMID:24566759

Martins, T. D., Ribeiro, A. C. C., de Camargo, H. S., da Costa Filho, P. A., Cavalcante, H. P. M., & Dias, D. L. (2013). New insights on optical biosensors: Techniques, construction and application. In T. Rinken (Ed.), *State of the art in biosensors - General aspects* (pp. 111–139). IntechOpen. doi:10.5772/52330

Marty, J. D., & Mauzac, M. (2005). Molecular imprinting: State of the art and perspectives. *Advances in Polymer Science*, *172*, 1–35. doi:10.1007/b97573

Medley, C. D., Smith, J. E., Tang, Z., Wu, Y., Bamrungsap, S., & Tan, W. (2008). Gold nanoparticle-based colorimetric assay for the direct detection of cancerous cells. *Analytical Chemistry*, *80*(4), 1067–1072. doi:10.1021/ac702037y PMID:18198894

Mehrotra, P. (2016). Biosensors and their applications - a review. *Journal of Oral Biology and Craniofacial Research*, *6*(2), 153–159. doi:10.1016/j.jobcr.2015.12.002 PMID:27195214

Metkar, S. K., & Girigoswami, K. (2019). Diagnostic biosensors in medicine - a review. *Biocatalysis and Agricultural Biotechnology*, *17*, 271–283. doi:10.1016/j.bcab.2018.11.029

Mitchell, S. J., & Wu, Y. (2010). Surface plasmon resonance biosensors for highly sensitive detection of small biomolecules. In P. A. Serra (Ed.), *Biosensors* (pp. 151–168). IntechOpen., doi:10.5772/7208

Mittal, S., Kaur, H., Gautam, N., & Mantha, A. K. (2017). Biosensors for breast cancer diagnosis: A review of bioreceptors, biotransducers and signal amplification strategies. *Biosensors & Bioelectronics*, *88*, 217–231. doi:10.1016/j.bios.2016.08.028 PMID:27567264

Moczko, E., Guerreiro, A., Cáceres, C., Piletska, E., Sellergren, B., & Piletsky, S. A. (2019). Epitope approach in molecular imprinting of antibodies. *Journal of Chromatography. B, Analytical Technologies in the Biomedical and Life Sciences*, *1124*, 1–6. doi:10.1016/j.jchromb.2019.05.024 PMID:31176265

Monošík, R., Streďanský, M., & Šturdík, E. (2012). Biosensors - classification, characterization and new trends. *Acta Chimica Slovenica*, *5*(1), 109–120. doi:10.2478/v10188-012-0017-z PMID:24061179

Morales, M. A., & Halpern, J. M. (2018). Guide to selecting a biorecognition element for biosensors. *Bioconjugate Chemistry*, *29*(10), 3231–3239. doi:10.1021/acs.bioconjchem.8b00592 PMID:30216055

Muhammad, T., Nur, Z., Piletska, E. V., Yimit, O., & Piletsky, S. A. (2012). Rational design of molecularly imprinted polymer: The choice of cross-linker. *Analyst (London)*, *137*(11), 2623. doi:10.1039/c2an35228a PMID:22534800

Nakamura, C., Hasegawa, M., Nakamura, N., & Miyake, J. (2003). Rapid and specific detection of herbicides using a self-assembled photosynthetic reaction center from purple bacterium on an SPR chip. *Biosensors & Bioelectronics*, *18*(5-6), 599–603. doi:10.1016/S0956-5663(03)00030-7 PMID:12706568

Ng, S. M. (2019). Carbon dots as optical nanoprobes for biosensors. In S. C. B. Gopinath & T. Lakshmipriya (Eds.), *Nanobiosensors for biomolecular targeting* (pp. 269–300). Elsevier., doi:10.1016/B978-0-12-813900-4.00012-9

Nikolovska-Coleska, Z. (2015). Studying protein-protein interactions using surface plasmon resonance. In C. L. Meyerkord & H. Fu (Eds.), *Methods in molecular biology* (Vol. 1278, pp. 109–138). Humana Press., doi:10.1007/978-1-4939-2425-7_7

Nylander, C., Liedberg, B., & Lind, T. (1982). Gas detection by means of surface plasmon resonance. *Sensors and Actuators*, *3*, 79–88. doi:10.1016/0250-6874(82)80008-5

Osman, B., Uzun, L., Beşirli, N., & Denizli, A. (2013). Microcontact imprinted surface plasmon resonance sensor for myoglobin detection. *Materials Science and Engineering C*, *33*(7), 3609–3614. doi:10.1016/j.msec.2013.04.041 PMID:23910256

Özgür, E., Topçu, A. A., Yılmaz, E., & Denizli, A. (2020). Surface plasmon resonance based biomimetic sensor for urinary tract infections. *Talanta*, *212*, 120778. doi:10.1016/j.talanta.2020.120778 PMID:32113541

Pandey, H., Khare, P., Singh, S., & Singh, S. P. (2020). Carbon nanomaterials integrated molecularly imprinted polymers for biological sample analysis: A critical review. *Materials Chemistry and Physics*, *239*, 121966. doi:10.1016/j.matchemphys.2019.121966

Patel, P., & Patel, J. (2017). Biosensors and biomarkers: Promising tools for cancer diagnosis. *International Journal of Biosensors & Bioelectronics*, *3*(4), 313–316. doi:10.15406/ijbsbe.2017.03.00072

Rich, R. L., & Myszka, D. G. (2002). Survey of the year 2001 commercial optical biosensor literature. *Journal of Molecular Recognition*, *15*(6), 352–376. doi:10.1002/jmr.598 PMID:12501157

Ritzefeld, M., & Sewald, N. (2012). Real-time analysis of specific protein-DNA interactions with surface plasmon resonance. *Journal of Amino Acids, 2012*, 1–19. doi:10.1155/2012/816032 PMID:22500214

Ruzzin, J. (2012). Public health concern behind the exposure to persistent organic pollutants and the risk of metabolic diseases. *BMC Public Health, 12*(1), 298. doi:10.1186/1471-2458-12-298 PMID:22520265

Sahoo, S. K., Parveen, S., & Panda, J. J. (2007). The present and future of nanotechnology in human health care. *Nanomedicine; Nanotechnology, Biology, and Medicine, 3*(1), 20–31. doi:10.1016/j.nano.2006.11.008 PMID:17379166

Sapsford, K. E., Bradburne, C., Delehanty, J. B., & Medintz, I. L. (2008). Sensors for detecting biological agents. *Materials Today, 11*(3), 38–49. doi:10.1016/S1369-7021(08)70018-X

Sari, E., Üzek, R., Duman, M., & Denizli, A. (2016). Fabrication of surface plasmon resonance nanosensor for the selective determination of erythromycin via molecular imprinted nanoparticles. *Talanta, 150*, 607–614. doi:10.1016/j.talanta.2015.12.043 PMID:26838449

Sari, E., Üzek, R., Duman, M., & Denizli, A. (2018). Detection of ciprofloxacin through surface plasmon resonance nanosensor with specific recognition sites. *Journal of Biomaterials Science. Polymer Edition, 29*(11), 1302–1318. doi:10.1080/09205063.2018.1457417 PMID:29607779

Saxena, S. K., Nyodu, R., Kumar, S., & Maurya, V. K. (2020). Current advances in nanotechnology and medicine. In S. K. Saxena & S. M. P. Khurana (Eds.), *NanoBioMedicine* (pp. 3–16). Springer., doi:10.1007/978-981-32-9898-9_1

Say, R., Ersöz, A., Türk, H., & Denizli, A. (2004). Selective separation and preconcentration of cyanide by a column packed with cyanide-imprinted polymeric microbeads. *Separation and Purification Technology, 40*(1), 9–14. doi:10.1016/j.seppur.2003.12.021

Saylan, Y., Akgönüllü, S., Çimen, D., Derazshamshir, A., Bereli, N., Yılmaz, F., & Denizli, A. (2017). Development of surface plasmon resonance sensors based on molecularly imprinted nanofilms for sensitive and selective detection of pesticides. *Sensors and Actuators. B, Chemical, 241*, 446–454. doi:10.1016/j.snb.2016.10.017

Saylan, Y., Yılmaz, F., Derazshamshir, A., Yılmaz, E., & Denizli, A. (2017). Synthesis of hydrophobic nanoparticles for real-time lysozyme detection using surface plasmon resonance sensor. *Journal of Molecular Recognition, 30*(9), e2631. doi:10.1002/jmr.2631 PMID:28322473

Selvolini, G., & Marrazza, G. (2017). MIP-based sensors: Promising new tools for cancer biomarker determination. *Sensors (Basel), 17*(4), 718. doi:10.339017040718 PMID:28353669

Sener, G., Uzun, L., Say, R., & Denizli, A. (2011). Use of molecular imprinted nanoparticles as biorecognition element on surface plasmon resonance sensor. *Sensors and Actuators. B, Chemical, 160*(1), 791–799. doi:10.1016/j.snb.2011.08.064

Situ, C., Mooney, M. H., Elliott, C. T., & Buijs, J. (2010). Advances in surface plasmon resonance biosensor technology towards high-throughput, food-safety analysis. *Trends in Analytical Chemistry, 29*(11), 1305–1315. doi:10.1016/j.trac.2010.09.003

Soper, S. A., Brown, K., Ellington, A., Frazier, B., Garcia-Manero, G., Gau, V., Gutman, S. I., Hayes, D. F., Korte, B., Landers, J. L., Larson, D., Ligler, F., Majumdar, A., Mascini, M., Nolte, D., Rosenzweig, Z., Wang, J., & Wilson, D. (2006). Point-of-care biosensor systems for cancer diagnostics/prognostics. *Biosensors & Bioelectronics*, *21*(10), 1932–1942. doi:10.1016/j.bios.2006.01.006 PMID:16473506

Steiner, G. (2004). Surface plasmon resonance imaging. *Analytical and Bioanalytical Chemistry*, *379*(3), 328–331. doi:10.100700216-004-2636-8 PMID:15127177

Stigter, E. C. A., De Jong, G. J., & Van Bennekom, W. P. (2005). An improved coating for the isolation and quantitation of interferon-γ in spiked plasma using surface plasmon resonance (SPR). *Biosensors & Bioelectronics*, *21*(3), 474–482. doi:10.1016/j.bios.2004.11.008 PMID:16076437

Syedmoradi, L., Daneshpour, M., Alvandipour, M., Gomez, F. A., Hajghassem, H., & Omidfar, K. (2017). Point of care testing: The impact of nanotechnology. *Biosensors & Bioelectronics*, *87*, 373–387. doi:10.1016/j.bios.2016.08.084 PMID:27589400

Szentirmay, Z. (1992). Surface plasmon spectroscopy of metal/dielectric structures. *Spectrochimica Acta. Part A: Molecular Spectroscopy*, *48*(1), 9–17. doi:10.1016/0584-8539(92)80192-Y

Taylor, A. D., Ladd, J., Yu, Q., Chen, S., Homola, J., & Jiang, S. (2006). Quantitative and simultaneous detection of four foodborne bacterial pathogens with a multi-channel SPR sensor. *Biosensors & Bioelectronics*, *22*(5), 752–758. doi:10.1016/j.bios.2006.03.012 PMID:16635568

Topçu, A. A., Özgür, E., Yılmaz, F., Bereli, N., & Denizli, A. (2019). Real time monitoring and label free creatinine detection with artificial receptors. *Materials Science and Engineering B*, *244*, 6–11. doi:10.1016/j.mseb.2019.04.018

Tothill, I. E. (2009). Biosensors for cancer markers diagnosis. *Seminars in Cell & Developmental Biology*, *20*(1), 55–62. doi:10.1016/j.semcdb.2009.01.015 PMID:19429492

Toumey, C. (2009). Plenty of room, plenty of history. *Nature Nanotechnology*, *4*(12), 783–784. doi:10.1038/nnano.2009.357 PMID:19966818

Tsai, W. C., & Hsu, Y. H. (2012). Development of a surface plasmon resonance-based DNA sensor and its application for screening DNA-targeted anticancer drugs. *Analytical Letters*, *45*(11), 1495–1505. doi:10.1080/00032719.2012.675496

Tsé, C., Gauchez, A. S., Jacot, W., & Lamy, P. J. (2012). HER2 shedding and serum HER2 extracellular domain: Biology and clinical utility in breast cancer. *Cancer Treatment Reviews*, *38*(2), 133–142. doi:10.1016/j.ctrv.2011.03.008 PMID:21549508

Türkoğlu, E. A., Yavuz, H., Uzun, L., Akgöl, S., & Denizli, A. (2013). The fabrication of nanosensor-based surface plasmon resonance for IgG detection. *Artificial Cells, Nanomedicine, and Biotechnology*, *41*(3), 213–221. doi:10.3109/10731199.2012.716066 PMID:23110360

ul Ain, N., Anis, I., Ahmed, F., Shah, M. R., Parveen, S., Faizi, S., & Ahmed, S. (2018). Colorimetric detection of amoxicillin based on querecetagetin coated silver nanoparticles. *Sensors and Actuators B*, *265*, 617-624. doi:10.1016/j.snb.2018.03.079

Uzun, L., Say, R., Ünal, S., & Denizli, A. (2009). Production of surface plasmon resonance based assay kit for hepatitis diagnosis. *Biosensors & Bioelectronics*, *24*(9), 2878–2884. https://doi.org/10.1016/j.bios.2009.02.021

Van Gosen, B. S., Blitz, T. A., Plumlee, G. S., Meeker, G. P., & Pierson, M. P. (2013). Geologic occurrences of erionite in the United States: An emerging national public health concern for respiratory disease. *Environmental Geochemistry and Health*, *35*(4), 419–430. https://doi.org/10.1007/s10653-012-9504-9

Vasilescu, A., Gáspár, S., Gheorghiu, M., David, S., Dinca, V., & Peteu, S. … Szunerits, S. (2017). Surface plasmon resonance based sensing of lysozyme in serum on Micrococcus lysodeikticus-modified graphene oxide surfaces. *Biosensors and Bioelectronics, 89,* 525-531. doi:10.1016/j.bios.2016.03.040

Verheyen, E., Schillemans, J. P., Van Wijk, M., Demeniex, M. A., Hennink, W. E., & Van Nostrum, C. F. (2011). Challenges for the effective molecular imprinting of proteins. *Biomaterials*, *32*(11), 3008–3020. https://doi.org/10.1016/j.biomaterials.2011.01.007

Wang, Q., Wen, X., & Kong, J. (2019). Recent progress on uric acid detection: A review. *Critical Reviews in Analytical Chemistry*, *50*(4), 359–375. https://doi.org/10.1080/10408347.2019.1637711

Wegner, G. J., Lee, H. J., Marriott, G., & Corn, R. M. (2003). Fabrication of histidine-tagged fusion protein arrays for surface plasmon resonance imaging studies of protein - protein and protein - DNA interactions. *Analytical Chemistry*, *75*(18), 4740–4746. https://doi.org/10.1021/ac0344438

Welford, K. (1991). Surface plasmon-polaritons and their uses. *Optical and Quantum Electronics*, *23*, 1–27. https://doi.org/10.1007/BF00619516

Wolf, A. M. D., Wender, R. C., Etzioni, R. B., Thompson, I. M., D'Amico, A. V., & Volk, R. J. … Smith, R. A. (2010). American cancer society guideline for the early detection of prostate cancer: Update 2010. *CA: A Cancer Journal for Clinicians, 60*(2), 70-98. doi:10.3322/caac.20066

Wood, R. W. (1902). XLII. On a remarkable case of uneven distribution of light in a diffraction grating spectrum. *The London, Edinburgh and Dublin Philosophical Magazine and Journal of Science*, *4*(21), 396–402. https://doi.org/10.1080/14786440209462857

Wulff, G. (1995). Molecular imprinting in cross-linked materials with the aid of molecular templates - A way towards artificial antibodies. *Angewandte Chemie International Edition in English*, *34*(17), 1812–1832. https://doi.org/10.1002/anie.199518121

Yan, H., & Row, K. H. (2006). Characteristic and synthetic approach of molecularly imprinted polymer. *International Journal of Molecular Sciences*, *7*(5), 155–178. https://doi.org/10.3390/i7050155

Yang, K., Zhang, L., Liang, Z., & Zhang, Y. (2012). Protein-imprinted materials: Rational design, application and challenges. *Analytical and Bioanalytical Chemistry*, *403*(8), 2173–2183. https://doi.org/10.1007/s00216-012-5840-y

Yao, T., Gu, X., Li, T., Li, J., Li, J., & Zhao, Z. … She, Y. (2016). Enhancement of surface plasmon resonance signals using a MIP/GNPs/rGO nano-hybrid film for the rapid detection of ractopamine. *Biosensors and Bioelectronics, 75,* 96-100. doi:10.1016/j.bios.2015.08.027

Yilmaz, E., Majidi, D., Ozgur, E., & Denizli, A. (2015). Whole cell imprinting based Escherichia coli sensors: A study for SPR and QCM. *Sensors and Actuators. B, Chemical, 209*, 714–721. https://doi.org/10.1016/j.snb.2014.12.032

Yılmaz, F., Saylan, Y., Akgönüllü, S., Çimen, D., Derazshamshir, A., Bereli, N., & Denizli, A. (2017). Surface plasmon resonance based nanosensors for detection of triazinic pesticides in agricultural foods. In A. M. Grumezescu (Ed.), New pesticides and soil sensors (pp. 679–718)., https://doi.org/10.1016/b978-0-12-804299-1.00019-9.

Yola, M. L., Atar, N., & Eren, T. (2014). Determination of amikacin in human plasma by molecular imprinted SPR nanosensor. *Sensors and Actuators. B, Chemical, 198*, 70–76. https://doi.org/10.1016/j.snb.2014.02.107

Yola, M. L., Eren, T., & Atar, N. (2014). Molecular imprinted nanosensor based on surface plasmon resonance: Application to the sensitive determination of amoxicillin. *Sensors and Actuators. B, Chemical, 195*, 28–35. https://doi.org/10.1016/j.snb.2014.01.011

Yu, J. Y., Jiao, S. Q., Nawaz, T., Wang, S. Q., & Wei, T. X. (2019). Surface plasmone resonance sensor for biomimetic detection of progesterone with macroporous molecularly imprinted polymers prepared by visible light. *IOP Conference Series. Materials Science and Engineering, 688*(3). https://doi.org/10.1088/1757-899X/688/3/033032

Yuan, X. C., Ong, B. H., Tan, Y. G., Zhang, D. W., Irawan, R., & Tjin, S. C. (2006). Sensitivity-stability-optimized surface plasmon resonance sensing with double metal layers. *Journal of Optics. A, Pure and Applied Optics, 8*(11), 959–963. https://doi.org/10.1088/1464-4258/8/11/005

Zhang, L., Zhu, C., Chen, C., Zhu, S., Zhou, J., Wang, M., & Shang, P. (2018). Determination of kanamycin using a molecularly imprinted SPR sensor. *Food Chemistry, 266*, 170–174. https://doi.org/10.1016/j.foodchem.2018.05.128

Zhang, Q., Jing, L., Wang, Y., Zhang, J., Ren, Y., & Wang, Y. … Liedberg, B. (2014). Surface plasmon resonance sensor for femtomolar detection of testosterone with water-compatible macroporous molecularly imprinted film. *Analytical Biochemistry, 463,* 7-14. doi:10.1016/j.ab.2014.06.014

KEY TERMS AND DEFINITIONS

Bioreceptor: It is the part of the biosensor that interacts with the target molecule.

Biosensor: Biosensor is an analytical device included a recognition part (bioreceptor) and transducers to detect target molecule.

Molecular Imprinting: Molecular imprinting is an emerging approach for creating and designing artificial recognition sites in a polymer matrix

Molecularly Imprinted Polymer (MIP): It is a polymer matrix designed for the 3D synthetic receptors of the desired molecule.

Nanomaterial: It is a kind of material in which at least particle size of the half of the nanoparticle number in the particle distribution is 100 nm and below.

Surface Plasmon Resonance: The excitation and propagation of electromagnetic waves in a layer between the metal surface and the analyte.

Transducer: It is the part of biosensor where the biointeractions turn into a measurable signal.

Chapter 2
Nanotechnology and Its Applications in Environmental Remediation

Joan Nyika
https://orcid.org/0000-0001-8300-6990
Technical University of Kenya, Kenya

ABSTRACT

Decontamination of pollutants from soil, air, and water is a challenging quest in contemporary society due to the recalcitrant, bioaccumulative, and bio-resistant nature of such contaminants. Remediation processes of these environmental contaminants relies on a number of processes including adsorption, photocatalysis, redox transformations, and filtration among other chemical reactions. The use of nanotechnology to enhance the performance of remediation processes has developed research interest in modern day due to the high reactivity and environmental friendliness associated with nanoparticles. This chapter explores the science behind the application of nanotechnology in environmental remediation, the processes used in decontaminating environmental media, and the various categories of nanomaterials. Various examples based on literature are used to enhance insight on the subject.

INTRODUCTION

Environmental pollution is a grave challenge in contemporary society worldwide. It is aggravated by increased urbanisation and industrialisation in the manufacturing, mining, refining, transportation and construction sectors (Nyika, 2020a). These processes deplete land and water resources and lead to generation of massive hazardous wastes and pollutants that are public health and environmental threats. Examples of resultant contaminants include organic compounds, sewage, industrial effluents, toxic gases, oil spills, fertilisers, herbicides, pesticides, heavy metals and particulate matter just to mention a few. In addition, they affect human health once inhaled, ingested or absorbed directly and indirectly through food chains (Mehndiratta et al., 2013). The capacity of these pollutants to bioaccumulate and persist in the environment increases their pollution capacity.

DOI: 10.4018/978-1-7998-5563-7.ch002

In recognition of these trends, the urgency to develop cost efficient and sustainable toxin monitoring and treatment approaches is indispensable. A number of novel technologies are often researched on for remediation of soil, air and water contaminants. Additionally, a variety of materials are being applied for remediation considering that the capture and metabolism of contaminants is challenging due to their low reactivity, high volatility and the complexity of their mixtures that are difficult to isolate (Guerra et al., 2018; Nyika, 2020b). Nanotechnology is one of the most promising of these approaches to environmental remediation and recent research has intensified its focus in pollutant management.

Nanotechnology is a technique to produce systems, devices and materials of nanoscale that have important characteristics and functions that regulate the shape and size of matter (Ibrahim et al., 2016). According to Guerra et al. (2018), nanomaterials are more effective compared to conventional bulkier products, which gives them enhanced reactivity advantage and potential use in remediation. Furthermore, their exceptional surface chemistry facilitates the addition of functional groups that target specific molecules of pollutants to enable their breakdown and subsequent depollution. The capacity to tune the physical characteristics of nanoparticles including their porosity, morphology, size and chemical components offers advantages that enable effective remediation (Guerra et al., 2018). Nanomaterials are also preferred as they can be introduced to polluted environs directly and their removal is highly effective owing to their enhanced reactivity. Nanomaterials and nanocomposites are biodegradable and in that way, they do not become pollutants during remediation processes. This makes them greener, cleaner, non-hazardous, eco-friendly and safer in addition to being target precise. Specific examples of nanoparticles' features include (Nyika, 2020a):

- They have the capacity to adsorb and absorb large quantities of contaminants due to their high surface energy and large surface area.
- They speed up reactions better than bulk material, which reduces energy consumption during degradation and impedes contaminant release in environs once absorbed or adsorbed.
- Nanotized particle forms enable easy access of contaminants in-situ as opposed to ex-situ during remediation processes.
- The particles can be coated with ligands to enhance surface area to volume ratio, modify the shape and design sensors of great specificity, sensitivity and selectivity to a given pollutant.

This book chapter explores the recent advances in nanotechnology use in environmental remediation using existent literature. The processes involved in nanotechnology-based remediation such as adsorption, catalysis and transformation and various materials used in the processes are highlighted.

The Science in Nanotechnology-Based Remediation

A number of reasons justify the use of nanomaterials in remediation (Rizwan et al., 2014). First, nanoscale materials increase the potential of coming into contact with surrounding materials owing to their large surface to unit mass ratio, which increases reactivity. Secondly, nanomaterials possess the quantum effect and hence, require less activation energy for chemical reactions to take place. Thirdly, nanoparticles have surface plasmon resonance properties that help in detection of contaminants. Their shapes and sizes are also varied, which makes them suitable in cleaning up a wide variety of contaminated materials. Nanomaterials can be metallic, bimetallic and non-metallic (such as carbon-based nanoparticles) and can penetrate in interior zones of polluted material where microparticles cannot access. They also have high affinity for redox-amenable contaminants.

For instance, Rizwan et al. (2014) noted that iron oxide coated (Fe^0) nanoparticles form outer-sphere complexes and bond weakly to carbon tetrachloride (CT) -based contaminants. In this case, reactivity through electron transfer is enhanced by oxide coating, which enables metabolism of CT to carbon monoxide, formate and methane. The same reaction using Fe^0 nanoparticles converts contaminants such as benzoquinone, chlorinated aliphatic hydrocarbons and bytrichloroethane to chemicals with reduced toxicity as a study by Nurmi et al. (2005) established using field assessments and batch experiments. Titanium (IV) oxide (TiO_2) nanotubes metabolised pentachlorophenol (PCP) in a photoelectrocatalytic reaction and at laboratory settings (Quan et al., 2005). Metal-based nanoparticles such as palladium, Pd (0) are applied in de-chlorination reactions as biocatalysts. Their deposition in *Shewanella oneidensis*' cytoplasm occur after the nanoparticles are charged positively with hydrogen radicals (H*) and by adding electron donors, which leads to chlorine removal in PCP (Windt et al., 2005). Electron donors used as substrates in this reaction include formate, acetate and hydrogen.

Nanomaterials are also used in recovery of and degradation of some chemicals in contaminants through microbial cell immobilisation. This procedure uses Fe_3O_4 magnetic nanoparticles by coating them on *Pseudomonas delafieldii* and through ammonium oelate functionalisation (Rizwan et al., 2014). Using an external magnetic field on the microbes, the magnetic nanoparticles are amassed in a bioreactor wall, which is detached from the bulk solution and reused to treat the same substrate. According to Shan et al. (2005), a bioreactor reaction confirmed that these microbes could desulfurize organic sulphur from dibenzothiophene better that non-coated nanoparticles. Nanotechnology materials used in specific environmental remediation processes will be discussed at a later stage of the chapter. However, a summary of the various nanotechnology applications in remediation processes is shown in Figure 1.

PROCESSES OF ENVIRONMENTAL REMEDIATION

Remediation of contaminants can occur through photocatalytic reactions, filtration, chemical reactions, adsorptive and absorptive processes according to Guerra et al. (2018). Das et al. (2018) summarises these processes into three: photocatalysis, transformation through chemical reactions and adsorption. Figure 2 best represents these three processes.

Adsorption

In adsorption, pollutants bind on an adsorbent's surface in an exothermic process orchestrated by ionic and surface interactions (Wang et al., 2019). For a mole of adsorbate to be attached as a thin film on a surface, the resultant heat produced is called enthalpy. Adsorption occurs spontaneously when pressure and temperature are constant leading to reduction of Gibb's free energy (Pan & Xing, 2008). It is from this principle that nanoscale adsorbents are produced biologically using named prokaryotic and eukaryotic species as factories and can remediate contaminants cost effectively and through eco-friendly processes (Das et al., 2018). These include bimetallic nanoparticles (BNPs), metal and metal oxide nanoparticles, multifunctional nanocomposites and modified nanomaterials.

BNPs are synthesised through plants, fungi, yeast and bacteria at room temperature extra- or intracellularly. These conditions make them biocompatible during nanoparticle synthesis. A case example are iron particles whose reactivity has been enhanced through their coating with noble metals (Das et al., 2018). Govindaraju et al. (2008) also studied the use of BNPs made from silver (Ag) and gold (Au) in contaminant remediation and their synthesis from *Spirulina platensis* (a cyanobacterium). Metal and metal oxide nanoparticles are important adsorbents in large-scale wastewater treatment. A case example is the use of Fe_3O_4 nanoparticles in adsorption of arsenic (As) (II) and (V) from tea waste (Lunge et al., 2014). Copper (Cu) oxide nanotubes were also used to adsorb organic dyes and lead (Pb) (II) from aqueous solutions (Mustafa et al., 2013).

Figure 1. Applications of nanotechnology in remediation processes.

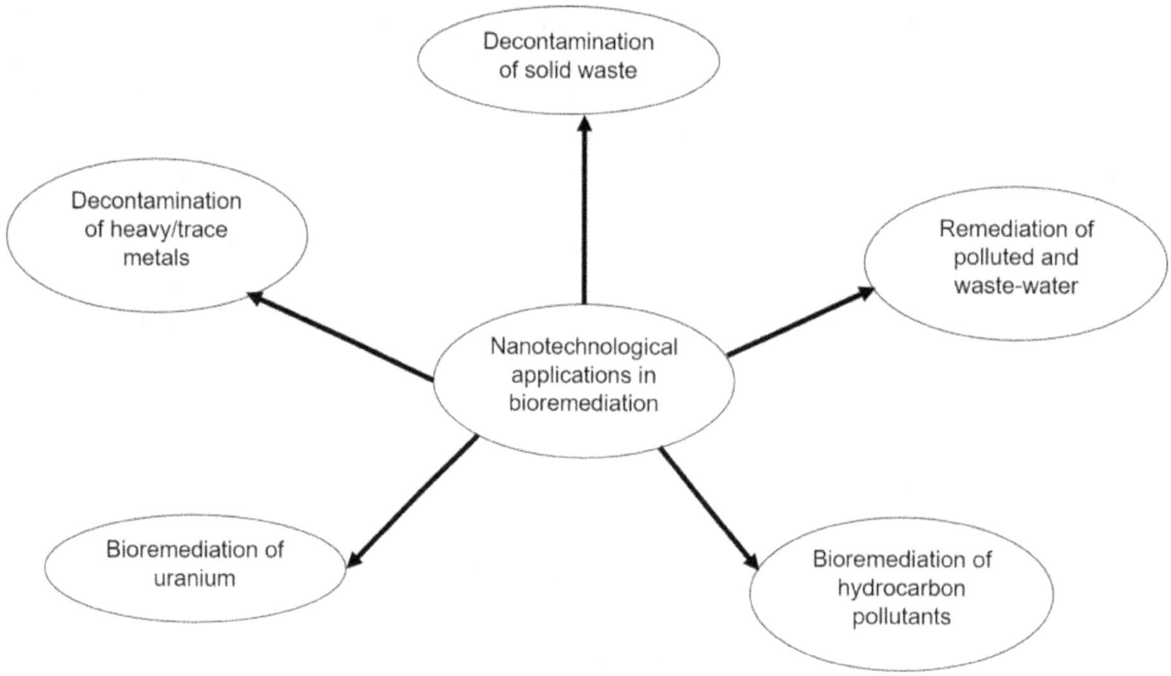

The use of multifunctional nano-composites is currently being explored to create smart remediation materials with multiple actions. A case example is the use of *Amaranthus tristis* (a plant) to biologically synthesize silver nanoparticles and embed them on polyvinyl alcohol documented by Nehru and Suvakumar (2012). This particle was tested for multiple functions including remediation of pharmaceutical, textile and tannery wastes among other industrial effluents. Modification of metal oxide nanoparticles and BNPs is being done in advanced nanotechnology processes to stabilize them and prevent their aggregation. According to Das et al. (2018), modification of nanoparticles regulates their high magnetic characteristics, surface energy and reactivity to prevent easy oxidation in water and air and disrupted adsorptive capacities. Modification is done through coating using inorganic and organic materials such as silica, metal sulphide, metal oxide, biomolecules, polymers and surfactants among others (Wang et al., 2019). Case examples are the modification of metal oxide nanoparticles with organic particles to increase cadmium (Cd) (II) adsorptive binding sites (Singh et al., 2014) and the addition of agarose in iron nanoparticles, which enabled the biodegradation of trichloroethylene and chromium (Luo et al., 2016).

Figure 2. Processes involved in remediation of environmental contaminants using nanotechnology. Me; represents metal while NO_X; nitrogen oxide gases, $(OH)_x$; a hydroxide compound.

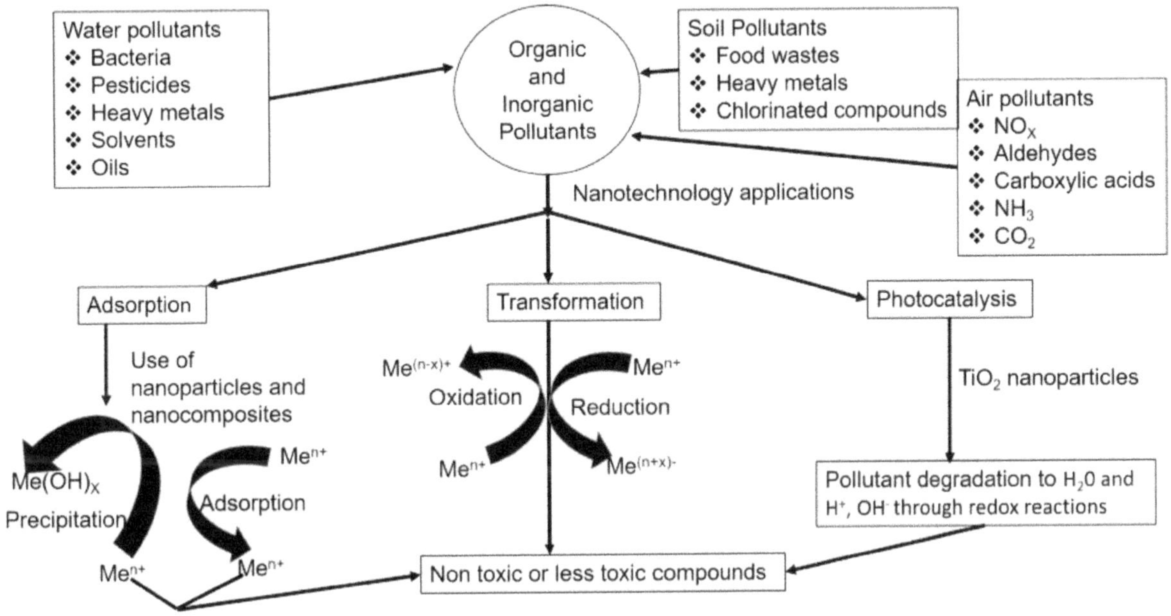

Transformation

Transformation reactions are redox-based processes of decontaminating pollutants and lead to reduced metal toxicity through their speciation (De Windt et al., 2005; White et al., 2009). Toxicity states or sites are modified through electron transfer reactions. Case examples are the use of zerovalent iron (ZVI) nanoparticles as electron donors to reduce chromium (VI) (Singh et al., 2012) and zinc (Liang et al., 2014) from wastewater. ZVI nanoparticle remediation through reduction of organic pollutants such as chlorinated solvents, nitro-aromatics, organophosphates and chlorinated pesticides has been reported (Rychoudhury & Scheytt, 2013).The focus of the process is to remove contaminants by modifying them to less toxic compounds through oxidative and reductive reactions.

Catalysis

Optimal catalysis requires that the proteins used have many active sites, a high surface area and a small size. Catalytic processes based on photocatalysis, which is an enhanced reaction in the presence of ultraviolet or visible light and a catalyst have been used in remediation (Wang et al., 2019). The procedure involves the use of a semi-conductor- based catalyst, which is initially exposed to visible or ultraviolet light to sensitize it and form holes and electrons (Khan et al., 2015). Irradiation continues until the semiconductor's bandgap energy is equal or greater than the incident light energy to prompt valence-band electron excitation, their transfer to the semiconductor's conduction band and subsequent creation of holes at the valence band (Khan et al., 2015; Fagan et al., 2016). Resultant electrons and holes transform water to hydroxyl radicals and hydrogen gas in a series of oxidative reactions and consequently, degrade organic contaminants oxidatively. Lu et al. (2016) documented the use of titanium, zinc and silver metal oxides in remediation of contaminants through photocatalysis. Nanoparticles made from silver and gold were used to degrade methylene blue dye in a photocatalytic reaction (Suvith & Phillip, 2014). Bacteria and plant synthesized TiO_2 nanoparticles were used to degrade organic and inorganic pollutants where they served as catalysts (Jayaseelan et al., 2013).

Fenton Reaction

Fenton reaction is an advanced oxidation process (AOP), which has attracted research attention due to its ability to degrade organic and inorganic pollutants that were previously resistant to metabolism (He et al., 2016). These pollutants include oil refinery waste, pharmaceutical products, phenols and phenolic compounds of wastewater and industrial effluents. A case example is the use of iron oxides as heterogeneous catalysts to convert iron (II) (Fe^{2+}) to iron (III) (Fe^{3+}) in a hydrogen peroxide (H_2O_2) oxidised reaction. This leads to the formation of a hydroxide anion (OH^-) and a hydroxyl radical (OH^*). In the second reaction phase, H_2O_2 oxidation leads to the formation of a proton (H^+) and a hydroperoxyl radical ($^*OOH$), which oxidise organic pollutants (He et al., 2016). Fenton reactions are widely researched on because of their ability to degrade recalcitrant wastewater pollutants compared to conventional techniques (Tisa et al., 2014; Wang et al., 2014; Garca-Segura et al., 2016).

NANOTECHNOLOGY MATERIALS USED IN ENVIRONMENTAL REMEDIATION

There are varieties of nanomaterials used in environmental remediation. These materials, the methods used to synthesize them and specific examples are summarised in Table 1. Each of these nanomaterials and their mechanism of action will be discussed in the following sections.

Metal and Metal Oxide-Based Nanomaterials

Varieties of metal- and metal oxide-based nanoparticles have been studied for remediation purposes particularly the removal of chlorinated organic pollutants and heavy metals in polluted water. Their suitability is pegged on their high adsorptive capacity and flexibility in ex- and in-situ applications for remediation of aqueous systems (Santhosh et al., 2016). Metal-based nanomaterials are classified into seven: 1) BNPs, 2) iron-based, 3) binary oxide mixtures, 4) titanate nanotubes, 5) TiO_2, 6) metal-doped TiO_2 and 7) Ag^+/Ag nanoparticles (Guerra et al., 2018).

Iron-based nanoparticles consist of elemental iron (Fe^0) also known as zerovalent in a core-shell structure mixed with Fe^{2+} and Fe^{3+} oxides (Kharisov et al., 2012). The zerovalent forms the core and the oxides form the shell. Through electron donation from the core, reduction of chlorinate compounds and heavy metals occurs. Pollutants that have higher reduction potential compared to the standard Fe/Fe^{2+} couple such as trace metals can be reduced at the shell. Nanoparticles of silver (Ag^+/Ag) are applied in disinfection of water due to their antiviral, antifungal and antibacterial properties. According to Pal et al. (2007), Ag nanoparticles with a diameter below 10 nm were toxic to *Pseudomonas aeruginosa* and *Escherichia coli*. The nanoparticles also bind on the glycoproteins of viruses preventing their binding to target hosts (Gogoi et al., 2006). The shape of these Ag nanoparticles determines their remediation efficacy as Pal et al. (2007) reported in a study where triangular particles exhibited superior antimicrobial properties in contaminated water compared to spherical and rod-shaped ones.

Table 1. Nanomaterials used in environmental remediation processes, methods used to synthesize them and their specific examples (Das & Ansari, 2009; Guerra et al., 2018).

Type of nanomaterial	Methods used to synthesize	Examples
Metal -based	Electro, thermal and bio-chemical processes	Ag, Au, CdSe, CdTe, Co, CoNi, Cu, Cu_3Au, FeNi, Ir, Pd, Pt, Rh and ZnS
Metal oxide-based	Electrochemical deposition, reverse micelles process, sol-gel, hydro- and solvo-thermal processes.	$BaCO_3$, $BaSO_4$, Fe_2O_3, Fe_3O_4, MgO, TiO_2 and ZnO
Carbon-based	Laser ablation, chemical vapour deposition and arc- discharge processes	Cylindrical nanotubes and fullerenes
Polymer-based	Electrochemical polymerisation	Polyamidoamine dendrimers, nanowires of polyaniline and polypyrrole.
Silica-based	Physical impregnation, in situ polymerisation and covalent tethering techniques	Amine-based xerogels, thiol-, amino-, carboxylic acid- functionalized mesoporous silica.
Bionanomaterials	Biological methods	Plasmids, bacterial, viruses, plants and protein-based nanoparticles
Nanocomposites	Innovative methods	Carbon nanotubes modified with polyester polyamides, polyethylene glycol, fluoropolymers and polycarbonates

TiO_2 nanoparticles are studied in environmental remediation studies aimed at photocatalytic treatment of contaminated water, air pollution, self-cleansing of surfaces and waste treatment. The versatility of these particles in these remediation processes is justified by their semi-conducting ability, non-toxicity, low cost, high energy converting and gas sensing abilities (Li et al., 2008). They have disinfectant properties against algae, viruses, fungi and bacteria owing to their ability to form reactive oxidants such as OH*. TiO_2 particles have low photocatalytic ability in their pristine form unless they are doped with other metals. This was established by Park and Lee (2014) using sol-gel electrospinning technique where doping of TiO_2 particles with silver proved successful in photocatalytic metabolism of 2-chlorophenol. The authors attributed the resultant higher efficacy compared to non-doped nanofibers to expanded response to irradiation at the visible region, effective photo-induction of electrons and holes, their prompt transfer to adsorptive surfaces and increased surface area for the activity of hydroxyl groups. Inorganic complexes of TiO_2 commonly known as titanates are also used in the form of nanotubes to for remediation purposes. Nitric oxide (NO) gas was catalytically reduced to ammonia using neutral, acidic and basic titanate nanotubes synthesized through hydrothermal processes (Chen et al., 2013). Manganese (Mn) doping of basic, acidic and neutral media titanate to form nanosheets, nanorods and nanotubes, respectively was done and the nanomaterials were used for redox remediation purposes to assay the effects of varied active species dispersion and surface area on the efficacy of the three particles (Chen et al., 2013). Results showed that high surface area and wide dispersion of active species were favourable characteristics to decontamination processes. Activity by neutral titanate nanotubes was negligible.

The use of binary mixed oxides such as TiO_2 and SiO_2 has been investigated in remediation studies. In an investigation conducted by Rasalingam et al. (2014), these binary oxides were prepared using silica sourced from bamboo and titanium butoxide and titanium isopropoxide. The materials showed significant photocatalytic activity to degrade methylene blue dye. After varying the treatment frequency and duration, the two oxides were found efficient in wastewater treatment of small-scale industries compared to exclusive TiO_2 nanomaterials (Rasalingam et al., 2014). Monometallic nanomaterials have high aggregation propensity and low stability. These limitations have facilitated the use of BNPs that are modified using surfactants and stabilisers in addition to doping them with a second metal to increase stability (Khin et al., 2012). With enhanced stability, the contaminant degradation rate and capacity of these nanomaterials can be enhanced. ZVI nanoparticle modification with metals such as palladium (Wu & Ritchie, 2006), nickel (Fang et al., 2011) and copper (Zhu et al., 2010) was documented for their improved stability. The use of noble metals such as palladium that resist moist air oxidation and corrosion in combination with ZVI nanoparticles enhanced hydrogenation and de-chlorination of wastewater contaminants as Karn et al. (2009) reported in an in-situ study. Some of the metal-based nanomaterials used in remediation of pollutants are summarized in Table 2.

Table 2. Examples of metal oxides used in remediation and their target pollutant

Metal Oxide	Targeted pollutant	Reference
Magnetite (Fe_3O_4)	Fluoride	Poursaberi et al., 2012
	Cu (II)	Hao et al., 2010
	Cd(II), Zn(II), Pb (II), Cu (III)	Ge et al., 2012
Titanate nanotubes (TNTs)	Pb (II), Cd (II), Cu (II), Cr (II)	Liu et al., 2011
Titanate nanoflowers (TNF)	Cd (II), Ni (II), Zn (II), Pb (II)	Huang et al., 2012
Iron oxide-alumina (Fe_2O_3-Al_2O_3)	Cu (II), Pb (II), Ni (II), Hg (II)	Ibrahim et al., 2016
Titanium oxide	Pb, Cd, Cu, Ni, Zn	
Hydrous cerium oxide (SCO)	As	
NiO nanoparticles	Cd (II) and Pb (II)	
Nanocomposite (GO-ZrO $(OH)_2$ magnetite (Fe_3O_4)	Pb (II)	
Iron (III) oxide	As (v)	
Magnetic nanoparticle impregnated with activated maize cob powder	Methylene blue	
Amorphous zirconium oxide (Am-ZrO_2)	Phosphate	
	As (III) (v)	
Nano ZnO	Pb (II)	
Mg and Zn oxide	Cu (II)	

Carbon-Based Nanomaterials

Carbonaceous materials have unique electronic, chemical and physical characteristics that emanate from the elemental carbon's changeable hybridization state and composition compared to metals (Ren et al., 2011). From these characteristics, different structural configurations such as graphene, fullerene C_{540}, fullerene C_{60}, single- and multiple-walled nanotubes can occur and be useful in nanotechnology-based remediation (Madima et al., 2020). The adsorptive properties of these materials make them suitable in decontaminating aqueous solutions and air pollutants though they require prior to functionalization, activation and surface treatment of pristine carbon (Mauter & Elimelech, 2008). Remediation using carbon-based nanomaterials can occur through photocatalysis. In the process ultraviolet radiation is used to generate photons of high energy compared to the band gap of nanomaterials that are then transformed to conduction band electrons (e^-) and valence band holes (h^+). The holes speed up the formation of hydroxyl radicals, which oxidise chlorinated organic pollutants while the electrons, enhance the formation of superoxide radicals that reduce heavy metals to less toxic compounds. In synthesizing these photocatalytic nanomaterials, graphene is preferred due to its enhanced conductivity as Zhang et al. (2010) observed in a study using TiO_2 graphene nanocomposites to metabolise volatile aromatic pollutants. The general mechanism of photocatalysis using carbon-based nanomaterials is summarised in Figure 3.

Figure 3. Photocatalytic degradation of pollutants using carbon-based nanomaterials (Ren et al., 2011).

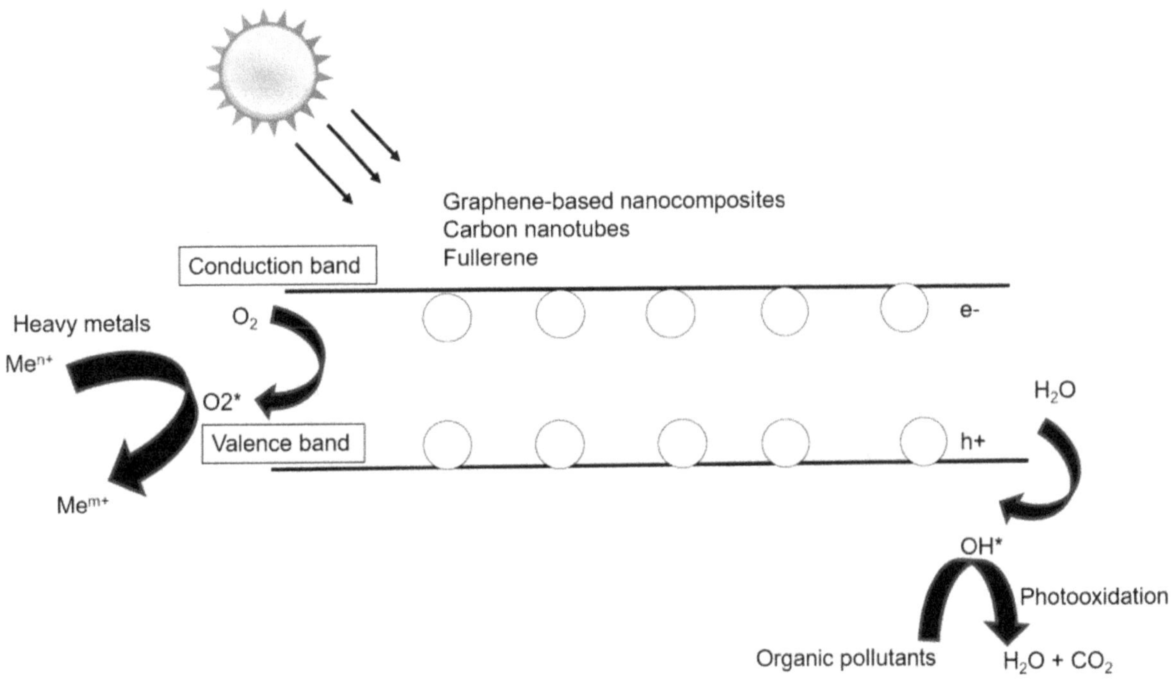

Carbon Nanotubes

Carbon nanotubes used in remediation processes are classified as either single-walled or multiple-walled (Ren et al., 2011). The former occurs in a hexagonal configuration with one tube surrounded by six other to form a bund that is porous structured and heterogeneous. In such an open-ended bundle, adsorption occurs in areas of high and low energy on the surface, between and within tubes (Lithoxoos et al., 2010; Madima et al., 2020). The latter do not exist as bundles but have aggregated and inner pores. Apart from the configuration of carbon nanotubes, their adsorptive efficacy is influenced by their oxygen content, which is a function of their purification and synthetic procedures. According to Ren et al. (2011), these nanotubes contain functional groups such as –COOH, –C=O and –OH that are oxidised by a number of chemicals including NaOH, NaOCL, KOH, H_2O_2, $KMnO_4$ and HNO_3. The functional groups and oxidising agents determine adsorptive properties that are a function of pH. Remediation is favoured in basic conditions due to increased electrostatic attraction of contaminants and nanotube surfaces as Khin et al. (2012) established in a study that reported high adsorptive properties for cationic dyes at high pH. Carbon nanotubes have been used in the degradation of ethylbenzene (Bina et al., 2012) and removal of metals such as Cu (Li et al., 2010) and Ni (Kandah & Meunier, 2007)

GRAPHENE MATERIALS

Four different types of graphene nanomaterials are used in remediation processes. They include pristine graphene, graphene oxide, TiO_2-graphene and ZnO/CdS- graphene (Guerra et al., 2014; Madima et al., 2020). Pristine graphene was used in removal of fluoride from aqueous solution via adsorption (Li et al., 2011). Even though, pristine graphene has adsorptive properties, it is prone to aggregation that decreases remediation efficacy through reduced surface area. This limitation necessitates the use of modified graphene. An example is the use of graphene oxide whose surface modifications were shown to enhance adsorption of water and air pollutants including volatile organic compounds, SO_X, H_2S, NH_3, pharmaceuticals, pesticides and heavy metals (Wang et al., 2013; Yang et al., 2019). Nanocomposites of graphene and TiO_2 were used in degradation of volatile aromatic contaminant such as benzene in a photocatalytic reaction (Zhang et al., 2010). Liu et al. (2011) reported the use of CdS graphene and ZnO-graphene nanocomposites in remediation of water contaminants. The two nanomaterials were used in photocatalytic reduction of chromium (IV). The used of these nanocomposites required the relative addition of graphene as high levels reduced the system's photoactive component and lowered the intensity of light, which negatively affected their remediation efficacy (Zhang et al., 2010; Liu et al., 2011).

Polymer-Based Nanomaterials

The use of host materials such as polymers to support nanomaterials is a researched alternative to their enhanced stability. Polymers are used to detect microorganisms such as viruses and bacteria, organic pollutants, gases and contaminant chemicals (Yang et al., 2019; Nyika, 2020b). Polymeric hosts such as surface functionalized ligands, stabilizing agents, surfactants and emulsifiers overcome the aggregation limitations of pristine nanoparticles in addition to having recyclability, thermal stability, mechanical strength and durability advantages (Guerra et al., 2018). The use of amphiphilic polyurethane (APU) nanoparticles to remove polynuclear aromatic hydrocarbons in soils was reported by Tungittiplakorn et al. (2004). These nanoparticles have a hydrophobic interior with high affinity for water-resistant organic pollutants while their surface is hydrophilic to enhance their mobility in soils among other environmental media. APU nanoparticles also have high affinity for phenanthrene found in pesticides, plastics and dyes. A study by Tungittiplakorn et al. (2004) confirmed these suggestions but expressed negativity on its use, as it could not biodegrade the pollutant.

Poly amidoamine (PAMAM) are dendritic polymers that contain hydroxamates, carboxylates and amines as functional groups. They bind on a wide range of metal ions including Ag, Au, Cu, Fe (II), Fe (III), Ni, U and Zn thereby acting as ultrafilters and chelators of water pollutants (Diallo et al., 2005). A study by Brinkmann et al. (1999) also established that these nanoparticles have antifungal and antibacterial properties. The globular shape and polydispersive characteristics of these nanopolymers makes them useful in micro- and ultra-filtration as they do not pass through such filtration membranes (Biricova & Laznickova, 2009). Guerra et al. (2018) documented the use of functionalised non-toxic and biodegradable polymeric nanomaterials in the capture of volatile organic compounds. In their study, the authors combined polyethyleneimine (PEI) functional groups into polymeric nanoparticles and found an almost ideal specificity for volatile organic compounds with carboxylic acid and aldehyde functional groups. Amine functionalized polymeric nanomaterials were used in the capture of aldehydes and carboxylic acid compounds in a laboratory study using gas chromatographic headspace analysis (Campbell et al., 2015).

Nanoparticles that have coated or interspersed polymers on their surface form nanocomposites (Yang et al., 2019). These polymeric nanomaterials exhibit high mechanical strength and have high reactivity because of a large surface area. They incorporate metal and metal oxides to make fabricated membranes used for remediation of gases associated with fouling (Campbell et al., 2015). Other nanocomposites consisting of polymers and inorganic hybrid nanoparticles have been used to adsorb microorganisms, dyes and trace metal ions in wastewater (Guerra et al., 2018; Nyika, 2020b). Another example is the use of chitosam-based carbon nanofibers together with polyvinyl alcohol nanofilms and iron oxide nanoparticles to reduce Cr (IV) in polluted water (Khare et al., 2016).

Silica-Based Nanomaterials

Mesoporous silica has tunable pore sizes, large pore volume, simplistic surface modifications and high surface area. The characteristics that make it suited for environmental remediation using nanotechnology (Tsai et al., 2016). Mesoporous silica is used in contaminant remediation in their gaseous phases and can also undergo surface modifications at its hydroxyl groups. Grafting functional groups enhances adsorbent characteristics and facilitates catalytic action of these nanoparticles during remediation. Huang and Yang (2003) reported the use of amine-surface modified mesoporous silica and xerogels to remove H_2S and CO_2 from polluted air. Amino modified aluminosilicates captured ketones, aldehydes and CO_2 through absorptive techniques, some of which were reversible (Bollini et al., 2011; Nomura & Jones, 2013). Functionalization of mesoporous silica with –COOH functional group improved its efficacy in cleaning wastewater off organic dyes (Tsai et al., 2016). Vunain et al. (2016) reported the use of thiol-functionalized, aminopropyl-functionalized and amino-functionalized silica nanomaterials in remediation of Al, Cd, Co, Cr, Cu, Hg, Ni, Pb, U and Zn ions from contaminated soils and water. *E.coli*, *Aeromonas hydrophila*, *P. aeruginosa*, *Staphylococcus aureus* and *Streptococcus pyogenes* microbial species were used together with TiO_2 nanoparticles to confer antibacterial activity (Jayaseelan et al., 2013).

Bionanomaterials

The high quantities of pollutants in the environment has forced microorganisms (bacteria, viruses, fungi, plasmids and actinomycetes) to develop adaptive responses. Bioremediation using bionanomaterials relies on transformation of harmful contaminants to less or non-harmful products (Nyika, 2020a). The target pollutants for bionanomaterials include chlorinated hydrocarbons, heavy metals, xenobiotics and pesticides. Usually, the materials increase pollutant sorption and through redox reactions bio-transform harmful compounds (Pandey et al., 2015). For instance, bacteria species such as *enterobacteriaceae* were associated with heavy metal resistance in humans (Yang et al., 2018). These microorganisms use mechanisms such as the formation of extracellular barriers, efflux of pollutants, genetically controlled resistance, oxido-reductive processes, intra- and extra- cellular sequestration to immobilize and decontaminate pollutants (Panday et al., 2015).

It is from these tendencies that nanotechnology is constructing nanoparticles equipped with pollutant-resistant microorganisms in bioremediation studies. A case example is the use of *Noaea mucronata* incorporated nanoparticles to cleanse contaminated water off heavy metals (Gupta & Joia, 2016). Gogoi et al. (2006) investigated the use of silver nanoparticles in a model integrating *E. coli* proteins to show their antimicrobial ability successfully. Rizwan et al. (2014) used the bacteria *Pseudomonas delafieldii* to modify iron (III) oxide magnetic nanoparticles and enhance their pollutant remediation efficacy in polluted water. Balagurunathan et al. (2011) documented the synthesis of gold nanoparticles using actinomycete species such as *Rhodococcus species* and *Streptomyces viridogens* for remediation purposes. Additionally, the use of fungi species such as *Fusarium oxysporum* and *Aspergillus fumigates* to construct, Au, Ag and Ti nanocomposites for bioremediation of chlorinated organic pollutants was reported (Pandey et al., 2015). The advantage of using these bionanomaterials over the other categories is their eco-friendly and non-hazardous nature. Their adoption promotes green synthesis in remediation processes (Pandey et al., 2015).

Microbes have high reducing ability to pollutants especially heavy metal ions hence their synthesis at nanoscale. They also secrete enzymes to speed up the process and can be produced in large quantities. Some of the nanoparticles used in bioremediation and the microorganisms from which they are produced are summarized in Table 3 (Pandey, 2018).

Table 3. Examples of nanoparticles used in bioremediation and the microorganisms used to produce them (Panday, 2018)

Nanoparticle	Producing microorganisms
Silver nanoparticles	*Actinomycete, Nocardiopsis sp.* MBRC-1, *Trichoderma reesei, Cladosporium cladosporiodes, Neurospora crassa, Stremptomyces sp. Brevibacterium casei, Staphylococcus aureus.*
Gold nanoparticles	*Aspergillus clavatus, Penicillium brevicompactum, Neueospora crassa, Aspergillus clavatus, Thermonospora sp. Rhodococcus sp., Streptomyces sp., Klebsiella pheumonia*
Palladium nanoparticles	*Fusarium oxysporum, Desulfovibrio desulfuricans, Shewanella oneidensis*
Titanium	*Aeromonas hydrophila, Bacillus amyloliquefaciens, Bacillus subtilis*
Copper nanoparticles	*S. oneidensis, Pseudomonas sp., Serrati asp., Stremptomyces sp., Hypocrea lixii, Sterium hirsutum*
Zinc nanoparticles	*Candida albicans, Stremptomyces sp., Lactobacillus*
Iron nanoparticles	*Plerotus sp. Escherichia coli, Chaetomium globosum*

The synthesis of nanobiomaterials involves fives steps:

1. The preparation of bio-reductant parts of microbes in addition to metal ions. The process involves conversion to solution at the right kinetics and pH.
2. The recovery and purification of nanoparticles through ultraviolet visible analyses.
3. The conversion of nanoparticles from solution to powder through a series of reactions including scanning electron microscopy (SEM), transmission electron microscopy (TEM), X-ray diffraction (XRD) and dynamic light scattering (DLS) analyses.
4. Physicochemical characterization through assessment of size, size distribution and shape analyses.
5. Biofunctionalization before the end use in bioremediation.

CONCLUSION

Nanotechnology is a promising tool in remediation of environmental pollutants found in soils and water among other samples. This ability is attributable to the outstanding characteristics of nanomaterials such as a high affinity for functional groups of pollutants and a high surface area. Examples of nanomaterials include polymer-, silica-, carbon-, metal- and metal oxide-based and bio- nanoparticles. The nanoparticles can be used in their pristine form or modified using other substances to enhance their stability and efficacy. The nanoparticles breakdown contaminants to lower toxic forms and enhance their degradation rates hence are effective and sustainable. The specific mechanisms of the various nanomaterials to decontaminate environmental media such as water, soil, solid waste and toxic gases in air from various pollutants were also examined. Mechanisms such as adsorption, photocatalysis and transformation applied by these nanomaterials are shown to be viable in decontaminating both organic and inorganic contaminants. Examples of various particles and the adsorbents they remediate were also provided. This discussion emphasized that nanotechnology has immense remediation applications and capabilities and its potential in enhancing sustainable environmental management is indispensable if research in the field is intensified.

REFERENCES

Balagurunathan, R., Radhakrishnan, M., Rajendran, B. R., & Velmurugan, D. (2011). Biosyntheis of gold nanoparticles by actinomycetes *Streptomyces viridogens* strain HM10. *Indian Journal of Biochemistry & Biophysics*, *48*, 331–335. PMID:22165291

Bina, B., Pourzamani, H., Rashidi, A., & Amin, M. M. (2012). Ethylbenzene removal by carbon nanotubes from aqueous solution. *Journal of Environmental and Public Health*, *817187*, 1–8. doi:10.1155/2012/817187 PMID:22187576

Biricova, V., & Laznickova, A. (2009). Dendrimers: Analytical characterization and applications. *Bioorganic Chemistry*, *37*(6), 185–192. doi:10.1016/j.bioorg.2009.07.006 PMID:19703699

Bollini, P., Didas, S. A., & Jones, C. W. (2011). Amine-oxide hybrid materials for acid gas separations. *Journal of Materials Chemistry*, *21*(39), 15100–15120. doi:10.1039/c1jm12522b

Brinkmann, N., Giebel, D., Lohmer, G., Reetz, M. T., & Kragl, U. (1999). Allylic substitution with dendritic palladium catalysts in a continuously operating membrane reactor. *Journal of Catalysis*, *183*(2), 163–168. doi:10.1006/jcat.1999.2462

Campbell, M. L., Guerra, F. D., Dhulekar, J., Alexis, F., & Whitehead, D. C. (2015). Target-Specific Capture of Environmentally Relevant Gaseous Aldehydes and Carboxylic Acids with Functional Nanoparticles. *Chemistry (Weinheim an der Bergstrasse, Germany)*, *21*(42), 14834–14842. doi:10.1002/chem.201502021 PMID:26331393

Chen, X., Cen, C., Tang, Z., Zeng, W., Chen, D., Fang, P., & Chen, Z. (2013). The key role of pH value in the synthesis of titanate nanotubes-loaded manganese oxides as a superior catalyst for the selective catalytic reduction of NO with NH_3. *Journal of Nanomaterials*, *871528*, 1–7. doi:10.1155/2013/871528

Das, I., & Ansari, S. A. (2009). Nanomaterials in science and technology. *Journal of Scientific and Industrial Research, 68*(8), 657–667.

Das, S., Chakraborty, J., Chatterjee, S., & Kumar, H. (2018). Prospects of biosynthesized nanomaterials for remediation of organic and inorganic environmental contaminants. *Environmental Science. Nano, 5*(12), 2784–2808. doi:10.1039/C8EN00799C

De Windt, W., Aelterman, P., & Verstraete, W. (2005). Bioreductive deposition of palladium (0) nanoparticles on *Shewanella oneidensis* with catalytic activity towards reductive dechlorination of polychlorinated biphenyls. *Environmental Microbiology, 7*(3), 314–325. doi:10.1111/j.1462-2920.2005.00696.x PMID:15683392

Diallo, M. S., Christie, S., Swaminathan, P., Johnson, J. H., & Goddard, W. A. (2005). Dendrimer enhanced ultrafiltration.1. Recovery of Cu (II) from aqueous solutions using PAMAM dendrimers with ethylene diamine core and terminal NH_2 groups. *Environmental Science & Technology, 39*(5), 1366–1377. doi:10.1021/es048961r PMID:15787379

Fagan, R., McComack, D., Dionysiou, D., & Pillai, S. (2016). A review of solar visible light active TiO2 photocatalysis for treating bacteria, cyanotoxins and contaminants of emerging concern. *Materials Science in Semiconductor Processing, 42*, 2–14. doi:10.1016/j.mssp.2015.07.052

Fang, Z., Qiu, X., Chen, J., & Qiu, X. (2011). Debromination of polybrominated diphenyl ethers by Ni/Fe bimetallic nanoparticles: Influencing factors, kinetics, and mechanism. *Journal of Hazardous Materials, 185*(2-3), 958–969. doi:10.1016/j.jhazmat.2010.09.113 PMID:21035251

Garca-Segura, S., Bellotindos, L. M., Huang, Y. H., Brillas, E., & Lu, M. C. (2016). Fluidized-bed Fenton process as alternative wastewater treatment technology—A review. *Journal of the Taiwan Institute of Chemical Engineers, 67*, 211–225. doi:10.1016/j.jtice.2016.07.021

Ge, F., Li, M.-M., Ye, H., & Zhao, B.-X. (2012). Effective removal of heavy metal ions Cd^{2+}, Zn^{2+}, Pb^{2+}, Cu^{2+} from aqueous solution by polymermodified magnetic nanoparticles. *Journal of Hazardous Materials, 211–212*, 366–372. doi:10.1016/j.jhazmat.2011.12.013 PMID:22209322

Gogoi, S. K., Gopinath, P., Paul, A., Ramesh, A., Ghosh, S. S., & Chattopadhyay, A. (2006). Green Fluorescent Protein-Expressing *Escherichia coli* as a Model System for Investigating the Antimicrobial Activities of Silver Nanoparticles. *Langmuir, 22*(22), 9322–9328. doi:10.1021/la060661v PMID:17042548

Govindaraju, K., Basha, S. K., Kumar, V. G., & Singaravelu, G. (2008). Silver, gold and bimetallic nanoparticles production using single-cell protein (*Spirulina platensis*) Geitler. *Journal of Materials Science, 43*(15), 5115–5122. doi:10.100710853-008-2745-4

Guerra, F., Attia, M., Whitehead, D., & Alexis, F. (2018). Nanotechnology for environmental remediation: Materials and applications. *Molecules (Basel, Switzerland), 23*(7), 1760. doi:10.3390/molecules23071760 PMID:30021974

Gupta, A., Joia, J., Sood, A., Sood, R., & Sidhu, C. (2016). Microbes as Potential Tool for Remediation of Heavy Metals: A Review. *Journal of Microbial & Biochemical Technology, 8*(4), 364–372. doi:10.4172/1948-5948.1000310

Hao, Y.-M., Man, C., & Hu, Z.-B. (2010). Effective removal of Cu (II) ions from aqueous solution by amino-functionalized magnetic nanoparticles. *Journal of Hazardous Materials, 184*(1-3), 392–399. doi:10.1016/j.jhazmat.2010.08.048 PMID:20837378

He, J., Yang, X., Men, B., & Wang, D. (2016). Interfacial mechanisms of Heterogenous Fenton reactions catalyzed by iron based materials: A review. *Journal of Environmental Sciences (China), 39*, 97–109. doi:10.1016/j.jes.2015.12.003 PMID:26899649

Huang, H. Y., Yang, R. T., Chinn, D., & Munson, C. L. (2003). Amine-Grafted MCM-48 and Silica Xerogel as Superior Sorbents for Acidic Gas Removal from Natural Gas. *Industrial & Engineering Chemistry Research, 42*(12), 2427–2433. doi:10.1021/ie020440u

Huang, J., Cao, Y., Liu, Z., Deng, Z., Tang, F., & Wang, W. (2012). Efficient removal of heavy metal ions from water system by titanate nanoflowers. *Chemical Engineering Journal, 180*, 75–80. doi:10.1016/j.cej.2011.11.005

Ibrahim, R., Hayyan, M., AlSaadi, M., Hayyan, A., & Ibrahim, S. (2016). Environmental application of nanotechnology: Air, soil and water. *Environmental Science and Pollution Research International, 23*(14), 13754–13788. doi:10.100711356-016-6457-z PMID:27074929

Jayaseelan, C., Rahuman, A. A., Roopan, S. M., Kirthi, A. V., Venkatesan, J., Kim, S. K., Iyappan, M., & Siva, C. (2013). Biological approach to synthesize TiO_2 nanoparticles using *Aeromonas hydrophila* and its antibacterial activity. *Spectrochimica Acta. Part A: Molecular and Biomolecular Spectroscopy, 107*, 82–89. doi:10.1016/j.saa.2012.12.083 PMID:23416912

Kandah, M. I., & Meunier, J. L. (2007). Removal of nickel ions from water bymulti-walled carbon nanotubes. *Journal of Hazardous Materials, 146*(1-2), 283–288. doi:10.1016/j.jhazmat.2006.12.019 PMID:17196328

Karn, B., Kuiken, T., & Otto, M. (2009). Nanotechnology and in situ remediation: A review of the benefits and potential risks. *Environmental Health Perspectives, 117*(12), 1813–1831. doi:10.1289/ehp.0900793 PMID:20049198

Khan, M. M., Adil, S. F., & Al-Mayouf, A. (2015). Metal oxides as photocatalysts. *Journal of Saudi Chemical Society, 19*(5), 462–464. doi:10.1016/j.jscs.2015.04.003

Khare, P., Yadav, A., Ramkumar, J., & Verma, N. (2016). Microchannel-embedded metal–carbon–polymer nanocomposite as a novel support for chitosan for efficient removal of hexavalent chromium from water under dynamic conditions. *Chemical Engineering Journal, 293*, 44–54. doi:10.1016/j.cej.2016.02.049

Kharisov, B. I., Rasika Dias, H. V., Kharissova, O. V., Manuel Jiménez-Pérez, V., Olvera Pérez, B., & Muñoz Flores, B. (2012). Iron-containing nanomaterials: Synthesis, properties, and environmental applications. *Royal Society of Chemistry Advances, 2*(25), 9325–9358. doi:10.1039/c2ra20812a

Khin, M. M., Nair, A. S., Babu, V. J., Murugan, R., & Ramakrishna, S. A. (2012). Review on nanomaterials for environmental remediation. *Energy & Environmental Science, 5*(8), 8075–8109. doi:10.1039/c2ee21818f

Li, Q., Mahendra, S., Lyon, D. Y., Brunet, L., Liga, M. V., Li, D., & Alvarez, P. (2008). Antimicrobial nanomaterials for water disinfection and microbial control: Potential applications and implications. *Water Research*, *42*(18), 4591–4602. doi:10.1016/j.watres.2008.08.015 PMID:18804836

Li, Y., Liu, F., Xia, B., Du, Q., Zhang, P., Wang, D., Wang, Z., & Xia, Y. (2010). Removal of copper from aqueous solution by carbon nanotube/calcium alginate composites. *Journal of Hazardous Materials*, *177*(1–3), 876–880. doi:10.1016/j.jhazmat.2009.12.114 PMID:20083351

Liang, C., Dai, X., Zhou, B., & Zhang, Y. (2014). Application of zero-valent iron nanoparticles for the removal of aqueous zinc ions under various experimental conditions. *PLoS One*, *9*(1), e85686. doi:10.1371/journal.pone.0085686 PMID:24416439

Lithoxoos, G. P., Labropoulos, A., Peristeras, L. D., Kanellopoulos, N., Samios, J., & Economou, I. G. (2010). Adsorption of N_2, CH_4, CO and CO_2 gases in single walled carbon nanotubes: A combined experimental and Monte Carlo molecular simulation study. *The Journal of Supercritical Fluids*, *55*(2), 510–523. doi:10.1016/j.supflu.2010.09.017

Liu, Y., Zhang, P., Du, Q., Peng, X., Liu, T., Wang, Z., Xia, Y., Zhang, W., Wang, K., & Zhu, H. (2011). Adsorption of fluoride from aqueous solution by graphene. *Journal of Colloid and Interface Science*, *363*(1), 348–354. doi:10.1016/j.jcis.2011.07.032 PMID:21821258

Lu, H., Wang, J., Stoller, M., Wang, T., Bao, Y., & Hao, H. (2016). An overview of nanomaterials for water and wastewater treatment. *Advances in Materials Science and Engineering*, *4964828*, 1–10. doi:10.1155/2016/4964828

Lunge, S., Singh, S., & Sinha, A. (2014). Magnetic iron oxide (Fe_3O_4) nanoparticles from tea waste for arsenic removal. *Journal of Magnetism and Magnetic Materials*, *356*, 21–31. doi:10.1016/j.jmmm.2013.12.008

Luo, F., Chen, Z., Megharaj, M., & Naidu, R. (2016). Simultaneous removal of trichloroethylene and hexavalent chromium by green synthesized agarose-Fe nanoparticles hydrogel. *Chemical Engineering Journal*, *294*, 290–297. doi:10.1016/j.cej.2016.03.005

Madima, N., Mishra, S., Inamuddin, I., & Mishra, A. (2020). Carbon-based nanomaterials for remediation of organic and inorganic pollutants from wastewater: A review. *Environmental Chemistry Letters*, *18*(4), 1169–1191. doi:10.100710311-020-01001-0

Mauter, M., & Elimelech, M. (2008). Environmental applications of carbon-based nanomaterials. *Environmental Science & Technology*, *42*(16), 5843–5859. doi:10.1021/es8006904 PMID:18767635

Mehndiratta, P., Jain, A., Srivastava, S., & Gupta, N. (2013). Environmental pollution and nanotechnology. *Environment and Pollution*, *2*(2), 49–58. doi:10.5539/ep.v2n2p49

Mustafa, G., Tahir, H., Sultan, M., & Akhtar, N. (2013). Synthesis and characterization of cupric oxide (CuO) nanoparticles and their application for the removal of dyes. *African Journal of Biotechnology*, *12*(47), 6650–6660. doi:10.5897/AJB2013.13058

Nehru, K., & Sivakumar, M. (2012). Biosynthesis of Ag nanoparticles using Amaranthus tristis extract for the fabrication of nanoparticle embedded PVA membrane. *Current Nanoscience*, *8*, 703–708. doi:10.2174/157341312802884436

Nomura, A., & Jones, C. W. (2013). Amine-functionalized porous silicas as adsorbents for aldehyde abatement. *ACS Applied Materials & Interfaces*, *5*(12), 5569–5577. doi:10.1021/am400810s PMID:23716505

Nurmi, J. T., Tratnyek, P. G., Sarathy, V., Baer, D. R., Amonette, J. E., Pecher, K., Wang, C., Linehan, J. C., Matson, D. W., Penn, R. L., & Driessen, M. D. (2005). Characterization and properties of metallic iron nanoparticles: Spectroscopy, electrochemistry, and kinetics. *Environmental Science & Technology*, *39*(5), 1221–1230. doi:10.1021/es049190u PMID:15787360

Nyika, J. M. (2020a). The use of microorganism derived enzymes for bioremediation of soils pollutants. In S. Dey & B. Acharya (Eds.), *Recent advances in bioremediation of metal contaminants*. IGI Global.

Nyika, J. M. (2020b). Tolerance of microorganisms to heavy metals. In S. Dey & B. Acharya (Eds.), *Recent advances in bioremediation of metal contaminants*. IGI Global.

Pal, S., Tak, Y. K., & Song, J. M. (2007). Does the antibacterial activity of silver nanoparticles depend on the shape of the nanoparticle? A study of the gram-negative bacterium *Escherichia coli*. *Applied and Environmental Microbiology*, *73*(6), 1712–1720. doi:10.1128/AEM.02218-06 PMID:17261510

Pan, B., & Xing, B. (2008). Adsorption mechanisms of organic chemicals on carbon nanotubes. *Environmental Science & Technology*, *42*(24), 9005–9013. doi:10.1021/es801777n PMID:19174865

Pandey, G. (2018). Prospects of nanobioremediation in environmental clean-up. *Oriental Journal of Chemistry*, *34*(6), 2828–2840. doi:10.13005/ojc/340622

Pandey, S., Kumari, M., Singh, S. P., Bhattacharya, A., Mishra, S. K., Chauhan, P. S., & Mishra, A. (2015). Bioremediation via Nanoparticles: An Innovative Microbial Approach. In S. Singh & K. Srivastava (Eds.), *Handbook of research on uncovering new methods for ecosystem management through bioremediation*. IGI Global. doi:10.4018/978-1-4666-8682-3.ch019

Park, J., & Lee, I. H. (2014). Photocatalytic degradation of 2-chlorophenol using Ag-doped TiO2 nanofibers and a near-UV light-emitting diode system. *Journal of Nanomaterials*, *250803*, 1–8.

Poursaberi, T., Hassanisadi, M., Torkestani, K., & Zare, M. (2012). Development of zirconium (IV)-metalloporphyrin grafted Fe3O4 nanoparticles for efficient fluoride removal. *Chemical Engineering Journal*, *189–190*, 117–125. doi:10.1016/j.cej.2012.02.039

Quan, X., Yang, S., Ruan, X., & Zhao, H. (2005). Preparation of Titania Nanotubes and Their Environmental Applications as Electrode. *Environmental Science & Technology*, *39*(10), 3770–3775. doi:10.1021/es048684o PMID:15952384

Rasalingam, S., Peng, R., & Koodali, R. T. (2014). Removal of hazardous pollutants from wastewaters: Applications of TiO2-SiO2 mixed oxide materials. *Journal of Nanomaterials*, *617405*, 1–10. doi:10.1155/2014/617405

Ren, X., Chen, C., Nagatsu, M., & Wang, X. (2011). Carbon nanotubes as adsorbents in environmental pollution management: A review. *Chemical Engineering Journal*, *170*(2-3), 395–410. doi:10.1016/j.cej.2010.08.045

Rizwan, M., Singh, M., Mitra, C. & Morve, R. (2014). Eco-friendly application of nanomaterials: nanobioremediation. *Journal of Nanoparticles*, 1-7.

Rychoudhury, T., & Scheytt, T. (2013). Potential of zerovalent iron nanoparticles for remediation of environmental organic contaminants in water: A review. *Water Science and Technology*, *68*(7), 1425–1439. doi:10.2166/wst.2013.358 PMID:24135090

Santhosh, C., Velmurugan, V., Jacob, G., Jeong, S. K., Grace, A. N., & Bhatnagar, A. (2016). Role of nanomaterials in water treatment applications: A review. *Chemical Engineering Journal*, *306*, 1116–1137. doi:10.1016/j.cej.2016.08.053

Shan, G., Xing, J., Zhang, H., & Liu, H. (2005). Biodesulfurization of Dibenzothiophene by Microbial Cells Coated with Magnetite Nanoparticles. *Applied and Environmental Microbiology*, *71*(8), 4497–4502. doi:10.1128/AEM.71.8.4497-4502.2005 PMID:16085841

Singh, D., Gautam, R. K., Kumar, R., Shukla, B. K., Shankar, V., & Krishna, V. (2014). Citric acid coated magnetic nanoparticles: Synthesis, characterization and application in removal of Cd (II) ions from aqueous solution. *Journal of Water Process Engineering*, *4*, 233–241. doi:10.1016/j.jwpe.2014.10.005

Singh, R., Misra, V., & Singh, R. P. (2012). Removal of hexavalent chromium from contaminated ground water using zerovalent iron nanoparticles. *Environmental Monitoring and Assessment*, *184*(6), 3643–3651. doi:10.100710661-011-2213-5 PMID:21769560

Suvith, V. S., & Philip, D. (2014). Catalytic degradation of methylene blue using biosynthesized gold and silver nanoparticles. *Spectrochimica Acta. Part A: Molecular and Biomolecular Spectroscopy*, *118*, 526–532. doi:10.1016/j.saa.2013.09.016 PMID:24091344

Tisa, A., Raman, A., & Daud, W. (2014). Applicability of fluidized bed reactor in recalcitrant compound degradation through advanced oxidation processes: A review. *Journal of Environmental Management*, *146*, 260–275. doi:10.1016/j.jenvman.2014.07.032 PMID:25190594

Tsai, C. H., Chang, W. C., Saikia, D., Wu, C. E., & Kao, H. M. (2016). Functionalization of cubic mesoporous silica SBA-16 with carboxylic acid via one-pot synthesis route for effective removal of cationic dyes. *Journal of Hazardous Materials*, *309*, 236–248. doi:10.1016/j.jhazmat.2015.08.051 PMID:26906434

Tungittiplakorn, W., Lion, L. W., Cohen, C., & Kim, J. Y. (2004). Engineered Polymeric Nanoparticles for Soil Remediation. *Environmental Science & Technology*, *38*(5), 1605–1610. doi:10.1021/es0348997 PMID:15046367

Vunain, E., Mishra, A. K., & Mamba, B. B. (2016). Dendrimers, mesoporous silicas and chitosan-based nanosorbents for the removal of heavy-metal ions: A review. *International Journal of Macromolecules*, *86*, 570–586. doi:10.1016/j.ijbiomac.2016.02.005 PMID:26851359

Wang, S., Sun, H., Ang, H. M., & Tadé, M. O. (2013). Adsorptive remediation of environmental pollutants using novel graphene-based nanomaterials. *Chemical Engineering Journal*, *226*, 336–347. doi:10.1016/j.cej.2013.04.070

Wang, T., Jin, X., Chen, Z., Megharaj, M., & Naidu, R. (2014). Green synthesis of Fe nanoparticles using eucalyptus leaf extracts for treatment of eutrophic wastewater. *The Science of the Total Environment*, *466–467*, 210–213. doi:10.1016/j.scitotenv.2013.07.022 PMID:23895784

Wang, Y., Pan, C., Chu, W., Vipin, A., & Sun, L. (2019). Environmental remediation applications of carbon nanotubes and graphene oxide: Adsorption and catalysis. *Nanomaterials (Basel, Switzerland)*, *9*(3), 439. doi:10.3390/nano9030439 PMID:30875970

White, B., Stackhouse, T., & Holcombe, J. (2009). Magnetic γ-Fe2O3 NPs coated with poly-L-cysteine for chelation of As (III), Cu (II), Cd (II), Ni (II), Pb (II) and Zn(II). *Journal of Hazardous Materials*, *161*(2-3), 848–853. doi:10.1016/j.jhazmat.2008.04.105 PMID:18571848

Windt, W. D., Aelterman, P., & Verstraete, W. (2005). Bioreductive deposition of palladium (0) nanoparticles on *Shewanella oneidensis* with catalytic activity towards reductive dechlorination of polychlorinated biphenyls. *Environmental Microbiology*, *7*(3), 314–325. doi:10.1111/j.1462-2920.2005.00696.x PMID:15683392

Wu, L., & Ritchie, S. (2006). Removal of trichloroethylene from water by cellulose acetate supported bimetallic Ni/Fe nanoparticles. *Chemosphere*, *63*(2), 285–292. doi:10.1016/j.chemosphere.2005.07.021 PMID:16226292

Yang, J., Hou, B., Wang, J., Tian, B., Bi, J., Wang, N., Li, X., & Huang, X. (2019). Nanomaterials for the removal of heavy metals from wastewater. *Nanomaterials (Basel, Switzerland)*, *9*(3), 424. doi:10.3390/nano9030424 PMID:30871096

Yang, Q., Agouri, S., Tyrrell, J., & Walsh, T. (2018). Heavy metal resistance genes are associated with blaNDM-1 and blaCTX-M15 carrying *enterobecteriaceae. Antimicrobial Agents and Chemotherapy*, *62*(5), e02614–e02642. doi:10.1128/AAC.02642-17 PMID:29507071

Zhang, Y., Tang, Z. R., Fu, X., & Xu, Y. J. (2010). TiO_2 Graphene Nanocomposites for Gas-Phase Photocatalytic Degradation of Volatile Aromatic Pollutant: Is TiO_2 Graphene Truly Different from Other TiO2 Carbon Composite Materials? *ACS Nanotechnology*, *4*(12), 7303–7314. doi:10.1021/nn1024219 PMID:21117654

Zhu, N., Luan, H., Yuan, S., Chen, J., Wu, X., & Wang, L. (2010). Effective dechlorination of HCB by nanoscale Cu/Fe particles. *Journal of Hazardous Materials*, *176*(1-3), 1101–1105. doi:10.1016/j.jhazmat.2009.11.092 PMID:19969417

KEY TERMS AND DEFINITIONS

Advanced Oxidative Process: A set of chemical protocols used in degradation of organic pollutants via oxidation of hydroxyl radicals during treatment of water/wastewater.

Dendritic Polymers: Multiple branched polymers with regulated structures that have many functional groups, good solubility, and low melt viscosity.

Electrospinning: A fibre production method that applies electrical force, high temperatures and coagulation chemistry to remove charged threads of polymeric solutions of nanoscale sizes.

Gibb's Free Energy: It is the highest amount of non-expansion work taken out of a closed thermodynamic system in its normal conditions. Also known as free enthalpy.

Headspace Analysis: A technology developed to analyse the odour of gases and gaseous compounds.

Quantum Effects: Any consequence of subatomic particle interactions with motion that accesses the quality of a wave-particle and quantization of its energy.

Surface Plasmon Resonance: The resonant oscillation resulting from electron conduction at the border between positive and negative charges and is induced by rays of light striking on a surface.

Chapter 3
Nanomaterials Useful in Health and Medicine to Improve Public Health

Manish Kumar Dwivedi
Indira Gandhi National Tribal University, Amamrakantak, India

Suvashish Kumar Pandey
https://orcid.org/0000-0001-6524-475X
School of Bio-Sciences and Technology, VIT University, Vellore, India

Prashant Kumar Singh
https://orcid.org/0000-0002-8117-4592
Indira Gandhi National Tribal University, Amarkantak, India

ABSTRACT

In modern research, nanotechnology is a very attractive technology and helps to reduce infectious diseases. Nanoparticles have gained significantly more important than the bulk counterparts due to their unique properties. This chapter gives knowledge about the general introduction of nanoparticles with classification and also discussed the effect of nanoparticles impact on public health. Nanotechnology is most widely used to reduced different types of infectious diseases such as bacterial, viral, parasitic diseases, etc. Nanotechnology is applied to detect different types of diseases such as cancer, diabetes, and other diseases. Nanotechnology is a useful technique to develop novel drug delivery systems due to their high specificity, high drug-carrying capacity, and high stability. Nanotechnology can be able to improve human health but on the other hand, we have seen a negative impact on human health and environmental health. The solubility and toxicity of nanoparticles is a major issue worldwide.

DOI: 10.4018/978-1-7998-5563-7.ch003

INTRODUCTION

Nanotechnology is a modern science that studies commercially produced materials having at least one dimension less than 100 nm. It is being widely used in modern medicines and pharmaceuticals modernizing the healthcare market of the twentieth century (Pautler, et al., 2010). "Norio Taniguchi" from Tokyo Science University, Japan first described the word 'nanotechnology' in 1974 (Taniguchi, 1974). Nanotechnology is referred to as the study of nanoparticles, including design, synthesis, structure characterization, and application of nanoparticles through monitoring the shapes and sizes at the nanoscale level. The word "nano" comes from the Latin word "*nanus*" which means "*dwarf*" and by extension '*very small*' (Yousaf, & Salamat, 2008). Nowadays, the word nanotechnology, nanomaterials, nanochemistry, or nanoscience are just a small number which often arises in scientific research articles, nanotechnology related books, and have become familiar to a wide public, even non-specialists too (Manavalan et al., 2011). The measurement of nanoparticles (NPs), according to the International System of Units (SI), is nanometers (1nm corresponding to 10^{-9}m) and includes systems whose sizes are beyond molecular dimensions and below macroscopic ones (>1nm and <100nm). Nanotechnology is a new field of science which studies the microscopic particles. "Nano" means one-billionth and one nanometer is one-billionth of a meter in science (Manavalan et al., 2011).

NPs have received excessive research attention because of their unique properties including size, shape, and the chemistry of molecules/materials used to coat their surface. NPs are engineered at the molecular level to accomplish superior properties compared to similar materials in larger size (Moffatt, 2016). During the last few years applications of nanotechnology and nanoscience have emerged rapidly in wide range of product domains. It is used in association with electronics, optics, biomedical and materials sciences (Sabir et al., 2014). NPs are actually modified form of basic elements obtained by changing their atoms as well as the molecular properties of elements.

BACKGROUND

Nanotechnology is one of the most rising arenas of science and technology with marvelous development. It is transforming the overwhelmed experiments of traditional drug delivery systems based on the development and manufacturing of NP's with novel characteristics (Zhang et al., 2013). The unique properties of NPs are responsible for enhanced drug efficiency, solidity, pharmacokinetics, drug monitoring activities and reduced toxicity. Local diseases such as infection and inflammation not only have perforated vasculature but also acquire some epitopes or receptors that can be used as targets. Nanomedicines can be actively targeted at such locations that may be beneficial in ameliorating the condition. A variety of NP based systems have been tried as potential drug delivery systems, including fullerenes, solid lipid nanoparticles (SLN), polymeric micelles, nanocapsules, nanogels, nanoliposomes, dendrimers, metal NPs, biodegradable polymeric NPs, carbon nanotubes (Hong et al. 2009) and quantum dots **(Figure 1)** (Cai et al., 2007).

Figure 1. Illustrate a different types nanoparticle

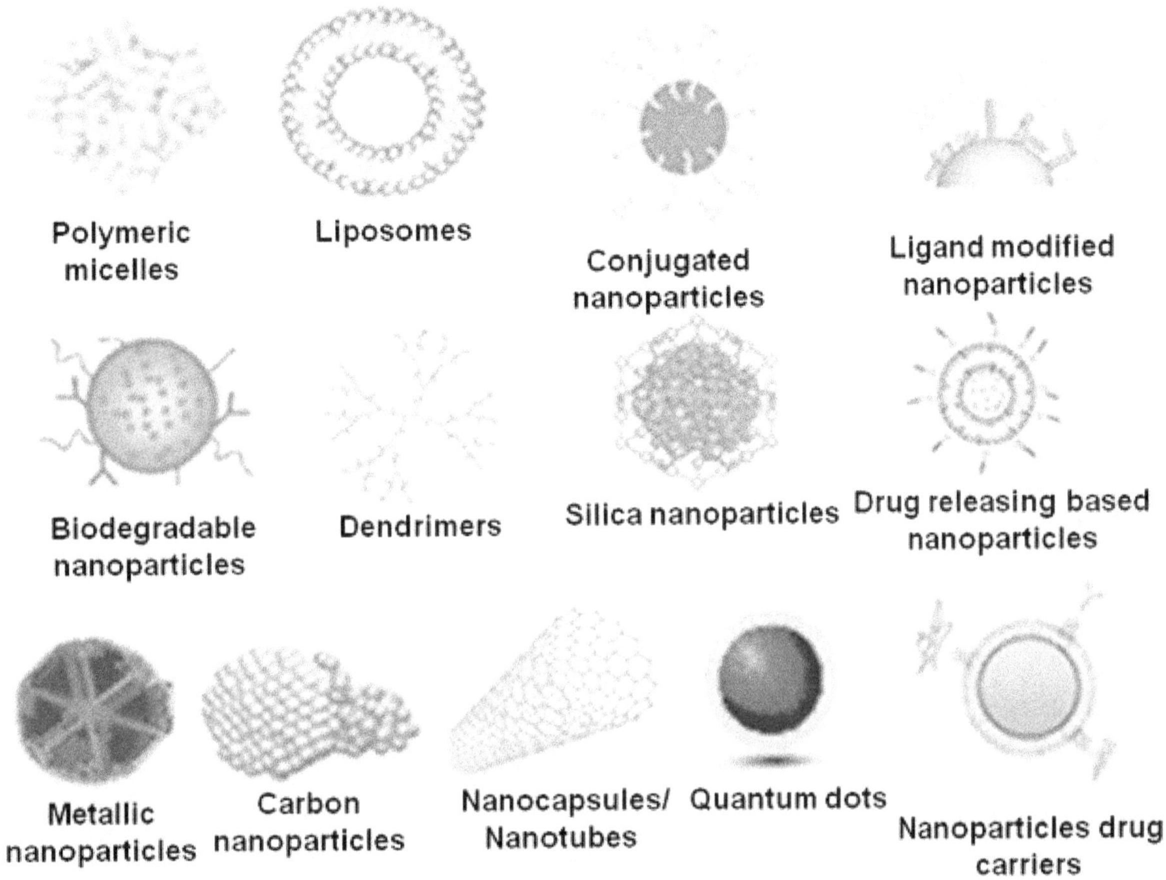

NPs have been utilized for the development of systemic, oral, pulmonary, trans-dermal and other administration routes for drug targeting. It is also an improvement of drug bioavailability and defense of drug bioactivity and constancy. In recent years, the encapsulation of antimicrobial drugs in the NP systems has emerged as an innovative and promising alternative that enhances therapeutic effectiveness and reduces the undesirable side effects of drugs. A major goal of designing NPs is the surface properties and the particle size of the delivery system that can regulate the pharmaceutically active agents for site-specific action at a clinically active rate.

There are several sectors where the NPs can be specifically utilized such as chemical engineering, biotechnology, biopesticides, cosmetics, aquaculture technology, sensor applications, environmental engineering, energy and electronics, manufacturing and materials, biological or medicine like fluorescent biological labels (Wang et al., 2002), drug and gene delivery (Panatarotto et al., 2003), pathogens detection (Edelstein et al., 2000), probing of DNA structures (Mahtab et al., 1995), proteins detection (Nam et al., 2003), tissue engineering (Ma et al., 2003), tumor engineering, pharmacokinetic studies (Parak et al., 2002), magnetic resonance imaging contrast enhancement (Weissleder et al., 1990), agriculture and plant sciences (Tripathi et al., 2016;Tiwari et al., 2017). Lately, biomedical NPs have gained more concerns due to their major biological characteristics and biomedical applications. NPs have also been generated to transform diagnostics, drug delivery, gene therapy and general therapeutics (Mishra, et al., 2017).

CLASSIFICATION OF NANOMATERIALS / NANOPARTICLES

Nanotechnology has emerged as a significant solution for the treatment of various types of diseases utilising different types of nanoparticle based drug delivery systems. NPs can be synthesized via two approaches namely top-down and bottom-up approach. The Bottom-up approach is the best method used by the biological system due to less energy utilization and minimal wastage. This approach depends on the molecular self-assembly related to physical and chemical interactions at the nanoscale which assemble primary building blocks atom by atom into macroscopic structures. The physical method use laser diodes and electricity and are being used for large scale manufacture of NPs such as carbon nanotubes that are the most commonly used nanomaterials in today's world. The chemical method works by chemical modifications changing the bulk materials during chemical synthesis using metal ions and organic solutions. The molecular interactions include non-covalent bonds, such as hydrogen and ionic bonds, van der Waals forces and water mediated hydrogen bonds. The green synthesis is a new method that is being used most commonly by the biological researchers for NPs synthesis using metal ions and plant extracts.

Different types of nanoparticles can be prepared using several methods of NPs synthesis (**Figure 2**). We have discussed some important and most commonly used methods for the synthesis of NPs.

(A) Material Based Nanoparticles

NPs are categorized based on their external morphology, size and chemical properties. On the basis of physical and chemical characteristics the major classification is as follows:

a) Carbon Nanoparticles

Carbon NPs (CBNs) are significant nanomaterials used in the field of medical therapy and other areas of science and technology that are being explored broadly for use in various applications. These are condensed octahedral structures with 2-8 nm diameter size (Zhang et al., 2009). CBNs are differently classified as amorphous carbon, graphite and diamonds to newly discovered promising carbon nanotubes (CNTs), graphene oxide (GO), graphene quantum (GQDs), fullerene, and carbon fibers (Mostofizadeh et al., 2011). CBNs are graphene sheets rolled into a tube which is 100 times stronger than steel. Based on the walls they can be single-walled or multi-walled CNTs. Another carbon NP based structures are fullerenes that are composed of carbon molecules forming pentagonal and hexagonal hollow cage structure contained sixty (C-60) or more carbon atoms. These are widely used commercially because of their structure, insolubility in water and organic solvents and its low tendency to form aggregates. Fullerenes have an electron deficient structure that favors its interactions with compounds possessing electron donor groups. Carbon NPs are broadly used in various biological applications including drug delivery, tissue engineering, biosensing, cancer therapy, diagnosis, and imaging (Bhattacharya et al., 2016).

Figure 2. Display different types of methods for the preparation of different types of nanoparticles

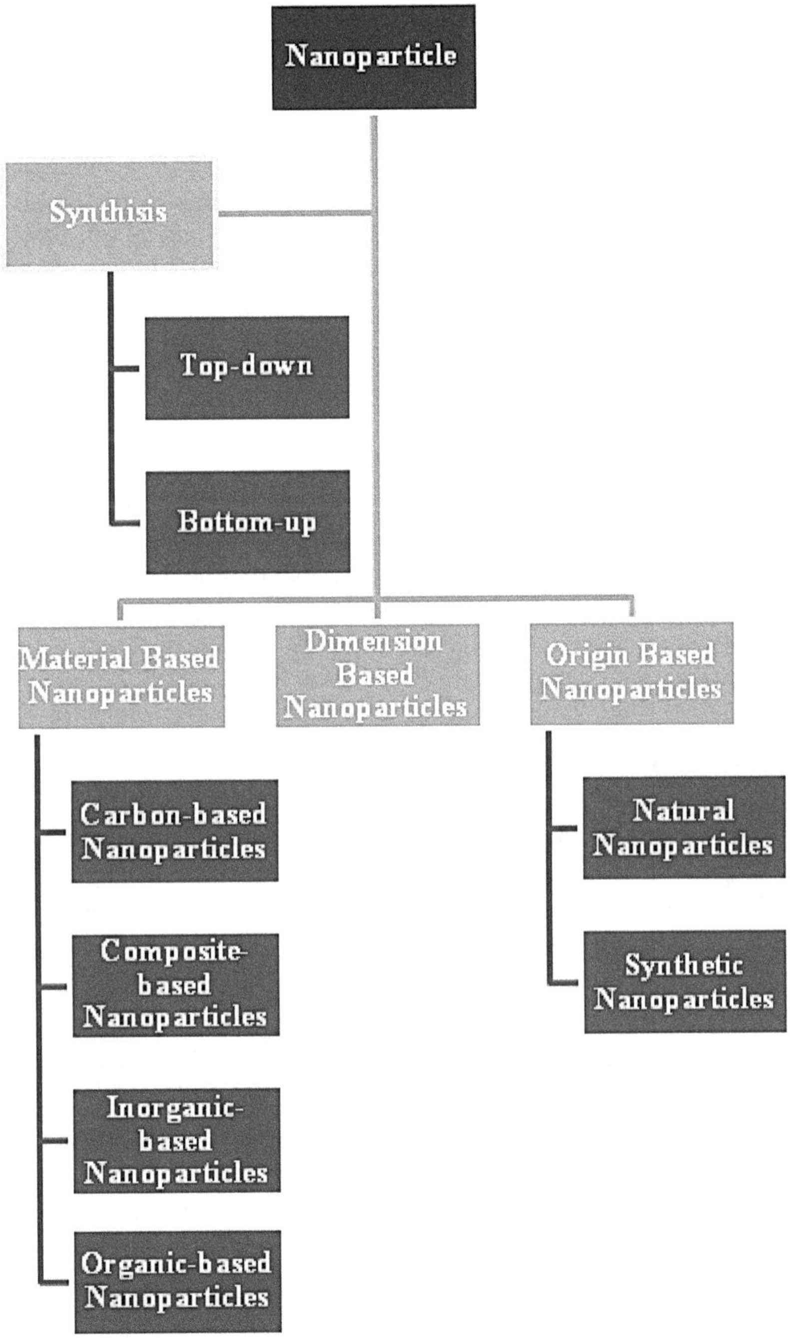

(b) Inorganic Metallic Nanoparticles

Inorganic metallic NPs represent a new type of NPs with unique physical and chemical properties that can be used in many physical, biological, biomedical, and pharmaceutical applications. Inorganic NPs cover broad range of substances including elemental metals, metal oxide, and metal salts (Chaloupka et al., 2010) and can be synthesized into metals such as Au, Ag (AgNPs), TiO_2 (TiO_2NPs), ZnO (ZnONPs), Cu (CuNPs), Fe (INPs) and semiconductors such as silicon and ceramics. These NPs can be synthesized and modified with various chemical functional groups that allow them to be conjugated with antibodies, ligands, and drugs of interest. These characteristics have opened a wide range of applications in biotechnology, magnetic separation, target analytes concentration, target based drug delivery, gene and drug delivery vehicles and for diagnostic imaging purposes. The advanced technologies such as magnetic resonance imaging, computed tomography, positron emission tomography, ultrasound, surface-enhanced Raman spectroscopy and optical imaging are dependent upon contrast as an aid to image various disease states. The availability of several NPs such as magnetic NPs (Fe3O4) gold, and silver NPs has helped in developing such technologies. Gold, silver and magnetic (iron oxide) NPs are being continuously used for diagnostic and therapeutic purposes.

(c) Organic Nanoparticles

Organic NPs have emerged as the excellent choice for biomedical applications. There are number of reports that focus on use organic NPs for bone, cartilage, skin or dental tissues regeneration. The use of natural or synthetic organic nanostructures have been found to be advantages in dental science for implantology, endodontics, and periodontics, regenerative dentistry and wound healing. The commonly researched organic NPs are nanoforms of chitosan, silk fibroin, synthetic polymers and their combinations (Virlan et al., 2016).

(d) Composite-Based Nanoparticles

Nowadays composite NPs are gaining much attention due to their scientific importance and application. These are structurally multiphase solid heterogeneous materials surrounded by more than one dimension of less than 100nm (Joshi & Adak, 2018). Composite NPs have at least two layers of coating, one a nanocrystalline phase and another an amorphous phase (Zhang et al., 2003). In recent years, composite NPs are characterized by attractive and cost-effective functional surface coating. By reason for this type of coating has shown increasing interest in many industries such as aerospace, automotive, electronics, and petroleum. The coatings of nanocomposites have improved weight reduction, mechanical strength, increased heat, improved barrier properties, and scratch resistance for endless performance. Composite NPs are used for different types of biomedical uses such as antimicrobial, anticorrosion, adhesive application, antifogging, drug delivery, tissue engineering, stem cell therapy, wound dressings, cardiac prosthesis, cancer therapy, artificial blood vessels, enzyme immobilization, and biosensors (Grande et al., 2009; Ullah et al., 2016).

(B) Dimension Based Nanoparticles

This classification of NPs is based on the number of dimensions of a material, which are outside the nanoscale (<100 nm) range. Four types of NPs are categorized based on the dimension (i) zero-dimensional (0D) NPs (ii) one-dimensional (1D) NPs, two-dimensional (2D) NPs and three-dimensional (3D) NPs (Jeevanandam et al., 2018). Zero-dimensional NPs are defined within the nanoscale (<100 nm) and are nanosized particles that have their length and width within the nanometer range. Most commonly 0D nanomaterials are nanoparticles. In 1D NPs one dimension is outside the nanoscale, for example nanotubes, nanorods, and nanowires. In 2D NPs, two dimensions are outside the nanoscale exhibiting plate-like shapes. The examples of this class are graphene, nanofilms, nanolayers, and nanocoatings. 3D NPs are materials that are not confined to the nanoscale in any dimension. This class can contain bulk powders, dispersions of nanoparticles, bundles of nanowires, and nanotubes as well as multi-nanolayers (Deshpande et al., 2009; Jeevanandam et al., 2018).

(C) Origin Based Nanoparticles

In addition to material and dimension based classification NPs can also be classified as natural or synthetic based on their origin.

(a) Natural Nanoparticles

Natural NPs are available from natural sources such as biological species, by geochemical or mechanical process prepared into micro and nanoscale templates without direct or indirect connection to human activity. Natural materials exist in huge quantities in the earth. In Earth, naturally formed nanomaterials are contained in the Earths circles such as the atmosphere (troposphere), the hydrosphere (oceans, lakes, rivers, groundwater, and hydrothermal vents), the lithosphere (rocks, soils, magma), and the biosphere (microorganisms, higher organisms-humans) (Hochella et al., 2015; Sharma et al., 2015). Kenaf, for example, is a natural tropical plant that has been fully-fledged commercially to produce a sub-ordinary source of income for emerging countries due to its high cellulose content (63%) (Jonoobi et al., 2009). The cellulose nanocrystals (CNC) and nanofibers (NFC) can be produced through acid hydrolysis and mechanical treatment of the Kenaf cellulose. CNC and NFC natural nanomaterials have been used in various applications such as filler in polymer composite to make a broad range of other functional materials (Kelly et al., 2013; Walther et al., 2011).

(b) Synthetic Nanoparticles

Synthetic NPs are basic and important components of nanoscience which are produced by a different processes such as mechanical grinding, chemical synthesis, green synthesis, physical, biological or hybrid methods (Wagner et al., 2014). Even though the hasty progress of nanotechnology, the association of humans and the environment of synthetic NPs are at probable risk. There are reports from diverse fields like epidemiology, occupational health and aerosols studies that ultrafine particles (< 100 nm) may have negative impact on human health (Wagner et al., 2014; Jeevanandam et al., 2018). The toxicological outcomes of some studies on ultrafine particles only cover a small part of the effects of the large chemical diversity of synthetic NPs. It has been expected that emissions of NPs into the environment will increase rapidly through multiple exposure ways. There is unequivocal need to form legislative safety guidelines to review waste disposal, emission limit values and environmental quality standards in air and water to adequately address the toxicity issues due to NPs (Ghaemi et al., 2017).

IMMUNE SYSTEM AND NANOPARTICLES

The immune system is the body's defense system against invading foreign organisms. It plays a vital role in the survival and well being of human beings. The Immune system is composed of various specialized cells, tissues and organs that are responsible for antigen identification and processing. As a foreign organism or antigen enters the body, it is spotted and the immune response is mounted against the foreign object. This process is known as the immune response. The immune system can be categorized into two major type innate and adaptive immune system. Innate immunity consists of cells such as macrophages and neutrophils which distinguishes pathogens through identifying pathogen surface moieties, phagocytosis, and the suppression of pathogens by activation of different effector functions **(Figure 3)** (Pati et al., 2018). Adaptive immunity functions by two most important T and B-cells that are essential for the activation of cell-mediated and humoral responses. T-cells are further classified as CD4+ helper cells and CD8+ cytotoxic cells. These cells secrete various cytokines that moderate the function of B-cells besides identifying and destroying virally infected cells respectively **(Figure 3)**. The global incidence of infectious diseases is rising and several new pathogenic diseases are emerging as a new challenge to the scientific community around the world.

Figure 3. Targeted delivery of antigenic molecules using nanoparticles into the antigen presenting cells (APCs)

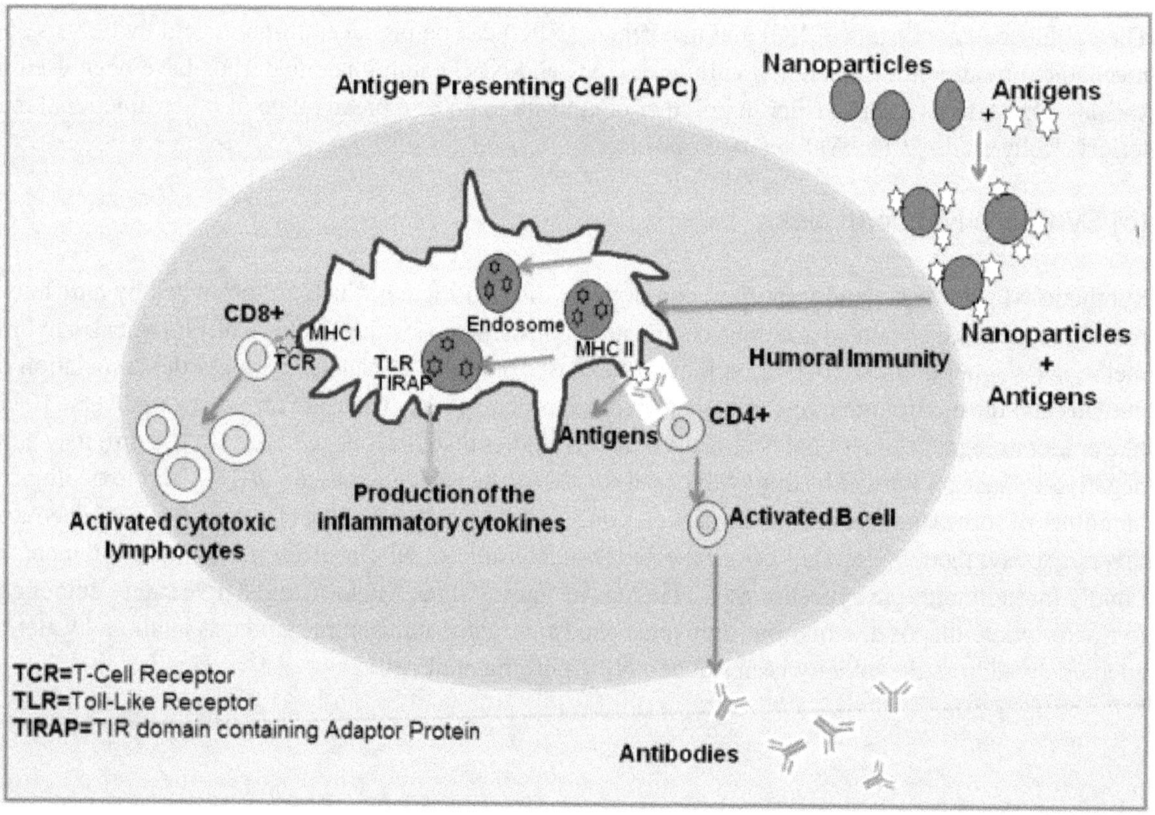

NPs are able to stimulate various immune cells and activate the host immune system. The unique characteristics of NPs such as size, shape and surface chemistry (binding ability) are important factors that can possibly activate the immune response by increasing the synthesis of resistance genes and inflammatory reactions (Smith et al., 2013). NPs are prepared by the use of different metal oxides. Materials such as gold, polymers, liposomes and carbon have the ability to induce immune reactive proteins such as cytokines and antibody mediated reactions (Mottram et al., 2007; Vallhov et al., 2006; Shvedova et al., 2005). This activity of NPs has been reported by several researchers. It has been observed that the empty PEGylated liposomes were capable to produce IgM response in *in vivo* animal models (Wang et al., 2007; Ishida, 2007). NPs are also used for the preparation of vaccines due to their size. The nanoparticles are the nanoscale (10-100nm) that can increase the vaccine efficiency *in vivo* better than huge molecules (Smith et al., 2013; Irvine et al., 2013) for the examples inorganic nanoparticles such as iron and silica-based nanoparticles (Pusic et al., 2013), polymeric nanoparticles such as chitosan, PLGA (32-37), liposomes such as cholesterol and lipids (Prego et al., 2010).

APPLICATIONS OF NANOTECHNOLOGY IN DISEASE DIAGNOSIS AND THERAPY

Infectious diseases are life-threatening infections that can spread from one person to another. They are caused by pathogenic microorganisms, such as bacteria, viruses, parasites or fungi (Dye, 2015). Such diseases are prevalent worldwide mostly in developing countries and are common amongst children and young adults. According to the, World Health Organization (WHO) lower respiratory infections caused 3.0 million deaths, diarrheal diseases caused 1.4 million deaths, tuberculosis was responsible for 1.3 million deaths, HIV/AIDS caused 1.0 million deaths and malaria accounted for a cause of death in low income countries (https://www.bcm.edu/departments/molecular-virology-and-microbiology/emerging-infections-and-biodefense/introduction-to-nfectious-diseases). These diseases are also called communicable diseases that are transmitted from person to person such as tuberculosis and also occasionally from species to another species such as influenza (Sundar et al., 2012). The chemotherapy for the infections caused by infectious agents that inhabit intracellularly presents several uncommon challenges. Microorganisms have initiated the approach to produce a silent infection inside the cells avoiding the immune responses. Several approaches for diagnosing and treatment of these infections presently exist but there is an essential need for developing the existing methods and development of novel therapeutic molecules. Infectious disease can be divided into three categories, firstly the known diseases such as malaria, tuberculosis etc. and secondly new and earlier unidentified diseases such as severe acute respiratory syndrome. Third category includes those infectious diseases that threaten to emerge shortly in the near future such as avian influenza (Tallury, et al., 2010). Malaria is an infectious disease infected an estimated 228 million cases worldwide in 2018 and was responsible for around 405000 global deaths (WHO, 2019). Another infectious disease, tuberculosis infects 10 million people killing about 1.5 million people per year (https://www.who.int/health-topics/tuberculosis#tab=tab_1). Typhoid is responsible for 11 to 21 million cases and around 128000-161000 people die due to typhoid annually (WHO, https://www.who.int/immunization/diseases/typhoid/en/; Sundar, et al., 2012).

(A) Use of Nanoparticles in Bacterial Infections

Bacteria are universally present and play a major role in maintaining the environment around us. A small percentage of the world's bacteria is responsible for causing infections and diseases. However, the impact of these bacterial infections is large enough on the global health. Structurally bacteria are prokaryotic microorganisms containing a double-stranded circular DNA with some bacterial species also possessing small circular plasmids. Preliminary bacterial infections usually require only a small number of organisms to cause potentially overwhelming infection. Bacterial infections can be treated with antibiotics but recently emergence of bacterial resistance to currently known antimicrobials is a major problem with potentially harmful consequences. In light of evolutionary perspective, bacteria utilizes two major genetic strategies to counter the antibiotic therapy (i) mutations in gene(s) often associated with the mechanism of action of the compound, and (ii) acquisition of foreign DNA coding for resistance determinants through horizontal gene transfer (HGT) (Munita JM et al., 2016; McManus, 1997; Kumar & Varela, 2013; Munita, 2016). Some important components are present in bacteria to avoid the antibiotics such as hair-like organelle structure which are present in selected Gram-negative and Gram-positive bacteria (Ribert & Cossart, 2015; Melville & Craig, 2013; Pizarro-Cerda & Cossart, 2006), pili, and biofilms (consist proteins, exopolysaccharides, eDNA) (Pizarro-Cerda & Cossart, 2006; Joo & Otto, 2012). There are reports that biofilm formation is responsible for resistance against antibiotics and reduced antimicrobial activity (Joo & Otto, 2012; Roberts, 2005; Ammons, 2010). Metal-based NPs have exclusive properties including high surface, and small size that are responsible for increased surface area leading to increased cellular interaction (**Figure 4**), generation of reactive oxygen species and ability to bind DNA or RNA that altogether may inhibiting microbial replication processes (Arvizo et al., 2012; Zain et al., 2014). Due to small size, NPs are capable of crossing membrane boundaries and are positively absorbed into the bloodstream thus antibiotics in conjugation with NPs may have improved antibacterial activities (Singh et al., 2011).

Silver Nanoparticles

Owing to effective antibacterial properties Silver (Ag) has been vastly used in therapeutic preparations. Silver NPs synthesized through nanotechnology have improved physical, chemical, and biological properties that can be utilized to treat several infectious diseases. Silver NPs are being synthesized in different shapes such as nanorods, nanoplates, nanospheres, nanoprisms, and nanocubes. There are reports that silver NPs can inhibit various types of bacterial infections such as *Staphylococcus aureus, Escherichia coli, Mycobacterium tuberculosis*, some urinary tract infection-causing bacteria such as *P. aeruginosa* and *Enterobacter*, a few sexually transmitted diseases such as chlamydia, gonorrhea and syphilis, etc. During silver NP treatment silver ions are released that may deactivate the cellular active enzymes by interacting with thiol groups, stall membrane permeability and at last lead to cell death (Prabhu & Poulose, 2012; Lu et al., 2013; Choi et al., 2008; Feng et al., 2000). There are some reports which propose that antibacterial activity might be due to release of free radicals that are able to destroy the cell membrane causing cell death (Prabhu & Poulose, 2012; Kim et al., 2007). Silver NPs may interact with sulfur and phosphorus atom of bacterial DNA, inhibit DNA replication and cause cell death (Prabhu & Poulose, 2012; Morones et al., 2005).

Figure 4. Display nanomedicine treated bacterial and viral infections

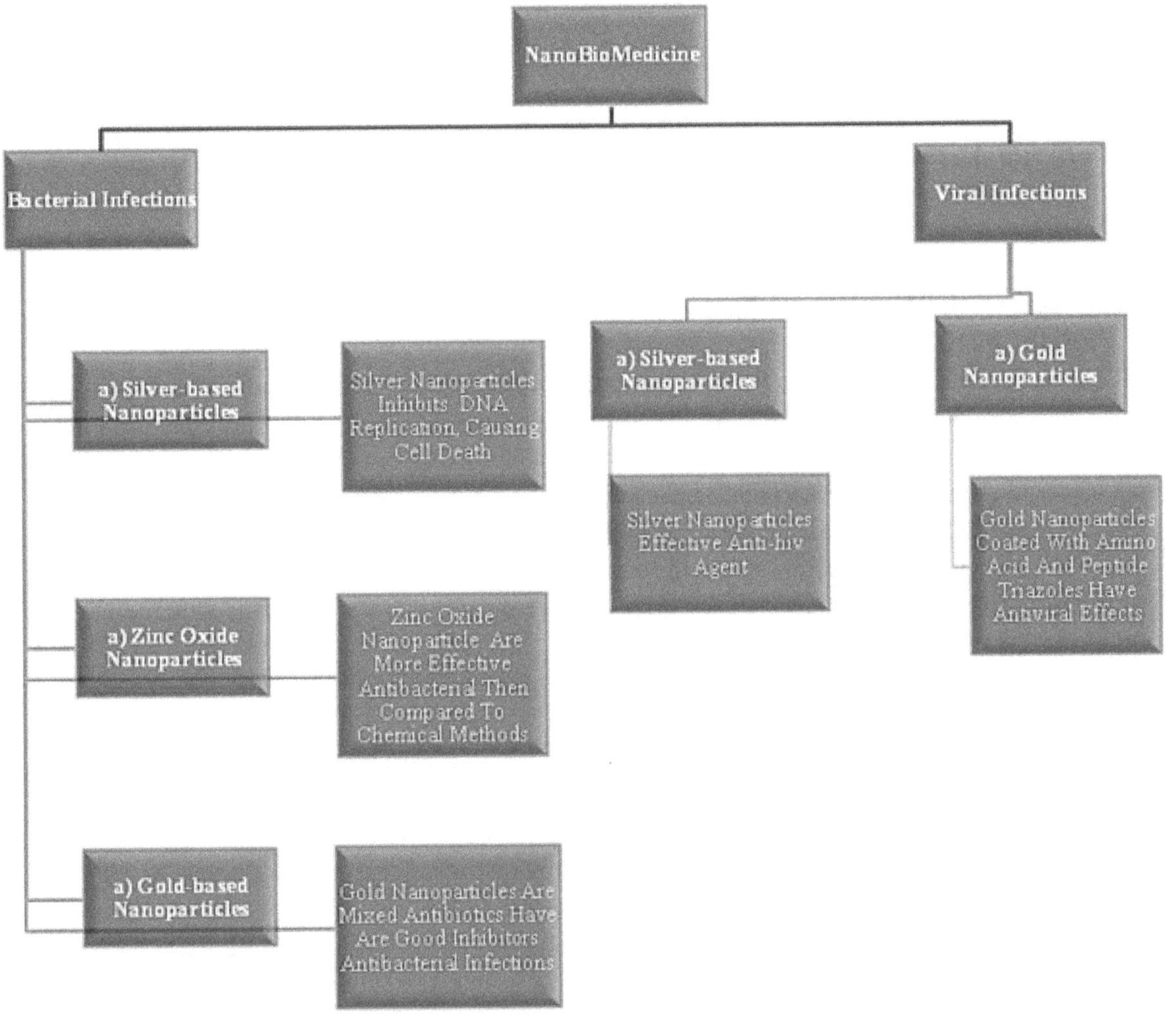

Sometimes even silver NPs are not able to treat bacterial infections due to drug-resistant properties, therefore cocktail of different NPs may be useful. For the treatment of drug resistance bacterial infections such as *M. tuberculosis*, silver NPs mixed with zinc oxide NPs have been used in the past. It was that cocktail of NPs displayed more effective antibacterial activity compared to either NP alone (Jafari et al., 2016). Silver NPs in conjugation with gold NPs displayed have been used for the treatment of tuberculosis and displayed potent anti-mycobacterial activities (Singh et al., 2015). The use of silver NPs with relevant antibiotics have been successful for the treatment of bacterial infections. Silver NPs were mixed with polymixin B and rifampicin antibiotics for the treatment of *Acinetobacter baumannii*, that were able to bind with outer cell membrane of the bacteria resulting into cell death (Wan et al., 2016). Silver NPs in conjugation with amoxicillin has been demonstrated for the treatment of E. coli infections (Li et al., 2005). Silver NP in combination with lactams, quinolones, aminoglycoside and polypeptides have been used against *Salmonella typhimurium* (Deng et al., 2016), gentamicin and penicillin for the treatment of *Actinobacillus pleuropneumoniae,* and *Pasteurella multocida* (Smekalova et al., 2016).

Recently the green synthesis silver NPs using plant extracts has been on the rise. Plant extracts contains various types of phytochemicals such as alkaloids, flavonoids, saponins, polyphenols, and other phytochemicals that are responsible for the formation of stable silver NPs that are used for the treatment of various types of bacterial infections and other infectious diseases. Few plant extracts such as *Azadirachta indica* leaves (Verma & Mehata, 2016), *aloe vera* (Tippayawat et al., 2016), *Malus domestica* extract (Ali et al., 2016), *Ocimum sanctum* (Singhal et al., 2011) have been reported for the synthesis of silver NPs with demonstrable antibacterial activities. The synthesis of silver using bacteria, viruses, and fungi is also demonstrated by several workers.

Zinc Oxide (ZnO) Nanoparticles

ZnO NPs are metal-based NPs that display good antibacterial activity against bacterial infections. Several researchers have developed ZnO NPs for the treatment of various types of bacterial infections such as *Klebsiella pneumonia, Bacillus subtilis, E. coli,* and *Staphylococcus aureus*. The synthesized NPs interact with bacterial cell wall membrane creating oxidative stress resulting in bacterial cell death (Reddy, et al., 2014; Hsueh, et al., 2015; Narasimha et al., 2014; Dobrucka & Długaszewska, 2016). The concentration of ZnO NPs also plays an important role in the treatment of bacterial infections. The antibacterial activity was found to be concentration dependent and increased inhibition was directly related to the concentration of the ZnO NPs (Liu et al., 2009). ZnO NPs has been combined with antibiotics like gentamicin and used for the treatment of *E. coli, Pseudomonas aeruginosa, S. aureus, Bacillus cereus*, and *Listeria monocytogenes* displaying significant results (Voicu et al., 2013).

Gold (Au) Nanoparticles

Au NPs have significant antibacterial properties. Several researchers have reported that Au NPs are capable to treat various types of bacterial infectious diseases such as *Corynebacterium pseudotuberculosis, E. coli, Gram-negative* and *Gram-positive* bacteria and also the drug resistance bacteria (Mohamed et al., 2017). Au NPs interact with cell wall membrane of bacteria and disrupt it causing cell death. Au NPs are known to have mild toxicity to mammalian cells (Li et al., 2014). Au NPs in combination with selected antibiotics such as gentamicin (Burygin et al., 2009), ampicillin (Saha et al., 2007), kanamycin (Saha et al., 2007), levofloxacin (Bagga et al., 2016), and streptomycin (Saha et al., 2007) have been used for the treatment of various types of bacterial infections. NPs mixed antibiotics are able to inhibit antibacterial infections compared to the antibiotics alone.

(B) Use of Nanoparticles in Viral Infections

Viruses not seen by the naked eye are the smallest microbes, microscopic microorganisms and have the capacity to reproduce themselves. They are capable of persisting and reproducing inside living cells called 'host cell'. Viruses contain DNA or RNA as genetic material enclosed in a protein shell called capsid. The capsid is occasionally enclosed through an extra spiked coat called an envelope. Viruses are transmitted through an infectious particle known as 'virion' which contains nucleic acids and proteins. Viruses are capable of infecting animals, plants and other organisms on the planet. Recently there has been an increase in the emergence of several viral infections such as HIV, Ebola virus, SARS-CoV, and MERS-CoV and the COVID-19. Increased human contact with animals basically due to the expansion of the human settlements is the cause for such new viruses infecting the human race. There are no drugs or vaccine for many of these viruses. The current known drugs that are used for the treatment or breakdown of the spread of viral infection are facing with the major problem of drug resistance leading to decreased activity, causing serious illnesses and death e.g. HIV, cervical cancer, influenza, herpes, hepatitis, and others. Thus, drug resistance is one of the major challenges to contain the extent of the virus and its effect on human health. According to WHO and United Nations AIDS (UNAIDS) HIV/AIDS infected 37.9 million people in 2019 (WHO, 2019; UNAIDS, 2019) marking HIV/AIDS as a severe public health problem. Several studies have done in the treated patient of HIV-1 viruses and result shown they were resistant to the least one of the accessible drugs (Vercauteren et al., 2008). Thus, there is an unambiguous need to develop new anti-HIV drugs with a novel mechanism of action. NPs have shown some hope in the treatment of viral infection and need to be explored further for anti viral drug development programs **(Figure 4)**.

Silver Nanoparticles

Silver NPs are effectively shown to treat HIV infections in both the early and post replication stages of the HIV-1 life cycle (Lara et al., 2010). They have been demonstrated to interact with gp120 and inhibit CD4 virion biding that prevents HIV-1 cell-free and cell-associated infection (Elechiguerra et al., 2005). Silver NPs also inhibit viral adsorption and inhibit viral entry to the cells thus preventing the infections. Fusion inhibitors such as Enfuvirtide inhibited the virus adsorption in the initial stage of HIV-1 infection and prevented the infection (Lara et al., 2010).

Gold Nanoparticles

Gold NPs are not much effective antiviral agent when applied alone but if coated with other materials display greater activity against HIV-1 infection (Garrido et al., 2015). Coated gold NPs are widely used for the treatment of viral infections (Kesarka et al., 2015). Some researchers have observed that coated NPs displayed effective results. Gold NPs when coated with polyethylene glycol displayed superior antiviral activity (Kesarkar et al., 2017). Gold NPs coated with raltegravir displayed good activity against HIV infections (Garrido et al., 2015). Similarly gold NPs coated with carbohydrates and conjugated with nucleoside reverse transcriptase inhibitors such as abacavir and lamivudine inhibited the viral replication (Chiodo et al., 2014). Gold NPs coated with amino acid and peptide triazoles displayed potent antiviral effects against HIV-1 when compared with free gold NPs and free peptide triazoles (Kesarka et al., 2015; Bastian et al., 2015).

Nanotechnology is not only limited to metal-based NPs but it is also used in wide fields such as devices, diagnosis, cell repair, biochemical sensors, and drug delivery systems. Nanotubes are used to detect cancer cells in the bloodstream by the identification of DNA changes associated with cancer cells. Carbon-based nanotubes embedded on a chip are used for the detection of cancer cells (Drabu et al., 2010). Kidney injury can be diagnosed using gold nanorods that are attached to the protein generated by the damaged kidney. Nanoshells are gold-coated beads that can absorb a specific wavelength of light and can simply enter a number of centimeters in human tissues. These nanoshells are used for the detection of human breast carcinoma cells (Martis Elvis et al., 2012). Liposomes are nanostructures composed of lipid bilayers that surround a central aqueous space. It can improve the pharmacodynamics and pharmacokinetics of associated drugs. Liposome based formulations are used for the treatment of metastatic breast cancer and Kaposi's sarcoma (Ravindran, 2011). The most important NPs function as biosensors which can detect various chemical reactions during catalytic activity. Various types of biosensors used for the detection of different types of diseases such as glucose nanosensors are used for the detection of glucose levels in diabetic's patients. Triglycerides nanosensors are used for the detection of hyperlipidemia (El-Ansary & Faddah, 2010). Nanotechnology is emerging as the most widely used technology in different fields of science for the improvement of human health. We have summarized some bacterial and viral infectious diseases treated with different nanoparticles **(Table 1)**.

Table 1.

Metal based-Nanoparticles	Biological activity	References
Silver nanoparticles	Effective against *Escherichia coli* and *Staphylococcus aureus*	(Prabhu & Poulose, 2012; Lu et al., 2013; Aderibigbe, 2017)
Sphere-shaped, and triangle shaped silver nanoparticles	Effective against *P. aeruginosa* bacteria	(Raza et al., 2016; Aderibigbe, 2017)
Rod-shaped silver nanoparticles	Inhibited the growth of *Mycobacterium tuberculosis*	(Jafari et al., 2016; Aderibigbe, 2017)
Silver nanoparticles	Effective against bacteria causing sexually transmitted disease (Chlamydia trachomatis)	(Yilma et al., 2013; Aderibigbe, 2017)
Silver nanoparticles conjugated with amoxicillin	Good synergistic effects against *Escherichia coli*	(Li et al., 2005; Aderibigbe, 2017)
Silver nanoparticles conjugated with other antibacterial compounds cefazolin, mupirocin, gentamycin, neomycin, tetracycline or vancomycin	Effective against *Staphylococcus aureus, Pseudomonas aeruginosa* and *Escherichia coli*	(Thirumurugan et al., 2015; Aderibigbe, 2017)
Zinc oxide nanoparticles	Effective against *Klebsiella pneumonia* that causes respiratory infection	(Reddy et al., 2015; Aderibigbe, 2017)
Zinc oxide nanoparticles	Effective against *Campylobacter jejuni*	(Xie et al., 2011; Aderibigbe, 2017)
Gold nanoparticles	Effective against *Escherichia coli, Staphylococcus aureus, Bacillus subtilis, Klebsiella pneumonia Salmonella typhi*	(Shamaila et al., 2016; Aderibigbe, 2017)
Gold nanoparticles capped with cefaclor	Effective against *Staphylococcus aureus* and *Escherichia coli*	(Rai et al., 2010; Aderibigbe, 2017)
Silver nanoparticles	HIV Inhibition of CD4-dependent virion binding, fusion, and infectivity	(Strasfeld & Chou, 2010; Aderibigbe, 2017)
Gold nanoparticles combined with Azidothymidine	HIV Inhibition of early stages of viral replication	(Kesarkar et al., 2015; Aderibigbe, 2017)
Silver nanoparticles	Herpes Virus replication was inhibited	(Hu et al., 2014)
Gold and silver nanoparticles	Influenza Effective against influenza A virus	(Feng et al., 2013; Aderibigbe, 2017)
Silver nanoparticles	Effective against influenza viruses resulting in damage to their morphological structure	(Li et al., 2016; Aderibigbe, 2017)

IMPACT OF NANOTECHNOLOGY ON PUBLIC HEALTH

Nanotechnology is now being extensively used in medicinal research for the treatment of different types of infectious diseases and non infectious diseases. However there are few studies that discuss the impact of nanotechnology on public health or human life. As a modern science, nanotechnology has important impact on day-to-day life of human beings with several positive and negative implications. Nano-materials/particles are prepared by using different chemicals and reacted with different types of molecules present in the body. The NPs are very small in size (nm) and even smaller than the physiological barrier present in the body, thus they can simply enter into our body and create an additional interaction, so that the association of NPs and human health cannot be avoided.

Molecular imaging has emerged as an evolutionary step in diagnostic imaging and therapy that can readily improve the diagnostic accuracy and sensitivity by providing an in vivo analog of immunocytochemistry or in situ hybridization. The technology can enhance the conspicuity of microscopic pathologies by targeting the molecular components or processes representing actual mechanisms of disease. The imaging technology will be an important aspect of in vivo analysis of the complex disease mechanisms depicting how many molecular processes are contributing to the disease progression and how the body is responding to the therapy.

Expansion of nanotechnology is playing a fundamental role in molecular imaging but is also having an important impact in biosensors, biomarkers, and drug delivery methods. NPs can be applied to in vivo activities as a probe (using organic dyes) that is capable of interacting with proteins, antibodies, and nucleic acid due to cellular reactions (Tian et. Al., 2009). Nanoparticles are used as drug delivery systems for site specific targeting that is effective for specific bioavailability, negligible lateral effects, and reducing toxicity to other organs. NPs finds potential uses in the treatment of cancer by the exploration of a tumor-specific thermal scalpel to heat and burn tumors. For example, gold nanoshells are coated with polyethylene that can be used to inhibit the growth of a tumor. Metal-based NPs such as silver and gold NPs have strong anti-microbial, and anti-inflammatory properties and have been formulated in the form of deodorants, burn medications, and anti-wrinkle creams. They are highly stable, inert, biosynthetic and non-cytotoxic (Yiwei et al., 2011). Nanotechnology is making our life easier due to widespread applications in pharmaceutical and cosmetic products, energy-related products, water treatment, air filtration, chemical and biological sensors, and defense products for military and medical applications. Nanotechnology is also playing an important role in the food industry by providing novel tastes and flavors in food preparations, disinfection of food handling processes, packing (lightweight and durable packing), and compact agrochemicals, colors, flavors, and preservatives (Nanotechnology and human health, 2013). Nanotechnology has made way into almost all the industries including health and diagnostics but there are not many reports on the toxicity of NPs on the environment and human health. Toxic analysis of NPs and their adverse effects on human health is of primary concern of the health industry. NPs can cross biological membranes, get access to cells, tissues and organs which is not possible in case of larger particles. There are some reports on the toxic effects of NPs on the respiratory system and lung injury (Handy & Shaw, 2007). Nanomaterials are entering the blood stream through different routes such as ingestion, implantation, injection and inhalation leading to genotoxicity and biochemical toxicity. NPs can also get access to skin through cosmetic products as cobalt and chromium-based NPs are commonly used in the cosmetics. NPs have a toxic effect on mammalian cells has been confirmed by several studies on mammalian cell lines. Some experiments have been conducted where NPs were directly delivered to the lung (intratracheal instillations) and observed for the development of lung injuries after the exposure of the NPs (Driscoll et al. 2000). The damage to the respiratory system and also lung epithelium was observed and symptoms such as coughing or throat irritation were recorded. Several researchers have tested CNT for toxicity evaluation in mice models and found that CNT was found to be more toxic in the lung than carbon black or ultrafine quartz particles (Lam et al. 2004; Warheit et al. 2004). Titanium dioxide (TiO_2) based NPs are used for the inhalation studies by several scientists and it was observed that TiO_2 NPs increased tumors in the lung and gets accumulated in the lung over the long term exposure (Heinrich et al. 1995). Several researchers have proposed mechanisms of the adverse effects which may lead to cardiopulmonary morbidity and mortality in populations exposed to NPs. NPs can stimulate the neurons in the lung affecting the central nervous system and cardiovascular autonomic function. Overall these studies suggest that oxidative stress (the production of damaging oxygen radicals) is one possible mechanism of toxicity. Several studies had tried to explain the injury caused by oxidative stress. The bovine serum-based carbon particles have demonstrated antioxidant properties and caused toxic oxidative stress (Barlow et al. 2005). Some workers have shown that oxidative stress is responsible for the formation of free radicals and the accumulation of peroxide products due to loss of cell viability (Shvedova et al. 2003).

FUTURE RESEARCH THRUST

Nanotechnology has emerged as an innovative tool for biomedicine and diagnostic applications and has led to incredible technological advancements in both the fields. NPs can interact with bio-molecules within the cells and on the cell surface to provide us with novel opportunities to study the cell surface, molecular trafficking, cell division and biochemical processes that can be utilized for the treatment of different types of conditions as well as for treatment of infectious diseases. NPs based drug delivery systems will continue to improve treatment of various types, particularly in life-threatening infections diseases for example malaria, tuberculosis, leishmania, and other infections. NPs have some limitations such as drug resistance, water solubility, and toxicity, so suitable NPs with improved character would be developed and will be used in nanomedicine. In target oriented research, nanotechnology shows a dynamic role and also plays a vital role in the detection of microorganisms or infectious agents. Nanomaterial based medical implants would be a routine procedure that will not only help in improving the overall health but will also help in monitoring the early infections. There are enormous hurdles for nanotechnology in the field of medicine but the outcomes outnumber such minor attributes. The effort required to commercially produce nanoscale biomedical or therapeutic devices is highly interdisciplinary and experts from diverse fields such as physiology, biotechnology, physics, chemistry, electrical engineering, and materials science will be required in a collaborative project. The dangers associated with such a powerful technology should be handled seriously as the technology can be applied in warfare and can have tremendous negative effects. Nanotechnology has emerged as an science with an meeting point of various disciplines.

CONCLUSION

Infectious diseases are caused by specific pathogens that are becoming resistant to several currently used drugs. With the emergence of several new infectious agents there is a need to design novel drugs and delivery systems with improved capabilities. Worldwide the health organizations and scientific institutes are focusing on the complete reduction of infectious diseases, reducing both human morbidity and associated financial costs. NPs having unique chemical and physical properties have provided the answers to these problems. NPs are small in size (nm) that can reduce drug dosage, improve the drug absorption and drug activities. Advancement in nanotechnology has helped in the development of unique drug delivery systems with enhanced molecular interactions allowing NPs to facilitate the immune response against foreign organisms. This has helped in overcoming the drug resistance mechanisms of the microorganisms. With the use of specific NPs, the immune system can be modulated to generate either Th1 or Th2 type immune response in the desired direction. The use of NPs in combination with traditional drugs allows for targeted drug delivery with increased activity. The large surface-to-volume ratio of NPs increases the rate of drug penetration by disrupting the cell walls or cytoplasmic membranes. However studies are required to study the effects of NPs and their interaction with genetic material. The growing concern of toxicity should be addressed so that the safety of the NPs and their use in several products may be established. The future of nanotechnology in the area of Infectious disease treatment, diagnosis and human health is not only bright but will be game changer as how the health care industry works today. The technology will outdate several current technologies providing low cost and effective treatment and diagnostic options.

REFERENCES

Aderibigbe, B. A. (2017). Metal-Based Nanoparticles for the Treatment of Infectious Diseases. *Molecules (Basel, Switzerland)*, *22*(8), 1370. doi:10.3390/molecules22081370 PMID:28820471

Ali, Z. A., Yahya, R., Sekaran, S. D., & Puteh, R. (2016). Green synthesis of silver nanoparticles using apple extract and its antibacterial properties. *Adv. Mater. Sci. Eng.*, *4102196*, 6. doi:10.1155/2016/4102196

Ammons, M. C. (2010). Anti-biofilm strategies and the need for innovations in wound care. *Recent Patents on Anti-infective Drug Discovery*, *5*(1), 10–17. doi:10.2174/157489110790112581 PMID:19807676

Arvizo, R. R., Bhattacharyya, S., Kudgus, R. A., Giri, K., Bhattacharya, R., & Mukherjee, P. (2012). Intrinsic therapeutic applications of noble metal nanoparticles: Past, present and future. *Chemical Society Reviews*, *41*(7), 2943–2970. doi:10.1039/c2cs15355f PMID:22388295

Bagga, P., Ansari, T. M., Siddiqui, H. H., Syed, A., Bahkali, A. H., Rahman, M. A., & Khan, M. S. (2016). Bromelain capped gold nanoparticles as the novel drug delivery carriers to aggrandize effect of the antibiotic levofloxacin. *EXCLI Journal*, *15*, 772–780. PMID:28337108

Barlow, P. G., Donaldson, K., MacCallum, J., Clouter, A., & Stone, V. (2005). Serum exposed to nanoparticle carbon black displays increased potential to induce macrophage migration. *Toxicology Letters*, *155*(3), 397–401. doi:10.1016/j.toxlet.2004.11.006 PMID:15649623

Bastian, A. R., Nangarlia, A., Bailey, L. D., Holmes, A., Sundaram, R. V., Ang, C., Moreira, D. R., Freedman, K., Duffy, C., Contarino, M., & .... (2015). Mechanism of multivalent nanoparticle encounter with HIV-1 for potency enhancement of peptide triazole virus inactivation. *The Journal of Biological Chemistry*, *290*(1), 529–543. doi:10.1074/jbc.M114.608315 PMID:25371202

Bhattacharya, K., Mukherjee, S. P., Gallud, A., Burkert, S. C., Bistarelli, S., & Bellucci, S. (2016). Biological interactions of carbon-based nanomaterials: from coronation to degradation. *Nanomedicine, 12*, 333–351. doi: .nano.2015.11.011 doi:10.1016/j

Burygin, G. L., Khlebtsov, B. N., Shantrokha, A. N., Dykman, L. A., Bogatyrev, V. A., & Khlebtsov, N. G. (2009). On the enhanced antibacterial activity of antibiotics mixed with gold nanoparticles. *Nanoscale Research Letters*, *4*(8), 794–801. doi:10.100711671-009-9316-8 PMID:20596384

Cai, W., & Hong, H. (2012). In a "nutshell": Intrinsically radio-labeled quantum dots. *American Journal of Nuclear Medicine and Molecular Imaging*, *2*, 136–140. PMID:23133808

Cai, W., Hsu, A. R., Li, Z. B., & Chen, X. (2007). Are quantum dots ready for in vivo imaging in human subjects? *Nanoscale Research Letters*, *2*(6), 265–281. doi:10.100711671-007-9061-9 PMID:21394238

Chaloupka, K. Y., Malam, A. M., & Seifalian, A. M. (2010). Seifalian, Nanosilver as a new generation of nanoproduct in biomedical applications. *Trends in Biotechnology*, *28*(11), 580–588. doi:10.1016/j.tibtech.2010.07.006 PMID:20724010

Chiodo, F., Marradi, M., Calvo, J., Yuste, E., & Penadés, S. (2014). Glycosystems in nanotechnology: Gold glyconanoparticles as carrier for anti-HIV prodrugs. *Beilstein Journal of Organic Chemistry*, *10*, 1339–1346. doi:10.3762/bjoc.10.136 PMID:24991287

Choi, O., Deng, K. K., Kim, N. J., Ross, L. Jr, Surampalli, R. Y., & Hu, Z. Q. (2008). The inhibitory effects of silver nanoparticles, silver ions, and silver chloride colloids on microbial growth. *Water Research*, *42*(12), 3066–3074. doi:10.1016/j.watres.2008.02.021 PMID:18359055

Deng, H., McShan, D., Zhang, Y., Sinha, S. S., Arslan, Z., Ray, P. C., & Yu, H. (2016). Mechanistic study of the synergistic antibacterial activity of combined silver nanoparticles and common antibiotics. *Environmental Science & Technology*, *50*(16), 8840–8848. doi:10.1021/acs.est.6b00998 PMID:27390928

Deshpande, V. V., Chandra, B., Caldwell, R., Novikov, D. S., Hone, J., & Bockrath, M. (2009). Mott Insulating State in Ultraclean Carbon Nanotubes. *Science*, *323*(5910), 106–110. doi:10.1126cience.1165799 PMID:19119228

Dobrucka, R., & Długaszewska, J. (2016). Biosynthesis and antibacterial activity of ZnO nanoparticles using Trifolium pratense flower extract. *Saudi Journal of Biological Sciences*, *23*(4), 517–523. doi:10.1016/j.sjbs.2015.05.016 PMID:27298586

Drabu, S., Khatri, S., Babu, S., & Verma, D. (2010). Nanotechnology: An introduction to future drug delivery system. *Journal of Chemical and Pharmaceutical Research*, *2*, 171–179.

Driscoll, K. E., Costa, D. L., Henderson, R., Oberdo¨ rster, G., Salem, H. Schlesinger, R. B. (2000). Intratracheal instillation as an exposure technique for the evaluation of respiratory tract toxicity: Uses and limitations, *Toxicological Sciences*, *55*, 24 – 35.

Dye, C. (2014). After 2015: Infectious diseases in a new era of health and development. *Philosophical Transactions of the Royal Society of London. Series B, Biological Sciences*, *369*(1645), 20130426. doi:10.1098/rstb.2013.0426 PMID:24821913

Edelstein, R. L., Tamanaha, C. R., Sheehan, P. E., Miller, M. M., Baselt, D. R., Whitman, L. J., & Colton, R. J. (2000). The BARC biosensor applied to the detection of biological warfare agents. *Biosensors & Bioelectronics*, *14*(10-11), 805–813. doi:10.1016/S0956-5663(99)00054-8 PMID:10945455

El-Ansary, A., & Faddah, L. M. (2010). Nanoparticles as biochemical sensors. *Nanotechnology, Science and Applications*, *3*, 65–76. doi:10.2147/NSA.S8199 PMID:24198472

Elechiguerra, J. L., Burt, J. L., Morones, J. R., Camacho-Bragado, A., Gao, X., Lara, H. H., & Yacaman, M. J. (2005). Interaction of silver nanoparticles with HIV-1. *Journal of Nanobiotechnology*, *3*(1), 6. doi:10.1186/1477-3155-3-6 PMID:15987516

Feng, F., Sakoda, Y., Ohyanagi, T., Nagahori, N., Shibuya, H., Okamastu, M., Miura, N., Kida, H., & Nishimura, S. I. (2013). Novel thiosialosides tethered to metal nanoparticles as potent influenza A virus haemagglutinin blockers. *Antiviral Chemistry & Chemotherapy*, *23*(2), 59–65. doi:10.3851/IMP2553 PMID:23425865

Feng, Q. L., Wu, J., Chen, G. Q., Cui, F. Z., Kim, T. N., & Kim, J. O. (2000). A mechanistic study of the antibacterial effect of silver ions on Escherichia coli and Staphylococcus aureus. *Journal of Biomedical Materials Research*, *52*(4), 662–668. doi:10.1002/1097-4636(20001215)52:4<662::AID-JBM10>3.0.CO;2-3 PMID:11033548

Garrido, C., Simpson, C. A., Dahl, N. P., Bresee, J., Whitehead, D. C., Lindsey, E. A., Harris, T. L., Smith, C. A., Carter, C. J., Feldheim, D. L., Melander, C., & Margolis, D. M. (2015). Gold nanoparticles to improve HIV drug delivery. *Future Medicinal Chemistry*, *7*(9), 1097–1107. doi:10.4155/fmc.15.57 PMID:26132521

Ghaemi, F., Abdullah, L. C., & Tahir, P. Md. (2017). Natural and synthetics nanomaterials: comparative study on their mechanical and thermal properties as nanofiller in polymer composite. *IOP Conf. Series: Journal of Physics: Conf. Series 914*. doi:10.1088/1742-6596/914/1/012014

Grande, C. J., Torres, F. G., Gomez, C. M., & Carmen Bañó, M. (2009). Bañó, Nanocomposites ofbacterial cellulose/hydroxyapatite for biomedical applications. *Acta Biomaterialia*, *5*(5), 1605–1615. doi:10.1016/j.actbio.2009.01.022 PMID:19246264

Handy, R. D., & Shaw, B. J. (2007). Toxic effects of nanoparticles and nanomaterials: Implications for public health, risk assessment and the public perception of nanotechnology. *Health Risk & Society*, *9*(2), 125–144. doi:10.1080/13698570701306807

Hochella, M. F. Jr, Spencer, M. G., & Jones, K. L. (2015). Nanotechnology: Nature's gift or scientists' brainchild? *Environmental Science. Nano*, *2*(2), 114–119. doi:10.1039/C4EN00145A

Hong, H., Gao, T., & Cai, W. (2009). Molecular imaging with single-walled carbon nanotubes. *Nano Today*, *4*(3), 252–261. doi:10.1016/j.nantod.2009.04.002 PMID:21754949

Hsueh, Y. H., Ke, W. J., Hsieh, C. T., Lin, K. S., Tzou, D. Y., & Chiang, C. L. (2015). ZnO nanoparticles affect Bacillus subtilis cell growth and biofilm formation. *PLoS One*, *10*(6), e0128457. doi:10.1371/journal.pone.0128457 PMID:26039692

Hu, R. L., Li, S. R., Kong, F. J., Hou, R. J., Guan, X. L., & Guo, F. (2014). Inhibition effect of silver nanoparticles on herpes simplex virus 2. *Genetics and Molecular Research*, *13*(3), 7022–7028. doi:10.4238/2014.March.19.2 PMID:24682984

Irvine, D. J., Swartz, M. A., & Szeto, G. L. (2013). Engineering synthetic vaccines using cues from natural immunity. *Nature Materials*, *12*(11), 978–990. doi:10.1038/nmat3775 PMID:24150416

Ishida, T., Wang, X., Shimizu, T., Nawata, K., & Kiwada, H. (2007). PEGylated liposomes elicit an anti-PEG IgM response in a T cell-independent manner. *Journal of Controlled Release*, *122*(3), 349–355. doi:10.1016/j.jconrel.2007.05.015 PMID:17610982

Jafari, A. R., Mosavi, T., Mosavari, N., Majid, A., Movahedzade, F., Tebyaniyan, M., & Arastoo, S. (2016). Mixed metal oxide nanoparticles inhibit growth of Mycobacterium tuberculosis into THP-1 cells. *International Journal of Mycobacteriology*, *5*, S181–S183. doi:10.1016/j.ijmyco.2016.09.011 PMID:28043541

Jeevanandam, J., Barhoum, A., Yen, S. C., Dufresne, A., & Danquah, M. K. (2018). Review on nanoparticles and nanostructured materials: History, sources, toxicity and regulations. *Beilstein Journal of Nanotechnology*, *9*, 1050–1074. doi:10.3762/bjnano.9.98 PMID:29719757

Jonoobi, M., Harun, J., Mishra, M., & Oksman, K. (2009). Chemical composition, crystallinity and thermal degradation of bleached and unbleached kenaf bast (*Hibiscus cannabinus*) pulp and nanofibers. *BioResources*, *4*(2), 626–639.

Joo, H. S., & Otto, M. (2012). Molecular basis of in vivo biofilm formation by bacterial pathogens. *Chemistry & Biology*, *19*(12), 1503–1513. doi:10.1016/j.chembiol.2012.10.022 PMID:23261595

Joshi, M., & Adak, B. (2018). *Advances in Nanotechnology Based Functional, Smart and Intelligent Textiles: A Review* (2nd ed.). Comprehensive Nanoscience and Nanotechnology., doi:10.1016/B978-0-12-803581-8.10471-0

Karmakar, P. (2007). In Vitro structural and functional evaluation of gold nanoparticles conjugated antibiotics. *Nanoscale Research Letters*, *2*(12), 614–622. doi:10.100711671-007-9104-2

Kelly, J. A., Shukaliak, A. M., Cheung, C. C., Shopsowitz, K. E., Hamad, W. Y., & MacLachlan, M. J. (2013). Responsive Photonic Hydrogels Based on Nanocrystalline Cellulose. *Angewandte Chemie International Edition*, *52*(34), 8912–8916. doi:10.1002/anie.201302687 PMID:23881841

Kesarkar, R., Oza, G., Pandey, S., Dahake, R., Mukherjee, S., Chowdhary, A., & Sharon, M. (2017). Gold nanoparticles: Effective as both entry inhibitors and virus neutralizing agents against HIV. *Journal of Microbiology and Biotechnology Research*, *2*, 276–283.

Kesarkar, R., Shroff, S., Yeole, M., Chowdhary, A. (2015). L-Cysteine Functionalized Gold Nanocargos Potentiates Anti-HIV Activity of Azidothymydine against HIV-1Ba-L Virus. *J. Immunol. Virol.*, *1*.

Kim, J. S., Kuk, E., Yu, K., Kim, J. H., Park, S. J., Lee, H. J., Kim, S. H., Park, Y. K., Park, Y. H., Hwang, C. Y., Kim, Y.-K., Lee, Y.-S., Jeong, D. H., & Cho, M.-H. (2007). Antimicrobial effects of silver nanoparticles. *Nanomedicine (London)*, *3*(1), 95–101. doi:10.1016/j.nano.2006.12.001 PMID:17379174

Kumar, S., & Varela, M. F. (2003). Molecular mechanisms of bacterial resistance to antimicrobial agents. In A. Méndez-Vilas (Ed.), *Microbial Pathogens and Strategies for Combating Them: Science, Technology and Education* (Vol. 1, pp. 522–534). Formatex Research Centre.

Lam, C. W., James, J. T., McCluskey, R., & Hunter, R. L. (2004). Pulmonary toxicity of single-wall carbon nanotubes in mice 7 and 90 days after intratracheal instillation. *Toxicological Sciences*, *77*(1), 126–134. doi:10.1093/toxsci/kfg243 PMID:14514958

Lara, H. H., Nilda, V. A., Liliana, I. T., & Cristina, R. P. (2010). Mode of antiviral action of silver nanoparticles against HIV-1. *Journal of Nanobiotechnology*, *8*(1), 1. doi:10.1186/1477-3155-8-1 PMID:20145735

Levsen, K. (1995). Chronic inhalation exposure of wistar rats and 2 different strains of mice to diesel-engine exhaust, carbon-black, titanium dioxide. *Inhalation Toxicology*, *7*(4), 533–556. doi:10.3109/08958379509015211

Li, P., Li, J., Wu, C., Wu, Q., & Li, J. (2005). Synergistic antibacterial effects of _-lactam antibiotic combined with silver nanoparticles. *Nanotechnology*, *16*(9), 1912–1917. doi:10.1088/0957-4484/16/9/082

Li, X., Robinson, S. M., Gupta, A., Saha, K., Jiang, Z., Moyano, D. F., Sahar, A., Riley, M. A., & Rotello, V. M. (2014). Functional gold nanoparticles as potent antimicrobial agents against multi-drug-resistant bacteria. *ACS Nano*, *8*(10), 10682–10686. doi:10.1021/nn5042625 PMID:25232643

Li, Y., Lin, Z., Zhao, M., Guo, M., Xu, T., Wang, C., Xia, H., & Zhu, B. (2016). Reversal of H1N1 influenza virus-induced apoptosis by silver nanoparticles functionalized with amantadine. *RSC Advances*, *6*(92), 89679–89686. doi:10.1039/C6RA18493F

Liu, Y., He, L., Mustapha, A., Li, H., Hu, Z. Q., & Lin, M. (2009). Antibacterial activities of zinc oxide nanoparticles against Escherichia coli O157: H7. *Journal of Applied Microbiology*, *107*(4), 1193–1201. doi:10.1111/j.1365-2672.2009.04303.x PMID:19486396

Lu, Z., Rong, K., Li, J., Yang, H., & Chen, R. (2013). Size-dependent antibacterial activities of silver nanoparticles against oral anaerobic pathogenic bacteria. *Journal of Materials Science. Materials in Medicine*, *24*(6), 1465–1471. doi:10.100710856-013-4894-5 PMID:23440430

Ma, J., Wong, H., Kong, L. B., & Peng, K. W. (2003). Biomimetic processing of nanocrystallite bioactive apatite coating on titanium. *Nanotechnology*, *14*(6), 619–623. doi:10.1088/0957-4484/14/6/310

Mahtab, R., Rogers, J. P., & Murphy, C. J. (1995). Protein-sized quantum dot luminescence can distinguish between "straight", "bent", and "kinked" oligonucleotides. *Journal of the American Chemical Society*, *117*(35), 9099–9100. doi:10.1021/ja00140a040

Manavalan, R., Lal Pal, S., Jana, U., Manna, P. K., & Mohanta, G. P. (2011). Nanoparticle: An overview of preparation and characterization. *Journal of Applied Pharmaceutical Science*, *01*(06), 228–234.

Martis Elvis, A., Badve Rewa, R., Degwekar Mukta, D. (2012). Nanotechnology based devices and applications in medicine: An overview. *Nanotechnology Devices and Applications, 3*(1), 68-73. . doi:10.4103/2229-5186.94320

McManus, M. C. (1995). Mechanisms of bacterial resistance to antimicrobial agents. *American Journal of Health-System Pharmacy*, *54*(12), 1420–1433. doi:10.1093/ajhp/54.12.1420 PMID:9194989

Melville, S., & Craig, L. (2013). Type IV pili in Gram-positive bacteria. *Microbiology and Molecular Biology Reviews*, *77*(3), 323–341. doi:10.1128/MMBR.00063-12 PMID:24006467

Mishra, P. K., Mishra, H., Ekielski, A., Talegaonkar, S., & Vaidya, B. (2017). Zinc oxide nanoparticles: A promising nanomaterial for biomedical applications. *Drug Discovery Today*, *22*(12), 1825–1834. doi:10.1016/j.drudis.2017.08.006 PMID:28847758

Moffatt, S. (2016). Nanotechnology to nanomedicine: Reconciling ethical implications and public health. *MOJ Proteomics Bioinform.*, *3*(4), 77–79. doi:10.15406/mojpb.2016.03.00090

Mohamed, M. M., Fouad, S. A., Elshoky, H. A., Mohammed, G. M., & Salaheldin, T. A. (2017). Antibacterial effect of gold nanoparticles against Corynebacterium pseudotuberculosis. *International Journal of Veterinary Science and Medicine*, *5*(1), 23–29. doi:10.1016/j.ijvsm.2017.02.003 PMID:30255044

Morones, J. R., Elechiguerra, J. L., Camacho, A., Holt, K., Kouri, J. B., Ramirez, J. T., & Yacaman, M. J. (2005). The bactericidal effect of silver nanoparticles. *Nanotechnology*, *16*(10), 2346–2353. doi:10.1088/0957-4484/16/10/059 PMID:20818017

Mostofizadeh, A., Li, Y., Song, B., & Huang, Y. (2011). Synthesis, properties, and applications of low-dimensional carbon-related nanomaterials. *Journal of Nanomaterials*, *685081*, 1–21. Advance online publication. doi:10.1155/2011/685081

Mottram, P. L., Leong, D., Crimeen-Irwin, B., Gloster, S., Xiang, S. D., Meanger, J., Ghildyal, R., Vardaxis, N., & Plebanski, M. (2007). Type 1 and 2 immunity following vaccination is influenced by nanoparticle size: Formulation of a model vaccine for respiratory syncytial virus. *Molecular Pharmaceutics*, *4*(1), 73–84. doi:10.1021/mp060096p PMID:17274665

Munita, J. M., & Arias, C. A. (2016). Mechanisms of antibiotic resistance. *Microbiology Spectrum*, *4*(2). Advance online publication. doi:10.1128/microbiolspec.VMBF-0016-2015 PMID:27227291

Nam, J. M., Thaxton, C. C., & Mirkin, C. A. (2003). Nanoparticles-based bio-bar codes for the ultrasensitive detection of proteins. *Science*, *301*(5641), 1884–1886. doi:10.1126cience.1088755 PMID:14512622

Nanotechnology and Human Health. (2013). Scientific evidence and risk governance. Report of the WHO expert meeting. *WHO Regional Office for Europe*.

Narasimha, G., Sridevi, A., Devi Prasad, B., & Praveen Kumar, B. (2014). Chemical synthesis of Zinc Oxide (ZnO) nanoparticles and their antibacterial activity against a clinical isolate Staphylococcus aureus. *International Journal of Nanodimension*, *5*, 337–340.

Panatarotto, D., Prtidos, C. D., Hoebeke, J., Brown, F., Kramer, E., Briand, J. P., Muller, S., Prato, M., & Bianco, A. (2003). Immunization with peptide-functionalized carbon nanotubes enhances virus-specific neutralizing antibody responses. *Chemistry & Biology*, *10*(10), 961–966. doi:10.1016/j.chembiol.2003.09.011 PMID:14583262

Parak, W. J., Boudreau, R., Gros, M. L., Gerion, D., Zanchet, D., Micheel, C. M., Willams, S. C., Alivisatos, A. P., & Larabell, C. A. (2002). Cell motility and metastatic potential studies based on quantum dot imaging of phagokinetic tracks. *Advanced Materials*, *14*(12), 882–885. doi:10.1002/1521-4095(20020618)14:12<882::AID-ADMA882>3.0.CO;2-Y

Pati, R., Shevtsov, M., & Sonawane, A. (2018). Nanoparticle Vaccines Against Infectious Diseases. *Frontiers in Immunology*, *9*, 2224. Advance online publication. doi:10.3389/fimmu.2018.02224 PMID:30337923

Pautler, M., & Sara, B. (2010). Nanomedicine: Promises and challenges for the future of public health. *International Journal of Nanomedicine*, *5*, 803–809. PMID:21042425

Pizarro-Cerda, J., & Cossart, P. (2006). Bacterial adhesion and entry into host cells. *Cell*, *124*(4), 715–727. doi:10.1016/j.cell.2006.02.012 PMID:16497583

Prabhu, S., & Poulose, E. K. (2012). Silver nanoparticles: Mechanism of antimicrobial action, synthesis, medical applications, and toxicity effects. *International Nano Letters*, *2*(1), 32. doi:10.1186/2228-5326-2-32

Prego, C., Paolicelli, P., Díaz, B., Vicente, S., Sánchez, A., González-Fernández, Á., & Alonso, M. J. (2010). Chitosan-based nanoparticles for improving immunization against hepatitis B infection. *Vaccine*, *28*(14), 2607–2614. doi:10.1016/j.vaccine.2010.01.011 PMID:20096389

Pusic, K., Aguilar, Z., McLoughlin, J., Kobuch, S., Xu, H., Tsang, M., Wang, A., & Hui, G. (2013). Iron oxide nanoparticles as a clinically acceptable delivery platform for a recombinant blood-stage human malaria vaccine. *The FASEB Journal*, *27*(3), 1153–1166. doi:10.1096/fj.12-218362 PMID:23195035

Rai, A., Prabhune, A., & Perry, C. C. (2010). Antibiotic mediated synthesis of gold nanoparticles with potent antimicrobial activity and their application in antimicrobial coatings. *Journal of Materials Chemistry*, *20*(32), 6789–6798. doi:10.1039/c0jm00817f

Ravindran, R. (2011). Nanotechnology in cancer diagnosis and treatment: An overview. *Oral Maxillofac Pathol J.*, *2*, 101–106.

Raza, M.A., Kanwal, Z., Rauf, A., Sabri, A.N., Riaz, S., Naseem, S. (2016). Size-and shape-dependent antibacterial studies of silver nanoparticles synthesized by wet chemical routes. *Nanomater., 6.*

Reddy, L. S., Nisha, M. M., Joice, M., & Shilpa, P. N. (2014). Antimicrobial activity of zinc oxide (ZnO) nanoparticle against Klebsiella pneumonia. *Pharmaceutical Biology*, *52*(11), 1388–1397. doi:10.3109/13880209.2014.893001 PMID:25026353

Ribet, D., & Cossart, P. (2015). How bacterial pathogens colonize their hosts and invade deeper tissues. *Microbes and Infection*, *17*(3), 173–183. doi:10.1016/j.micinf.2015.01.004 PMID:25637951

Roberts, M. C. (2005). Update on acquired tetracycline resistance genes. *FEMS Microbiology Letters*, *245*(2), 195–203. doi:10.1016/j.femsle.2005.02.034 PMID:15837373

Sabir, S., Muhammad, A., & Chaudhari, S. K. (2014). Zinc Oxide Nanoparticles for Revolutionizing Agriculture: Synthesis and Applications, *Scientific World Journal. Article ID*, *925494*, 8. doi:10.1155/2014/925494 PMID:25436235

Saha, B., Bhattacharya, J., Mukherjee, A., Ghosh, A., Santra, C., Dasgupta, A. K., & Karmakar, P. (2007). In Vitro Structural and Functional Evaluation of Gold Nanoparticles Conjugated Antibiotics. *Nanoscale Research Letters*, *2*(12), 614–622. doi:10.100711671-007-9104-2

Shamaila, S., Zafar, N., Riaz, S., Sharif, R., Nazir, J., & Naseem, S. (2016). Gold nanoparticles: An efficient antimicrobial agent against enteric bacterial human pathogen. *Nanomater, 6.*

Sharma, V. K., Filip, J., Zboril, R., & Varma, R. S. (2015). Natural inorganic nanoparticles—Formation, fate, and toxicity in the environment. *Chemical Society Reviews*, *44*(23), 8410–8423. doi:10.1039/C5CS00236B PMID:26435358

Shvedova, A. A., Castranova, V., Kisin, E. R., Schwegler-Berry, D., Murray, A. R., Gandelsman, V. Z., Maynard, A., & Baron, P. (2003). Exposure to carbon nanotube material: Assessment of nanotube cytotoxicity using human keratinocyte cells. *Journal of Toxicology and Environmental Health. Part A.*, *66*(20), 1909–1926. doi:10.1080/713853956 PMID:14514433

Shvedova, A. A., Kisin, E. R., Mercer, R., Murray, A. R., Johnson, V. J., & Potapovich, A. I. (2005). Unusual inflammatory and fibrogenic pulmonary responses to singlewalled carbon nanotubes in mice. *Am J Physiol Cell Mol Physiol., 289*, L698–708. . doi:10.1152/ajplung.00084.2005

silver-polyvinyl pyrrolidone (Ag-PVP) nanoparticles in mouse macrophages infected with live Chlamydia trachomatis. *Int. J. Nanomed., 8*, 2421–2432.

Singh, M., Manikandan, S., & Kumaraguru, A. K. (2011). Nanoparticles: A new technology with wide applications. *Res. J. Nanosci. Nanotechnol.*, *1*(1), 1–11. doi:10.3923/rjnn.2011.1.11

Singh, R., Nawale, L. U., Arkile, M., Shedbalkar, U. U., Wadhwani, S. A., Sarkar, D., & Chopade, B. A. (2015). Chemical and biological metal nanoparticles as antimycobacterial agents: A comparative study. *International Journal of Antimicrobial Agents*, *46*(2), 183–188. doi:10.1016/j.ijantimicag.2015.03.014 PMID:26009020

Singhal, G., Bhavesh, R., Kasariya, K., Sharma, A. R., & Singh, R. P. (2011). Biosynthesis of silver nanoparticles using Ocimum sanctum (Tulsi) leaf extract and screening its antimicrobial activity. *Journal of Nanoparticle Research*, *13*(7), 2981–2988. doi:10.100711051-010-0193-y

Smekalova, M., Aragon, V., Panacek, A., Prucek, R., Zboril, R., & Kvitek, L. (2016). Enhanced antibacterial effect of antibiotics in combination with silver nanoparticles against animal pathogens. *Veterinary Journal (London, England)*, *209*, 174–179. doi:10.1016/j.tvjl.2015.10.032 PMID:26832810

Smith, D. M., Simon, J. K., & Baker, J. R. Jr. (2013). Applications of nanotechnology for immunology. *Nature Reviews. Immunology*, *13*(8), 592–605. doi:10.1038/nri3488 PMID:23883969

Strasfeld, L., & Chou, S. (2010). Antiviral drug resistance: Mechanisms and clinical implications. *Infectious Disease Clinics of North America*, *24*(3), 809–833. doi:10.1016/j.idc.2010.07.001 PMID:20674805

Sundar, S., Prajapati, V. K. (2012). Drug targeting to infectious diseases by nanoparticles surface functionalized with special biomolecules. *Curr Med Chem.*, *1*(19), 3196–3202.

Tallury, P., Malhotra, A., Byrne, L., & Santra, S. (2010). Nanobioimaging and sensing of infectious diseases. *Advanced Drug Delivery Reviews*, *62*(4-5), 424–437. doi:10.1016/j.addr.2009.11.014 PMID:19931579

Taniguchi, N. (1974). On the basic concept of nano-technology. *Proc. Intl. Conf. Prod. Eng. Tokyo, Part II, 10*, 5-10.

Thirumurugan, G., Rao, J. S., & Dhanaraju, M. D. (2016). Elucidating pharmacodynamic interaction of silver nanoparticle-topical deliverable antibiotics. *Scientific Reports*, *6*(1), 29982. doi:10.1038rep29982 PMID:27427207

Tian, X., Ning, L., & Andre, E. (2009). Potential health impact of nanoparticles. *Annual Review of Public Health*, *30*(1), 137–150. doi:10.1146/annurev.publhealth.031308.100155 PMID:19705557

Tippayawat, P., Phromviyo, N., Boueroy, P., & Chompoosor, A. (2016). Green synthesis of silver nanoparticles in aloe vera plant extract prepared by a hydrothermal method and their synergistic antibacterial activity. *PeerJ*, *4*, 4. doi:10.7717/peerj.2589 PMID:27781173

Tiwari, M., Sharma, N. C., Fleischmann, P., Burbage, J., Venkatachalam, P., & Sahi, S. V. (2017). Nanotitania exposure causes alterations in physiological, nutritional and stress responses in tomato (Solanum lycopersicum). *Front. Plant Sci.*, *8*, 8. doi:10.3389/fpls.2017.00633 PMID:28484486

Tripathi, S., Singh, D. K., Singh, S., Dubey, S., & Chauhan, N. K. (2016). Impact of nanoparticles on photosynthesis: Challenges and opportunities. *Mater. Focus*, *5*(5), 405–411. doi:10.1166/mat.2016.1327

Ullah, H., Wahid, F., Santos, H. A., & Khan, T. (2016). Advances in biomedical and pharmaceutical applications of functional bacterial cellulose-based nanocomposites. *Carbohydrate Polymers*, *150*, 330–352. doi:10.1016/j.carbpol.2016.05.029 PMID:27312644

UNAIDS. (2019). *Global HIV & AIDS statistics — 2019 fact sheet*. https://www.unaids.org/en/resources/fact-sheet

Vallhov, H., Qin, J., Johansson, S. M., Ahlborg, N., Muhammed, M. A., Scheynius, A., & Gabrielsson, S. (2006). The importance of an endotoxin-free environment during the production of nanoparticles used in medical applications. *Nano Letters*, *6*(8), 1682–1686. doi:10.1021/nl060860z PMID:16895356

Venkataraju, J. L., Sharath, R., Chandraprabha, M. N., Neelufar, E., Hazra, A., & Patra, M. (2014). Synthesis, characterization and evaluation of antimicrobial activity of zinc oxide nanoparticles. *Journal of Biochemical Technology*, *3*, 151–154.

Vercauteren, J., Deforche, K., Theys, K., Debruyne, M., Duque, L. M., Peres, S., Carvalho, A. P., Mansinho, K., Vandamme, A.-M., & Camacho, R. (2008). Mansinho K, Vandamme AM, Camacho R: The incidence of multidrug and full class resistance in HIV-1 infected patients is decreasing over time (2001-2006) in Portugal. *Retrovirology*, *5*(1), 12. doi:10.1186/1742-4690-5-12 PMID:18241328

Verma, A., & Mehata, M. S. (2016). Controllable synthesis of silver nanoparticles using Neem leaves and their antimicrobial activity. *J. Radiat. Res. Appl. Sci.*, *9*(1), 109–115. doi:10.1016/j.jrras.2015.11.001

Virlan Maria, J. R., Daniela, M., Radu, R., Cristina, M. S., Alexandra, T., Bogdan, C., & Maria, G. (2016). Organic Nanomaterials and Their Applications in the Treatment of Oral Diseases. *Molecules (Basel, Switzerland)*, *21*(2), 207. doi:10.3390/molecules21020207 PMID:26867191

Voicu, G., Oprea, O., Vasile, B. S., & Andronescu, E. (2013). Antibacterial activity of zinc oxide-gentamicin hybrid material. *Digest Journal of Nanomaterials and Biostructures*, *8*, 1191–1203.

Wagner, S., Gondikas, A., Neubauer, E., Hofmann, T., & von der Kammer, F. (2014). Spot the Difference: Engineered and Natural Nanoparticles in the Environment—Release, Behavior, and Fate. *Angewandte Chemie International Edition*, *53*, 12398–12419. doi:10.1002/anie.201405050

Walther, A., Timonen, J. V., Díez, I., Laukkanen, A., & Ikkala, O. (2011). Multifunctional high-performance biofibers based on wet-extrusion of renewable native cellulose nanofibrils. *Advanced Materials*, *23*(26), 2924–2928.

Wan, G., Ruan, L., Yin, Y., Yang, T., Ge, M., & Cheng, X. (2016). Effects of silver nanoparticles in combination with antibiotics on the resistant bacteria Acinetobacter baumannii. *International Journal of Nanomedicine*, *11*, 3789–3800.

Wang, S., Mamedova, N., Kotov, N. A., Chen, W., & Studer, J. (2002). Antigen/antibody immunocomplex from CdTe nanoparticle bioconjugates. *Nano Letters*, *2*, 817–822.

Wang, X., Ishida, T., & Kiwada, H. (2007). Anti-PEG IgM elicited by injection of liposomes is involved in the enhanced blood clearance of a subsequent dose of PEGylated liposomes. *Journal of Controlled Release*, *119*, 236–244. doi:10.1016/j.jconrel.2007.02.010

Warheit, D. B., Laurence, B. R., Reed, K. L., Roach, D. H., Reynolds, G. A. M., & Webb, T. R. (2004). Comparative pulmonary toxicity assessment of single-wall carbon nanotubes in rats. *Toxicological Sciences*, *77*, 117–125.

Weissleder, R., Elizondo, G., Wittenburg, J., Rabito, C. A., Bengele, H. H., & Josephson, L. (1990). Ultrasmall superparamagnetic iron oxide: Characterization of a new class of contrast agents for MR imaging. *Radiology*, *175*, 489–493.

WHO. (2016). *Global Tuberculosis Report*. World Health Organization.

WHO. (2019). *Number of people (all ages) living with HIV Estimates by WHO region*. https://apps.who.int/gho/data/view.main.22100WHO?lang=en

Xie, Y., He, Y., Irwin, P. L., Jin, T., & Shi, X. (2011). Antibacterial activity and mechanism of action of zinc oxide nanoparticles against Campylobacter jejuni. *Applied and Environmental Microbiology*, *77*(7), 2325–2331. doi:10.1128/AEM.02149-10 PMID:21296935

Yilma, A.N., Singh, S.R., Dixit, S., & Dennis, V.A. (2013). Anti-inflammatory effects of

Yiwei, T. (2011). Health impact and safety of engineered nanomaterials. *Chemical Communications*, *47*(25), 7025–7038. doi:10.1039/c0cc05271j PMID:21479319

Yousaf, S. A., & Salamat, A. (2008). *Effect of heating environment on fluorine doped tin oxide (f: SnO/sub 2/) thin films for solar cell applications*. Faculty of Engineering & Technology.

Zain, N. M., Stapley, A. G., & Shama, G. (2014). Green synthesis of silver and copper nanoparticles using ascorbic acid and chitosan for antimicrobial applications. *Carbohydrate Polymers*, *112*, 195–202.

Zhang, B., Li, Y., & Fang, C. Y. (2009a). Receptor- mediated cellular uptake of folate conjugated fluorescent nanodiamonds: A combined ensemble and single- particle study. *Small*, *5*, 2716–2721.

Zhang, S., Sun, D., Fu, Y., & Du, H. (2003). Recent Advances of Superhard Nanocomposite Coatings: A Review. *Surface and Coatings Technology*, *167*(2–3), 113–119.

Zhang, Y., Tapas, R. N., Hao, H., & Weibo, C. (2013). Biomedical Applications of Zinc Oxide Nanomaterials. *Current Molecular Medicine*, *13*(10), 1633–1645.

Chapter 4
Nanomaterials for Food and Agriculture

Mintu Maan Dutta
Gauhati University, India

ABSTRACT

Nanotechnology has emerged as one of the most promising tools for the present revolution in the field of agri-food sector. Engineered nano materials (ENMs) are a part of nanotechnology which has led to the invention of smart and active materials such as nanosensors, nanofertilizers, nanopesticides, etc. Bioinspired and biosynthesis approach for the synthesis of nanomaterials using various eco-friendly green chemistry methods has overcome the various problem associated with the use of toxic chemicals and harsh reaction conditions. Thus, use of these nanomaterial in this sector has tremendously increased the crop yield and quality thereby reducing the use of toxic crop protecting agents.

INTRODUCTION

The present scenario of population rise presumes the world population to reach 9.8 billion in 2050 and 11.2 billion in 2100. (Sekhon, 2014; Marchiol, 2018) Conventional inputs such as land, water, energy, fertilizers and pesticides used in traditional agriculture practices are not able to meet the need of the target. (Marchiol, 2018) Chemical fertilizers used in agriculture provide plants with essential nutrients for optimal growth and productivity, but this method is also not able to fulfill the growing demand of food to feed this increasing population. (Zulfiqar *et al.*, 2019) Furthermore, excess use of chemical fertilizers causes severe environmental related problems including climatic changes, urbanization, accumulation of pesticides, insecticides and fertilizers, water eutrophication, soil quality degradation and pollution. (Yadav, 2017; Zulfiqar *et al.*, 2019)

To meet the increase in demand for food, there is an need to increase approximately 60% of the world agricultural production. Food security can be achieved by following new systems for food, water and energy. Literature search reveals that researchers have emphasized more on use of nanotechnology i.e. towards the development of herbicides, nano-pesticide, nano-fertilizers, insect repellants, or genes that can increase the yield and quality of agricultural products manifold with lower cost, energy and waste.

DOI: 10.4018/978-1-7998-5563-7.ch004

(Servin & White, 2016; Robles-García *et al.,* 2016; Mishra *et al.,* 2019) Some strategies includes the use of precision fertilization, fertigation and use of Nanofertilizer. (Zulfiqar *et al.,* 2019)

Nanotechnology is a newly emerging branch of science that deals with the study of matter (1-100 nm) that has the potential to increase the quality and quantity of agricultural production with the minimum damage of agro ecology. (Manjunatha *et al.,* 2016) Recently, reports have been found which explains the use of nanotechnology in solving various social problems that persists worldwide. (Adisa *et al.,* 2019) Materials in nanometer scale possess specific physical, chemical and biological properties that differs from properties of bulk. Potential application of nanotechnology includes its use in cosmetic industry, catalysis, scientific tools, electronics, biomedical application, food science, agriculture, environmental remediation and many industrial applications. (Adisa *et al.,* 2019; Kumar *et al.,* 2019) In particular, the application of nanotechnology in the plant production systems in plant science is defined with the term "**Phytonanotechnology**". Thus, green nanotechnology aims towards the use of biodegradable nanomaterials with reduced effects on the environment or human beings by minimizing the emissions of greenhouse gases such as carbon dioxide (CO_2), nitrous oxide (N_2O) and methane (CH_4) from agricultural land into the atmosphere (Sohail *et al.,* 2019). Further, green synthesis approach minimizes the cost and limits the use of hazardous chemicals during the synthesis of nanoparticles. (Chaudhry *et al.,* 2018) Thus, **Figure 1** represents the various application of nanotechnology and nanomaterials in food and agriculture sectors.

Figure 1. Application of nanotechnology and nanomaterials in food and agriculture sectors (Kaphle et al., 2018)

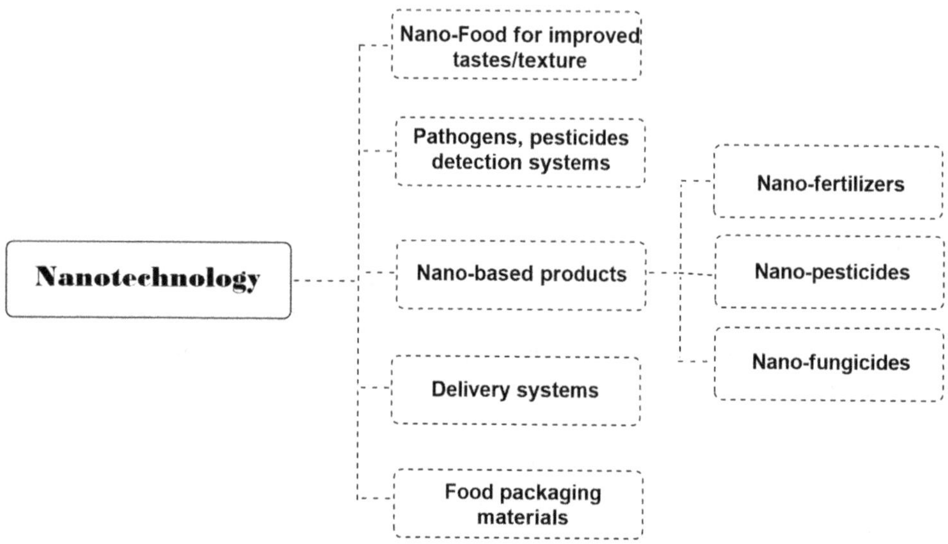

For a nanomaterial to be used in agriculture effectively, it must possess the following characteristics (Sohail *et al.,* 2019):

a. High solubility
b. Highly specific

c. Component controlled release
d. Non self-decomposition.

Aim of nanotechnology in the Agriculture (Yadav, 2017):

a. Reduces pollution from agrochemicals.
b. Improves resistivity to climatic conditions.
c. Ability to add valuable nutrients to plants.
d. Helps in detection and remediation of heavy metals from soil.
e. Increase yields through genetic improvement.

Nanomaterials used in agri/feed/food may be either of natural origin or engineered material. Several definitions have been proposed for the term "Nanomaterial" during various period. Out of which, definition proposed by European Union in 2015 describes the engineered material as "*Any intentionally produced material that has one or more dimensions of the order of 100 nm or less or that is composed of discrete functional parts, either internally or at the surface, many of which have one or more dimensions of the order of 100 nm or less, including structures, agglomerates or aggregates, which may have a size above the order of 100 nm but retain properties that are characteristic of the nanoscale*." (European Parliament and Council, 2015)

Based on composition Engineered Nanomaterials (ENMs) can be classified into three categories: (Peters *et al.,* 2016):

(A) Inorganic, (B) Organic and (C) Combined materials.

A. **Inorganic nanomaterials** comprises of metals, metal oxides, salts, full carbon-based materials such as carbon nanotubes, fullerenes, carbon black and clay. (Sonkaria *et al.,* 2012) Surface functionalization of inorganic nanomaterials such as clays with an organic coating, definitely improves its dispersion in polymer matrices. (Peters *et al.,* 2016) Since last several decades, these materials have been used to solve the food-related problems. Few examples includes the use of Silicon dioxide as synthetic amorphous silica (SAS) in food processing industries as anti-caking agent; use of nano-sized metal particles such as nano selenium and colloidal suspensions e.g. gold, platinum and silver as food or health supplements. (Peters *et al.,* 2016)
B. **Organic nanomaterials** includes natural products. **Nano encapsulates** is made up of an organic shell and a core containing the (bio) active ingredient. Thus, nano encapsulation method is used to entrap bioactive molecules. (Yadav, 2017) (Phospho)Lipid-based nanomaterials, comprising of micelles and liposomes. These are most commonly used organic nanomaterials because of its wide solubility range (hydrophilic or lipophilic surface), i.e. they can be "tuned" to an application. Nano-encapsulation increases the solubility, stability, delivery and bioavailability of nutrients (vitamins, minerals, anti-oxidants and micronutrients), agrochemicals or pharmaceuticals. Further, nano encapsulation will also increase the bioavailability and biodistribution of bioactives.
C. **Combined nanomaterials** refers to the synthesis of metallic nanoparticles via. environmentally benign procedures by using some bio templates. These nanomaterials exhibits biocide

potency against broad spectrum of pathogens, biosensing applications and wastewater treatment. (Holzinger *et al.*, 2017, Eltarahony *et al.*, 2018)

Remarkable properties of metal nanoparticles (NPs) makes it a suitable material for the development of new materials for several application. Metal nanoparticles has been widely engaged in food and agriculture science. Further, its application has been extended to its use as bio sensors, food packaging materials, food and beverage storage etc. (Kaphle *et al.,* 2018) Few examples of metal nanoparticles includes gold nanoparticles and silver nanoparticles. These nanoparticles have widely been used in diagnostics, therapeutics, antimicrobial and drug delivery applications. Nano metal oxides includes zinc oxide (ZnO), cerium oxide (CeO_2) and titanium dioxide (TiO_2) nanoparticles. TiO_2 acts as disinfecting agent, food additive (white color pigment) and flavor enhancer. There are various synthetic methods for the synthesis of these nanoparticles. These nanoparticles possess ''surface plasmon resonance (SPR)'' property which is an important criterion for the development of sensors. In addition to this, these nanoparticles also used in surface enhanced Raman spectroscopy (SERS) for single molecule detection. (Kaphle *et al.,* 2018) For example tryptophan-capped gold particles was used to detect Hg(II) ions. (Kaphle *et al.,* 2018, Senapati *et al.,* 2011)

INSIGHTS OF BIOINSPIRED MATERIALS AND BIOSYNTHESIZED MATERIALS

Bioinspired Nanomaterials

Bioinspired approach for the synthesis of nanomaterials generally deals with the design of novel nanomaterials with similar morphologies and functions that resembles with some biological template such as mussel, cilia, insect tentacles, etc. This approach has been widely used in the design and application of various advanced materials in the field of nanofluidics (Feng *et al.*, 2017), drug delivery in biomedical researches (Yoo *et al.*, 2011) and has immense potential towards the development of soft robotics and smart devices in near future (Zong et al, 2017; Feng *et al.*, 2017) Table 1 below represents the use of bioinspired nanomaterials in food and agriculture sectors for various applications such as environmental sensing, pathogen detection, bioanalysis in nutritional and dietary supplements.

Table 1. Bioinspired nanomaterials in food and agriculture

Bioinspired template	Nanomaterials	Application	Reference
Mussel	Mussel avermectin NPs [P(St-MAA)-Av-Cat]	As nanocarrier: Controlled release of avermectin; protection against UV light. Higher toxicity towards aphids.	Liang *et al.*, 2018
	Polydopamine (PDA)-coated molecularly imprinted SiO_2 NPs	Detection of Papain; Nutritional and dietary supplement	Yang *et al.*, 2016
Cactus	$ZnSnO_3/TiO_2$ Nanostructures	Humidity nanosensors	Zhang *et al.*, 2015
Zwitterion	Fluorescent biomimetic carbon quantum dots	Bioanalaysis in nutritional and dietary supplement; detection of vitamin-B12 in cell system.	Wang *et al.*, 2018
Insect tentacles	Porous antenna like Prussian blue (PB) nanocube heads/TiO_2 nanowire (NW) arms (PB-TiO_2)	3D cellular interfacial sensing and molecular recognition	Kong *et al.*, 2014
Cactus and spider silk	ZnO wire; poly(vinylacetate) (PVAc), poly(methyl methacrylate) (PMMA), polystyrene (PS), and poly(vinylidene fluoride) (PVDF); Poly-(methyl methacrylate) (PMMA) electrospinning, Fog of titanium tetrachloride ($TiCl_4$) hydrolyzed nanoparticles	Water collecting abilities; Fog collection	Zhu *et al.*, 2016

Biosynthesized nanomaterials: Biosynthesis refers to the synthesis of nanomaterials via. various Eco-friendly green chemistry methods. These methods includes the use of several biological systems that comprises of bacteria, fungi, yeasts, enzymes, actinomycetes and various plants extracts. **Table 2** below includes the synthesis of nanoparticles using various biological systems.

Biosynthesized nanomaterials have several advantages that are as follows (Xiaojia He, 2019):

a. Biological systems may act as capping agent, stabilizer and reducing agents.
b. Synthesis takes place under ambient temperature, pressure and neutral pH.
c. Biocompatible and less toxic.

Table 2. Biosynthesized nanomaterials using various biological systems (Xiaojia He, 2019)

	Biological Systems	Biogenic nanoparticles (NPs)	Remarks	References
Bacteria	*Pichia fermetas JA2*	Silver and ZnO NPs	Synergistic effect with antibiotics	
	Bacillus cereus strain HMH1	Magnetic iron oxide NPs	Capping and stabilizing agents	
	Serraita sp. BHU-S4	Silver NPs	Reduction and stabilization	
Fungi	*Saccharomyces cerevisiae*	Silver NPs	Reducing agent and capping agent	
	Aspergillus flavus TFR 7	TiO_2 NPs	Fungi directly isolated from Rhizosphere soil	
	Aspergillus flavus and *Emericella nidulans*	Silver NPs	Reducing and capping agent	
Yeast	*Candida lusitaniae*	Silver/silver chloride NPs	Yeast isolated from termite gut	
	Magnusiomyces ingens LH-F1	Gold NPs	Reducing, stabilizing/ capping agents	
	Cryptococcus laurentii and *Rhodotorula glutinis*	Silver NPs	Yeast isolated from apple peal	
Actinomycetes	Isolate VITBN4	CuO NPs	Isolated from soil samples. Reduction, capping and stabilization	(Xiaojia He, 2019)
	Streptomyces sp. Strain NH21	Silver and gold NPs	Isolated from acidic salt. Capping agent	
Enzyme	Alpha amylase	TiO_2 NPs	Reducing, capping agents	
Plant extracts	*Coffee arabica* seed	Silver NPs		
	Red ginseng root	Silver and gold NPs	Reduction and stabilization	
	Aloe vera plant	Nano-scale zero valent iron	Plant extract as reducing agent	
	Cassia tora leaf	Silver NPs	Plant extract as reducing agent	
	Nigella sativa leaf	Silver NPs	Plant extract as reducing and capping agent	
	Pineapples and orange fruits	Silver NPs	Reducing agent	
	Longan fruit	Silver NPs	Reducing, stabilizing and capping agent	
	Melia azedarach L.	TiO_2 NPs	Reducing and capping agent	Muhammad Rafque, 2019
	Onion extract *(Allium cepa L.)*	Silver NPs and gold NPs	Reducing agents	Pratibha Acharya, 2019
	Aegle marmelos	ZnO NPs	Stabilizing agent	J. Fowsiya, 2019
	Argyeria nervosa leaf extract	Silver NPs	capping agent	Rijuta Ganesh Saratale, 2018, Saratale *et al.*, 2017b
	Nephelium lappaceum L peel extract	MgO NPs	precipitant and capping agent	Rijuta Ganesh Saratale, 2018,
Marine algae	*Macroalga sargassum* muticum	ZnO NPs		
	Brown alga Crystoseria trinodis	CuO NPs	Reducing, stabilizing agent	(Xiaojia He, 2019)
Microalgae		Silver NPs	Reducing agent	Ana Luiza Machado Terra, 2019

Application of nanomaterials in various areas of food and agriculture: (Sonkaria *et al.,* 2012)

A. **Agriculture:**
   a. Nanocapsules for delivery of pesticides, fertilizers, vaccines and other agrochemicals.
   b. Nanosensors for monitoring soil conditions and crop growth; detection of animal and plant pathogens. Nanosensors are also used for flavor/color enhancement or texture modification. (Jain *et al.,* 2018)
   c. Nanochips for preservation of identity and tracking.
   d. Nanomaterials are used to deliver DNA to plants (targeted genetic engineering.)

B. **Food processing:**
   a. Nanocapsules to improve the bioavailability of neutraceuticals in standard ingredients.
   b. Nanoencapsulates are flavor enhancer.
   c. Nanotubes acts as gelation and viscosifying agents.
   d. Nanoemulsion and nanoparticles for better availability and dispersion of nutrients.

C. **Food Packaging:**
   a. Biodegradable nanosensors for temperature, moisture and time monitoring.
   b. Antibodies attached to fluorescent nanoparticles helps in the detection of chemicals and foodborne pathogens.
   c. Nanoclays and nanoflims acts as a barrier material to prevent spoilage and oxygen adsorption.
   d. Surface coating with metal nanoparticles (silver, magnesium and zinc) acts as antimicrobial and antifungal agents.
   e. Silicate nanoparticles are lighter, stronger and used as heat resistant films.

D. **Supplements:**
   a. Nanosize powder increases absorption and targeted delivery of nutrients.
   b. Cellulose nano crystal composites acts as drug carrier.
   c. Nanocochleates (coiled nanoparticles) helps in the delivery of nutrients to the cells.
   d. Nanodroplets for vitamin spray for better adsorption.

Besides the application mentioned above, there are also some other distinctive properties of nanomaterials (such as Au NPs, Ag NPs, quantum dots, magnetic nanoparticles etc.) that makes it appropriate for its application in various fields i.e., represented in **Table 3**.

Table 3. Properties and application of nanomaterials

Sl No.	Types of nanomaterials	Function/property	Applications (Yadav, 2017)
1	Gold nanoparticles	Fluorescence, anti-bacterial nature, SERS effect	Used in Nanosensors for detection of pesticides in water, gold nanoparticles attached with nanomatrix can be used for absorption of pesticides, used in development of food packaging materials, can induce plant growth and yield, help in detection of bacteria in food samples
2	Silver nanoparticles	Surface Plasmon resonance, anti-microbial nature	Used in food packaging, filtration media, pesticide detection, absorption, larvicidal and antifouling nature of silver can be used in agriculture to prevent foul smell in stagnant waters.
3	Quantum dots	Fluorescent property	Used to detect food borne pathogen and toxicants
4	Cellulose nanocrystals	High water uptake capacity, biocompatible	Can be used in food packaging, development of nanocomposites, for enhancing seed germination, immobilization of enzymes, vitamins and minerals and their delivery to target plant part, used in absorption of heavy metal ions in water
5	Magnetic nanoparticles	Large specific surface area	Gene delivery, plant disease diagnostics, removal of heavy metals, food analysis, enzyme immobilization, protein purification, pathogen monitoring
6	Polymeric nanoparticles	Biodegradable nature, ease of surface modification	Development of nanoformulations of pesticides, fertilizers, food additives, bioactive molecules, nutraceuticals and phytochemicals
7	Carbon nanotubes	Optical, electrical and mechanical properties, thermal conductivity	Used in delivery of pesticides, fertilizers and other chemicals, can penetrate the membrane, act as plant growth modulators, can stimulate seed germination, can enhance water and ionic nutrients, used in food inspection and vacuum proof food packaging

Perspectives of Nanomaterials in Various Food Products (Xiaojia He, 2019)

Nanomaterials possess unique physicochemical properties such as melting point, solubility, electrical conductivity, or changes in the crystalline structure of the materials that makes it different from their bulk counterparts. (Jain *et al.,* 2018; Elder *et al.,*, 2009; Savolainen *et al.,*, 2010). These properties makes is apposite for the formation of new, high-performance materials, which shall have high applicability on food manufacturing, packaging and storage (**Table 4**). (Sekhon, 2010) Reports have been found in the literature, which explains the applications of nanomaterials as nanocoating, nanocapsules, and nanocans for surface coating, control release, packaging, storage and transportation respectively. (Jain *et al.,* 2018; Ravichandran, 2010; Cushen *et al.,* 2012) Storage conditions and temperature greatly affects the stability of nanomaterials in food. This may change the characteristics of the food such as texture, taste, coloring strength and stability during shelf life after their interactions with the nanoparticles. (Jain *et al.,* 2018; Selin, 2007; Monica and Calster, 2010; Dasgupta *et al.,*, 2015a; Ranjan *et al.,*, 2016).

Literature search reveals that synthetic amorphous silica (SAS) as the most common food additives. SAS is formed as precipitated or fumed silica, which is made up of aggregates of primary particles, which size ranges within few nanometers. SAS is most commonly used as clarifying agent for beverages and anti-caking agent. Some of the other anti-caking agent includes the use of calcium silicate, sodium aluminosilicate, dicalcium phosphate, sodium ferricyanide and microcrystalline cellulose but there is no information whether the particles are in nano range. (Peters *et al.,* 2016)

Titanium dioxide (E171) appears as an important food additive and flavor enhancer in variety foods, including dairy products, dried vegetables, mustard, beer and wine, which helps to enhance the white

Table 4. Use of nanomaterials in Food Industries

Sector	Nanomaterials	Application	Permissible amount	References
Food processing	TiO_2	Color additives	<1% by weight of food	(Xiaojia He *et al.*, 2019)
	Synthetic iron oxides		<0.25% for dogs and cats and 0.1% by weight for humans	
	ZnO	Additive or polymer production aid	Authorization based on particle size	The European Commission, Commission Regulation (EU) No 10/2011
	Iron oxide			
	Aluminium oxide			
	Silicon oxide			
	Cobalt oxide			
	Manganese oxide (E530)			
	Titanium nitride		Upto 20 mg/Kg in PET bottles	
	Carbon black		<2.5% w/w in polymer	
	Silica-silver	Preservatives	<4 ppm by weight of silver as anti-microbial agents blended into polymers	U.S. FDA Inventory of effective food contact substance (FCS)
	Silicon dioxide (E551)	Flavor carrier	<10,000 mg/Kg	(Xiaojia He *et al.*, 2019)
	Silicon dioxide (E551)	Marking fruit and vegetables	<2% of ink solids	(Xiaojia He *et al.*, 2019)
	Silicon dioxide (E551)	Anticaking agent	<2% by weight of food	(Xiaojia He *et al.*, 2019)
	Copper oxide, Iron oxide, ZnO	Nutritional dietary supplement	Approved for animal feed	(Xiaojia He *et al.*, 2019)
Food contact packaging	Zin oxide QDs	Pesticides detection		D. Sahoo *et al.*, 2018
	AuAg nanochains	Pesticides detection		Anxin Jiao, 2019
	Magnetic nanosensors, Plasmonic nanosensors, Fluorescent nanosensors	Pathogens detection		Y. Sun *et al.*, 2018; H. Kearns *et al.*, 2017; I. Perçin *et al.*, 2017; T. Banerjee *et al.*, 2016.
	Fluorescent nanosensors, Plasmonic nanosensors, Phosphorescent QDs	Toxins detection		A. Sun *et al.*, 2018; C.H. Zhang *et al.*, 2016; W. Zhang *et al.*, 2017.
	Chitosan/ Nano silica coating	Edible film/coating	Tested on Longan fruit	S. Shi *et al.*, 2013
	Chitosan based nanomaterials	Pharmaceuticals and biomedical engineering; medicine, tissue engineering, drug delivery, gene therapy and cancer therapy		Balsam R. Rizeq, 2019
	Poly-ε-carolactone		Tested on "Red-delicious" apples	M. L. Zambrano-Zaragoza *et al.*, 2014
	Nanoemulsion/Quinoa protein/Chitosan		Tested on fresh strawberries	N. Robledo *et al.*, 2018
	Bio-nano hybrid pectins and LDH-salicylate		Tested on fresh apricots	G. Gorrasi *et al.*, 2016
	Nanoemulsion with lemon grass essential soil		Tested on Fuji-apples	L. Salvia-Trujillo *et al.*, 2015
	Montmorillonite	Flame retardation additives, gas barrier etc. Prevent abrasive wear		U.S. FDA Inventory of effective food contact substance (FCS)
	Montmorillonite Chromium (III) oxide			G. Gorrasi *et al.*, 2016
	Nanoemulsion with lemon grass essential soil			L. Salvia-Trujillo *et al.*, 2015
	Titanium aluminium nitride	Prevent abrasive wear Heating enhancer in polyethylene terephthalate (PET) polymers	Maximum thickness of surface coating shall not exceed 5 µm.	(Xiaojia He *et al.*, 2019)
	Tin antimony oxide		<0.05% by weight of the polymer.	U.S. FDA Inventory of effective food contact substance (FCS)
Food storage	Silver, zinc oxide NPs	Inhibition of yeast, and bacterial growth		(Jaspreet Singh, 2019)
	Polyurethane	inhibition of *E. coli* and *S. aureus* growth		(Jaspreet Singh, 2019)
	Silver NPs	Inhibition of aerobic bacterial growth		(Jaspreet Singh, 2019)
	Silver, TiO_2 NPs	Inhibition of *Penicillium*, *Lactobacillus* growth		(Jaspreet Singh, 2019)
	Silver, TiO_2 NPs	Inhibition of *S. aureus*, *Coliforms*, *E. coli*, *Listeria* growth		(Jaspreet Singh, 2019)
	Silver NPs	Inhibition of total aerobic bacteria, lactic acid bacteria, *Pseudomonas* spp., *Enterobacteriaceae*		(Jaspreet Singh, 2019)

color of certain foods. In addition to this nano TiO_2 in combination with other compounds or elements such as nickel oxide and cobalt is used as antimicrobial agent against various foodborne pathogens. (Peters *et al.*, 2016)

Polymer nanocomposites has emerged as a better alternative to traditional packaging materials such as glass, paper and metals for packaging of industrial, food and agricultural products. These nanocomposites possess superior properties including barrier, mechanical, electrical, and thermal properties. (Idumah *et al.*, 2019) These properties makes it suitable for its use as food packaging material for ethylene absorption, oxygen scavenging, removal of water vapor and ethanol absorption. (Idumah *et al.*, 2019)

Table 5. Function of nanomaterials in various agricultural products

Application	Nanomaterial composition	Function of nanomaterials	Current status	References
Nanofertilizer	Unknown materials	Fertilizer	Commercialized	(Xiaojia He, 2019)
Nanopesticides	$Cu(OH)_2$ NPs	Fungicide	R&D	
	Silica NPs	Controlled release	R&D	
	Polymeric NPs	Controlled release	R&D	
	ZnO NPs	Bactericide	R&D	
	Copper NPs	Fungicide and Bactericide	Commercialized	
Nanoherbicides	Poly-$_{\varepsilon}$-caprolactone (PCL) nanocapsules	Controlled release	R&D	
Nanosensors	Copper doped montmorillonite	Propineb fungicide detection in aquatic environment	R&D	
	Graphene	Pathogen detection in wastewater	R&D	

Current Perspectives of Nanotechnology in Agriculture (Xiaojia He, 2019)

There has always been high demand of various agricultural products due to the gradual increase in global population. Green revolution took place during 1970's, since then it has targeted the four basic elements of the production system that helped in significant increase in the agricultural production. (Agrawal & Rathore, 2014) However, this has become static these days, which has effected the livelihood of the farming community. (Agrawal & Rathore, 2014) This limitation has been overcomed-using nanotechnology. Nanotechnology deals with nanomaterials that have exceptionally unique properties such as high reactivity, enhanced bioavailability and bioactivity, adherence effects and surface effects of nanoparticles. (Gutiérrez *et al.*, 2011) Thus, nanotechnology has been able to create many new materials (such as nanofertilizers, smart polymers, nanoadditives) and devices (nano-chips, nano-sensors, solar cells, and light trapping photovoltaic). (Lu and Bowles 2013) Details of its function and application are represented in **table 5**. Further nanotechnology can be used for the genetic improvement of plants, delivery of genes and drug molecules to the target in plants and animals, delivery of agrochemicals like fertilizers and pesticides. (Mukhopadhyay, 2014) The progress of nanotechnology helps in addressing various areas of agriculture such as environmental remediation, crop protection, food production, toxin and pathogen exposure, water purification, wastewater treatment and food packaging. (Idumah *et al.*, 2019)

Table 6. Application of nanoparticles for controlling plant diseases

Nanomaterials	Application	References
Silver Ions and Nanoparticles	Antifungal	(S. W. Kim *et al.*, 2009)
AgNPs and GO (graphene oxide)	Antibacterial agent against *Xanthomonas perforans* which causes bacterial spots in tomatoes	I. Ocsoy *et al.*, 2013
Nano-silver liquid	Inhibited *Sclerotium cepivorum*, which causes white rot disease in the green onion	J. H. Jung *et al.*, 2010
Ag NPs	Antifungal agent against rose powdery mildew	H. S. Kim *et al.*, 2008
	Killing root-knot nematodes (*Meloidogyne spp.*)	W. A. Cromwell *et al.*, 2014
	Excellent antibacterial activity against agricultural plant pathogens	K. Paulkumar *et al.*, 2014
CuNPs	Antifungal agent, Effective against plant pathogenic fungi *Fusarium* spp.	P. Van Viet *et al.*, 2016
	The antifungal activity was evaluated against three common crop pathogenic *Fusarium* spp.	K. Bramhanwade *et al.*, 2016
AgNPs, CuNPs, Ag/CuNPs	Novel fungicide used for the management of red root-rot disease in tea plantations	S.M. Ouda, 2014
ZnO, MgO	Effective against variety of pathogens	Wani & Shah, 2012
ZnO NPs	Antimicrobial activity of Zinkicide for protection of leaves and fruit	J. H. Graham *et al.*, 2016
	ZnO NPs in the presence of visible light exhibit strong antibacterial and antifungal activity	K. Kairyte *et al.*, 2013
TiO_2	Antibacterial property against *Xanthomonas perforans*	M. L. Paret *et al.*, 2013
	Titanium dioxide nanoparticles prevents the fungal colonization of wood samples over long time	G. De Filpo *et al.*, 2013
CeO_2	Potential to suppress Fusarium wilt disease in tomato and increased yield	I.O. Adisal *et al.*, 2017

Nanofertilizer

Nanofertilizers are referred to Engineered Nanomaterials (ENMs) that can directly deliver one or more required nutrients to the plants that can boost the performance, availability and utilization of conventional fertilizers. (Adisa *et al.,* 2019) Thus, Nanofertilizer are formed as of interaction between nanomaterials and fertilizers due to the increased reactivity of nanomaterials (i.e. high specific surface area, small size). Some of the commonly used nanomaterials includes single or multiwalled nanotubes, magnetized iron nanoparticles, copper (Cu), silver (Ag), gold (Au), zinc (Zn) and zinc oxide (ZnO), cerium oxide (Ce_2O_3), and titanium dioxide (TiO_2) etc. (Zulfiqar *et al.,* 2019) Nanofertilizer can feed plants gradually in a controlled manner, which help in increasing the fertilizer use efficiency thereby minimizing environmental hazards. Nanofertilizer boosts the crop productivity by enhancing seed germination, helps in seedling growth, photosynthesis, nitrogen metabolism, protein and carbohydrate synthesis, improving stress tolerance. (Zulfiqar *et al.,* 2019) These nanofertilizers minimizes its use, transport expenditures and thus an increase in overall application. (Zulfiqar *et al.,* 2019)

Based on the nutrient categorization nanofertilizers can be classified into two i.e., macronutrient nanofertilizers and micronutrient nanofertilizers. (Liu and Lal, 2015) In addition to these nanobiofertilizers are also emerging as an additional category. (Liu and Lal, 2015; A. A. Feregrino-Pérez *et al.,* 2018)

Macronutrient Nanofertilizers

Fertilizers that are synthesized by the combination of essential macronutrients (such as nitrogen (N), phosphorus (P), potassium (K), magnesium (Mg), sulphur (S) and calcium (Ca) have with nanomaterials for the deliver an precise amount of nutrients to the crops. This reduces the bulk requirements thereby reducing the purchasing and transportation costs. Some of the examples of macronutrient nanofertilizers includes urea-modified zeolites, hydroxyapatite and mesoporous silica nanomaterials that have shown promising results. (Liu and Lal, 2015; Monreal *et al.,* 2016)

Micronutrient Nanofertilizers

Fertilizers that are synthesized by the combination of essential micronutrients (such as Zinc, Boron, Iron, Manganese, Copper etc.) with nanomaterials for the synthesis of carbohydrates, protein metabolism, regulation of auxins, and makes the plants resistant against harmful pathogen. (Broadley *et al.,* 2007) For example: Zn nanoparticles as nanofertilizer helps in increasing the crop production, iron oxide nanoparticles considerably enhanced the chlorophyll contents and root activity. (Zulfiqar *et al.,* 2019)

Nanobiofertilizers

Fertilizers that are synthesized by the combination of biofertilizers (commonly microorganisms) with nanostructures or nanoparticles to improve the plant growth. For example: Gold nanoparticles and rhizobacteria. (Malusá *et al.,* 2012; Shukla, *et al.,* 2015) One of the vital problem of nanobiofertilizers is that, since size of the nanoparticles are smaller than cells, macroscopic filters made of carbon nanotube walls aids in the absorption of *Escherichia coli* which sequentially collects other microorganisms from fermentation processes and deliver it to the plants. (T. Simarmata *et al.,* 2016; J. Vandergheynst *et al.,* 2007; Zulfiqar *et al.,* 2019)

Limitations of nanofertilizers:

a. Nanomaterial phytotoxicity: Plants are dose-dependent and respond in a different way to various nanomaterials. (P. Ashkavand, *et al.,* 2018; Zulfiqa *et al.,* 2019)
b. High reactivity and variability: Due to small size and high surface area, it may harm farm workers on its continuous exposure. Thus, it has become an important matter of concern. (A. Konate, *et al.,* 2018; Zulfiqar *et al.,* 2019)

Nano and Biosensors

Nanosensors are substances that are made up of nanomaterials combined with various sensors. (Singh *et al.,* 2019) These sensors are very sensitive and can monitor various soil conditions (such as moisture content, soil fertility, availability of nutrients etc.) as well as detect the presence of pathogens, insects, and weeds in the soil in food ensuring food safety and security. In addition to this, nanosensors are also able to provide information about the irrigation level, ideal timing of sowing and harvesting, accurate rate of pesticide, herbicide and fertilizer required. (Baruah and Dutta, 2009; Sohail *et al.,* 2019) Based on that, it provides information about when and how much pesticide or herbicide needs to be administered, thereby avoiding the overuse and unnecessary exposure of non-target organisms. (Bartolucci, 2017) Nanosensors used in food sector have been used to detect metabolites from microbial growth and byproducts obtained after food degradation. Different types of Nanosensors used in food sector are as follows (Muthu *et al.,* 2018):

a. Electronic Nose: Wine discrimination
b. Array biosensors: Detection of food-borne contaminants
c. Microfluidics sensors: Lab-on-a-chip
d. NEMS: Detection of pathogens
e. Carbon-nanotube based sensors: Capsaicinoids in chilli peppers.

Application of Nanosensors (Singh *et al.,* 2019):

 a. Detection of bacterial contaminants (such as Salmonella, Escherichia coli, Vibrio cholera, Staphylococcal Enterotoxin B.)
 b. Detection of fungal contaminants (such as aflatoxin B1- AF B1, Ochratoxin A-OTA.)
 c. Detection of chemical contaminants (such as melamine, carbofuran, ampicillin, 2,4-Dinitrophenol etc.)

Nano-Coatings

Nanomaterials plays a major role in food safety during both processing and packaging. Several application of nano-coatings includes its use in food production machinery (e.g., biofilm formation), nanostructured sieves, filters and membranes (e.g. enabling cold sterilization), nanostructured as well as nanoscale adsorbents, which provides benefits in food processing. (Bartolucci, 2017)

Reports have been found which explains the use of different nanomaterials as therapeutic and diagnostic tool to prevent the blind usage of pesticides to control plant diseases and overcome the shortcomings with the conventional pesticides. (Gour *et al.,* 2019) The activity of these nanoparticles are similar to that of conventional pesticides but they act at a lower concentration thereby causing less toxicity. **Table 6** below explains the application of nanoparticles for controlling plant diseases.

METHODS TO IMPROVE THE QUALITY OF SOIL

In addition to all the above-mentioned application of various nanomaterials to enhance the productivity and quality of agricultural products, quality of soil also plays an important role. Various reports have been found in the literature, which reports the use of hydrogels, nanoclays, and nano zeolites to enhance the water-holding capacity of soil. (Sekhon, 2014) This will assist the slow release of water from soil during dry seasons and help in retaining the quality of soil throughout the year. Another important application of nanomaterials includes the use of various organic nanomaterials (polymer and carbon nanotubes) and inorganic nanomaterials (metals and metal oxides nanomaterials) for the adsorption of environmental contaminants. (Fraceto *et al.,* 2016)

Benefits of Nanomaterials in Food and Agriculture

I. Increased Quality and Quantity of Yields

a. **Sustainable use of water:** Water can be replaced with nano-hydrogels, which will enhance the absorption and release of water and other nutrients in cycles, leading to more efficient use of water. Example: Silver coated hydrogels.
b. **Treatment of seeds:** Seeds treated with nanoparticles germinate faster with higher capabilities to withstand environmental stress.
c. **Pest and disease detection:** Nano-biosensors provide a very precise tool that can be used to prevent pest outbreaks and monitor soil quality, which enhances quality and quantity of yields.
d. **Enhanced delivery of nutrients and plant protection products (ppp):** Nano biosensors can enhance this process by enabling smart delivery systems to precisely release nutrients and ppp's in response to environmental triggers and biological demands. This provides opportunities for real-time monitoring and control.

II. Decreased Pollution
a. **Reduced runoff:** Smart delivery systems reduces pollution, environmental and health risks resulting from fertilizers, ppp's and agrochemicals.
b. **Remediation:** Nanomaterial based soil remediation techniques are proclaimed to be effective because of its low cost and environmentally friendly nature. Example: Iron nanoparticles used for reduction of Trichloroethane (a solvent in pesticides).

Toxicity of Nanomaterials

In addition, to the positive impact of nanomaterials, continuous research in this field affirms that prolonged exposure of these nanomaterials may also have detrimental effect to the environment. Humic acid (organic matter) present in the soil helps to prevent adhesion and decreases its toxicity. However, the abiotic factors and living organism intervention changes the properties of nanomaterials. (Makarenko & Makarenko, 2019) According to the Organization for Economic Co-operation and Development (OECD) chemicals coming to the environment because of human activity must have Eco toxicological assessment.

Nanomaterials may also be toxic to the plants. Its influence on different plants are explained in **Table 7**. These nanomaterials from Nanofertilizer enter to the plant and causes changes in the metabolism of plants, stress and cause damage at cell level. Therefore, it is always necessary to study the dependence-dose effect. (Makarenko & Makarenko, 2019)

Table 7. Toxicity of nanomaterials towards various plants

Nanoparticles	Influence on	References
ZnO NPs	Test plant: *Pisum sativum* L.; influence on photosynthesis, colouring agents, proteins and carbohydrates	Makarenko & Makarenko, 2019
ZnO and TiO_2 NPs	Test plant: Rice root system (*Oryza satyva* L.); influence on development of root system	P. Boonyanitipong *et al.,* 2011
TiO_2 NPs	Test plant: *Anabaena variabilis;* depressed the process of nitogen fixation	Cherchi & Gu, 2010;(Feizi *et al.,*, 2012)
	Test plant: *Triticum aestivum;* reduced the energy of germination	
Al NPs	Test plant: *Lolium perenne*; influences root growth, reduced seed germination	Lin & Xing, 2007
Ag NPs	Test plant: *Allium cepa;* Changed passing metaphases, changed chromosomes, destroyed cell walls.	Kumari *et al.,*, 2009; Stampoulis *et al.,*, 2009
	Test plant: *Cucurbita pepo*; changed the process of transpiration	
Zn NPs	Test plant: *Zea mays, Lactuca sativus*; influences root growth and development	Lin & Xing, 2007
Cu NPs	Test plant: *Phaseolus radiates*; hinders seed germination	Lee *et al.,*, 2008

CONCLUSION

Nanotechnology has the immense potential for being used in the field of food and agriculture sectors. Various nanomaterials such as metal nanoparticles, metal oxide nanomaterials, carbon based materials have been used in food manufacturing, packaging, storage, water purification, plant protection, therapeutics, antimicrobial and drug delivery applications. These will help to enhance the quality and quantity of agricultural products, which will help to overcome the growing demand of food to feed this increasing population. In addition, to the positive influence of nanomaterials, nanomaterials may also be toxic depending upon the size, aggregation, composition, crystallinity and surface functionalization. These may causes changes in the metabolism of body tissue/organs and cause damage at cell level.

List of Abbreviations

Av: avermectin
ENMs: Engineered Nanomaterials
NPs: Nanoparticles
NW: Nanowire
OECD: Organization for Economic Co-operation and Development
ppp: plant protection products
PDA: Polydopamine
PB: Prussian blue
PVAc: poly(vinylacetate)
PMMA: poly(methyl methacrylate)
PS: polystyrene
PVDF: poly(vinylidene fluoride)

PMMA: Poly-(methyl methacrylate)
R&D: Research and Development
SPR: surface plasmon resonance
SERS: surface enhanced Raman spectroscopy
SAS: synthetic amorphous silica

REFERENCES

Acharya, P., Jayaprakasha, G. K., Crosby, K. M., Jifon, J. L., & Patil, B. S. (2019). Green-Synthesized Nanoparticles Enhanced Seedling Growth, Yield, and Quality of Onion (*Allium cepa* L.). *ACS Sustainable Chemistry & Engineering*, *7*(17), 14580–14590. doi:10.1021/acssuschemeng.9b02180

Adisa, I. O., Pullagurala, V. L. R., Peralta-Videa, J. R., Dimkpa, C. O., Elmer, W. H., Gardea-Torresdey, J. L., & White, J. C. (2019). Recent advances in nano-enabled fertilizers and pesticides: A critical review of mechanisms of action. *Environmental Science. Nano*, *6*(7), 2002–2030. doi:10.1039/C9EN00265K

Agrawal, S., & Rathore, P. (2014). Article. *International Journal of Current Microbiology and Applied Sciences*, *3*, 43–55.

Ashkavand, P., Zarafshar, M., Tabari, M., Mirzaie, J., Nikpour, A., Bordbar, S. K., Struve, D., & Striker, G. G. (2018). Application of SiO2 nanoparticles as pretreatment alleviates the impact of drought on the physiological performance of Prunus mahaleb (Rosaceae). *Boletín de la Sociedad Argentina de Botánica*, *53*(2), 207–219. doi:10.31055/1851.2372.v53.n2.20578

Banerjee, T., Sulthana, S., Shelby, T., Heckert, B., Jewell, J., Woody, K., Karimnia, V., McAfee, J., & Santra, S. (2016). Multiparametric Magneto-fluorescent Nanosensors for the Ultrasensitive Detection of *Escherichia coli* O157:H7. *ACS Infectious Diseases*, *2*(10), 667–673. doi:10.1021/acsinfecdis.6b00108 PMID:27737552

Bartolucci, C. (2017). Nanotechnology in Agriculture and Food Science. Academic Press.

Baruah, S., & Dutta, J. (2009). Nanotechnology applications in pollution sensing and degradation in agriculture: A review. *Environmental Chemistry Letters*, *7*(3), 191–204. doi:10.100710311-009-0228-8

Boonyanitipong, P., Kositsup, B., Kumar, P., Baruah, S., & Dutta, J. (2011). Toxicity of ZnO and TiO2 Nanoparticles on Germinating Rice Seed Oryza sativa L. *International Journal of Bioscience, Biochemistry, Bioinformatics*, *1*, 282–285. doi:10.7763/IJBBB.2011.V1.53

Bramhanwade, K., Shende, S., Bonde, S., Gade, A., & Rai, M. (2016). Article. *Environmental Chemistry Letters*, 14.

Broadley, M. R., White, P. J., Hammond, J. P., Zelko, I., & Lux, A. (2007). Zinc in plants. *The New Phytologist*, *173*(4), 677–702. doi:10.1111/j.1469-8137.2007.01996.x PMID:17286818

Chaudhry, N., Dwivedi, S., Chaudhry, V., Singh, A., Saquib, Q., Azam, A., & Musarrat, J. (2018). Bio-inspired nanomaterials in agriculture and food: Current status, foreseen applications and challenges. *Microbial Pathogenesis*, *123*, 196–200. doi:10.1016/j.micpath.2018.07.013 PMID:30009970

Cherchi, C., & Gu, A. Z. (2010). Impact of Titanium Dioxide Nanomaterials on Nitrogen Fixation Rate and Intracellular Nitrogen Storage in *Anabaena variabilis*. *Environmental Science & Technology*, *4*(21), 8302–8307. doi:10.1021/es101658p PMID:20853867

Cromwell, W. A., Yang, J., Starr, J. L., & Jo, Y. K. (2014). Article. *Journal of Nematology*, *46*, 261–266. PMID:25275999

Cushen, M., Kerry, J., Morris, M., Cruz-Romero, M., & Cummins, E. (2012). Nanotechnologies in the food industry – Recent developments, risks and regulation. *Trends in Food Science & Technology*, *24*(1), 30–46. doi:10.1016/j.tifs.2011.10.006

Dasgupta, N., Ranjan, S., Mundekkad, D., Ramalingam, C., Shanker, R., & Kumar, A. (2015a). Nanotechnology in agro-food: From field to plate. *Food Research International*, *69*, 381–400. doi:10.1016/j.foodres.2015.01.005

De Filpo, G., Palermo, A. M. F., Rachiele, F. P., & Nicoletta, F. P. (2013). Preventing fungal growth in wood by titanium dioxide nanoparticles. *Int. Biodeter. Biodegr.*, *85*, 217–222. doi:10.1016/j.ibiod.2013.07.007

Eltarahony, M., Zaki, S., ElKady, M., & Abd-El-Haleem, D. (2018). Article. *Journal of Nanomaterials*, *2018*, 1–16.

European Parliament and Council. (2015). Regulation (EC) 2015/2283 of the European parliament and of the Council of 25 November 2015 on novel foods. Author.

Feizi, H., Moghaddam, P. R., Shahtahmassebi, N., & Fotovat, A. (2012). Impact of Bulk and Nanosized Titanium Dioxide (TiO2) on Wheat Seed Germination and Seedling Growth. *Biological Trace Element Research*, *146*(1), 101–106. doi:10.100712011-011-9222-7 PMID:21979242

Feng, Y., Zhu, W., Guo, W., & Jiang, L. (2017). Bioinspired Energy Conversion in Nanofluidics: A Paradigm of Material Evolution. *Advanced Materials*, *29*(45), 1702773. doi:10.1002/adma.201702773

Feregrino-Pérez, A. A., Magaña-López, E., Guzmán, C., & Esquivel, K. (2018). A general overview of the benefits and possible negative effects of the nanotechnology in horticulture. *Scientia Horticulturae*, *238*, 126–137. doi:10.1016/j.scienta.2018.03.060

Fowsiya, J., Asharani, I. V., Mohapatra, S., Eshapula, A., Mohi, P., Thakar, N., Monad, S., & Madhumitha, G. (2019). Aegle marmelos phytochemical stabilized synthesis and characterization of ZnO nanoparticles and their role against agriculture and food pathogen. *Green Process Synth.*, *8*(1), 488–495. doi:10.1515/gps-2019-0017

Fraceto, L. F., Grillo, R., de Medeiros, G. A., Scognamiglio, V., Rea, G., & Bartolucci, C. (2016). Nanotechnology in Agriculture: Which Innovation Potential Does It Have? *Frontiers in Environmental Science*, *4*. Advance online publication. doi:10.3389/fenvs.2016.00020

Ganachari, S. V., Yaradoddi, J. S., Somappa, S. B., Mogre, P., Tapaskar, R. P., Salimath, B., Venkataraman, A., & Viswanath, V. J. (2018). *Handbook of Ecomaterials*. Springer International Publishing AG., doi:10.1007/978-3-319-48281-1_184-1

Gorrasi, G., & Bugatti, V. (2016). Edible bio-nano-hybrid coatings for food protection based on pectins and LDH-salicylate: Preparation and analysis of physical properties. *Lebensmittel-Wissenschaft + Technologie*, *69*, 139–145. doi:10.1016/j.lwt.2016.01.038

Graham, J. H., Johnson, E. G., Myers, M. E., Young, M., Rajasekaran, P., Das, S., & Santra, S. (2016). Potential of Nano-Formulated Zinc Oxide for Control of Citrus Canker on Grapefruit Trees. *Plant Disease*, *100*(12), 2442–2447. doi:10.1094/PDIS-05-16-0598-RE PMID:30686171

Idumah, C. I., Zurina, M., Ogbu, J., Ndem, J. U., & Igba, E. C. (2019). A review on innovations in polymeric nanocomposite packaging materials and electrical sensors for food and agriculture. *Composite Interfaces*, *27*(1), 1–72. doi:10.1080/09276440.2019.1600972

Jain, A., Ranjan, S., Dasgupta, N., & Ramalingam, C. (2018). Nanomaterials in food and agriculture: An overview on their safety concerns and regulatory issues. *Critical Reviews in Food Science and Nutrition*, *58*(2), 297–317. doi:10.1080/10408398.2016.1160363 PMID:27052385

Jiao, A., Dong, X., Zhang, H., Xu, L., Tian, Y., Liu, X., & Chen, M. (2019). Construction of pure worm-like AuAg nanochains for ultrasensitive SERS detection of pesticide residues on apple surfaces. *Spectrochimica Acta. Part A: Molecular and Biomolecular Spectroscopy*, *209*, 241–247. doi:10.1016/j.saa.2018.10.051

Jung, J. H., Kim, S. W., Min, J. S., Kim, Y. J., Lamsal, K., Kim, K. S., & Lee, Y. S. (2010). The Effect of Nano-Silver Liquid against the White Rot of the Green Onion Caused by *Sclerotium cepivorum*. *Mycobiology*, *38*(1), 39–45. doi:10.4489/MYCO.2010.38.1.039 PMID:23956623

Kairyte, K., Kadys, A., & Luksiene, Z. (2013). Antibacterial and antifungal activity of photoactivated ZnO nanoparticles in suspension. *Journal of Photochemistry and Photobiology. B, Biology*, *128*, 78–84. doi:10.1016/j.jphotobiol.2013.07.017 PMID:24035847

Kaphle, A., Navya, P. N., Umapathi, A., & Daima, H. K. (2018). Nanomaterials for agriculture, food and environment: Applications, toxicity and regulation. *Environmental Chemistry Letters*, *16*(1), 43–58. doi:10.100710311-017-0662-y

Kearns, H., Goodacre, R., Jamieson, L. E., Graham, D., & Faulds, K. (2017). SERS Detection of Multiple Antimicrobial-Resistant Pathogens Using Nanosensors. *Analytical Chemistry*, *89*(23), 12666–12673. doi:10.1021/acs.analchem.7b02653 PMID:28985467

Kim, H. S., Kang, H. S., Chu, G. J., & Byun, H. S. (2008). Antifungal Effectiveness of Nanosilver Colloid against Rose Powdery Mildew in Greenhouses. *Diffusion and Defect Data, Solid State Data. Part B, Solid State Phenomena*, *135*, 15–18. doi:10.4028/www.scientific.net/SSP.135.15

Konate, A., Wang, Y., He, X., Adeel, M., Zhang, P., Ma, Y., Ding, Y., Zhang, J., Yang, J., Kizito, S., Rui, Y., & Zhang, Z. (2018). Comparative effects of nano and bulk-Fe3O4 on the growth of cucumber (Cucumis sativus). *Ecotoxicology and Environmental Safety*, *165*, 547–554. doi:10.1016/j.ecoenv.2018.09.053 PMID:30223168

Kong, B., Tang, J., Wu, Z., Selomulya, C., Wang, H., Wei, J., Wang, Y., Zheng, G., & Zhao, D. (2014). Bio-inspired porous antenna-like nanocube/nanowire heterostructure as ultra-sensitive cellular interfaces. *NPG Asia Materials*, *6*(8), e117. doi:10.1038/am.2014.56

Kumar, A., Gupta, K., Dixit, S., Mishra, K., & Srivastava, S. (2019). A review on positive and negative impacts of nanotechnology in agriculture. *International Journal of Environmental Science and Technology, 16*(4), 2175–2184. doi:10.100713762-018-2119-7

Kumari, M., Mukherjee, A., & Chandrasekaran, N. (2009). Genotoxicity of silver nanoparticles in Allium cepa. *The Science of the Total Environment, 407*(19), 5243–5246. doi:10.1016/j.scitotenv.2009.06.024 PMID:19616276

Lee, W. M., An, Y. J., Yoon, H., & Kwbon, H. S. (2008). Toxicity and bioavailability of copper nanoparticles to the terrestrial plants mung bean (phaseolus radiatus) and wheat (triticum aestivum): plant agar test for water-insoluble nanoparticles. *Environmental Toxicology and Chemistry, 27*(9), 1915–1921. doi:10.1897/07-481.1 PMID:19086317

Liang, J., Yu, M., Guo, L., Cui, B., Zhao, X., Sun, C., Wang, Y., Liu, G., Cui, H., & Zeng, Z. (2018). Bioinspired Development of P(St–MAA)–Avermectin Nanoparticles with High Affinity for Foliage To Enhance Folia Retention. *Journal of Agricultural and Food Chemistry, 66*(26), 6578–6584. doi:10.1021/acs.jafc.7b01998 PMID:28727420

Lin, D., & Xing, B. (2007). Phytotoxicity of nanoparticles: Inhibition of seed germination and root growth. *Environmental Pollution, 150*(2), 243–250. doi:10.1016/j.envpol.2007.01.016 PMID:17374428

Liu, R., & Lal, R. (2015). Potentials of engineered nanoparticles as fertilizers for increasing agronomic productions. *The Science of the Total Environment, 514*, 131–139. doi:10.1016/j.scitotenv.2015.01.104 PMID:25659311

Liu, R., & Lal, R. (2015). Potentials of engineered nanoparticles as fertilizers for increasing agronomic productions. *The Science of the Total Environment, 514*, 131–139. doi:10.1016/j.scitotenv.2015.01.104 PMID:25659311

Lu, J., & Bowles, M. (2013). Article. *Int. Food Agribus. Manag. Assoc., 16*, 21–42.

Makarenko, N. A., & Makarenko, V. V. (2019). Nanotechnologies in crop cultivation: Ecotoxicological aspects. *Biosystems Diversity, 27*(2), 148–155. doi:10.15421/011920

Malusá, E., Sas-Paszt, L., & Ciesielska, J. (2012). *Transfus.* Apher. Sci.

Manjunatha, S. B., Biradar, D. P., & Aladakatti, Y. R. (2016). Article. *J. Farm Sci., 29*, 1–13.

Marchiol, L. (2018). *New Visions in Plant Science*. doi:10.5772/intechopen.74425

Mishra, M., Dashora, K., Srivastava, A., Fasake, V. D., & Nag, R. H. (2019). Prospects, challenges and need for regulation of nanotechnology with special reference to India. *Ecotoxicology and Environmental Safety, 171*, 677–682. doi:10.1016/j.ecoenv.2018.12.085 PMID:30658303

Monica, J. C. (2010). *G. V. CalsterMatthew Hull and Diana Bowman publisher*. Elsevier.

Mukhopadhyay, S. S. (2014). Nanotechnology in agriculture: Prospects and constraints. *Nanotechnology, Science and Applications, 7*, 63–71. doi:10.2147/NSA.S39409 PMID:25187699

Ocsoy, I., Paret, M. L., Ocsoy, M. A., Kunwar, S., Chen, T., You, M., & Tan, W. (2013). Nanotechnology in Plant Disease Management: DNA-Directed Silver Nanoparticles on Graphene Oxide as an Antibacterial against *Xanthomonas perforans*. *ACS Nano*, *7*(10), 8972–8980. doi:10.1021/nn4034794 PMID:24016217

Ouda, S. M. (2014). Antifungal Activity of Silver and Copper Nanoparticles on Two Plant Pathogens, Alternaria alternata and Botrytis cinerea. *Res. J. Microbiol.*, *9*(1), 34–42. doi:10.3923/jm.2014.34.42

Paret, M. L., Vallad, E. G., Averett, R. D., Jones, B. J., & Olson, M. S. (2013). Photocatalysis: Effect of Light-Activated Nanoscale Formulations of TiO_2 on *Xanthomonas perforans* and Control of Bacterial Spot of Tomato. *Phytopathology*, *103*(3), 228–236. doi:10.1094/PHYTO-08-12-0183-R PMID:23190116

Perçin, I., Idil, N., Bakhshpour, M., Yılmaz, E., Mattiasson, B., & Denizli, A. (2017).. . *Sensors and Actuators. B, Chemical*, *17*, 1375.

Peters, R. J. B., Bouwmeester, H., Gottardo, S., Amenta, V., Arena, M., Brandhoff, P., Marvin, H. J. P., Mech, A., Moniz, F. B., Pesudo, L. Q., Rauscher, H., Schoonjans, R., Undas, A. K., Vettori, M. V., Weigel, S., & Aschberger, K. (2016). Nanomaterials for products and application in agriculture, feed and food. *Trends in Food Science & Technology*, *54*, 155–164. doi:10.1016/j.tifs.2016.06.008

Rafque, M., Jahangir, J., Amin, B. A. Z., Tahir, M. B., Nabi, G., Khan, M. I., Khalid, N. R., Gillani, S. S. A., & Sadaf, I. (2019). Article. *Journal of Inorganic and Organometallic Polymers and Materials*, *29*, 2133–2144. doi:10.100710904-019-01173-5

Ranjan, S., Dasgupta, N., Ganesh, S. A., Ramalingam, C., & Kumar, A. (2016). Microwave-irradiation-assisted hybrid chemical approach for titanium dioxide nanoparticle synthesis: Microbial and cytotoxicological evaluation. *Environmental Science and Pollution Research International*, *23*(12), 12287–12302. doi:10.100711356-016-6440-8 PMID:26976013

Ravichandran, R. (2010). Nanotechnology Applications in Food and Food Processing: Innovative Green Approaches, Opportunities and Uncertainties for Global Market. *Int. J. Green Nanotechnol. Phys. Chem.*, *1*(2), 72–P96. doi:10.1080/19430871003684440

Rizeq, B. R., Younes, N. N., Rasool, K., & Nasrallah, G. K. (2019). Article. *International Journal of Molecular Sciences*, *20*(5776), 1–24.

Robledo, N., López, L., Bunger, A., Tapia, C., & Abugoch, L. (2018). Effects of Antimicrobial Edible Coating of Thymol Nanoemulsion/Quinoa Protein/Chitosan on the Safety, Sensorial Properties, and Quality of Refrigerated Strawberries (Fragaria × ananassa) Under Commercial Storage Environment. *Food and Bioprocess Technology*, *11*(8), 1566–1574. doi:10.100711947-018-2124-3

Robles-García, M. A., Rodríguez-Félix, F., Márquez-Ríos, E., Aguilar, J. A., Barrera Rodríguez, A., Aguilar, J., Ruiz-Cruz, S., & Lizette Del-Toro-Sánchez, C. (2016). Applications of Nanotechnology in the Agriculture, Food, and Pharmaceuticals. *Journal of Nanoscience and Nanotechnology*, *16*(8), 8188–8207. doi:10.1166/jnn.2016.12925

Sahoo, D., Mandal, A., Mitra, T., Chakraborty, K., Bardhan, M., & Dasgupta, A. K. (2018). Nanosensing of Pesticides by Zinc Oxide Quantum Dot: An Optical and Electrochemical Approach for the Detection of Pesticides in Water. *Journal of Agricultural and Food Chemistry*, *66*(2), 414–423. doi:10.1021/acs.jafc.7b04188 PMID:29239610

Salvia-Trujillo, L., Rojas-Graü, M. A., Soliva-Fortuny, R., & Martín-Belloso, O. (2015). Use of antimicrobial nanoemulsions as edible coatings: Impact on safety and quality attributes of fresh-cut Fuji apples. *Postharvest Biology and Technology*, *105*, 8–16. doi:10.1016/j.postharvbio.2015.03.009

Saratale, R. G., Saratale, G. D., Shin, H. S., Jacob, J. M., Pugazhendhi, A., Bhaisare, M., & Kumar, G. (2018). New insights on the green synthesis of metallic nanoparticles using plant and waste biomaterials: Current knowledge, their agricultural and environmental applications. *Environmental Science and Pollution Research International*, *25*(11), 10164–10183. doi:10.100711356-017-9912-6 PMID:28815433

Savolainen, K., Alenius, H., Norppa, H., Pylkkänen, L., Tuomi, T., & Kasper, G. (2010). Risk assessment of engineered nanomaterials and nanotechnologies—A review. *Toxicology*, *269*(2-3), 92–104. doi:10.1016/j.tox.2010.01.013 PMID:20105448

Sekhon, B. S. (2010). *Nanotechnology, Science and Applications*. Academic Press. PMID:24198465

Sekhon, B. S. (2014). Nanotechnology in agri-food production: An overview. *Nanotechnology, Science and Applications*, *7*, 31–53. doi:10.2147/NSA.S39406 PMID:24966671

Selin, C. (2007). Expectations and the Emergence of Nanotechnology. *Human Values*, *32*(2), 196–220. doi:10.1177/0162243906296918

Senapati, T., Senapati, D., Singh, A. K., Fan, Z., Kanchanapally, R., & Ray, P. C. (2011). Highly selective SERS probe for Hg(ii) detection using tryptophan-protected popcorn shaped gold nanoparticles. *Chemical Communications (Cambridge)*, *47*(37), 10326–10328. doi:10.1039/c1cc13157e

Servin, A. D., & White, J. C. (2016). Nanotechnology in agriculture: Next steps for understanding engineered nanoparticle exposure and risk. *NanoImpact*, *1*, 9–12. doi:10.1016/j.impact.2015.12.002

Shi, S., Wang, W., Liu, L., Wu, S., Wei, Y., & Li, W. (2013). Effect of chitosan/nano-silica coating on the physicochemical characteristics of longan fruit under ambient temperature. *Journal of Food Engineering*, *118*(1), 125–131. doi:10.1016/j.jfoodeng.2013.03.029

Shukla, S. K., Kumar, R., Mishra, R. K., Pandey, A., Pathak, A., Zaidi, M. G. H., Srivastava, S. K., & Dikshit, A. (2015). Prediction and validation of gold nanoparticles (GNPs) on plant growth promoting rhizobacteria (PGPR): A step toward development of nano-biofertilizers. *Nanotechnology Reviews*, *4*(5), 439–448. doi:10.1515/ntrev-2015-0036

Sohail, M. I., Waris, A. A., Ayub, M. A., Usman, M., Rehman, M. Z., Sabir, M., & Faiz, T. (2019). Article. *Comprehensive Analytical Chemistry*, 1–54.

Sonkaria, S., Ahn, S.-H., & Khare, V. (2012). *Recent Patents on Food, Nutrition & Agriculture*. Academic Press. PMID:22316269

Stampoulis, D., Sinha, S. K., & White, J. C. (2009). Assay-Dependent Phytotoxicity of Nanoparticles to Plants. *Environmental Science & Technology*, *43*(24), 9473–9479. doi:10.1021/es901695c PMID:19924897

Sun, A., Chai, J., Xiao, T., Shi, X., Li, X., Zhao, Q., Li, D., & Chen, J. (2018). Development of a selective fluorescence nanosensor based on molecularly imprinted-quantum dot optosensing materials for saxitoxin detection in shellfish samples. *Sensors and Actuators. B, Chemical*, *258*, 408–414. doi:10.1016/j.snb.2017.11.143

Sun, Y., Fang, L., Wan, Y., & Gu, Z. (2018). Pathogenic detection and phenotype using magnetic nanoparticle-urease nanosensor. *Sensors and Actuators. B, Chemical, 259*, 428–432. doi:10.1016/j.snb.2017.12.095

The European Commission, Commission Regulation (EU) No 10/2011 of 14 January. (2011). 2011 on plastic materials and articles intended to come into contact with food Text with EEA relevance Official J. *European Union, 12*, 1–89.

U.S. FDA Inventory of effective food contact substance (FCS) notifications Administration USFaD (2018).

Van Viet, P., Nguyen, H. N., Cao, T. M., & Van Hieu, L. (2016). Article. *Nanomaterials (Basel, Switzerland), 2016*, 1957–612.

Vandergheynst, J., Scher, H., Guo, H. Y., & Schultz, D. (2007). Water-in-oil emulsions that improve the storage and delivery of the biolarvacide Lagenidium giganteum. *BioControl, 52*(2), 207–229. doi:10.100710526-006-9021-9

Wang, M., Liu, Y., Ren, G., Wang, W., Wu, S., & Shen, J. (2018). Bioinspired carbon quantum dots for sensitive fluorescent detection of vitamin B12 in cell system. *Analytica Chimica Acta, 1032*, 154–162. doi:10.1016/j.aca.2018.05.057 PMID:30143213

Wani, A. H., & Shah, M. A. (2012). Article. *Journal of Applied Pharmaceutical Science, 2*, 40–44.

Yadav, S. K. (2017). Realizing the Potential of Nanotechnology for Agriculture and Food Technology. *Journal of Tissue Science & Engineering, 8*(01), 195. doi:10.4172/2157-7552.1000195

Yang, B., Lv, S., Chen, F., Liu, C., Cai, C., Chen, C., & Chen, X. (2016). A resonance light scattering sensor based on bioinspired molecularly imprinted polymers for selective detection of papain at trace levels. *Analytica Chimica Acta, 912*, 125–132. doi:10.1016/j.aca.2016.01.030 PMID:26920781

Zambrano-Zaragoza, M. L., Mercado-Silva, E., Gutiérrez-Cortez, E., Cornejo Villegas, M. A., & Quintanar-Guerrero, D. (2014). The effect of nano-coatings with α-tocopherol and xanthan gum on shelf-life and browning index of fresh-cut "Red Delicious" apples. *Innovative Food Science & Emerging Technologies, 22*, 188–196. doi:10.1016/j.ifset.2013.09.008

Zhang, C. H., Liu, L. W., Liang, P., Tang, L. J., Yu, R. Q., & Jiang, J. H. (2016). Article. *Analytical Chemistry, 88*, 447–452.

Zhang, W., Han, Y., Chen, X., Luo, X., Wang, J., Yue, T., & Li, Z. (2017). Surface molecularly imprinted polymer capped Mn-doped ZnS quantum dots as a phosphorescent nanosensor for detecting patulin in apple juice. *Food Chemistry, 232*, 145–154. doi:10.1016/j.foodchem.2017.03.156 PMID:28490057

Zhang, Z., Huang, J., Dong, B., Yuan, Q., He, Y., & Wolfbeis, O. S. (2015). Rational tailoring of $ZnSnO_3/TiO_2$ heterojunctions with bioinspired surface wettability for high-performance humidity nanosensors. *Nanoscale, 7*(9), 4149–4155. doi:10.1039/C4NR07559E PMID:25665734

Zhu, H., Guo, Z., & Liu, W. (2016). Biomimetic water-collecting materials inspired by nature. *Chemical Communications (Cambridge), 52*(20), 3863–3879. doi:10.1039/C5CC09867J

Zong, L., Li, M., & Li, C. (2017). Bioinspired Coupling of Inorganic Layered Nanomaterials with Marine Polysaccharides for Efficient Aqueous Exfoliation and Smart Actuating Hybrids. *Advanced Materials*, *29*(10), 1604691. doi:10.1002/adma.201604691

Zulfiqar, F., Navarro, M., Ashraf, M., Akram, N. A., & Munné-Bosch, S. (2019). Nanofertilizer use for sustainable agriculture: Advantages and limitations. *Plant Science*, *289*, 110270. doi:10.1016/j.plantsci.2019.110270 PMID:31623775

Chapter 5
Magnesium Oxide (MgO): A Viable Agent for Antimicrobial Activity

Ashaq Hussain Sofi
https://orcid.org/0000-0003-4279-5481
National Institute of Technology, Srinagar, India

Shabir Ahmad Akhoon
Institute of Technology, University of Kashmir, India

Jaffar Farooq Mir
National Institute of Technology, Srinagar, India

Mehraj Ud Din Rather
Department of Physics, University of Kashmir, India

ABSTRACT

Bacterial contamination is an unusual menace for human well-being. Nanotechnology proposes diverse techniques to nurture new inorganic antibacterial agents. Nano-inorganic metal oxides possess an auspicious potential to diminish bacterial effluence. Magnesium oxide (MgO) is a significant inorganic oxide and has been widely employed in numerous arenas such as catalysis, ceramics, toxic waste remediation, antibacterial activity, and as an additive in paint and superconductor products by virtue of its distinctive properties. Numerous studies have shown that magnesium oxide nanostructures possess remarkable antibacterial activity. Therefore, in this direction, few synthesis methods such as hydrothermal method, sol-gel method, etc., antibacterial activity, and antibacterial mechanisms of magnesium oxide nanostructures have been incorporated in this chapter.

DOI: 10.4018/978-1-7998-5563-7.ch005

INTRODUCTION

In the span of two or three decades, the distinguishing properties of nanomaterials created an enormous interest amongst the researchers to develop simple and economical procedures, technologically imperative and productive, to fabricate nanostructures with diverse morphology. Nanomaterials, metal oxide nanomaterials in particular, with high surface area to volume ratio have attracted keen interest of scientific community on account of their prospective applications in numerous areas such as nanoelectronics, optoelectronics, sensing devices etc. A new class of antimicrobial agents are the metal oxide nanomaterials (Rajendra, 2010; Bindhu, 2016; Zhu, 2016). These metal oxides, such as zinc oxide (ZnO), magnesium oxide (MgO), copper oxide (CuO), calcium oxide (CaO), silver oxide (Ag_2O), and titanium dioxide (TiO_2) are believed to possess potential applications in food, healthcare and the environment, with the result these have been increasingly studied for their antibacterial properties. In the nanoregime, metal oxide nanomaterials display remarkable features such as antibacterial activity, large surface area to volume ration, large available surface area of interaction with cell, versatile morphology and tunable sizes, unparalleled surface properties, little chances for bacteria to develop resistance, extraordinary stability even under severe conditions, which pave the ways for abundant possibilities to develop nanomaterials as effective antimicrobial agents (He, 2016; Gold, 2018; Pugazhendhi, 2019). Among these, nanostructured MgO is particularly interesting by virtue of its strong antibacterial activity, cost effective and extraordinary thermal stability. It finds wide-range of applications in catalysis, ceramics, toxic waste remediation, antibacterial activity, paint industry and superconductor products (Yang, 2018; El-Sayyad, 2018; Sudakaran, 2017).

Magnesium oxide (MgO), a source of magnesium, is a hygroscopic solid mineral with a shiny white color, energy band gap, E_g=4.1–6.2eV, lattice parameters a=b=c=4.24nm, boiling point = 3,870 K, melting point = 3,098 K, and density = 3.6 gm/cm^3. In nature, it occurs in the form of periclase from which it is extracted using different metallurgical processes. Its empirical formula is MgO. MgO is composed of lattice of Mg^{2+} ions and O^{2-} ions and these constituents are held together by ionic bonding (Karthik, 2017; Fu, 2005).

Figure 1. The crystal structure of MgO showing the octahedral co-ordination of the Mg and O ions.

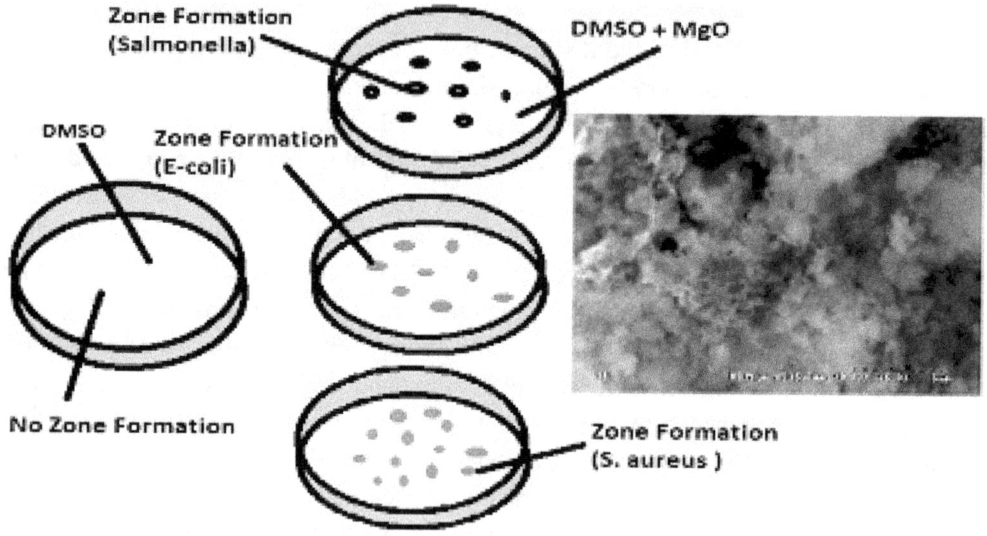

Graphical Abstract

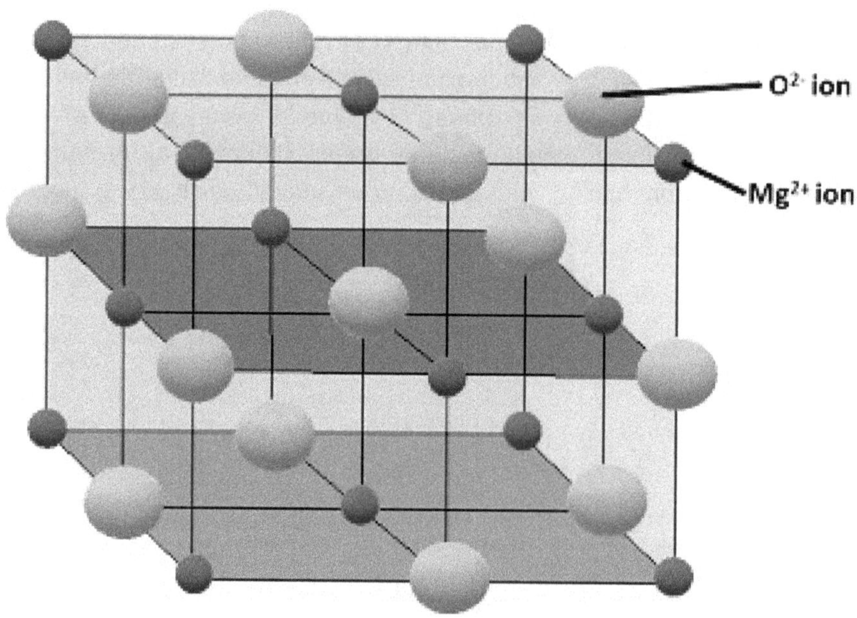

Figure 1 depicts the pictorial representation of MgO unit cell. The structure of MgO may be characterized as a cubic close packed arrangement of oxygen ions having magnesium ions at the octahedral sites. The Mg^{2+} ions as well as the O^{2-} ions are organized in a face-centred cubic (F.C.C.) pattern with lattice parameters. Each ion in the structure is octahedrally surrounded by six similar ions of other type. A regular three-dimensional array is formed with coordination number of six for both the types of ions.

Among the family of metal oxides, magnesium oxide has a simple stoichiometry, simple crystal structure and owes good ionic character. On account of the high concentration of edge/corner sites and structural imperfections on surface, magnesium oxide nanostructures retain high specific surface and reactivity (Makhluf, 2005; Xu, 2004). For antibacterial activity, several methods have been employed to fabricate MgO nanostructures with different morphology and particle size. We have utilized two different methods namely hydrothermal method and sol-gel method for the fabrication of MgO nanoparticles.

EXPERIMENT

To synthesize the magnesium oxide nanoparticles through hydrothermal method, an autoclave (a closed cylindrical Teflon lined stainless steel chamber) of 60 ml capacity was used. The autoclave was cleaned with de-ionized water several times followed by cleaning with acetone. Fine magnesium metal powder (0.4 g), 14 ml de-ionized water and 1 ml hydrogen peroxide were used as starting materials. The reaction mixture was taken in a glass veil and then sonicated for about 20 min. The reaction mixture was transferred to an autoclaved. An autoclave, sealed under inert conditions, was placed in a preheated box furnace at a temperature of 200 °C for 48 hrs. After 48 hrs, the furnace was switched-off and allowed to cool for next 24 hrs. To recover the product, the resulting sample was centrifuged for 15 min followed by washing multiple times with de-ionized water. . Finally, obtained product was vacuum dried at 130 °C for 12 hrs. The complete experimental procedure is depicted in Figure 2.

Figure 2. Synthesis of MgO via hydrothermal method.

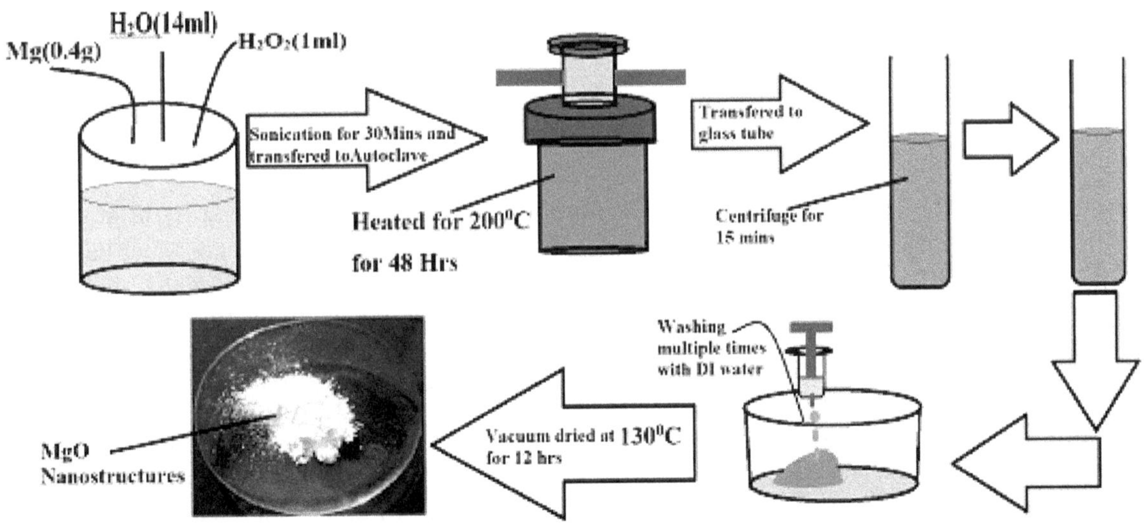

To produce the magnesium oxide nanoparticles via sol-gel method, magnesium nitrate (99.99%, Alpha Aesar) and anhydrous citric acid were used as starting materials. 1 molar (M) solution of magnesium nitrate and de-ionized was prepared. A separate solution of citric acid and deionized water, having molarity of 3.6 M, was also prepared. The molar ratio of 1:3.6 was chosen after number of trials in order to avoid precipitation. Citric acid acted as a complexant agent. Figure-2 depicts the schematic representation of the synthesis process. Prepared separate solutions were stirred for about 10 min. After stirring these were mixed and then heated at 70 ^{0}C for 1 hr followed heating at 300 ^{0}C to obtain precursor powder. The obtained powder was grinded into fine particles using mortar-pestle. In order to remove the impurities and to attain a good crystalline phase of MgO, the achieved powder was calcinated at a temperature of 500 ^{0}C for 5 hrs.

Figure 3. Synthesis of MgO via sol-gel method.

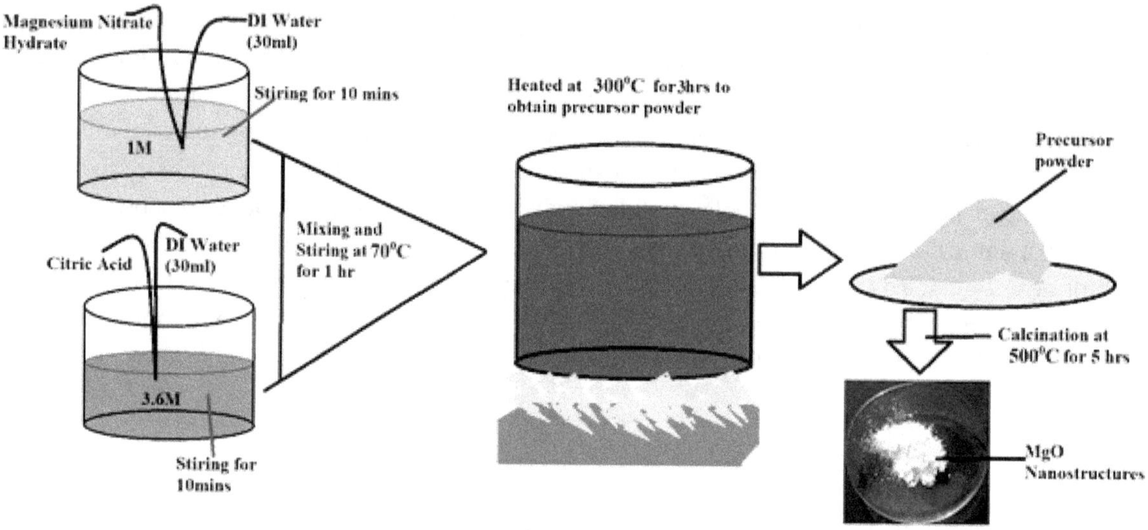

ANTIBACTERIAL ACTIVITY

To test the antibacterial action of the magnesium oxide nanoparticles prepared via two different methods, following set of tools were used; test sample, Mueller Hinton agar (MHA), hot water bath 45°C, sterile petri dishes, flame, colony counter with magnifying glass, sterile capped test tubes and pipettes of various sizes e.g. 01, 1.0 and 2.0 ml. Three different bacteria like Staphylococcus aureus (S. Aureus), Escherichia coli (E. coli) and Salmonella were chosen. Disc Diffusion Method, proposed by Rahman and Rashid, was employed to check the antimicrobial activity of the prepared samples (Rahman, 2008; Sikder, 2011). The test materials were in discs and then positioned on nutrient agar medium homogeneously seeded with the test microorganisms. To permit maximum diffusion of the test materials, the plates were kept at low temperature of 4 ^{0}C for 24 hours followed by an incubation at a temperature of 37 ^{0}C for 24 hours with the aim of permitting maximum growth of the organisms. Surrounding the discs, distinct zones of inhibition were observed because the test material possessing antimicrobial activity inhibited the growth of the micro-organisms. To determine the antimicrobial activity of the test agents the diameter of zone of inhibition triplicate was measured and the mean value of the observations was taken into consideration. Table-1 depicts the diameters of the various inhibition zones in test materials prepared via different methods.

Table 1. Diameters of zones of inhibition of different bacteria in mm

Item	E-coli	Salmonella	S. aureus
Pure DMSO	0.0 mm	0.0 mm	0.0 mm
MgO (hydrothermal method)	2.0 mm	1.0 mm	1.0 mm
MgO (sol-gel method)	1.0 mm	6.0 mm	8.0 mm

No inhibition zones were observed in case of Dimethyl sulfoxide (DMSO) as DMSO served as Positive control. The inhibition zones of diameters; (2.0, 1.0) mm, (1.0, 6.0) mm and (1.0, 8.0) mm were observed in case of E. Coli, Salmonella and S. aureus prepared via hydrothermal method and sol-gel method. In case of MgO nanoparticles, the zone formation was witnessed. However, the zone formation was limited to few millimeters for the reason that the nanoparticles penetrated and blocked the cell walls. The cell walls were blocked when nanoparticles attached themselves at the surface of the microorganisms. With the result, the microorganisms were prevented to accomplish the natural activity and eventually their growth was restricted to certain millimeters. Moreover, at the nanoscale, increase in the surface area of prepared magnesium oxide caused increase in the concentration of O^{2-} ions in the solution and subsequently lead to the annihilation of the cell wall of the bacteria effectively and in the end death of the micro-organisms (Rukh, 2020; Gokulakrishnan, 2012; Rohmawati, 2019; Yamamoto, 2010).

CONCLUSION

This chapter investigated the possibility of engineering structural properties of MgO by employing various synthesis methods like hydrothermal method and sol-gel method. The effect of synthesis conditions on the antibacterial activity have been examined. Major findings revealed that the highest diameter was observed in case of Salmonella and S aureus when treated with MgO prepared by sol-gel method. However, in case of E. Colie the highest value of diameter was obtained in case of MgO prepared by hydrothermal method. It will an efficient material against bacteria provided the synthesis condition must be optimized to achieve the smallest possible grain sizes and appropriate dopants have to be explored to enhance its efficiency

It would be interesting to check the antibacterial activity of MgO by optimizing the synthesis conditions in order to attain the feasible particle size (below 17 nanometers). Further, to enhance its efficiency antibacterial activity dopants like cobalt, nickel, etc., with optimized concentration may play a crucial role.

ACKNOWLEDGMENT

The authors are highly thankful to NIT Srinagar and University of Kashmir for providing experimental facilities.

REFERENCES

Bindhu, M. R., Umadevi, M., Micheal, M. K., Arasu, M. V., & Al-Dhabi, N. A. (2016). Structural, morphological and optical properties of MgO nanoparticles for antibacterial applications. *Materials Letters*, *166*, 19–22. doi:10.1016/j.matlet.2015.12.020

El-Sayyad, G. S., Mosallam, F. M., & El-Batal, A. I. (2018). One-pot green synthesis of magnesium oxide nanoparticles using Penicillium chrysogenum melanin pigment and gamma rays with antimicrobial activity against multidrug-resistant microbes. *Advanced Powder Technology*, *29*(11), 2616–2625. doi:10.1016/j.apt.2018.07.009

Fu, L., Liu, Z. H. I. M. I. N., Liu, Y., Han, B., Hu, P., Cao, L., & Zhu, D. A. O. B. E. N. (2005). Beaded cobalt oxide nanoparticles along carbon nanotubes: Towards more highly integrated electronic devices. *Advanced Materials*, *17*(2), 217–221. doi:10.1002/adma.200400833

Gokulakrishnan, R., Ravikumar, S., & Raj, J. A. (2012). In vitro antibacterial potential of metal oxide nanoparticles against antibiotic resistant bacterial pathogens. *Asian Pacific Journal of Tropical Disease*, *2*(5), 411–413. doi:10.1016/S2222-1808(12)60089-9

Gold, K., Slay, B., Knackstedt, M., & Gaharwar, A. K. (2018). Antimicrobial activity of metal and metal-oxide based nanoparticles. *Advanced Therapeutics*, *1*(3), 1700033. doi:10.1002/adtp.201700033

He, Y., Ingudam, S., Reed, S., Gehring, A., Strobaugh, T. P. Jr, & Irwin, P. (2016). Study on the mechanism of antibacterial action of magnesium oxide nanoparticles against foodborne pathogens. *Journal of Nanobiotechnology*, *14*(1), 54. doi:10.118612951-016-0202-0 PMID:27349516

Karthik, K., Dhanuskodi, S., Kumar, S. P., Gobinath, C., & Sivaramakrishnan, S. (2017). Microwave assisted green synthesis of MgO nanorods and their antibacterial and anti-breast cancer activities. *Materials Letters*, *206*, 217–220. doi:10.1016/j.matlet.2017.07.004

Makhluf, S., Dror, R., Nitzan, Y., Abramovich, Y., Jelinek, R., & Gedanken, A. (2005). Microwave-assisted synthesis of nanocrystalline MgO and its use as a bacteriocide. *Advanced Functional Materials*, *15*(10), 1708–1715. doi:10.1002/adfm.200500029

Pugazhendhi, A., Prabhu, R., Muruganantham, K., Shanmuganathan, R., & Natarajan, S. (2019). Anticancer, antimicrobial and photocatalytic activities of green synthesized magnesium oxide nanoparticles (MgONPs) using aqueous extract of Sargassum wightii. *Journal of Photochemistry and Photobiology. B, Biology*, *190*, 86–97. doi:10.1016/j.jphotobiol.2018.11.014 PMID:30504053

Rahman, M. S., & Rashid, M. A. (2008). Antimicrobial activity and cytotoxicity of Eclipta prostrata. *Oriental Pharmacy and Experimental Medicine*, *8*(1), 47–52. doi:10.3742/OPEM.2008.8.1.047

Rajendra, R., Balakumar, C., Ahammed, H. A. M., Jayakumar, S., Vaideki, K., & Rajesh, E. (2010). Use of zinc oxide nano particles for production of antimicrobial textiles. *International Journal of Engineering Science and Technology*, *2*(1), 202–208. doi:10.4314/ijest.v2i1.59113

Rohmawati, L., Sholicha, S. P., Holisa, S. S., & Setyarsih, W. (2019, December). Identification of Phase CaCO3/MgO in Bangkalan Dolomite Sand as An Antibacterial Substance. *Journal of Physics: Conference Series*, *1417*(1), 012001. doi:10.1088/1742-6596/1417/1/012001

Rukh, S., Sofi, A. H., Shah, M. A., & Yousuf, S. (2019). Antibacterial activity of magnesium oxide nanostructures prepared by hydrothermal method. *Asian Journal of Nanosciences and Materials, 2*(4), 425–430.

Sikder, M. A. A., Kaisar, M. A., & Parvez, M. M., Hossian, A. N., Akhter, F., & Rashid, M. A. (2011). Preliminary antimicrobial activity and cytotoxicity of leaf extracts of Mesua nagassarium (Burm. f.). *Boletín Latinoamericano y del Caribe de Plantas Medicinales y Aromáticas, 10*(1), 83–87.

Sudakaran, S. V., Venugopal, J. R., Vijayakumar, G. P., Abisegapriyan, S., Grace, A. N., & Ramakrishna, S. (2017). Sequel of MgO nanoparticles in PLACL nanofibers for anti-cancer therapy in synergy with curcumin/β-cyclodextrin. *Materials Science and Engineering C, 71*, 620–628. doi:10.1016/j.msec.2016.10.050 PMID:27987753

Xu, H., Wang, H., Zhang, Y., He, W., Zhu, M., Wang, B., & Yan, H. (2004). Hydrothermal synthesis of zinc oxide powders with controllable morphology. *Ceramics International, 30*(1), 93–97. doi:10.1016/S0272-8842(03)00069-5

Yamamoto, O., Ohira, T., Alvarez, K., & Fukuda, M. (2010). Antibacterial characteristics of $CaCO_3$–MgO composites. *Materials Science and Engineering B, 173*(1-3), 208–212. doi:10.1016/j.mseb.2009.12.007

Yang, K., Han, Q., Chen, B., Zheng, Y., Zhang, K., Li, Q., & Wang, J. (2018). Antimicrobial hydrogels: Promising materials for medical application. *International Journal of Nanomedicine, 13*, 2217–2263. doi:10.2147/IJN.S154748 PMID:29695904

Zhu, X., Wu, D., Wang, W., Tan, F., Wong, P. K., Wang, X., & Qiao, X. (2016). Highly effective antibacterial activity and synergistic effect of Ag-MgO nanocomposite against Escherichia coli. *Journal of Alloys and Compounds, 684*, 282–290. doi:10.1016/j.jallcom.2016.05.179

Chapter 6
Nanotechnology as an Emerging Field in the Arena of Medicine

Nisar A. Dangroo
National Institute of Technology, Srinagar, India

Asif Ahmad Malik
National Institute of Technology, Srinagar, India

Tabassum Ara
National Institute of Technology, Srinagar, India

Gazunfor Ali
National Institute of Technology, Srinagar, India

ABSTRACT

Nanotechnology as an emerging scientific field has enabled humanity to manipulate the environment at molecular and atomic level and has touched and even revolutionized all scientific fields due to its characteristic features. Medicine is one of the important fields that witnessed a nanotechnological revolution that guided medical scientists to device new approaches to study pathologies and explore genuine therapeutic tricks by exploring nanotechnology to operate on more specific molecular targets and to reduce the adverse risks and side effects imposed by the conventional approaches. By manipulating drugs and other materials, the fundamental properties and bioactivity of the materials can be altered at the nano scale. These tools can led to the different characteristics of drugs or agents such as a) modulation in solubility and blood pool retention time, b) controlled release over short or long durations, c) environmentally triggered controlled release or highly specific site-targeted deliver.

INTRODUCTION

The field of nanotechnology is dedicated to research and technology advancement which enables the creation of useful materials, devices, and systems through the controlled manipulation of properties of matter on atomic and molecular levels. Jeevanandam, et al., (2018). From last two decades, the field of

DOI: 10.4018/978-1-7998-5563-7.ch006

nanotechnology has progressed tremendously with hundreds and thousands of publications in this field. Nanotechnology is the interdisciplinary research programme involving scientists from many different fields, including physics, chemistry, engineering, and biology. Although, the word nanotechnology seems to be relatively new for us, but the nature has already set its foundation with the creation of life millions of years ago. The constructing and basic units of life are having unique properties determined by the size, folding and patterns at nanoscale. The size of nucleotide bases in deoxyribonucleic acid (DNA) range in the sub-nanometre scale, and the diameter of the double helix structure of DNA is in the nanometre range. Likewise, cell membranes which consist of lipids and proteins are beautifully designed by nature at nanoscale. (Abu-Salah, et al., 2010). Thus exploiting this property, nanomedicine can be considered to be an ultimate therapeutics to interact with cells having dimensions (microns) that allow them to interact efficiently with nanoparticles (10–200 nm). Thus the basic knowledge and understanding of biological processes on the nanoscale level can be a strong attempt for the development of successful nanomedicine. In essence, nanomedicine is the medical use of nano-sized particles, nanofiber and nanodevices to deliver drugs, heat, light or other substances to specific cells in the human body and for the detection and treatment of diseases or injuries within the targeted cells, thereby minimizing the damage to healthy cells in the body. Application and uses of nanotechnology in screening, diagnosis and treatment of diseases are collectively referred to as 'Nanomedicine'. (Hu, Ye, et al. 2011)

The properties of nanomaterials are midway between molecular and bulk regimes. Whether nature or synthetic, nanoscale properties exist in all materials. Nevertheless, only synthetic materials are actually considered part of "nanoscience and engineering", while the study of bio- nanoscale structures are often studied as a part of characterization without taking into considering biological properties. Due to the midway properties of nanomaterials, it becomes difficult to limit a material's reach and confine its boundary by applying strict rules of definitions and solid numbers (e.g., bigger than atoms or small molecules, but smaller than 100 nm). More significantly, these nano-sized particles can display new and unique properties by virtue of which these can be explored for the design of new remedial benefits and diagnostics.

Because of their distinctive properties, it is likely that nanomedicine will guide for the development of highly specific, efficient, and modified nano-devices, drugs, and other possible applications which will be highly useful for early diagnoses or treatment of a variety of diseases which will improve patient's quality of life, figure 1.

In macro-materials vast majority of atoms lie inside the volume of the material rather than on the surface which makes the surface to-volume ratio very small. While in case of nanomaterials, atoms respond to their environment quite differently because the surrounded atoms are much smaller than the atoms on the surface and therefore the surface-to-volume ratio is much larger. The relative amount of atoms on the surface can significantly influence the properties of the material as a whole. This is one of the unique properties of nanoparticles which increase their performance for their applicability in biomedical fields.

Figure 1. Some major developments in the field of nanomedicine

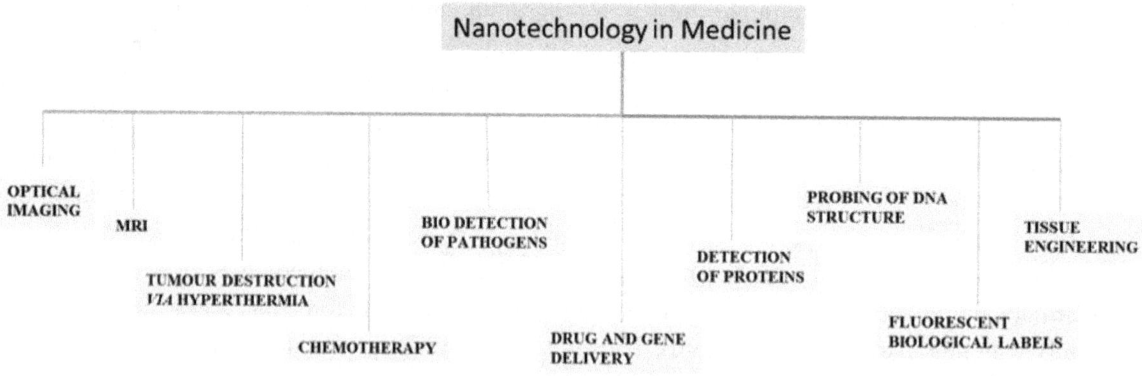

SYNTHESIS AND CHARACTERIZATION OF NANOPARTICLES

There are two approaches for the synthesis of NPs *viz* "Top-down" and "Bottom-up". Top-down approach involves suitable splitting of bulk material into fine particles by size reduction with different techniques such as Pulse laser ablation, evaporation – condensation, ball milling, pulse wire discharge method *etc*. In bottom-up approach, NPs can be synthesized using chemical and biological methods by self-assembly phenomenon. Biological methods involve the use microorganisms, enzymes, fungus, and plants or plant extracts. Biological methods are considered eco friendly and developing into an important branch of nanotechnology especially silver nanoparticles, which have many applications in medicine. (Dhand, et al., 2015)

The preparation of the nanoparticles is a crucial step for the production of nanostructure of desired qualities. Development of newer techniques, such as transmission electron microscope (TEM) including low- and high-resolution TEM (LRTEM and HRTEM), photon-correlation spectroscopy (PCS), scanning electron microscopy (SEM), atomic force microscopy (AFM), laser Doppler anemometry (LDA) have greatly facilitated the use of nanomaterials and their characterization. (Pal, et al. 2011).

Nanoparticles can be made from a vast range of materials, such as metals (gold/silver), metal oxides (e.g. Magnetic nanoparticles like Fe_3O_4 (magnetite) and Fe_2O_3 (maghemite) titanium dioxide -TiO_2, Silicon dioxide SiO_2), Inorganic materials (carbon nanotubes, quantum dots), polymeric materials and lipids. The other new sets of tools is available in nanotechnology are nanocrystals (Quantum dots), cantilevers, dendrimers, nanoshells and nanowires. Figure 2 shows some engineered nanoparticles used in medical sciences. These particles range from few to several hundreds of nanometres in diameter. Products made from each of these tools can be used for diagnosis (as biomarkers) and therapy. Many nanoparticle systems

Figure 2 represents engineered nanoparticles used in medical sciences

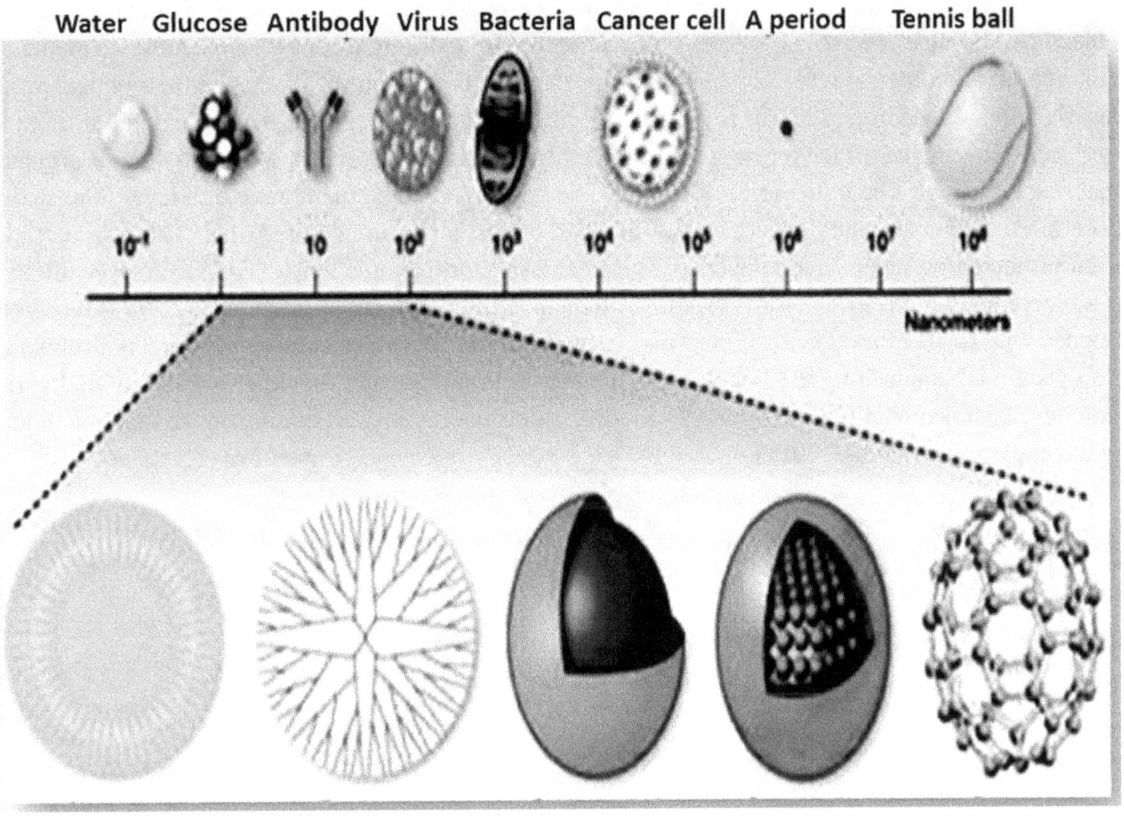

have found application in the formulation, encapsulation and release of active compounds extracted or derived from natural sources. (Dhand, Chetna, et al., 2015)

NANODEVICES AND THEIR INTERACTION WITH BIO-MOLECULES

Nanodevices match the typical size of naturally occurring functional units or components of living organisms and therefore enable more effective interaction with biological systems. Most of the animal cells are 10,000 to 20,000 nanometres in diameter. This indicates that nanoscale devices (less than 100 nanometers) can enter cells and even the organelles inside them to interact with DNA and proteins. (Auría-Soro, et al. 2019)

Nanodevices are able to detect disease in a very small amount of cells or tissue and can monitor cells within a living body. By virtue of their small size and larger surface area relative to their volume, nanodevices can readily interact with enzymes and receptors not only present on the cell surface but inside the cell as well. This property of the nanodevices has potential applications to detect diseases at the micro level. It is now possible to provide therapy at a molecular level with the help of nanotechnology. Temperature, magnetic fields, ultrasonic waves, pH, and light have been examined to act as useful stimuli to use in response release systems and this is very helpful for successful release of bioactive compounds at the target sites. Karimi, et al. 2016). In order to interact with biological receptor, a biomolecular coating or layer acting as a bioinorganic interface should be attached to the nanoparticle. These biological coatings may include antibodies, biopolymers like collagen, or monolayers of small molecules that make the nanoparticles biocompatible. In addition, as optical detection techniques are wide spread in biological research, nanoparticles should either fluoresce or change their optical properties. Samanta & Medintz, (2016). Nano-particle usually forms the core of nano-biomaterial. It can be used as a convenient surface for molecular assembly, and may be composed of inorganic or polymeric materials. It can also be in the form of nanovesicle surrounded by a membrane or a layer. The shape is more often spherical but cylindrical, plate-like and other shapes are also possible. The core particle is often protected by several monolayers of inert material, for example silica. The same layer might act as a biocompatible material. However, more often an additional layer of linker molecules is required to proceed with further functionalization. This linear linker molecule has reactive groups at both ends. One group is aimed at attaching the linker to the nanoparticle surface and the other is used to bind various moieties like biocompatibles (dextran), antibodies, fluorophores *etc.*, depending on the function required by the application. Idrees, (2015).

- **Liposomes**
- **Quantum dots (Nanocrystals)**
- **Nanoshells**
- **Cantilevers- A Nanoelectromechanical Sensor (NEMS)**
- **Dendrimers**
- **Nanowires**

LIPOSOMES

Liposomes are vesicles (a fluid filled sac) of spherical shape composed of phospholipids and steroids usually in the 50–450 nm size range. They are eco-friendly, biocompatible and non-immunogenic in nature, which makes them ideal drug carrier systems in therapeutics. Liposomes are made of concentric spheres, one sphere inside of another and each forming half of a bilayered wall. A bilayer is composed of two sheets of phospholipid. Liposomes are drug carrier loaded with great variety of molecules such as small drug molecules, proteins, nucleotides and even plasmids. Liposomes are lipid based nanoparticles used extensively in pharmaceutical and cosmetic industries because of their ability for breaking down inside cells, once their delivery function has been met. (Gao, et al., 2013) Almost half of the anticancer nano-drugs approved by the FDA are based on liposomal formulations of cytostatic drugs: daunorubicin (Daunoxome) for human immunodeficiency virus (HIV)-associated Kaposi's sarcoma, doxorubicin (Doxil/Caelyx) monotherapy for HIV-associated Kaposi's sarcoma and ovarian cancer, as well as in combined therapy with bortezomib for multiple myeloma, cytarabine (Depocyt) for lymphatic meningitis, vincristine (Margibo) for acute lymphoblastic leukaemia, and irinotecan (Onivyde), which was recently approved for metastatic pancreatic cancer. Yue, X., & Dai, Z. (2018), (Madamsetty, Mukherjee & Mukherjee, 2019).

QUANTUM DOTS

Quantum dots (QD) are tiny (~2-10 nanometers or ~10-50 atoms in diameter) light emitting (fluorescent NPs) semiconductor/nanocrystals with vast applications in medical sciences. They possess many advantageous features over organic fluorophores, such as high photostability, narrow emission band, and large two photon excitation cross sections. (Deerinck, 2008). They are so small that they can even enter in the cell. They obey quantum mechanical principle of quantum confinement. These can be used to detect cancer in the body. Quantum dots when used in conjunction with magnetic resonance imaging can produce exceptional images of tumor sites. They are water-soluble, can be functionalized by conjugation with a number of bioactive molecules, produced economically, and have excellent cell permeability and biocompatibility, making them attractive for intracellular sensing. (Matea, et.al., 2017). Quantum dots glow when they are stimulated by ultraviolet light. The wavelength, or color, of the light depends on the size of the crystal. By combining different sized quantum dots within a single bead, scientists can create probes that release distinct colours and intensities of light. When the crystals are stimulated by UV light, each bead emits light that serves as a sort of spectral bar code, identifying a particular region of DNA. Another advantage of quantum dots is that they can be used in the body, eliminating the need for biopsy. Quantum dots are 20 times brighter & 100 times more stable than traditional dyes. (Bailey, et.al., 2004).

NANOSHELLS

Nanoshells are tiny spheres of glass coated with gold in the form of beads that can absorb near infrared region in a size dependent manner to generate intense heat that can be used to kill target cells. Metal nanoshells particularly gold are brilliant optical absorbers. (Loo, 2005). Nanoshell size and thickness play an imperative role in optical tuning of certain wavelength. Nanoshells can be can be functionalised with antibodies, fluorophores, oligonucleotides, targeting ligands, polymers, therapeutic agents, and radioisotope to attain better efficacy, diagnostic and therapeutic objectives. Nanoshells (especially gold nanoshells) show promise application in biomedical imaging, target therapy, gene delivery, tissue welding, drug delivery systems, therapeutic applications especially in cancer imaging and treatment. For treatment, a cancer patient receives intravenously, and over the course of a day about 1% accumulate in a tumor site. Most of the rest wash out being so small in size. A physician then shines an infrared light over the tumor. After reaching the target site, nanoshells absorb light which creates an intense heat leading the burning tumor cells as known as Hyperthermia, while healthy cells nearby remain unharmed. Unlike chemotherapy and radiotherapy nanoshells have zero toxic effects and no involvement of ionizing radiation. (Hirsch, 2006). The improvement in micro- and nanofabrication technologies facilitate the preparation of progressively more smaller mechanical transducers competent of detecting the forces, motion, mechanical properties and masses that emerge in biomolecular interactions and fundamental biological processes. Thus, biosensors based on nanomechanical systems (NMS) have gained considerable relevance in the last decade. Due to the biological adsorption or interactions between the analyte (substance of interest, e.g. a particular chemical component, virus or micro-organism) and surface of cantilever some mechanical phenomena occur which shows a biological response. Nanoscale cantilevers work on this principle. The surface of cantilever is coated with bioreceptor/biorecognition element. Nanoscale cantilevers - microscopic, flexible beams resembling a row of diving boards - are built using semiconductor lithographic techniques. A biosensor consists of two components, a bioreceptor and a transducer. (Kim, et al., 2006). .The bioreceptor is a biomolecule that recognizes the target analyte thereby generating a comprehensive surface stress which causes a downwards bending of the cantilever whereas the transducer converts the recognition event into a measurable signal. They are also known as Nanoelectromechanical Systems (NEMS).

The physical properties of the cantilevers change as a result of the binding event. Researchers can read this change in real time and provide not only information about the presence and the absence but also the concentration of different molecular expressions. Nanoscale cantilevers, constructed as part of a larger diagnostic device, can provide rapid and sensitive detection of cancer-related molecules. (Hassanzadeh, etal., 2011).

DENDRIMERS

The word dendrimer originates from the Greek dendron, meaning 'tree' and meros, meaning 'part'. A dendrimer consists of molecular chains that branch out from a common center (like a tree), and there is no entanglement between each dendrimer molecules. Biodendrimers comprised of repeating units known to be biocompatible or biodegradable *in vivo* to natural metabolites. Dendrimers consist of three parts; a central core, an interior dendritic structure (the branches), and an exterior surface with functional surface groups. The interior of the dendrimer provide nano-sized cavities that can readily accept small molecules or particles, which make them ideally suitable for encapsulation, isolation from external media or active catalytic sites. The surface of the dendrimer can be modified with a wide variety of function, allowing to finely tuning the chemical, physical and topological properties of the molecule. The ends of the dendrimer molecule can be attached with other molecules for transport. These molecules give the dendrimers various functional applications. Roszek, et al., 2005). They are used in medical sciences for targeted drug delivery and contrast agent in MRI.

NANOWIRES

A nanowire is a narrow wire with typical width in the range of forty to fifty nanometres, whereas their length can be made as long as required by simple lengthening or by attaching more wires end to end. The nanowires have unique metallic, semiconducting, and insulating properties with extremely high surface-to-volume ratio which makes them best constructing blocks for the development of biosensor. They are highly biocompatible with comparable size with that of the host (biomolecules), with emphasis on novel electron transport properties. (Garnett, et al., 2019). Nanowires can detect even slight disturbances from the nearby surroundings and can generate electrical signals in the system. The nanowires are smaller than the smallest capillary in the circulatory system and thus can be threaded through the circulatory system to any point in the body without interfering in the normal blood flow or gases and nutrients exchange through the blood-vessel. Consequently, when guided to the brain the nanowires would spread out branching into smallest blood vessels would be used to record the electrical activity of single nerve cells, furnishing the capability to locate the damage caused by injury or stroke, localize the cause of seizures, and other brain abnormalities. (Salata, 2004).

Positron emission tomography (PET) is an imaging technique that is used to reveals the functioning of tissues and organs in the body. It uses a radioactive drug/tracer which may be injected, swallowed or inhaled depending on upon the organ or tissue being studied by PET scan. The tracer assembles in the body at areas of disease (sites which usually have higher levels of chemical activity). Upon PET scanning, the affected region appears as bright spots. Likewise, functional magnetic resonance imaging (fMRI) is a procedure used to determine brain activity. This technique detects the changes that occur in blood oxygenation and flow which take place in response to neural activity. The part of the brain which is more active demands more oxygen which in turn increases the demand of blood flow in the active region. fMRI can be used to produce activation brain maps of the specific region of the brain involved in mental process. It is known that people with Parkinson's disease there is a gradual development in the disorder of the nervous system that affects the movement, can experience significant improvement from direct stimulation of the affected area of the brain with electrical pulses. Indeed, that is now a common treatment for patients who do not respond to medication. But the stimulation is currently carried out by inserting nanowires through the skull and into the brain, a process that causes scarring of brain tissue. The hope is, by stimulating the brain with nanowires threaded through pre-existing blood vessels, doctors could give patients the benefits of the treatment without the damaging side effects. The small size of nanoparticles can be very useful in oncology, particularly in imaging. (Jena, 2013). There are numerous ways by which nanotechnology is currently being developed for many applications in different areas such as medical field, including drug delivery, biosensors and medical imaging. These nanomaterials are highly useful and offer much more targeted treatments for the deadly diseases such as cancers. Nano-antibiotics are being developed as alternative to conventional antibiotics for the treatment of infectious diseases. (Khurana, & Chudasama, 2018). A list of some of the applications of nanomaterials to biology or medicine is given below and heighted in figure 1:

- Drug and gene delivery
- Fluorescent biological labels
- Bio detection of pathogens
- Probing of DNA structure
- Detection of proteins
- Tissue engineering
- Separation and purification of biological molecules and cells
- Tumour destruction *via* hyperthermia
- MRI contrast enhancement
- Phagokinetic studies

BENEFITS OF USING NANOMATERIALS

It is beyond doubt that the great benefits of nanotechnology are in numerous fields particularly in medical field. These advantages can be attributed to their:

- Smaller devices are less invasive.
- They can be implanted inside body.
- Biochemical reaction time is much shorter.
- Devices are faster & more sensitive than typical drug delivery.

There is no doubt that various applications for nanomaterials as diagnostic agents, some thoughtfulness have to be made with regard to their pharmacokinetic properties. Diagnostic agents must be of high accuracy with respect to the target site, with low toxicity, and rapid elimination of the unbound portion of the material. The size management of the nanomaterial is also an imperative aspect. For agents with size greater than 5 nm, the renal clearance will be much slower than smaller counterparts. Conversely, for nanomaterials with size >1 μm it will be much difficult to undergo renal clearance and the unbound agents need to be cleared.

Since different combinations of materials are used to produce nanomaterials of different shapes and structures, there is a critical prerequisite to monitor the properties of these nanoparticles that they may generate adverse side reactions in the patients receiving these materials as part of diagnosis or treatment. For instance, quantum dots are used to advance medical imaging in cancer diagnosis as discussed in the previous section. However, quantum dots can contain heavy metals such as cadmium, selenium, arsenic, and lead. Although, these particles have significant advantages in diagnostics and imaging by virtue of their unique properties but are toxic metals which is well documented in the literature. Thus there must be a thorough examination that these nanomaterials did not create unexpected adverse effects.

There must be a proper balance between the safety of the materials and the efficiency related to the particular treatment. Toxicology related issues should be taken into consideration when suggesting the given nanoparticle for a treatment of stage four cancer as compared to one to be used for a routine diagnostic medical imaging. Therefore, a proper situational approach should be followed when considering the merits and negative aspects to using nanoparticles in therapeutic diagnosis and cure.

REFERENCES

Jeevanandam, J. (2018). Review on nanoparticles and nanostructured materials: history, sources, toxicity and regulations. *Beilstein Journal of Nanotechnology*, *9*(1), 1050-1074.

Abu-Salah. (2010). DNA-based applications in nanobiotechnology. *Journal of Biomedicine & Biotechnology*.

Hu, Y. (2011). Nanodevices in diagnostics. *Wiley Interdisciplinary Reviews. Nanomedicine and Nanobiotechnology*, *3*(1), 11–32.

Dhand, C. (2015). Methods and strategies for the synthesis of diverse nanoparticles and their applications: A comprehensive overview. *RSC Advances*, *5*(127), 105003–105037.

Pal, S. L. (2011). Nanoparticle: An overview of preparation and characterization. *Journal of Applied Pharmaceutical Science*, *1*(6), 228–234.

Auría-Soro, C. (2011). Interactions of nanoparticles and biosystems: microenvironment of nanoparticles and biomolecules in nanomedicine. *Nanomaterials*, *9*(10), 1365.

Karimi, M. (2016). Smart micro/nanoparticles in stimulus-responsive drug/gene delivery systems. *Chemical Society Reviews*, *45*(5), 1457–1501.

Samanta, A., & Medintz, I. L. (2016). Nanoparticles and DNA – a powerful and growing functional combination in bionanotechnology. *Nanoscale*, *8*(17), 9037–9095.

Idrees, M. (2015). Role of nanotechnology in medical sciences: A review. *Int. J. Drug Discovery*, *5*, 14–24.

Gao, W., Hu, C. M. J., Fang, R. H., & Zhang, L. (2013). Liposome-like nanostructures for drug delivery. *Journal of Materials Chemistry. B, Materials for Biology and Medicine*, *1*(48), 6569–6585.

Yue, X., & Dai, Z. (2018). Liposomal nanotechnology for cancer theranostics. *Current Medicinal Chemistry*, *25*(12), 1397–1408.

Madamsetty, V. S., Mukherjee, A., & Mukherjee, S. (2019). Recent trends of the bio-inspired nanoparticles in cancer theranostics. *Frontiers in Pharmacology*, 10.

Deerinck, T. J. (2008). The application of fluorescent quantum dots to confocal, multiphoton, and electron microscopic imaging. *Toxicologic Pathology*, *36*(1), 112–116.

Bailey, R. E., Smith, A. M., & Nie, S. (2004). Quantum dots in biology and medicine. *Physica E, Low-Dimensional Systems and Nanostructures*, *25*(1), 1–12.

Matea, C. T., Mocan, T., Tabaran, F., Pop, T., Mosteanu, O., Puia, C., ... Mocan, L. (2017). Quantum dots in imaging, drug delivery and sensor applications. *International Journal of Nanomedicine*, *12*, 5421.

Loo, C., Lowery, A., Halas, N., West, J., & Drezek, R. (2005). Immunotargeted nanoshells for integrated cancer imaging and therapy. *Nano Letters*, *5*(4), 709–711.

Hirsch, L. R., Gobin, A. M., Lowery, A. R., Tam, F., Drezek, R. A., Halas, N. J., & West, J. L. (2006). Metal nanoshells. *Annals of Biomedical Engineering*, *34*(1), 15–22.

Kim, T. S., Lee, J. H., & Yoon, D. S. (2006). Nanomechanical cantilever devices for biological sensors. In Micromanufacturing and Nanotechnology (pp. 299–321). Academic Press.

Hassanzadeh, P., Fullwood, I., Sothi, S., & Aldulaimi, D. (2011). Cancer nanotechnology. *Gastroenterology and Hepatology from Bed To Bench*, *4*(2), 63.

Roszek, B., De Jong, W.H., & Geertsma, R.E. (2005). *Nanotechnology in medical applications: state-of-the-art in materials and devices*. Academic Press.

Garnett, E., Mai, L., & Yang, P. (2019). *Introduction: 1D nanomaterials/nanowires*. Academic Press.

Salata, O. V. (2004). Applications of nanoparticles in biology and medicine. *Journal of Nanobiotechnology*, *2*(1), 3.

Jena, M., Mishra, S., Jena, S., & Mishra, S. S. (2013). Nanotechnology-future prospect in recent medicine: A review. *International Journal of Basic and Clinical Pharmacology*, *2*(4), 353.

Khurana, C., & Chudasama, B. (2018). Nanoantibiotics: strategic assets in the fight against drug-resistant superbugs. *International Journal of nanomedicine, 13*, 3.

Chapter 7
Applications of Organic Chemistry in Nano-Medicine:
Current and Future Prospects

Asif Ahmad Malik
National Institute of Technology, Srinagar, India

Nisar A. Dangroo
National Institute of Technology, Srinagar, India

Rabia Amin
National Institute of Technology, Srinagar, India

Zubaid Ul Khazir
National Institute of Technology, Srinagar, India

Tabassum Ara
National Institute of Technology, Srinagar, India

ABSTRACT

Nanotechnology offers multiple benefits. Nanomedicine and nanodelivery systems are relatively new areas in nanotechnology. There are number of outstanding applications of the nanomedicine in diagnosing diseases, delivering drugs to its target location, and thus treating human diseases. Here materials in the nanoscale range are employed to serve as means of diagnostic tools and also to deliver precise medicines to specific targeted sites in a controlled manner. Also, metal nanoparticles offer great interest in modern chemistry and materials research because of their applications in diverse fields such as photochemistry, nanoelectronics, optics, and catalysis. Chemistry provides various nanostructured materials either synthetic or isolated from natural sources offers opportunities and challenges in drug delivery and their applications including biomedical imaging, biosensing, diagnostic, and therapy. Thymoquinone, a bioactive compound in Nigella sativa, after encapsulation in lipid nanocarrier, has been found to show six-fold increase in bioavailability in comparison to free thymoquinone. In addition to this, organic nanomaterials have recently become of great interest for photovoltaic applications also.

DOI: 10.4018/978-1-7998-5563-7.ch007

INTRODUCTION

Science of the new era in nanomedicine has lot of application. It is used in drug designing, drug delivery, electronics and in various other industries. It involves manipulating matter at the atomic or molecular scale. A nano particle is generally of 100 nm or less in size. But usually the nano particles utilized in drug delivery are 100- 200 nm. Materials are designed at the atomic or molecular level by changing their dimensions, surface properties, compositions etc. their physiochemical properties can also be changed. Nanoparticles have different surface to volume ratios. Through nanotechnology diseases are diagnosed early. The medicines used at nanoscale leads it to the early and required treatment of the diseases at the micro level. Since nano-materials are common in the organic, inorganic, and biological fields therefore, modern smart nano structured systems are broadly divided into organic and inorganic nanocarriers.

Nanomedicine research is one of the fastest growing areas of research in nanotechnology and it revolutionise healthcare and medicine through transformative new diagnostic and therapeutic tools. Chemistry provides advances in nanomedicine and new functional materials as well as state-of-the art biochemical and analytical techniques. Various nanostructured materials have been synthesized for diverse applications, including biomedical imaging, biosensing, diagnostics and therapy. Their size-dependent physical properties and nanometer-scale dimensions play important roles in biological systems. Also various types of highly sensitive nanosensors are synthesized for biomarker detection. A variety of organic or inorganic nanoparticles have been synthesized with sizes ranging from several to several hundred nanometers, and many of them have shown important role in biomedical applications due to their tunable sizes, high agent loadings, prominent surface chemistry, controllable drug release kinetics, improved biocompatibility, and enhanced tumor accumulation through passive tumor targeting, the enhanced permeability and retention (EPR) effect, or active tumor targeting (Davis et al., 2010; Kim et al., 2013). Nanoscale materials allow the implementation of highly effective imaging techniques, such as magnetic resonance imaging (MRI), positron emission tomography (PET), computed tomography, and optical imaging () as Shown in figure1.

Figure 1.

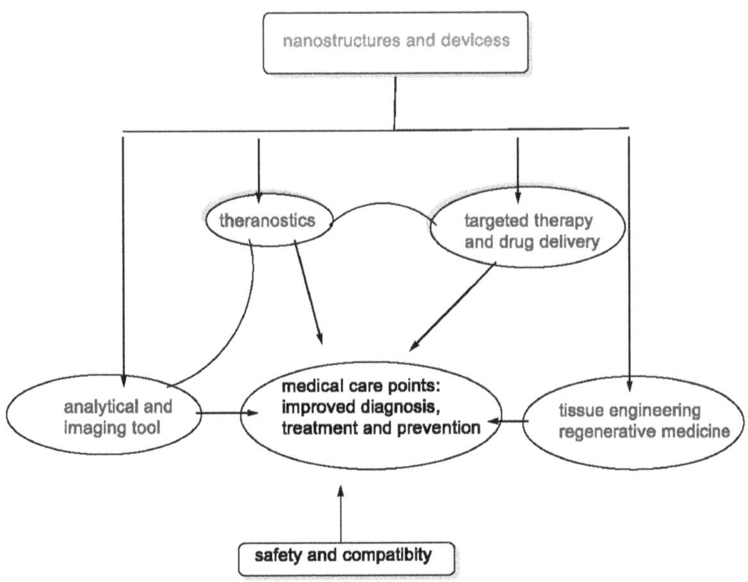

Nanotechnology employs curative agents at the nanoscale level to develop nanomedicines. The field of biomedicine comprising nanobiotechnology, drug delivery, biosensors, and tissue engineering has been powered by nanoparticles (Rudramurthy et al., 2016). They can move more freely in the human body as compared to bigger materials. Nanoscale sized particles exhibit unique structural, chemical, mechanical, magnetic, electrical, and biological properties. Nanomedicines have become well appreciated in recent times due to the fact that nanostructures could be utilized as delivery agents by encapsulating drugs or attaching therapeutic drugs and deliver them to target tissues more precisely with a controlled release (Lam et al., 2017).

CURRENT APPLICATIONS

Conventional methods of drug delivery have lot of disadvantages like toxicity, poor specificity, and drug resistance. More over their large size does not allow them to reach the targeted location. These disadvantages lead to the decrease efficiency of many drugs. In order to increase the efficacy of a drug, nanomedicine and nanodelivery systems are of great interest. Nano-medicine is a branch of nano technology in the medical field used for the benefit of human health. A nano meter is a billionth of a meter and thus involves intervention of the drug at the molecular scale for repairing of damaged tissues and of curing diseases. Nano medicines are more advantageous than conventional drugs. They can be used as delivery agents by encapsulating drugs or attaching therapeutic drugs to them then they deliver the drugs to target tissues more precisely and with a controlled release. The nanostructures penetrate in the tissue system and the cells take them easily thus they have an efficient drug delivery and that too at the targeted location. They also treat the diseased cells efficienciently with negligible side effects. Nanoscale sized particles exhibit unique properties like structural, chemical, mechanical, magnetic, electrical, and biological. The European Union (EU) Technology defines nanomedicine as 'the application of nanotechnology to achieve breakthroughs in healthcare' (Bregoli et al., 2016). Nanomaterials have a relatively larger surface area and, therefore, are more chemically reactive. They have more effective interaction with biological systems. Most animal cells are 10,000 to 20,000 nanometers in diameter. The nano devices of less than 100 nanometers can enter cells and interact with DNA and proteins.

A red blood cell is approximately 7000 nm wide. Many molecules including some proteins range between 1nm and larger the size of nano materials is similar to that of most biological molecules and structures. Thus nano materials can be useful for biomedical research and the materials designed from nano particles are usually small sized nano spheres therefore they can move more freely in the human body. On the basis of traditional practices and knowledge modern medicines are mainly derived from herbs. Extracts from plants were used by humans as medicines against various diseases from earlier times. They have excellent curative power with less toxicity, side effects, and price. Compounds obtained from these extracts are now being screened for treating diseases, like cancer, diabetes, cardiovascular, inflammatory and microbial etc. These natural compounds also act as leads in the discovery of novel drugs (Souery & Bishop, 2018).

Today most of the available pharmaceutical compounds and their derivatives are obtained from natural resources. Novel drugs are obtained from natural compounds with different molecular backgrounds. In drug discovery synthetically amenable lead molecules which mimic the natural product are designed. Further, computational studies have helped envisage molecular interactions of these drugs and develop next-generation drug inventions such as target-based drug discovery and drug delivery. If these drugs are encapsulated in nanoscale they offer more specificity, biocompatibility and site specific because of their nanosized.

Thus Organic chemistry is very advantageous in this field of nanotechnology through this building blocks can be designed as nanomedicine. It also programs their interaction among themselves or with their surroundings to generate new products and materials with different properties, which will be then exploited in the specific applications they were designed for. Organic nanoparticles are solid particles composed of organic compounds (mainly Lipids or polymeric) ranging in diameter from 10nm to1µm. The organic nanocarriers are carbon-based nanomaterials that are generally characterized by a high biocompatibility and improved drug loading capacity. They allow a versatile control of both morphology and chemical composition, while their colloidal stability and relatively large size allow in corporating and carrying a wide combination of different hydrophilic or hydrophobic drugs.

Tea polyphenols are a series of compounds found in tea. AFDA approved tea polyphenol, epigallocatechin gallate (EGCG), is found to surmount drug resistance. The most employed synthetic polymeric biomaterials for drug delivery are the saturated poly (α-hydroxyesters) like poly (lactic acid) (PLA), Poly (glycolic acid) (PGA), and poly (lactic-co-glycolide) (PLGA), copolymers.

US Food and Drug Administration (FDA) and European Medicines Agency (EMA) have approved these polymers for drug delivery as they are safe and effective. Thus the delivery of therapeutic biomacromolecules PLGA nanocarriers is able to maintain their colloidal stability and maximize their loading efficiency even in the harsh physiological environment condition of the diseased tissues. Thus organic nano particles either natural or synthetic have been found to be safe and therefore, often used for food applications and drug delivery. On the basis of their safety they can further be sub-divided into three categories as lipid based, protein based and polysaccharide based.

Lipid based systems are often made of phosphor lipids, lipid based nano encapsulation systems have advantages like, target ability and the ability to entrap compounds with different solubility and of being produced using natural ingredients on an industrial scale. Protein based systems are excellent for the encapsulation of bioactive compounds because have the ability to form gel sand emulsions. Protein hydro gels are widely used in food applications (Assadpour & Mahdi Jafari, 2019; Fathi et al., 2012).

Polysaccharide based systems: Monosaccharide is joined by glycosidic bonds to form large molecules called Polysaccharides. They are present in plants and animals. Plants have Pectin, Guar gum and Insulin where as animals have chitosan etc. These polymers are generally very large, and often branched (Kosaraju, 2005) and play an important role in biological processes. Chitosan is a copolymer of glucosamine and N-acetylated glucosamine. It is biodegradable, non toxic and biocompatible. Hence it is considered to be one of the most valuable polysaccharide for drug delivery (des Rieux et al., 2006). Pectin's which are non starch, linear polysaccharides extracted from plant cell walls are also important for drug delivery purposes.

Health care is one of the most significant fields in nano-biotechnology. The passage of molecules between the bloodstream and the brain are regulated by blood-brain barrier. Harmful substances are prevented from entering into the brain but at the same time it regulates the uptake and efflux of ions, nutrients, and metabolites. Physiological barriers are thus vital to homeostasis at the tissue, organ, and organism levels. Neurodegenerative diseases, like Parkinson's and Alzheimer's, are related to brain disorders. Here progressive degeneration of the structure and function of the central or peripheral nervous system takes. Effectiveness and bioavailability of curcumin, flavonoids, such as quercetin, Gingko biloba, and folic acid are being explored in order to prevent these diseases. Delivering drugs to specific areas of the brain is a major challenge. Peptides can be used as specialized coatings able to transport nanoparticles with specific properties, such as targeting. The nanoparticles can also carry a peptide drug. The combined use of peptides and nanotechnology offers tremendous hope in the treatment of brain disorders.

Liposomes discovered in early 1960's by Bangham and collegue (Salata, 2004) are lipid based nanoparticles. They are biodegradable and biocompatible. Thus they are safe and good as drug carriers. They also have the capacity to break down inside cells. Liposomes are loaded with great variety of molecules for example proteins, small drug molecules, nucleotides and even plasmids. Since liposomes are bilayered they transport water soluble drugs inside the core and water insoluble but lipid soluble drugs between the bilayer.

Nanotechnology in CANCER THERAPY

The applications of nanotechnology in cancer therapy have been developed recently. Loading of bioactive molecules into nano carriers increases the in vivo activity, stability, increase compounds blood circulation time and allow the drug for sustainable release. Designing of a bioactive cancer molecule into its nano particles increases the efficacy of treatment and reduces the side effects. The molecules isolated from natural products have also been found to be highly effective against cancer like resveratrol, curcumin etc. have been extensively studied as anticancer agents, and the incorporation of these

Figure 2.

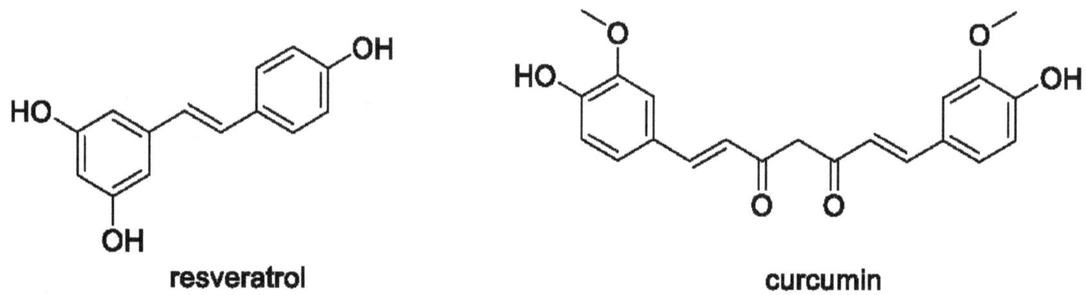

compounds into nano particles resulted in significant inhibition of cancer growth and induces apoptosis (Siddiqui & Sanna, 2016).

The nanoparticles (NPs) design parameters can be optimized to maximize their performances by tailoring their particle size, shape and surface properties, to increase the efficacy of treatment, reduce side effects, and overcome drug resistance (Fig. 1). The advantages of using nanocarriers such as NPs as drug delivery systems include (i) the possibility to manipulate particle size and surface, (ii) the control and sustained release of the drug, (iii) the site-specific targeting; and (iv) the use of various routes of administration (Kamaly et al., 2012). More specifically, attractive features for drug delivery by NPs are described below.

Organic Photovoltaic Applications

Organic materials have recently become of great interest for photovoltaic applications, due to their potential to utilize high through put, solution phase processing, which will lead to low cost electricity production. So large energy through photovoltaic energy conversion is the most promising for long term sustainable energy production in view of its low cost, large scale and ''green'' energy technology. Organic photovoltaics (OPVs) hold the promise for a cost-effective, light weight solar energy conversion plat form particularly for the provision of off grid electricity (Forrest, 2004) and portable consumer electronics. Memory organic field – effect transistor (FET) devices with ferroelectric insulators have been fabricated by *Schroeder et al. (*2004*),* efforts to demonstrate flash-type memory devices that replace the channel with an organic semiconductor have been produced. It is expected more and more new results will appear. There is lot of future for investigating organic materials for use as the semi conductive channel and also for the tunneling and control insulators

CONCLUSION AND FUTURE PROSPECTS

Nanomedicine and nano materials are currently among the most fascinating areas of research. Cancer found to be the best example of diseases where both its diagnosis and therapy have been treated from nonmedical technologies. By using various types of nanoparticles for the delivery of the accurate amount of drug to the affected cells such as the cancer/tumour cells, without disturbing the physiology of the normal cells, the application of nanomedicine and nano-drug delivery system is certainly the trend that will remain to be the future arena of research and development for decades to come. Also in the last ten years, the highest efficiency obtained from organic photovoltaics (OPVs), such as bulk hetero junction polymer, fullerene solar cells, has risen from 2.5 to 11%. This rapid progress suggests that the commercialization of OPVs should be realized so on if we can solve some technical issues. Inspite of the remarkable developments of recent methodologies in nanomedicine a number of unwanted side effects have been observed that diminish their efficient use in nanomedicine as well as in organic nanomaterials. Efforts are being made by scientists to overcome them. Nanomedicine, being only two decands old, there is a lot of future for research and development in the area of nanotechnology. Nanotechnology has already powerful implications in knowledge foundation, molecular medicine, energy conversion and storage. In the next decade nano based design of fundamentally new products based on complex nano systems and serving new areas of survelance such as quantum information system. Nanotechnologies play several important roles in developing sensor technology. First, the ideal sensor will be minimally invasive and therefore as small as possible. This includes the power supply, the sensing action, whereby the detected property is converted into an electrical signal, and the transmission of the sensing signal to a remote detector. Future bio-nanotechnology and nanomedicine devices may exploit many classes of functional biological materials. One particular group of proteins that is attracting attention is the membrane proteins; these are another class of protein-based machine that regulate many physiological processes. They include ion channels that enable rapid yet selective flux of ions across the cell membrane, hormone receptors that behave as molecular triggers and photoreceptors that switch between different conformational states by the absorption of a single photon of light, the process that is the basis of vision and photosynthesis.

REFERENCES

Assadpour, E., & Mahdi Jafari, S. (2019). A systematic review on nanoencapsulation of food bioactive ingredients and nutraceuticals by various nanocarriers. *Critical Reviews in Food Science and Nutrition, 59*(19), 3129–3151. doi:10.1080/10408398.2018.1484687 PMID:29883187

Bregoli, L., Movia, D., Gavigan-Imedio, J. D., Lysaght, J., Reynolds, J., & Prina-Mello, A. (2016). Nanomedicine applied to translational oncology: A future perspective on cancer treatment. *Nanomedicine; Nanotechnology, Biology, and Medicine, 12*(1), 81–103. doi:10.1016/j.nano.2015.08.006 PMID:26370707

Davis, M. E., Chen, Z., & Shin, D. M. (2010). Nanoparticle therapeutics, an emerging treatment modality for cancer: in Nanoscience and technology. In A collection of reviews from nature journals, (pp. 239-250). Academic Press.

des Rieux, A., Fievez, V., Garinot, M., Schneider, Y. J., & Préat, V. (2006). Nanoparticles as potential oral delivery systems of proteins and vaccines: A mechanistic approach. *Journal of Controlled Release, 116*(1), 1–27. doi:10.1016/j.jconrel.2006.08.013 PMID:17050027

Fathi, M., Mozafari, M. R., & Mohebbi, M. (2012). Nanoencapsulation of food ingredients using lipid based delivery systems. *Trends in Food Science & Technology, 23*(1), 13–27. doi:10.1016/j.tifs.2011.08.003

Forrest, S. R. (2004). The path to ubiquitous and low-cost organic electronic appliances on plastic. *Nature, 428*(6986), 911–918. doi:10.1038/nature02498 PMID:15118718

Jang, H., Lee, C., Nam, G. E., Quan, B., Choi, H. J., Yoo, J. S., & Piao, Y. (2016). In vivo magnetic resonance and fluorescence: Dual imaging of tumor sites by using dye-doped silica-coated iron oxide nanoparticles. *Journal of Nanoparticle Research, 18*(2), 41. doi:10.100711051-016-3353-x

Kamaly, N., Xiao, Z., Valencia, P. M., Radovic-Moreno, A. F., & Farokhzad, O. C. (2012). Targeted polymeric therapeutic nanoparticles: Design, development and clinical translation. *Chemical Society Reviews, 41*(7), 2971–3010. doi:10.1039/c2cs15344k PMID:22388185

Kim, C. S., Duncan, B., Creran, B., & Rotello, V. M. (2013). Triggered nanoparticles as therapeutics. *Nano Today, 8*(4), 439–447. doi:10.1016/j.nantod.2013.07.004 PMID:24159362

Kosaraju, S. L. (2005). Colon targeted delivery systems: Review of polysaccharides for encapsulation and delivery. *Critical Reviews in Food Science and Nutrition, 45*(4), 251–258. doi:10.1080/10408690490478091 PMID:16047493

Lam, P. L., Wong, W. Y., Bian, Z., Chui, C. H., & Gambari, R. (2017). Recent advances in green nanoparticulate systems for drug delivery: Efficient delivery and safety concern. *Nanomedicine (London), 12*(4), 357–385. doi:10.2217/nnm-2016-0305 PMID:28078952

Lee, S. B., Kim, H. L., Jeong, H. J., Lim, S. T., Sohn, M. H., & Kim, D. W. (2013). Mesoporous silica nanoparticle pretargeting for PET imaging based on a rapid bio-orthogonal reaction in a living body. *Angewandte Chemie, 125*(40), 10743–10746. doi:10.1002/ange.201304026

Nahrendorf, M., Keliher, E., Marinelli, B., Waterman, P., Feruglio, P. F., Fexon, L., Pivovarov, M., Swirski, F. K., Pittet, M. J., Vinegoni, C., & Weissleder, R. (2010). Hybrid PET-optical imaging using targeted probes. *Proceedings of the National Academy of Sciences of the United States of America*, *107*(17), 7910–7915. doi:10.1073/pnas.0915163107 PMID:20385821

Rudramurthy, G. R., Swamy, M. K., Sinniah, U. R., & Ghasemzadeh, A. (2016). Nanoparticles: Alternatives against drug-resistant pathogenic microbes. *Molecules (Basel, Switzerland)*, *21*(7), 836. doi:10.3390/molecules21070836 PMID:27355939

Salata, O. V. (2004). Applications of nanoparticles in biology and medicine. *Journal of Nanobiotechnology*, *2*(1), 3. doi:10.1186/1477-3155-2-3 PMID:15119954

Siddiqui, I. A., & Sanna, V. (2016). Impact of nanotechnology on the delivery of natural products for cancer prevention and therapy. *Molecular Nutrition & Food Research*, *60*(6), 1330–1341. doi:10.1002/mnfr.201600035 PMID:26935239

Souery, W. N., & Bishop, C. J. (2018). Clinically advancing and promising polymer-based therapeutics. *Acta Biomaterialia*, *67*, 1–20. doi:10.1016/j.actbio.2017.11.044 PMID:29246651

1Wang, K., Peng, H., Thurecht, K. J., Puttick, S., & Whittaker, A. K. (2015). Segmented highly branched copolymers: Rationally designed macromolecules for improved and tunable 19f mri. *Biomacromolecules*, *16*(9), 2827–2839. doi:10.1021/acs.biomac.5b00800 PMID:26218187

Zhao, Y., Sultan, D., Detering, L., Cho, S., Sun, G., Pierce, R., Wooley, K. L., & Liu, Y. (2014). Copper-64-alloyed gold nanoparticles for cancer imaging: Improved radiolabel stability and diagnostic accuracy. *Angewandte Chemie*, *126*(1), 160–163. doi:10.1002/ange.201308494 PMID:24272951

Chapter 8
Role of Gold Nanoparticles in Drug Delivery and Cancer Therapy

Mohammad Nadeem Lone
Department of Chemistry, School of Physical and Chemical Sciences, and Department of Biotechnology, School of Life Sciences, Central University of Kashmir, India

Irshad Ahmad Wani
Department of Chemistry, Government Degree College, Anantnag, India

Gulam Nabi Yatoo
Department of Chemistry, National Institute of Technology, Srinagar, India

Zubaid U-Khazir
Department of Chemistry, National Institute of Technology, Srinagar, India

Javid Ahmad Banday
Department of Chemistry, National Institute of Technology, Srinagar, India

ABSTRACT

Among various nanoparticles (NPs), gold nanoparticles (GNPs) gained valuable attention in the field of medicine because of some unique properties like small size and high surface area-to-volume ratio, inert nature, stability, high dispersity, non-cytotoxicity, and biocompatibility. These NPs are evolving as promising agents especially in drug carriers, cancer therapy, and constantly being exploring as photo-thermal agents, contrast agents, and radiosensitisers. Besides, GNPs interact with thiols that provides an effective and selective means of controlled intracellular release. At the present, cancer patients are increasing rapidly at national and international levels. In this chapter, efforts have taken to highlight the importance of GNPs, their critical mediation in drug delivery, as sensors for probing and imaging tumors and anti-angiogenesis. More importantly, this short piece of analysis highlights the photothermal effect of GNPs in therapy and as radiosensitizers. Finally, the current challenges and future perspectives of GNP's in cancer management are also discussed.

DOI: 10.4018/978-1-7998-5563-7.ch008

1. INTRODUCTION

Nanotechnology: the multidisciplinary field, the recent era of science have witnessed unprecedented use of nanocarriers as an emerging class of therapeutics for the treatment of cancer that has emerged recently as one of the most promising fields in the cancer treatment (Sengupta et al., 2005). Nanodrug has broad prospective for modernising cancer therapeutics and diagnostics by mounting creative biocompatible nanocomposites for drug delivery purposes (Parveen et al., 2008). The two nanodrugs Doxil (liposomal doxorubicin) and Abraxane1 (albumin bound paclitaxel) approved by US-FDA for breast cancer chemotherapy with the implications of an enhanced permeability and retention (EPR) (Bharali et al., 2009; Sparreboom et al., 2005). Basically, these nanosystems have four unique properties that distinguish them from other cancer therapeutics: (i) the nanosystems can themselves have therapeutic or diagnostic properties and can be designed to carry a large therapeutic 'payload'; (ii) nanosystems can be attached to multivalent targeting ligands, which yield high affinity and specificity for target cells; (iii) nanosystems can be made to accommodate multiple drug molecules that simultaneously enable combinatorial cancer therapy and (iv) nanosystems can bypass traditional drug resistance mechanisms. By using both passive and active targeting strategies, the nanocarriers can achieve increased intracellular concentration of drugs in cancer cells while minimizing toxicity in normal cells, simultaneously enhancing anticancer effects and reducing systemic toxicity (Acharya et al., 2009). Till date, many metal based nanomaterials have been developed so far as nanomedicines. But, due to several reasons gold nanoparticles (GNPs) has gained popularity in the area of research and medicinal chemistry. As these are considered to be biologically non-reactive and are more suitable for *in vivo* applications in comparison to other toxic metal nanoparticles (NPs) (Lewinski et al., 2008). Besides, these NP's are having strong optical properties (Jain, 2005), easily controllable surface chemistry that helps in adding surface functional groups (DeLong et al., 2010), and the ease in control over particle size and shape during synthesis (Kim et al., 2009). GNPs may be considered to be fully multifunctional, with the possibility of combining different desired functionalities in one molecular-sized package. All these factors contribute to the strong interest and preference for the use of GNPs over other nanomaterials (Cobley et al., 2011). Additional benefits of using GNPs for diagnosis of cancer is simple, less invasive, provides increased contrast for diagnosis. Besides, these NPs are nontoxic to human beings, with no photo bleaching or blinking which is inherent to many other fluorophores (Cai et al., 2008) and lastly, these NPs had important implications in stem cell proliferation and *in vitro* experiments to monitor differentiation (Nagesha et al., 2007).

As the case of cancer therapy, the key issue is to achieve the desired concentration of therapeutic agent in tumor sites and destroying cancerous cells with minimum harm to normal cells. Therefore, it is imperative to create potent single agents for the prevention, detection and treatment of cancer. Moreover, several ligand-targeted therapeutic strategies (immunotoxins, radioimmuno therapeutics and drug immune conjugates) are being developed to overcome the problems associated with the conventional drugs (Vasir & Labhasetwar, 2007). Although, these conjugated agents have shown promising efficacy, but target delivery still remains a major problem. Recent era of science suggests that nanomaterials have a profound impact on the target delivery, diagnosis, prevention and treatment of disease. Cancer nanotechnology in general is emerging as a new field of interdisciplinary research cutting across the disciplines of biology, chemistry, engineering and medicine. This book chapter is confined to GNPs that is expected to lead to major advances in cancer detection, diagnosis and treatment (Ferrari, 2005) (**Fig. 1**). The idea of crafting more effective cancer treatments by engineering matter at the nanoscale provides a compelling panacea for preferential elimination of cancer cells without serious damage to normal cells. Keeping in view of the above facts and knowledge of cancer therapy, this book chapter highlights the importance of GNPs, their critical mediation in drug delivery. More importantly, this short piece of analysis acme the role GNPs in cancer treatment. Finally, the current challenges and future perspectives of GNPs in cancer management have been discussed.

Figure 1. GNP architecture and drug delivery modalities a) Active targeting involves receptor mediated b) Passive targeting involves size mediated.

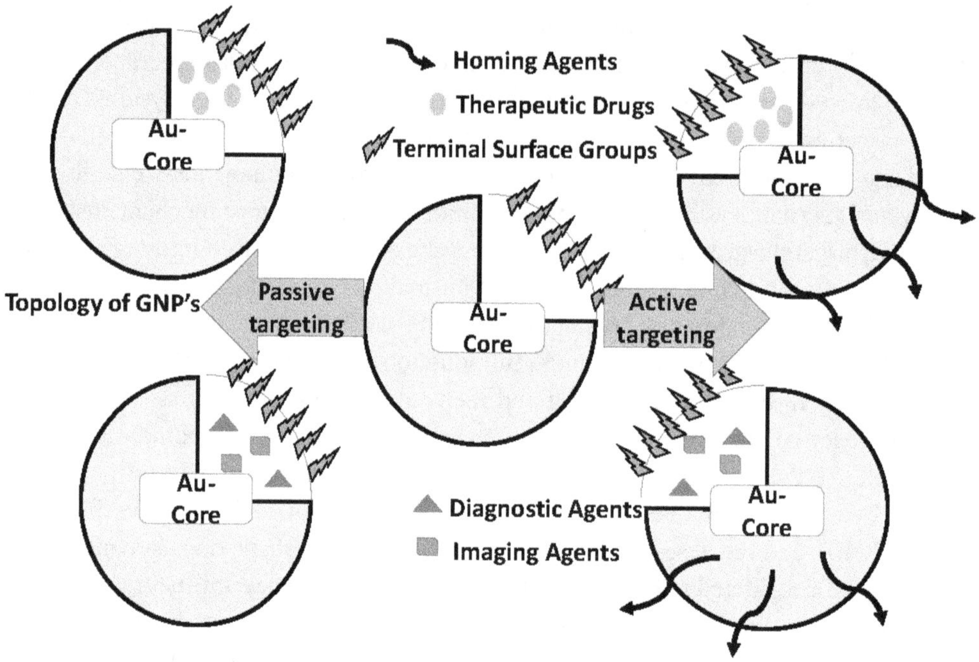

2. GNPs MEDIATION IN DRUG DELIVERY

Drug delivery systems (DDS's) provide positive attributes to a 'free' drug by improving solubility, *in vivo* stability, biodistribution and can also alter unfavourable pharmacokinetics of some free' drugs. Moreover, huge loading of pharmaceuticals on DDS's can render 'drug reservoirs' for controlled and sustained release to maintain the drug level within therapeutic window. For example, GNP with 2 nm core diameter could be, in principle, conjugated with ~100 molecules to available ligands (n=~108) in the monolayer (Hostetler et al., 1998). Gibson et al., (2007) have recently succeeded in coupling of ~70 molecules of paclitaxel, to a GNPs with 2 nm core diameter. An important demonstration of the potential of multifunctional GNPs for drug delivery was the use of 5-nm GNPs as a delivery vehicle, covalently bound to cetuximab, as an active targeting agent and gemcitabine as a therapeutic payload in pancreatic cancer (Jain et al., 2012). The epidermal growth factor receptor (EGFR) is overexpressed in up to 60% of pancreatic cancers and the combination of cetuximab and gemcitabine has been investigated in Phase-II trials of this disease (Kullmann et al., 2009). Patra et al., (2008) demonstrated that high intratumoural gold concentrations (4500 μg) could be achieved using this approach compared with

600 μg with untargeted GNPs with minimal accumulation in the liver or kidney. The GNP–cetuximab–gemcitabine nanocomplex was superior to any of the agents alone or in combination *in vitro* and *in vivo*. Low doses of complex gemcitabine (2 mg kg) led to >80% tumour growth inhibition in an orthotopic pancreatic cancer model compared with 30% inhibition using the non-conjugated agents in combination. Jiang et al., (2008) synthesised citrate-coated GNPs of controlled sizes ranging from 2 to 100 nm bound with multiple trastuzumab antibodies to enable targeting and cross-linking of human epidermal growth factor receptor (HER)-2 in human SK-BR-3 breast cancer cells. Larger NPs had a greater protein-to-nanoparticle ratio than smaller, more curved particles, with more avid trastuzumab binding. In this study, the optimal size for nanoparticle cellular entry was 40-50 nm. Smaller particles dissociated from the cell membrane and larger particles appeared to reduce the membrane wrapping necessary for RME to occur. Furthermore, with 40 nm GNP–HER particles, the HER-2 receptor complex was noted to internalise to the cytoplasm, leading to a 40% reduction in surface HER-2, a process that does not occur with trastuzumab binding alone. This led to a reduced expression of downstream kinases including protein kinase B (Akt) and mitogen-activated protein kinase (MAPK) and a twofold increase in trastuzumab cytotoxicity. The concentration of GNPs used in this study was extremely low (fM concentrations), yet GNP–HER was clearly visualised in cytoplasmic lysosomes. This important work demonstrated that GNPs may not simply act as passive drug carriers, but may also influence drug–cell interactions and enhance therapeutic effects (Jiang et al., 2008).

Targeted drug delivery is better than conventional drug therapy because in targeted drug delivery, drugs target the main effected area and deliver drug locally to minimize the side effects caused by conventional drugs (Rezende et al., 2010). Primary goal of developing anticancer agents is to minimize the various side effects caused by the conventional drugs and to improve selectivity and efficiency of drugs (Chen et al., 2010). Recently, and a lot of work has been done in the synthesis part for the targeted drug delivery systems (Lee et al., 2010). GNPs have the ability of bio-imaging of the effected cancerous cells for therapy (Pal et al., 2013). For effective drug delivery system or drug therapy it is important to investigate about the biological effects of the NPs (Chithrani et al., 2010) as GNPs have unique physical and chemical properties and have strong binding attraction for thiols, proteins (Lee et al., 2010), carboxylic acid (Deb et al., 2011) aptamers (Tarnawski et al., 2011) and disulfides so they have been extensively used in the field of biosciences especially in drug delivery for cancer therapy. Gold NPs followed three main pathways for the cellular uptake which includes receptor mediated endocytosis, phagocytosis and fluid phase endocytosis (Nalawade et al., 2012). The toxicity of GNPs depends on the size, shape, synthesis method, surface charge, surface coating and functionalized molecules but overall cytotoxicity of GNPs is inacceptable level as GNPs are considered to be non-toxic agents (Benkovicova et al., 2013). There are two factors, i.e. drug release and transport, which are very important for the efficient drug delivery system. Drugs are loaded on nanocarriers by noncovalent interaction or through covalent conjugation with the help of pro-drug, which is treated by the cell. GNPs have functional flexibility due to their monolayers so they provide efficient system (Yu et al., 2013).

2.1. Glutathione-Mediated Release of Small Molecules

GSH-mediated release represents an alternative non-enzymatic strategy for the selective intracellular activation of prodrugs. This methodology relies on the dramatic differential in intracellular GSH concentration (1–10 mM) (Anderson et al., 1998; Sies et al., 1999) versus extracellular thiol levels (Jones et al., 2000), where the predominant thiols in blood plasma are glutathione (2 μM) and cysteine (8 μM) (Jones et al., 1998). Current methodologies rely on disulphide linkages between the drugs and carriers (Saito et al., 2003; Huang et al., 1998; Weerapreeyakul et al., 2000; Wei-Chiang et al., 1989; Bernkop-Schnürch et al., 2005; Gunnarsdottir et al., 2002). While this approach can be effective, including an example currently in the clinic (Saito et al., 2003), it is difficult to tune the reactivity of the disulfide linkage. Additionally, thiol–disulfide exchange can occur with surface cysteines of proteins in the bloodstream, potentially creating protein–carrier conjugates with altered bioavailability and pharmacokinetic profiles. Ghosh et al., (2008) expected these NPs to be resistant to exchange with proteins due to the steric shielding of the gold–thiol interface. In recent studies, we have demonstrated cellular delivery and GSH mediated release of a hydrophobic dye (BODIPY), as a model of hydrophobic drugs, using functionalized GNPs (fGNPs) (Hong et al., 2006). The particles (core d=~2 nm) featured a mixed monolayer composed of tetra(ethylene glycol)ylated cationic ligands (TTMA) and fluorogenic ligands (HSBDP) (**Fig. 2a**). The cationic nature facilitates the crossing of cell-membrane barrier, and the fluorophore probes possible drug release mechanism. BODIPY-conjugated GNPs are nonfluorescent as the gold core quenches fluorescence via energy and/or electron transfer processes (Sapsford et al., 2006; Dulkeith et al., 2002]. The fluorescence signal emanates upon triggering the GNPs with GSH in cuvette, or cellular thiols in human liver cells (HepG2) (**Fig. 2b**). Controlled release of the dye was verified by treating mouse embryonic fibroblast cells (MEF, having ~50% lower intracellular GSH levels than HepG2) with varying concentration of glutathione monoester (GSH-OEt: 0, 5 and 20 mM) (**Fig. 2c**). GSH-OEt is rapidly internalized into cells and hydrolysed to GSH, and hence transiently manipulates cellular GSH levels.

Figure 2. **a**) *Schematic representation of GSH-mediated payload release via place-exchange reaction.* **b**) *Fluorescence and bright field micrographs of human Hep G2 cells after incubation with GNPs for 96 h.* **c**) *Showing dose-dependent release of the payloads via fluorescence images (Ghosh et al, 2008).*

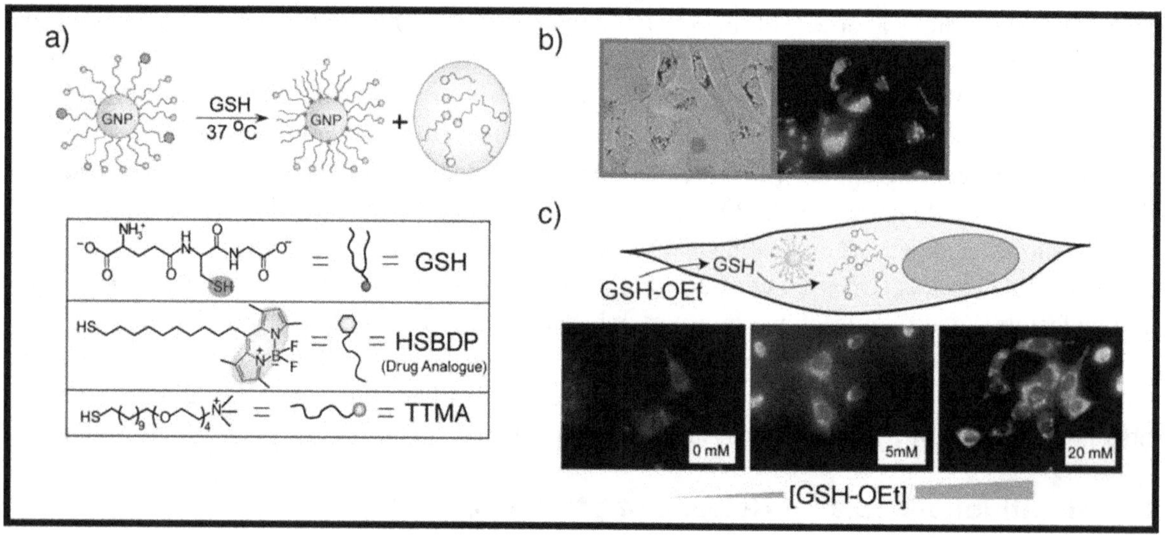

2.2. Release of Nitric Oxide and Singlet Oxygen from GNPs

GNPs could possibly be employed in delivery of diatomic therapeutic agents, like singlet oxygen, or nitric oxide. Singlet oxygen (1O2), a cytotoxic species, involves in photodynamic therapy of cancer (Weishaupt et al., 1976). Russell and co-workers decorated the surface of MPCs with phthalocyanines (PC's), a photosensitizer to generate singlet oxygen with good quantum yield (**Fig. 3A**) (Hone et al., 2002). The quantum yield of free PC's was increased by 50% (from 0.45 to 0.65) upon conjugation to MPCs. Moreover, the conjugation promoted solubility of hydrophobic PCs in polar solvent (from toluene to ethanol). Nitric oxide (NO) regulates multiple cellular processes including angiogenesis, vasodilation, and the immune response (Mocellin et al., 2007). Controlled release of NO could be an effective therapy for hypoxic respiratory failure associated with pulmonary hypertension. Schoenfisch et al. explained the storage efficiency of *via* covalent linking with polyamine stabilized MPCs by formation of acid labile N-diazeniumdiolate (**Fig. 3B**) (Polizzi et al., 2007). They showed effective release of NO from the water soluble nanocontainers in acidic condition (pH=3). pH-responsive materials are applicable for drug delivery due to presence of mild acidic environment inside inflammatory and tumor tissues (pH~6.8), or cellular vesicles like endosomes (pH ~5.5–6) and lysosomes (pH ~4.5–5.0) (Mellman et al., 1986; Engin et al., 1995; Yang et al., 2005).

Figure 3. **A**) *Phthalocyanine-fGNPs for generation of singlet oxygen* **B**) *Nanocontainer for NO storage.*

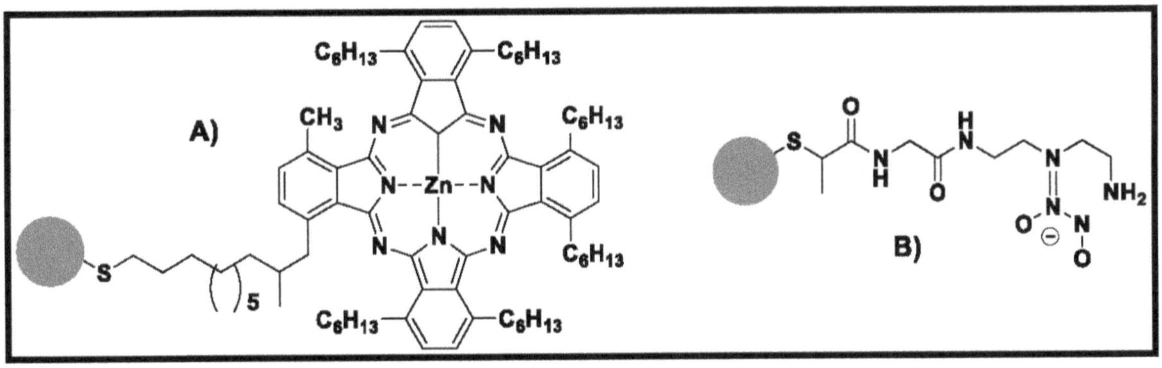

3. GNPs AS SENSORS FOR PROBING AND IMAGING TUMOR CELLS

GNPs are good candidates for labelling applications because of their ability to interact strongly with visible light. Upon exposure to light, free electrons in gold atoms are excited to a state of collective oscillation known as surface plasmon resonance (SPR), conferring gold the ability to absorb and scatter visible light (Kumar et al., 2007). In labelling applications, GNPs are targeted and accumulated at the site of interest and based on their optical scattering properties, they enable visualization of the region under study. GNPs may then be detected by any of the following ways: phase contrast optical microscopy, dark field microscopy, photothermal imaging, and photoacoustic imaging (Sperling et al., 2008). In addition, owing to its high atomic weight, GNPs remain the preferred label for visualization and immuno-staining at the ultra-structural level using transmission electron microscopy (Taatjes et al., 2019). A crucial step in successful cancer therapy involves early diagnosis. The strong optical scattering properties of GNPs, coupled with their relative biocompatibility, make them suitable as probes for cancer imaging. Through the conjugation of antibodies specific for antigens overexpressed on tumor cells, GNPs can be directed to tumor cells, thus pin pointing their precise location in the body (**Fig. 4**). It has been demonstrated that antibody-conjugated hollow gold nanospheres can be used for the surface-enhanced Raman spectroscopy (SERS) imaging of tumor biomarkers which are overexpressed in MCF-7 breast cancer cells (Lee et al., 2009). Raman scattering is a phenomenon that results from the inelastic collision of photons with molecules where energy, which is either lost or gained, translates to a change in the frequency of the scattered photons. This unique shift of frequency depends on the characteristic energy of molecular vibrations constituting the signal, hence a Raman spectrum consisting of different signals from molecular vibrations forms a "vibrational fingerprint" of a molecule (Kneipp et al., 2010). In SERS, these Raman signals are amplified several folds by nanostructures present in the vicinity of the molecules. Gold and silver have been shown to cause significant enhancement (Kneipp et al., 2006) and are favoured nanostructures used as sensors (Li jiaen et al., 2011). By attaching a reporter to SERS sensors, targeted sensitive probing of molecules within cells may be achieved (Kneipp et al., 2010). Recent studies have demonstrated the potential use of GNPs for *in vivo* targeted imaging of cancer using Raman spectroscopy. Large optical enhancements can possibly be achieved in the detection of tumors in live animals owing to the 14-15 orders of magnitude signal amplification by GNPs (Qian et al., 2008). The conjugation of GNPs with appropriate ligands, cancer markers such as EPGR present on the surface of human cancer cells and in xenograft tumor models could be targeted for detection. This shows the potential of using GNPs for biomedical imaging in live subjects. However, it is important to note that the successful optical imaging performed in mice cannot be directly scaled up for *in vivo* imaging of human subjects because the optical signals possess limited tissue penetration ability (Cai et al., 2008). At present, optical imaging only appears useful for tissues close to the skin surface or accessible by endoscopy. Hence, technological improvements are needed before Raman scattering by GNPs can be used in a clinical setting.

The utility of GNPs as novel biosensors for the detection of tumor cells can be demonstrated through the use of a screen printed carbon electrode (SPCE) coupled with a NP-based electrocatalytic method (de la et al., 2009). Using this technique tumor cell proliferation was detected and quantifed via the reaction of cell surface proteins, *in situ* with specific antibodies conjugated to GNPs. Human tumor HMy2 cells (human leukocyte antigen (HLA-DR) class II positive B cells) and human tumor PC-3 cells (HLA-DR class II negative prostrate carcinoma) were first

grown on the surface of SPCEs, following which they were incubated with a commercial monoclonal antibody (mAb) specific to DR molecules conjugated to GNPs (direct method) or

un-conjugated mAb followed by secondary antibodies conjugated to GNPs (indirect method). When hydrogen ions were catalytically reduced to hydrogen in the presence of GNPs, the amount of GNPs (and thus a corresponding indication of the quantity of attached tumor cells) could be quantifed. In both methods, the GNPs immune sensor was able to distinguish DR-positive tumor cells from DR-negative tumor cells, showing the efficiency of this novel biosensor in detecting specific tumor cells.

Figure 4. The localization of antibody conjugated gold to receptors present on the plasma membrane of cells.

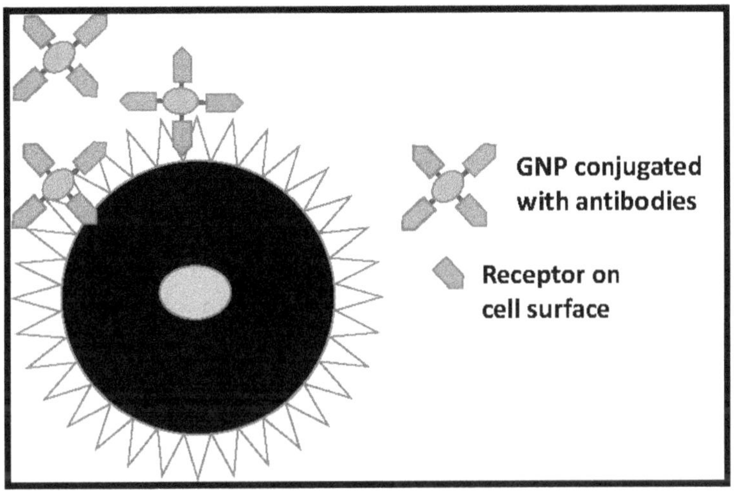

4. GNPs AS ANTI-ANGIOGENIC AGENTS

Fascinatingly, Mukherjee et al. (2005) claimed the anti-angiogenic property of GNPs. However, the exact mechanism of action is still unclear but, during experimentation it was witnessed that GNPs bind preferentially to VPF/VEGF-165 and bFGF (vascular permeability factor/vascular endothelial growth factor and basic fibroblast growth factor) mainly through the heparin-binding domain. This observation suggest researchers that GNPs are able to inhibit angiogenesis by preventing the downstream signalling effects of these mitogens on angiogenesis in cancer cells (Bhattacharya et al., 2008).

5. PHOTOTHERMAL EFFECT OF GNPs IN THERAPY

In addition to the surface chemistry of GNPs, their physical properties could be exploited for delivery applications (Jain et al., 2007). GNPs cause local heating when they are irradiated with light in the "water window" (800-1200 nm). El-Sayed et al. (2007) have recently reported about potential use of GNPs in photothermal destruction of tumors. Citrate-stabilized GNPs (core d=30 nm) were coated with anti-EGFR to target human oral squamous cell carcinoma. GNPs enhanced the efficacy of photothermal therapy by 20 times. In another approach, optically responsive delivery systems have been designed by incorporation of Au nanospheres into the shells of capsules. Caruso et al. prepared microcapsules *via* layer-by-layer technique to encapsulate macromolecules like fluorescein-labelled dextrans (**Fig. 5**) (Angelatos et al., 2005). The capsule shells were doped with GNPs, which response against near infrared light. FITC-dextran was released upon laser (1064 nm) treatment due to rupture of the shell. Skirtach, Parak and co-workers have extended this strategy to deliver encapsulated materials from polyelectrolyte-multilayer capsules inside living cancer cells (Skirtach et al., 2006).

Traditionally, heat has been used in the treatment of cancer via the induction of hyperthermia, a condition in which cells are subjected to high temperatures which kill them. While the sources of heat varies from microwaves, radiowaves, ultrasound waves to laser light in the past, such approaches to cancer therapy have not been widely used because of the consequential damage to normal tissues surrounding the targeted tumor. With the advent of nanotechnology, diverse nanostructures have been manufactured for the purpose of photothermal therapeutics. Noble metal NPs such as GNPs (and including Au nanospheres, nanorods, and nanocages) attract particular interest because they possess enhanced absorption cross-sections (Huang et al., 2008; Liu et al., 2009). Their strong absorbance enables effective laser therapy with minimal "collateral damage" to the surrounding healthy tissue. The mechanism by which GNPs exert their photothermal effect is through SPR. This leads to the formation of a heated electron gas which then cools rapidly within about 1 ps through exchanging energy with the NP lattice. The NP lattice in turn heats up the surrounding environment through the rapid transfer of energy spanning only about 100 ps (Link et al., 2000). The speed at which energy is converted and dissipated to the surrounding environment presents an efficient means of rapidly inducing hyperthermia in the vicinity of GNPs following irradiation with light. Irreversible cell damage resulting from denaturation of proteins and disruption of cell membrane will occur in the areas subjected to high temperatures. The underlying concept of using antibody-conjugated GNPs hinges on the necessity of tumor cells in expressing characteristic biomarkers, which are otherwise absent or expressed in significantly lower levels in normal cells. The successful detection and eradication of breast carcinoma cells overexpressing human epidermal growth factor receptor 2 (HER2) through the usage of anti-HER2 immunotargeted gold nanoshells with subsequent irradiation by near infra-red light to potentiate the gold nanoshells induced photothermal effect has been reported (Loo et al., 2005). The antibody-mediated targeting of GNPs to tumor cells was considered to be the more specific and efficient of the two approaches to tumor targeting. It is apparent from here that plasmonic GNPs exhibit vast potential in photothermal cancer therapy by providing a means to specifically target tumor cells.

Figure 5. Photothermal effect of gold NPs for releasing encapsulated materials. a) Preparation of a microcapsule by layer-by-layer process, b) Encapsulation of therapeutic agents, c) Doping of GNPs in the capsule–shells, d) Rupture of the shell upon light irradiation.

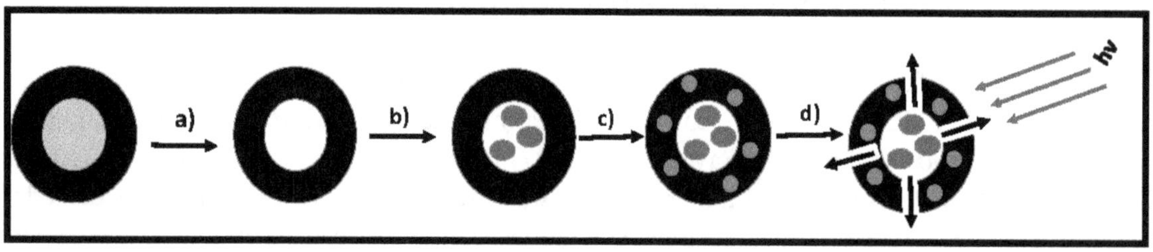

6. GNPs AS RADIOSENSITIZERS

Many studies have revealed that GNPs may have important applications as radiosensitizers (which are drugs that potentiate the effect of radiation for cancer therapy). A study on mice bearing subcutaneous EMT-6 mammary carcinomas showed that not only were GNPs (1.9 nm in diameter) non-toxic in nature and cleared from the body via the kidneys, they possessed the ability to enhance the effect of X-ray therapy leading to a remarkable survival rate of 86% as opposed to 20% with X-rays alone and 0% with GNPs alone (Hainfeld et al., 2005). However, it is crucial to note that while 1.9 nm GNPs seem to show potential as radiation enhancing agents, a recent study discovered evidence for acute cytotoxicity, DNA damage and apoptosis mediated by oxidative stress induced by cellular uptake of 1.9 nm GNPs (Butterworth et al., 2010). There is a need for further understanding of cellular responses to GNPs when exploring their potential to be used in radiation therapy to cure cancer. The effectiveness of GNPs as radiosensitizers seems to be closely related to their surface functionality. While the above studies utilized uncoated GNPs, another study showed that 5 nm GNPs coated with the gadolinium chelating agent dithiolated diethylenetriaminepentaacetic gadolinium (Au@ DTDTPA:Gd) did not exhibit radiosensitizing effect in both tumor cells in vitro and in vivo models (MC7-L1 tumor-bearing mice) (Hébert et al., 2010). Instead, a chemotherapeutic effect was observed, which warrants further investigation. The authors suggest that the radiosensitizing properties of GNPs could possibly be strongly reliant on the nature of their coating. However, the discrepancy over the radiosensitizing effects of GNPs may also be attributed to the different dimensions of GNPs used as well as the type of tumor cells under study.

7. CURRENT CHALLENGES AND FUTURE OUTLOOK

Despite the advances in the era of science, the cure for cancer remains a leading threat to human beings and a serious challenge to scientists and society. The uses of the presently available anticancer drugs are limited due to their side effects, and other drug issues and higher numbers of deaths are reported compared to the cases of survival. Moreover, these drugs are too expensive and cannot be afforded by everyone. Until now, there have been significant advances in the understanding of the molecular etiology of cancer, but ultimate therapeutic strategies are still largely missing. Therefore, it is very crucial to develop new therapeutic agents against this vulnerable disease. Nanotechnology, the creation of new objects in nanoscale dimensions, is a cutting edge technology having important applications in modern biomedical research for cancer detection, diagnosis, and therapy. Looking into the future, there are a number of research themes or directions that are particularly promising but require concerted effort for success. The first direction is the design and development of NPs with monofunctions, dual functions, three functions, or multiple functions. For example, DDS can be varied with one drug or a combination of two drugs or multiple drugs, with one targeting agent or multiple targeting agents along with an imaging agent etc. Therefore, this type of drug delivery system will have multifunctional activities that will be more effective for the treatment of cancer. Multifunctional NPs (targeting, imaging, sensing, therapy) will be more appropriate for clinical translational. We believe that in next few years we will see numerous applications of nanotechnology-based therapeutics and diagnostics in clinics. In addition, individualized medicine is another important area where nanotechnology can play a pivotal role. Due to cancer

heterogeneity and development of drug resistance any particular targeted therapy may not be effective for every population of patients. Therefore, identification of new molecular markers/targets that will only be present on cancer cells would be ideal for nanotechnology based targeted therapy. Similarly, smarter packaging technology is also essential to overcome the challenges posed by the physiologic barrier and by the cancer cells. Thus, basic research both in the field of cancer biology and nanotechnology are essential to meet the challenges that the deadly disease cancer poses to human beings.

8. CONCISE SUMMARY

GNPs, have been attractive in cancer therapy for long time due to small size and many more properties. As they can penetrate widely throughout the body and specifically the accumulation occurs at tumour sites owing to the EPR effect. More importantly, GNPs can bind drugs, proteins and gets dynamically targeted to cancer cells overexpressing cell surface receptors. Additionally, GNPs are biocompatible, it is clear that GNPs preparations can be toxic in *in vitro* and *in vivo* systems. GNPs have a high atomic number, which leads to greater absorption of kilovoltage X-rays and provides greater contrast than standard agents. They resonate when exposed to the light of specific energies, producing heat that can be used for tumour selective photothermal therapy. GNPs have been shown to cause radiosensitisation at kilovoltage and megavoltage photon energies. The exact mechanism remains to be seen but it may be physical, chemical or biological. Many questions need to be answered before GNP complexes enter routine clinical use. The factors that affect GNP pharmacokinetics, biodistribution and *in vivo* toxicity need to be clarified. Targeted GNPs need to exit tumour vasculature, cross the tumour interstitium, enter cells and potentially exit lysosomes to be effective in vivo. They must be able to reach hypoxic cells, which lie far from the vasculature, because these cells are known to be both chemoresistant and radioresistant. Long-term studies are required to evaluate the toxicity and mutagenic potential of GNP-RES uptake, because particles may remain in cells for many months. A standard approach for physicochemical characterisation and pre-clinical testing needs to be implemented, and this process is being aided by the NCL. Rigorous quality assurance needs to ensure minimal batch-to-batch variation, especially when production is scaled up for clinical use. There is huge potential to use NPs in cancer therapy. With intense global interest in nanotechnology and particularly in nanomedicine, it is likely that many of these questions will be addressed in the near future.

REFERENCES

Acharya, S., Dilnawaz, F., & Sahoo, S. K. (2009). Targeted epidermal growth factor receptor nanoparticle bioconjugates for breast cancer therapy. *Biomaterials*, *30*(29), 5737–5750. doi:10.1016/j.biomaterials.2009.07.008 PMID:19631377

Anderson, M. E. (1998). Glutathione: An overview of biosynthesis and modulation. *Chemico-Biological Interactions*, *111*, 1–14. doi:10.1016/S0009-2797(97)00146-4 PMID:9679538

Angelatos, A. S., Radt, B., & Caruso, F. (2005). Light-responsive polyelectrolyte/gold nanoparticle microcapsules. *The Journal of Physical Chemistry B*, *109*(7), 3071–3076. doi:10.1021/jp045070x PMID:16851322

Benkovicova, M., Vegso, K., Siffalovic, P., Jergel, M., Luby, S., & Majkova, E. (2013). Preparation of gold nanoparticles for plasmonic applications. *Thin Solid Films*, *543*, 138–141. doi:10.1016/j.tsf.2013.01.048

Bernkop-Schnürch, A., Pinter, Y., Guggi, D., Kahlbacher, H., Schöffmann, G., Schuh, M., Schmerold, I., Del Curto, M. D., D'Antonio, M., Esposito, P., & Huck, C. (2005). The use of thiolated polymers as carrier matrix in oral peptide delivery—Proof of concept. *Journal of Controlled Release*, *106*(1-2), 26–33. doi:10.1016/j.jconrel.2005.04.004 PMID:15939501

Bharali, D. J., Khalil, M., Gurbuz, M., Simone, T. M., & Mousa, S. A. (2009). Nanoparticles and cancer therapy: A concise review with emphasis on dendrimers. *International Journal of Nanomedicine*, *4*, 1. PMID:19421366

Bhattacharya, R., & Mukherjee, P. (2008). Biological properties of "naked" metal nanoparticles. *Advanced Drug Delivery Reviews*, *60*(11), 1289–1306. doi:10.1016/j.addr.2008.03.013 PMID:18501989

Butterworth, K. T., Coulter, J. A., Jain, S., Forker, J., McMahon, S. J., Schettino, G., Prise, K. M., Currell, F. J., & Hirst, D. G. (2010). Evaluation of cytotoxicity and radiation enhancement using 1.9 nm gold particles: Potential application for cancer therapy. *Nanotechnology*, *21*(29), 295101. doi:10.1088/0957-4484/21/29/295101 PMID:20601762

Cai, W., Gao, T., Hong, H., & Sun, J. (2008). Applications of gold nanoparticles in cancer nanotechnology. *Nanotechnology, Science and Applications*, *1*, 17–32. doi:10.2147/NSA.S3788 PMID:24198458

Cai, W., Gao, T., Hong, H., & Sun, J. (2008). Applications of gold nanoparticles in cancer nanotechnology. *Nanotechnology, Science and Applications*, *1*, 17–32. doi:10.2147/NSA.S3788 PMID:24198458

Chen, K. S., Hung, T. S., Wu, H. M., Wu, J. Y., Lin, M. T., & Feng, C. K. (2010). Preparation of thermosensitive gold nanoparticles by plasma pretreatment and UV grafted polymerization. *Thin Solid Films*, *518*(24), 7557–7562. doi:10.1016/j.tsf.2010.05.043

Chithrani, D. B., Dunne, M., Stewart, J., Allen, C., & Jaffray, D. A. (2010). Cellular uptake and transport of gold nanoparticles incorporated in a liposomal carrier. *Nanomedicine; Nanotechnology, Biology, and Medicine*, *6*(1), 161–169. doi:10.1016/j.nano.2009.04.009 PMID:19447206

Cobley, C. M., Chen, J., Cho, E. C., Wang, L. V., & Xia, Y. (2011). Gold nanostructures: A class of multifunctional materials for biomedical applications. *Chemical Society Reviews*, *40*(1), 44–56. doi:10.1039/B821763G PMID:20818451

de la Escosura-Muñiz, A., Sánchez-Espinel, C., Díaz-Freitas, B., Gonzalez-Fernandez, A., Maltez-da Costa, M., & Merkoçi, A. (2009). Rapid identification and quantification of tumor cells using an electrocatalytic method based on gold nanoparticles. *Analytical Chemistry*, *81*(24), 10268–10274. doi:10.1021/ac902087k PMID:19911778

Deb, S., Patra, H. K., Lahiri, P., Dasgupta, A. K., Chakrabarti, K., & Chaudhuri, U. (2011). Multistability in platelets and their response to gold nanoparticles. *Nanomedicine; Nanotechnology, Biology, and Medicine*, *7*(4), 376–384. doi:10.1016/j.nano.2011.01.007 PMID:21310267

DeLong, R. K., Reynolds, C. M., Malcolm, Y., Schaeffer, A., Severs, T., & Wanekaya, A. (2010). Functionalized gold nanoparticles for the binding, stabilization, and delivery of therapeutic DNA, RNA, and other biological macromolecules. *Nanotechnology, Science and Applications*, *3*, 53. doi:10.2147/NSA.S8984 PMID:24198471

Dulkeith, E., Morteani, A. C., Niedereichholz, T., Klar, T. A., Feldmann, J., Levi, S. A., van Veggel, F. C. J. M., Reinhoudt, D. N., Möller, M., & Gittins, D. I. (2002). Fluorescence quenching of dye molecules near gold nanoparticles: Radiative and nonradiative effects. *Physical Review Letters*, *89*(20), 203002. doi:10.1103/PhysRevLett.89.203002 PMID:12443474

Engin, K., Leeper, D. B., & Cater, J. R. (1995). a J. Thistlethwaite, L. Tupchong and JD McFarlane. *International Journal of Hyperthermia*, *11*, 211–216. doi:10.3109/02656739509022457 PMID:7790735

Ferrari, M. (2005). Cancer nanotechnology: Opportunities and challenges. *Nature Reviews. Cancer*, *5*(3), 161–171. doi:10.1038/nrc1566 PMID:15738981

Ghosh, P., Han, G., De, M., Kim, C. K., & Rotello, V. M. (2008). Gold nanoparticles in delivery applications. *Advanced Drug Delivery Reviews*, *60*(11), 1307–1315. doi:10.1016/j.addr.2008.03.016 PMID:18555555

Gibson, J. D., Khanal, B. P., & Zubarev, E. R. (2007). Paclitaxel-functionalized gold nanoparticles. *Journal of the American Chemical Society*, *129*(37), 11653–11661. doi:10.1021/ja075181k PMID:17718495

Gunnarsdottir, S., Rucki, M., & Elfarra, A. A. (2002). Novel glutathione-dependent thiopurine prodrugs: Evidence for enhanced cytotoxicity in tumor cells and for decreased bone marrow toxicity in mice. *The Journal of Pharmacology and Experimental Therapeutics*, *301*(1), 77–86. doi:10.1124/jpet.301.1.77 PMID:11907160

Hainfeld, J. F., Slatkin, D. N., & Smilowitz, H. M. (2005). *The use of gold nanoparticles to enhance radiotherapy in mice*. Academic Press.

Hébert, E. M., Debouttière, P. J., Lepage, M., Sanche, L., & Hunting, D. J. (2010). Preferential tumour accumulation of gold nanoparticles, visualised by Magnetic Resonance Imaging: Radiosensitisation studies in vivo and in vitro. *International Journal of Radiation Biology*, *86*(8), 692–700. doi:10.3109/09553001003746067 PMID:20586540

Hone, D. C., Walker, P. I., Evans-Gowing, R., FitzGerald, S., Beeby, A., Chambrier, I., Cook, M. J., & Russell, D. A. (2002). Generation of cytotoxic singlet oxygen via phthalocyanine-stabilized gold nanoparticles: A potential delivery vehicle for photodynamic therapy. *Langmuir*, *18*(8), 2985–2987. doi:10.1021/la0256230

Hong, R., Han, G., Fernández, J. M., Kim, B. J., Forbes, N. S., & Rotello, V. M. (2006). Glutathione-mediated delivery and release using monolayer protected nanoparticle carriers. *Journal of the American Chemical Society*, *128*(4), 1078–1079. doi:10.1021/ja056726i PMID:16433515

Hostetler, M. J., Wingate, J. E., Zhong, C. J., Harris, J. E., Vachet, R. W., Clark, M. R., ... Glish, G. L. (1998). Alkanethiolate gold cluster molecules with core diameters from 1.5 to 5.2 nm: Core and monolayer properties as a function of core size. *Langmuir*, *14*(1), 17–30. doi:10.1021/la970588w

Huang, S. Y., Pooyan, S., Wang, J., Choudhury, I., Leibowitz, M. J., & Stein, S. (1998). A polyethylene glycol copolymer for carrying and releasing multiple copies of cysteine-containing peptides. *Bioconjugate Chemistry*, *9*(5), 612–617. doi:10.1021/bc980038p PMID:9736495

Huang, X., Jain, P. K., & Ivan, H. (2008). El-Sayed and Mostafa A. El-Sayed, Plasmonic photothermal therapy (PPTT). *Lasers in Medical Science*, *23*, 217–228. doi:10.100710103-007-0470-x PMID:17674122

Jain, K. K. (2005). The role of nanobiotechnology in drug discovery. *Drug Discovery Today*, *10*(21), 1435–1442. doi:10.1016/S1359-6446(05)03573-7 PMID:16243263

Jain, P. K., El-Sayed, I. H., & El-Sayed, M. A. (2007). Au nanoparticles target cancer. *Nano Today, 2*(1), 18-29.

Jain, S., Hirst, D. G., & O'sullivan, J. M. (2012). Gold nanoparticles as novel agents for cancer therapy. *The British Journal of Radiology, 85*(1010), 101–113. doi:10.1259/bjr/59448833 PMID:22010024

Jiang, W., Kim, B. Y., Rutka, J. T., & Chan, W. C. (2008). Nanoparticle-mediated cellular response is size-dependent. *Nature Nanotechnology, 3*(3), 145–150. doi:10.1038/nnano.2008.30 PMID:18654486

Jones, D. P., Carlson, J. L., Mody, V. C. Jr, Cai, J., Lynn, M. J., & Sternberg, P. Jr. (2000). Redox state of glutathione in human plasma. *Free Radical Biology & Medicine, 28*(4), 625–635. doi:10.1016/S0891-5849(99)00275-0 PMID:10719244

Jones, D. P., Carlson, J. L., Samiec, P. S., Sternberg, P. Jr, Mody, V. C. Jr, Reed, R. L., & Brown, L. A. S. (1998). Glutathione measurement in human plasma: Evaluation of sample collection, storage and derivatization conditions for analysis of dansyl derivatives by HPLC. *Clinica Chimica Acta, 275*(2), 175–184. doi:10.1016/S0009-8981(98)00089-8 PMID:9721075

Kim, C. K., Ghosh, P., & Rotello, V. M. (2009). Multimodal drug delivery using gold nanoparticles. *Nanoscale, 1*(1), 61–67. doi:10.1039/b9nr00112c PMID:20644861

Kneipp, J., Kneipp, H., Wittig, B., & Kneipp, K. (2010). Novel optical nanosensors for probing and imaging live cells. *Nanomedicine; Nanotechnology, Biology, and Medicine, 6*(2), 214–226. doi:10.1016/j.nano.2009.07.009 PMID:19699322

Kneipp, K., Kneipp, H., & Kneipp, J. (2006). Surface-enhanced Raman scattering in local optical fields of silver and gold nanoaggregates from single-molecule Raman spectroscopy to ultrasensitive probing in live cells. *Accounts of Chemical Research, 39*(7), 443–450. doi:10.1021/ar050107x PMID:16846208

Kullmann, F., Hollerbach, S., Dollinger, M. M., Harder, J., Fuchs, M., Messmann, H., Trojan, J., Gäbele, E., Hinke, A., Hollerbach, C., & Endlicher, E. (2009). Cetuximab plus gemcitabine/oxaliplatin (GEMOXCET) in first-line metastatic pancreatic cancer: A multicentre phase II study. *British Journal of Cancer, 100*(7), 1032–1036. doi:10.1038j.bjc.6604983 PMID:19293797

Kumar, S., Harrison, N., Richards-Kortum, R., & Sokolov, K. (2007). Plasmonic nanosensors for imaging intracellular biomarkers in live cells. *Nano Letters, 7*(5), 1338–1343. doi:10.1021/nl070365i PMID:17439187

Lee, K., Lee, H., Bae, K. H., & Park, T. G. (2010). Heparin immobilized gold nanoparticles for targeted detection and apoptotic death of metastatic cancer cells. *Biomaterials, 31*(25), 6530–6536. doi:10.1016/j.biomaterials.2010.04.046 PMID:20537379

Lee, S., Chon, H., Lee, M., Choo, J., Shin, S. Y., Lee, Y. H., Rhyu, I. J., Son, S. W., & Oh, C. H. (2009). Surface-enhanced Raman scattering imaging of HER2 cancer markers overexpressed in single MCF7 cells using antibody conjugated hollow gold nanospheres. *Biosensors & Bioelectronics, 24*(7), 2260–2263. doi:10.1016/j.bios.2008.10.018 PMID:19056254

Lewinski, N., Colvin, V., & Drezek, R. (2008). Cytotoxicity of nanoparticles. *Small, 4*(1), 26-49.

Li Jia'en. (2011). *Cytotoxicity of Gold Nanoparticles in vitro* (Doctoral dissertation).

Link, S., & El-Sayed, M. A. (2000). Shape and size dependence of radiative, non-radiative and photothermal properties of gold nanocrystals. *International Reviews in Physical Chemistry*, *19*(3), 409–453. doi:10.1080/01442350050034180

Liu, C., Li, B. Q., & Mi, C. C. (2009). Fast transient thermal analysis of gold nanoparticles in tissue-like medium. *IEEE Transactions on Nanobioscience*, *8*(3), 271–280. doi:10.1109/TNB.2009.2028885 PMID:20051339

Loo, C., Lowery, A., Halas, N., West, J., & Drezek, R. (2005). Immunotargeted nanoshells for integrated cancer imaging and therapy. *Nano Letters*, *5*(4), 709–711. doi:10.1021/nl050127s PMID:15826113

Mellman, I., Fuchs, R., & Helenius, A. (1986). Acidification of the endocytic and exocytic pathways. *Annual Review of Biochemistry*, *55*(1), 663–700. doi:10.1146/annurev.bi.55.070186.003311 PMID:2874766

Mocellin, S., Bronte, V., & Nitti, D. (2007). Nitric oxide, a double edged sword in cancer biology: Searching for therapeutic opportunities. *Medicinal Research Reviews*, *27*(3), 317–352. doi:10.1002/med.20092 PMID:16991100

Mukherjee, P., Bhattacharya, R., Wang, P., Wang, L., Basu, S., Nagy, J. A., ... Soker, S. (2005). Antiangiogenic properties of gold nanoparticles. *Clinical Cancer Research*, *11*(9), 3530–3534. doi:10.1158/1078-0432.CCR-04-2482 PMID:15867256

Nagesha, D., Laevsky, G. S., Lampton, P., Banyal, R., Warner, C., DiMarzio, C., & Sridhar, S. (2007). In vitro imaging of embryonic stem cells using multiphoton luminescence of gold nanoparticles. *International Journal of Nanomedicine*, *2*(4), 813. PMID:18203448

Nalawade, P., Mukherjee, T., & Kapoor, S. (2012). High-yield synthesis of multispiked gold nanoparticles: Characterization and catalytic reactions. *Colloids and Surfaces. A, Physicochemical and Engineering Aspects*, *396*, 336–340. doi:10.1016/j.colsurfa.2012.01.018

Oyelere, A. K., Chen, P. C., Huang, X., El-Sayed, I. H., & El-Sayed, M. A. (2007). Peptide-conjugated gold nanorods for nuclear targeting. *Bioconjugate Chemistry*, *18*(5), 1490–1497. doi:10.1021/bc070132i PMID:17630680

Pal, R., Panigrahi, S., Bhattacharyya, D., & Chakraborti, A. S. (2013). Characterization of citrate capped gold nanoparticle-quercetin complex: Experimental and quantum chemical approach. *Journal of Molecular Structure*, *1046*, 153–163. doi:10.1016/j.molstruc.2013.04.043

Parveen, S., & Sahoo, S. K. (2008). Polymeric nanoparticles for cancer therapy. *Journal of Drug Targeting*, *16*(2), 108–123. doi:10.1080/10611860701794353 PMID:18274932

Patra, C. R., Bhattacharya, R., Wang, E., Katarya, A., Lau, J. S., Dutta, S., ... Yaszemski, M. J. (2008). Targeted delivery of gemcitabine to pancreatic adenocarcinoma using cetuximab as a targeting agent. *Cancer Research*, *68*(6), 1970–1978. doi:10.1158/0008-5472.CAN-07-6102 PMID:18339879

Polizzi, M. A., Stasko, N. A., & Schoenfisch, M. H. (2007). Water-soluble nitric oxide-releasing gold nanoparticles. *Langmuir*, *23*(9), 4938–4943. doi:10.1021/la0633841 PMID:17375944

Qian, X., Peng, X. H., Ansari, D. O., Yin-Goen, Q., Chen, G. Z., Shin, D. M., Yang, L., Young, A. N., Wang, M. D., & Nie, S. (2008). In vivo tumor targeting and spectroscopic detection with surface-enhanced Raman nanoparticle tags. *Nature Biotechnology*, *26*(1), 83–90. doi:10.1038/nbt1377 PMID:18157119

Rezende, T. S., Andrade, G. R., Barreto, L. S., Costa, N. B. Jr, Gimenez, I. F., & Almeida, L. E. (2010). Facile preparation of catalytically active gold nanoparticles on a thiolated chitosan. *Materials Letters*, *64*(7), 882–884. doi:10.1016/j.matlet.2010.01.051

Saito, G., Swanson, J. A., & Lee, K. D. (2003). Drug delivery strategy utilizing conjugation via reversible disulfide linkages: Role and site of cellular reducing activities. *Advanced Drug Delivery Reviews*, *55*(2), 199–215. doi:10.1016/S0169-409X(02)00179-5 PMID:12564977

Sapsford, K. E., Berti, L., & Medintz, I. L. (2006). Materials for fluorescence resonance energy transfer analysis: Beyond traditional donor–acceptor combinations. *Angewandte Chemie International Edition*, *45*(28), 4562–4589. doi:10.1002/anie.200503873 PMID:16819760

Sengupta, S., Eavarone, D., Capila, I., Zhao, G., Watson, N., Kiziltepe, T., & Sasisekharan, R. (2005). Temporal targeting of tumour cells and neovasculature with a nanoscale delivery system. *Nature*, *436*(7050), 568–572. doi:10.1038/nature03794 PMID:16049491

Sies, H. (1999). Glutathione and its role in cellular functions. *Free Radical Biology & Medicine*, *27*(9-10), 916–921. doi:10.1016/S0891-5849(99)00177-X PMID:10569624

Skirtach, A. G., Munoz Javier, A., Kreft, O., Köhler, K., Piera Alberola, A., Möhwald, H., Parak, W. J., & Sukhorukov, G. B. (2006). Laser-induced release of encapsulated materials inside living cells. *Angewandte Chemie International Edition*, *45*(28), 4612–4617. doi:10.1002/anie.200504599 PMID:16791887

Sparreboom, A., Scripture, C. D., Trieu, V., Williams, P. J., De, T., Yang, A., ... Desai, N. (2005). Comparative preclinical and clinical pharmacokinetics of a cremophor-free, nanoparticle albumin-bound paclitaxel (ABI-007) and paclitaxel formulated in Cremophor (Taxol). *Clinical Cancer Research*, *11*(11), 4136–4143. doi:10.1158/1078-0432.CCR-04-2291 PMID:15930349

Sperling, R. A., Gil, P. R., Zhang, F., Zanella, M., & Parak, W. J. (2008). Biological applications of gold nanoparticles. *Chemical Society Reviews*, *37*(9), 1896–1908. doi:10.1039/b712170a PMID:18762838

Taatjes, D. J., Schrader, M., Koji, T., & Roth, J. (2019). *Histochemistry and Cell Biology: 61 years and not tired at all*. Academic Press.

Tarnawski, R., & Ulbricht, M. (2011). Amphiphilic gold nanoparticles: Synthesis, characterization and adsorption to PEGylated polymer surfaces. *Colloids and Surfaces. A, Physicochemical and Engineering Aspects*, *374*(1-3), 13–21. doi:10.1016/j.colsurfa.2010.10.027

Vasir, J. K., & Labhasetwar, V. (2007). Biodegradable nanoparticles for cytosolic delivery of therapeutics. *Advanced Drug Delivery Reviews*, *59*(8), 718–728. doi:10.1016/j.addr.2007.06.003 PMID:17683826

Weerapreeyakul, N., Hollenbeck, R. G., & Chikhale, P. J. (2000). Stability of bioreductive drug delivery systems containing melphalan is influenced by conformational constraint and electronic properties of substituents. *Bioorganic & Medicinal Chemistry Letters*, *10*(21), 2391–2395. doi:10.1016/S0960-894X(00)00496-0 PMID:11078186

Wei-Chiang, S., Xiantang, D., Feener, E. P., & Ryser, H. J. P. (1989). The intracellular release of methotrexate from a synthetic drug carrier system targeted to Fc receptor-bearing cells. *Journal of Controlled Release*, *10*(1), 89–96. doi:10.1016/0168-3659(89)90020-5

Weishaupt, K. R., Gomer, C. J., & Dougherty, T. J. (1976). Identification of singlet oxygen as the cytotoxic agent in photo-inactivation of a murine tumor. *Cancer Research*, *36*(7 Part 1), 2326–2329. PMID:1277137

Yang, Q., Wang, S., Fan, P., Wang, L., Di, Y., Lin, K., & Xiao, F. S. (2005). pH-responsive carrier system based on carboxylic acid modified mesoporous silica and polyelectrolyte for drug delivery. *Chemistry of Materials*, *17*(24), 5999–6003. doi:10.1021/cm051198v

Yu, L., Qiu, J. J., Cheng, H., & Luo, Z. H. (2013). Facile preparation of gold nanoparticles using the self-assembled ABC non-amphiphilic fluorosilicone triblock copolymer template. *Materials Chemistry and Physics*, *138*(2-3), 780–786. doi:10.1016/j.matchemphys.2012.12.060

Chapter 9
Nanostructured Electromagnetic Metamaterials for Sensing Applications

Man Seng Sim
https://orcid.org/0000-0001-7776-2239
Universiti Teknologi Malaysia, Malaysia

Kok Yeow You
https://orcid.org/0000-0001-5214-7571
Universiti Teknologi Malaysia, Malaysia

Fahmiruddin Esa
Universiti Tun Hussein Onn Malaysia, Malaysia

Yi Lin Chan
Universiti Tun Hussein Onn Malaysia, Malaysia

ABSTRACT

Metamaterials are novel artificial materials with periodic arrangement of structural meta-atoms which exhibit unique properties. Field localization and enhancement at the surface of the meta-atoms allow the structure to be an effective tool for sensing applications. This chapter discusses the emerging field of nanostructured electromagnetic metamaterials in sensing applications. The first section introduces nanostructured metamaterials based on their structures, properties, and fabrication techniques. The following section encompasses the applications of metamaterial-based nano-sensors in medicine and food science. For biomedical sensing, the applications of metamaterial-based nano biosensors in medical field are highlighted. For food science sensing, the applications of nano metamaterials in food contamination detection and food quality control are discussed. The last section discusses the future trends of nanostructured metamaterials in shifting towards reconfigurable, controllable, and multi-functional meta-devices.

DOI: 10.4018/978-1-7998-5563-7.ch009

INTRODUCTION TO NANOSTRUCTURED ELECTROMAGNETIC METAMATERIALS

In this section, electromagnetic metamaterials are introduced in term of their structure, properties and applications. Furthermore, nanostructured electromagnetic metamaterials are discussed.

Electromagnetic Metamaterials

Electromagnetic metamaterials are engineered structures which are made of periodic arrangement of meta-atoms, exhibit unique properties not usually found in natural materials, and have unusual electromagnetic responses at certain frequency range (Tretyakov et al., 2010). The definition of metamaterials usually covers several aspects including their structure, properties and functionality. These aspects are further explained in details.

Structure of Electromagnetic Metamaterials

The structural organisation of metamaterials are periodic arrangement of unit cells (also known as meta-atoms or resonators). The unit cells are geometrical structures such as split rings (Geng et al., 2015; Ozden et al., 2016; Sim et al., 2018), thin wires (Landy et al., 2008; Zhao et al., 2011) and chiral structures (Helgert et al., 2011; Klimov & Guzatov, 2012). There are also hybrid structures which combine several geometrical structures in a unit cell (Shi et al., 2018; S. Wang et al., 2017). The properties of metamaterials are mainly originated from the structural design of the unit cell. Normally, the metallic unit cells are arranged in repeated pattern with periodicity, p on a planar dielectric substrate. There are also 3-dimensional design being engineered to achieve wide-angle of incidence and polarisation insensitive (Soheilifar & Sadeghzadeh, 2015; Wu et al., 2016). The unit cells have sub-wavelength unit cell size (Zheludev & Kivshar, 2012). This means that the unit cell size is much smaller than the wavelength of the operating frequency. The periodic arrangement of unit cells provide effective collective behaviour in response to the incoming electromagnetic waves. For a rough size comparison, the unit cell size of a metamaterial structure is in mm for gigahertz waves, µm for terahertz waves, and nm for infrared, visible light and ultraviolet.

Properties of Electromagnetic Metamaterials

Metamaterials exhibit unique bulk electromagnetic properties, which is not usually found in classical materials. The properties are originated from the unit cell structure due to both of its structural design and constituent material. The properties of a metamaterial can be categorised into two types, which are enhancement properties and novel properties (Tretyakov et al., 2010). Metamaterials can exhibit enhancement properties such as enhanced electric and magnetic properties, better conductivity, or stronger field enhancement and localisation (Kobljanskyj et al., 2012). Metamaterials can possess novel unusual properties such as negative refraction index (Shelby et al., 2001), reverse Doppler Effect (S. H. Lee et al., 2010), negative permittivity (Schurig et al., 2006), and negative permeability (Ishikawa & Tanaka, 2006). The permittivity and permeability of a metamaterial can be simultaneously negative at a specific frequency range (Hossain et al., 2015). These materials with double negative properties are known as double negative materials, left-handed materials, negative index materials or backward-wave materials. Some examples of the artificial structures and their properties are tabulated in Table 1.

Table 1. Examples of metamaterial structures and their unique properties

Metamaterial structure	Properties	Ref.
Artificial dielectrics (array of thin conducting wires)	• Possess macroscopic properties similar to dielectric medium • Effective permittivity smaller than unity • Permittivity and permeability can be tuned	(Brown, 1953)
Artificial magnetics (split ring)	• Negative permeability • Negative index of refraction • Strong magnetic moment when current is induced on the loop	(Ishikawa & Tanaka, 2006)
Bi-isotropic material (chiral structure)	• Rotate the polarization state of light • Magnetoelectric coupling	(Klimov & Guzatov, 2012)
Hyperbolic material (metal-dielectric super-lattice, metallic nanowires within a dielectric medium)	• Hyperbolic iso-frequency curves • Enhancement of spontaneous emission • Negative refraction	(Sreekanth et al., 2016a; Wong et al., 2017)

Applications of Electromagnetic Metamaterials

Metamaterials are artificial electromagnetic media that manipulates and controls the electromagnetic waves. This leads to new functionality of metamaterial structures in various applications (Zheludev, 2011). Based on Table 2, some common applications of metamaterials are perfect absorbers, cloaking or invisibility devices, sensors, and super lens. Metamaterial structures are sub-wavelength, which means that the operating wavelength is larger than the unit cell size. This allows metamaterials to have a smaller size compared to conventional devices. The structural design of metamaterial structure can be geometrically scaled to be adjusted to function at different frequency range of the electromagnetic spectrum including infrared (T. Xie et al., 2017), microwave (Sim et al., 2017), ultraviolet (Khansili et al., 2018), and visible light (X. Zhang et al., 2016). However, the choice of metal is one of the important design aspects for different frequency range. For instance, gold and silver are normally chosen at visible range due to their low optical losses or high DC conductivity (Naik et al., 2013). The fabrication techniques are also different as the metamaterials which operate at higher frequency range require higher precision in fabrication due to smaller geometries.

Table 2. Applications of electromagnetic metamaterials

Applications	Applications	Ref.
Perfect absorbers	• absorb all the wave energy of specific wavelength and dissipates the absorbed energy using its dissipation mechanisms • can be applied in thermal emitters and optical filters	(Landy et al., 2008; Naser-moghadasi et al., 2017; X. Zhang et al., 2016)
Cloaking devices	• bend the waves around an object and allow it to be undetectable	(S. He et al., 2009; Wong et al., 2017)
Sensors	• detect the changes of effective dielectric constant (or refractive index) due to the change of sensing parameters such as moisture content, temperature, concentration, or composition	(Jin, 2012; Ren et al., 2013; P. Wang et al., 2019)
Super lens	• go beyond the diffraction limit which improve fineness of the image resolution	(Kim & Rho, 2015)

Nanostructured Electromagnetic Metamaterials

The first electromagnetic metamaterial was experimentally demonstrated in microwave region of the electromagnetic spectrum (Smith et al., 2000). The microwave metamaterials can be scaled geometrically in size to operate at another frequency range. With current advance of nanofabrication technology, nanostructured electromagnetic metamaterials which have unique responses to the terahertz wave have been actively studied in recent research (Tretyakov et al., 2010).

Definition of Nanostructured Electromagnetic Metamaterials

Nanostructured electromagnetic metamaterials are metamaterial structures with at least one nano-sized dimension for electromagnetic applications. They are artificial materials composed of noble metals and exhibit surface plasmon resonance properties (Hedayati et al., 2014). Some of the commonly used metamaterial nano-structures including split rings (X. Xu et al., 2011), fishnets (Sharp et al., 2014), dots (Budak et al., 2012), clusters (J. H. Lee et al., 2009), pyramids (Gu et al., 2015), rods (Chung et al., 2011), wires in host (Y. He et al., 2013), and helices or chiral structures (Klimov & Guzatov, 2012) are illustrated in Figure 1. They are able to manipulate electromagnetic waves of nano-scale wavelength. The properties of metamaterial are geometry dependent. Therefore, high resolution fabrication are required to have good control of the size and shape without producing significant defects (Yoon et al., 2016).

Fabrication of Nanostructured Electromagnetic Metamaterials

Nanostructured metamaterials can be fabricated by both top-down and bottom up approaches (Jin, 2012; Tanaka & Ishikawa, 2017). Top-down approaches involve lithography techniques (such as photolithography, electron beam lithography, ion beam lithography and X-ray lithography) which reduce and carve a large pieces of materials down to a nano-scale structure (Walia et al., 2015). Bottom-up approaches involve chemical synthesis which arrange or stack atoms, molecules or nano-particles to form a bigger nano-scale structure (Yoon et al., 2016). Some examples of the metamaterial structures and their fabrication techniques are tabulated in Table 3.

Figure 1. Graphical illustration of some examples of nano-structures in metamaterials

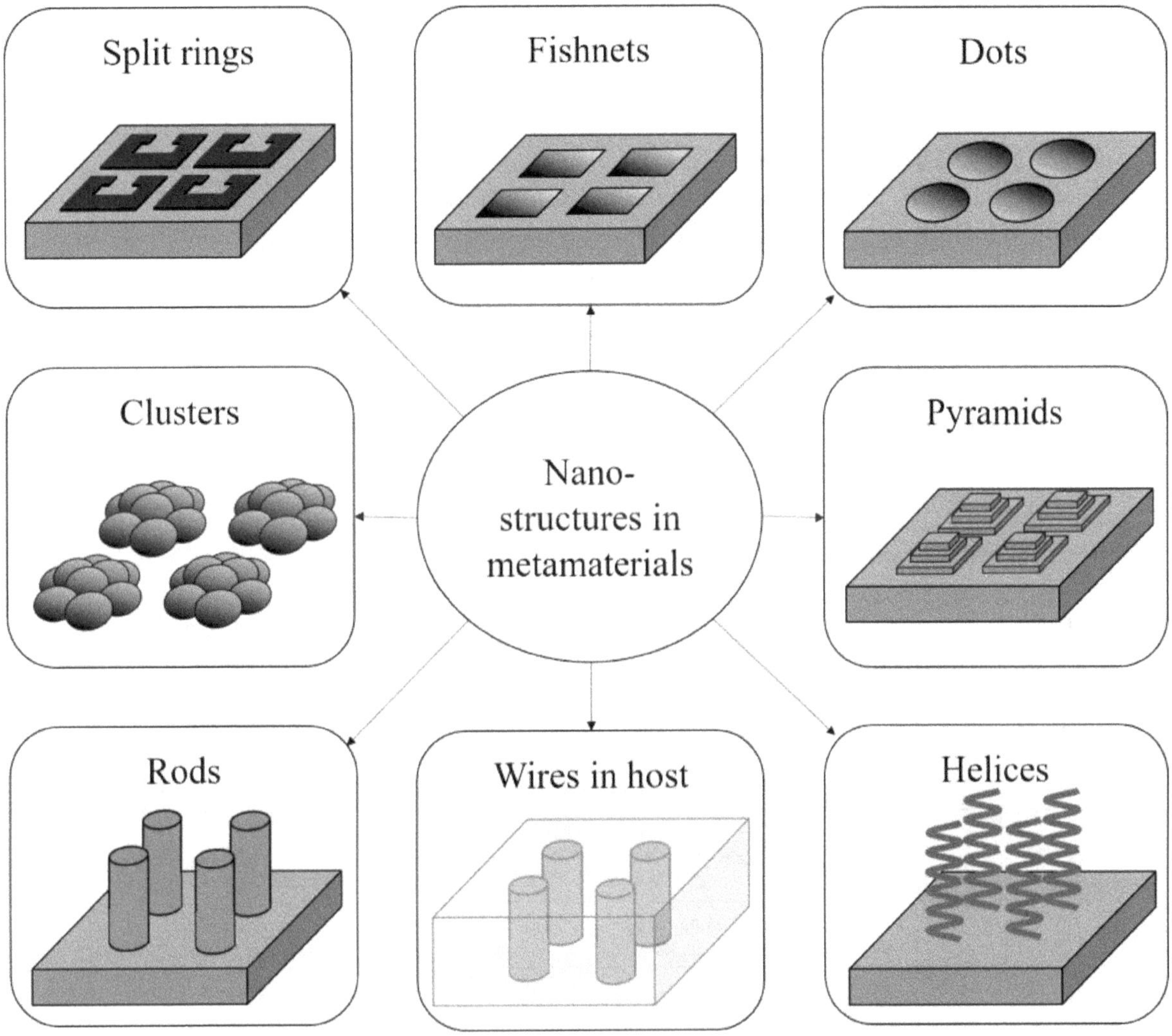

Table 3. Top-down and bottom-up fabrication approaches of nanostructured metamaterials

Approaches	Advantages	Disadvantages	Examples of metamaterial structures
Top-down (lithography)	• better control over size, shape, and inter-particle spacing • lower fabrication cost	• surface imperfection due to crystallographic damage during etching process • precision or resolution limitation	• nano-fishnets using electron beam lithography (Sharp et al., 2014) • nano discs using electron beam lithography (Hokari et al., 2019) • split rings using focus ion beam lithography (Pander et al., 2017)
Bottom-up (chemical self-assembly)	• better uniformity with less defects	• failure prone	• nano-rods using thin film deposition (Huang et al., 2019) • nano-dots using thermal dewetting process (Yoshino et al., 2019) • Carbon nanotubes forest using thermal chemical vapour deposition (Pander et al., 2017)

Properties of Nanostructured Electromagnetic Metamaterials

Nanostructured metamaterials exhibit enhanced electromagnetic properties because the designed structures can localise and enhance the electromagnetic field (Cao et al., 2013). The field is enhanced when the surface plasmons are excited when the plasmon frequency is resonant with the incident electromagnetic waves (Jin, 2012). There are two types of surface resonance phenomena, which are surface plasmon resonance (SPR) and localised surface plasmon resonance (LSPR) (T. Chen et al., 2012). The detailed comparison of both phenomena are given in Table 4. Nanostructured metamaterials comprising periodic arrays of unit cell structures can excite both surface plasmons and localised surface plasmons (Du et al., 2010). SPR and LSPR resonate with the incident electromagnetic waves at a specific wavelength depending on the geometrical design of the metamaterial structure (Zayats & Smolyaninov, 2003). The highly intense electromagnetic fields induced at the metamaterial surfaces allow the detection of refractive index changes at the surrounding.

Table 4. Differentiation between surface plasmon resonance and localised surface plasmon resonance in nanostructured metamaterials

Phenomena	Surface plasmon resonance (SPR)	Localised surface plasmon resonance (LSPR)
Description	• The incident electromagnetic waves are guided along the interface between a dielectric material (positive permittivity material) and a plasmonic material (negative permittivity material) (Patskovsky et al., 2004) • Propagative excitation of the plasmon	• The incident electromagnetic waves cause the localised electron in the conduction band to oscillate and strong surface waves are created on a material (negative permittivity material). (Khansili et al., 2018) • Non-propagative excitation of the plasmon
Properties	• enhanced field (Zeng et al., 2014)	• enhanced field • enhanced surface Raman scattering (Lai et al., 2017)
Applications	• sensing (Y. Chen & Ming, 2012) • switching (X. Yang et al., 2006)	• sensing (N. Liu et al., 2010) • heat generation (Nisar et al., 2020)
Structures	Metal-dielectric composites	Geometries which involves bound electron plasmas such as metal nanoparticles

Sensing Applications of Nanostructured Electromagnetic Metamaterials

Nanostructured electromagnetic metamaterials are applied in sensing applications in the fields of medicine, food science and industry (Monticone & Alu, 2017). A good nano-sensor gives measurable signals, pertains the linearity of sensing and sensitive. Resonance amplification which leads to stronger field confinement can enhance the sensing capability of a nano-sensor (Dong et al., 2010). The advantages of using nanostructured metamaterials as nano-sensors are label-free, non-destructive, sensitive and real-time. The nano-sensor can be calibrated according to the sensing parameters (Sreekanth et al., 2016b).

Sensitivity and figure of merit are used to characterise the performance of a nano-sensor. Sensitivity of a nano-sensor is the ratio of resonant wavelength shift to the refractive index variation (Chung et al., 2011). Sensitivity, S is expressed as:

Table 5. List of biosensors and their basic operating principle

Biosensors	Basic operating principle	Features	Ref.
Electrochemical Impendence Spectroscopy (EIS) biosensors	Detect variations in resistance and capacitance caused by biological events at the sensing electrode surface	• simplicity • inexpensive electrodes • suitable for glucose monitoring • low limit of detection can be achieved if integrated with nanomaterials such as carbon nanotubes and graphene	(Hammond et al., 2016)
Amperometric biosensors	Measure the electron flow generated during interaction between analyte and bio-probe	• high stability • high sensitivity • low specificity	(Stasyuk et al., 2019)
Bioluminescence biosensors	Detect waves in the visible region generated from the oxidation of certain organic molecules by enzymes (bio-luminescent reaction)	• high sensitivity • fast detection	(Erzinger et al., 2018)
Fluorescent biosensors	Detect the molecules which are labelled using fluorescent compounds	• time-consuming • expensive • infeasible for certain applications • may affect certain biological reactions	(Ma et al., 2016)
Surface plasmon resonance (SPR) biosensors	Detect the refractive index shift due to variable molecular interactions	• real-time	(Zeng et al., 2014)

$$S = \frac{\partial \lambda_{shift}}{\partial n} \qquad [1]$$

where $\partial\lambda_{\text{shift}}$ is the resonant wavelength shift (due to the change of refractive index), and ∂n is the variation of refractive index of the surrounding environment (due to the change of sensing parameter). The unit of sensitivity is nm/RIU (RIU is refractive index unit). The shift of resonant wavelength is usually the attribute used to evaluate nano-sensors. For metamaterials for microwave applications, the shift of resonant frequency is used. Furthermore, there are also sensing systems which use angle or phase of the resonant waves to detect the variation of surrounding refractive index (Danilov et al., 2018). Figure of merit of a nano-sensor is the ratio of the sensitivity to the full width at half maximum (FWHM). Figure of merit, *FOM* is expressed as (Chung et al., 2011):

$$FOM = \frac{S}{FWHM} \qquad [2]$$

The unit of *FOM* is RIU^{-1}.

NANOSTRUCTURED METAMATERIAL-BASED SENSORS IN BIOMEDICINE

In this section, conventional biosensors and nanostructured metamaterial-based biosensors are discussed.

Conventional Biosensors

A biosensor is a device with a biological recognition system to detect particular biomolecules and further quantify them through signal processing (Tiwari & Turner, 2014). Biosensors consist of a bio-probe to have specific interaction with analytes and a transducer to convert chemical information into a measurable signal. In medical field, biosensors are important for disease diagnostics, disease progression monitoring, and treatment assessment (T. Chen et al., 2012). Some examples of biosensors are listed in Table 5. Based on Table 5, the biosensors operate by detecting different variations in the sensing environment caused by the target analytes (Singh et al., 2020).

Nanostructured Metamaterial-Based Biosensors

Nanomaterials can be integrated in the design of biosensors to modify the sensing surface. Nanomaterial-modified sensing surfaces have higher surface area for the immobilization of biomolecules (Carrara et al., 2014). Nanomaterials are reported to increase the performance of the biosensors and lower the limit of detection (Hammond et al., 2016). For example, multi-walled carbon nanotubes which are deposited onto the electrode of a cholesterol biosensor enhance the enzyme activity at the electrode surface and improve the electron transfer up to 17.8 times larger compared to bare electrodes (Carrara et al., 2008). Graphene increases the refractive index sensitivity of a biosensor about 4 times compared to the structure without graphene (El et al., 2020).

Nanomaterials can be also structured to form array of meta-atoms which exhibit resonance at a particular wavelength. Based on the size of the meta-atoms, metamaterial-based biosensors can be classified into three types, which are milli-sized metamaterial biosensors (also known as microwave biosensors), micro-sized metamaterial biosensors (also known as terahertz biosensors), and nano-sized metamaterial biosensors (also known as plasmonic biosensors) (T. Chen et al., 2012). All three types of biosensors consist of periodic arrangement of meta-atoms which localizes and enhances field to detect the minor changes in the surrounding environment. The main difference is the size of their meta-atoms, which is associated with their ability to detect different bio-analytes or biological events. For instance, nanostructured metamaterials are used to detect biomolecules and chemical compounds such as cancer markers (biomolecules made by the cancer cells) (Cao et al., 2013), antibiotics (L. Xie et al., 2015) and viruses (Park et al., 2014). The resonance wavelength of nanostructured metamaterials can be tuned to match the specific vibrational modes of a particular molecule (Cao et al., 2013).

The basic working principle of most nanostructured metamaterial biosensors is based on the shift of resonance wavelength which is caused by the change of local refractive index. This allows the biosensors to detect bio-analytes such as proteins (X. Xu et al., 2011), DNA (Cao et al., 2013) and antigens (Presnova et al., 2017). These target bio-analytes bind to the receptor on the metallic nanostructures on the metamaterial surface. This environmental change due to mass accumulation at the surface of the plasmon-supporting metal will lead to a refractive index change. The resonant wavelength which is a dependence of refractive index is shifted to a new resonant wavelength (Kabashin et al., 2009). The presence of analytes can be detected by monitoring the resonant wavelength shift. The following are some examples of events which can lead to local refractive index changes: -

1. concentration change (Z. Zhang et al., 2018)
2. presence of bio-analytes (D. Lee et al., 2017)

3. structural changes after the chemical reaction between nanostructure and molecules (Nasir et al., 2014)
4. binding affinity and kinetic rate from molecules (Cao et al., 2013)

Table 6 shows some examples of the nanostructured metamaterials which are used in bio-sensing applications. Metamaterial can be function as a refractometer to detect changes in the refractive index of the body tissue. Imaging of the body tissue is realised by using contour plot of the refractive index at different points of a particular body part. This imaging technique helps detect tumour as the refractive index of tumour is different from the healthy tissue. This is due to abnormal uncontrolled cell growth, increment of blood supply and water content in the tumour. By doing refractive index analysis between healthy and tumour tissues, tumour can be detected and early cancer detection is possible (Yu et al., 2012). Keshavarz and Vafapour (2019) reported that skin cancer can be detected using metamaterial-based water rods on indium antimony film.

Besides imaging, metamaterials also detect cancer markers in early cancer diagnosis (Strangi et al., 2017; Sugumaran et al., 2018). Geng et al. (2017) reported that glutamine transferase isozymes II and alpha-fetoprotein can be detected using split ring metamaterials for early liver cancer diagnosis. Presnova et al. (2017) showed that prostate specific antigen can be detected using gold nanoparticles with average diameter of 5 nm for prostate cancer diagnosis. Compared to the conventional cancer detection techniques, metamaterial-based detection method is label-free, sensitive, real-time, and non-ionizing. Conventional cancer detection techniques which involves high ionization electromagnetic radiations such as X-ray and gamma rays affect health. Besides refractive index imaging or cancer markers detection, metamaterials have potential applications in heat generation for photothermal cancer therapy due to their resonance behaviour (Tang et al., 2018).

Table 6. Applications of nanostructured metamaterials in biosensing

Nanostructured metamaterials	Device features	Applications	Ref.
Chromium (thickness = 3 nm) and gold (thickness = 97 nm) electric-field-coupled (ELC) resonator with nano-gaps on a quartz substrate	• Operate based on shift of effective dielectric constant in the metamaterial nano-gap surrounding environment • Resonance at 0.8 THZ	• Detect bacteriophage PRD1 and MS2	(Park et al., 2017)
Split ring resonator (width = ~45 nm) on indium tin oxide (ITO) glass substrate	• Operate based on wavelength shift due to refractive index changes • Exhibits two resonance at visible and near infrared	• Probe the binding affinity of G-quadruplex • Detect the cancer biomarker which binds to G-quadruplex	(Cao et al., 2013)
Gold (thickness = 100 nm) array of square apertures on silicon substrate	• Operate based on transmission change due to the change of dielectric properties of antibiotics • Resonance at ~0.3 THz	• Detect the concentration of kanamycin sulphate (Sensitivity up to 100 pg/L)	(L. Xie et al., 2015)
Split ring resonator (thickness = 30 nm) on poly(ethylene naphthalate) substrate	• Operate based on wavelength shift due to change of strain and dielectric environment (Sensitivity = 436 nm/RIU) • Electric resonance at 542 nm and magnetic resonance at 756 nm. • Flexible substrate	• Detect bovine serum albumin (BSA) protein concentration (Sensitivity = ~4.5 nm/nM)	(X. Xu et al., 2011)

Table 7. Comparison of biosensors using micro-metamaterials, nano-materials and nano-metamaterials

	Micro-metamaterials	Nano-materials	Nano-metamaterials
Structure	Periodic artificial meta-atoms	Nano-particles	Periodic artificial nanostructured meta-atoms
Dimension	mm	nm	nm
Operating frequency	GHz	THz	THz
Properties	• Properties are derived mainly from the geometrical structure	• Able to immobilize biomolecules to form bioconjugate	• Properties are derived mainly from the geometrical structure • Strong signal enhancement • Strong field localisation
Detection	Detect effective dielectric constant	Detect biomolecular composition	Detect refractive index
Working principles	Shift of resonance frequency due to local dielectric constant change	Increase the surface area to volume ratio for the detection of bio-analytes	Exhibit evanescent field to detect the shift of resonance wavelength due to local refractive index change
Advantages	• Low fabrication cost • No complex chemistry involved	• Sensitive	• Label-free • The resonance can be tuned to match the vibrational modes of the biological molecules by changing the dimension of the meta-atoms
Disadvantages	• Large geometrical size • Lower sensitivity compared to nano biosensors	• Aqueous solution is required to stabilise biomolecules • Dependent on proximity and orientation of the biomolecules with respect to the substrate surface	• High fabrication cost • Fabrication complexity • Geometry dependent

Compared with biosensors without metamaterials, nanostructured metamaterial-based biosensors show better and improved performance. In a research work carried out by Xie et al. (2015), the minimal detectable concentration of kanamycin sulfate is estimated to be about 100 times higher for silicon substrate with metasurfaces compared to silicon substrate without metasurfaces. Nano-slot metamaterial sensing chip for Avian Influenza (AI) viruses detection in the work by D. Lee et al. (2017) shows 50 times THz field enhancement which lead to sensitivity and selectivity enhancement. Park et al. (2017) reported that the sensitivity of metamaterial with nano-gap (gap width = 200 nm) is approximately 13 times higher than metamaterial with micro-gap (gap width = 3 μm) for bacteriophage PRD1 detection.

The comparison between micro-metamaterials, nano-materials and nano-metamaterials as biosensors are listed in Table 7. The main difference between micro-metamaterials and nano-metamaterials lies in the size of their meta-atoms (T. Chen et al., 2012). Both consists of array of meta-atoms which is sensitive to the changes in the local environment. The unit cell size of the meta-atom is usually about an order of magnitude less than the operating wavelength of the incoming electromagnetic wave. Therefore, micro-metamaterials work in GHz frequency range and nano-metamaterials work in THz frequency range. Due to the size difference, their sensing capability also varies. For the comparison between normal nano-materials and nanostructured metamaterials, the main difference is their structure. Nanostructured metamaterials are nano-materials which are structured to make meta-atoms which exhibits resonance and produce evanescent field (Kim & Rho, 2015).

NANOSTRUCTURED METAMATERIAL-BASED SENSORS IN FOOD SCIENCE

In this section, conventional sensors and nanostructured metamaterial-based sensors in the field of food science are discussed.

Conventional Sensors in Food Science

Detection of microorganisms (*i.e.* bacteria, moulds and yeasts) and toxic chemicals (*i.e.* pesticides and fertilisers) in food helps ensure the food safety for consumers. The pathogens in food samples can be identified using culture dependent and culture-independent methods (Singh et al., 2020). Table 8 shows the list of pathogens detection methods in food science. Culture-dependent methods are microscopic visualisation, biochemical test, and microbiological plating whereas culture-independent methods are molecular methods, immunoassay and biosensors. The culture-dependent detection methods requires several days to give results as they requires time for the pathogens to multiply (Temmerman et al., 2004). Besides that, these conventional methods are labour intensive and require trained individuals to perform the laboratory works including culture medium preparation, colony observation, and biochemical testing.

Table 8. List of pathogens detection methods in food science

Methods		Explanation
Culture-dependent	Microscopic visualisation	The pathogens are observed through microscopy instruments
	Biochemical test	Identification of pathogens through bio-chemical test
	Microbiological plating	Colony counting after isolation and enumeration of pathogens on a nutrient medium
Culture-independent	Molecular methods • DNA microarrays (H. Liu et al., 2017) • Polymerase Chain Reaction (Holzhauser & Röder, 2015)	Detect DNA
	Immunoassay (Li et al., 2016)	Detect specific proteins by stimulating immune response using antigens or antibodies
	Biosensors • Amperometric (Mirela & Apetrei, 2013) • Bioluminescence (G. Cheng et al., 2014) • Fluorescent (Mcgrath et al., 2013) • Surface-enhanced Raman Scattering (Chao et al., 2016)	Investigate molecular or biophysical properties such as molecular weight, refractive index, and molecular charge (Khansili et al., 2018)

Nanostructured Metamaterial-Based Sensors in Food Science

Nanotechnology further enhances the performance of sensors in determining molecular or biophysical properties such as molecular weight, refractive index, and molecular charge (Khansili et al., 2018). Table 9 shows some examples of nanostructured metamaterials which are used for sensing applications in the field of food science. Nanostructured metamaterials can be applied in sensors to detect microorganisms in food since the microorganisms have comparable size to the size of a nanostructured meta-atom. Park et al. (2014) studied a nanostructured metamaterial with gold electric-field-coupled resonators which possesses resonance at ~0.8 THz and is able to detect microorganisms such as moulds, yeasts and bacteria. Yang et al. (2020) developed a metamaterial biosensor based on gold nanoparticles to detect *Staphylococcus aureus* with detection limit of 0.08 pg/μL.

Besides microorganisms, toxic chemicals from pesticides and fertilisers also affect the food safety. Utilisation of pesticides and fertilisers in growing crops increases risks in the contamination of water and food sources. Conventional techniques to detect chemical residue are high-performance liquid chromatography (HPLC) (Masiá et al., 2016) and gas chromatography (GC) (Sapozhnikova & Lehotay, 2015). These methods are highly sensitive but expensive and involve complex steps. Terahertz spectroscopy with meta-atoms enables them to localise and detect a small amount of chemical compounds on the nanostructured metamaterial surface. D. Lee et al. (2016) employed a slot-based metamaterials in a terahertz time-domain spectroscopy (THz-TDS) to detect methomyl. W. Xu et al. (2017) developed a THz-TDS integrated with gold patches metamaterial to detect chlorpyrifos-methy with a limit of detection of 0.204 mg/L. Qin et al. (2018) developed a THz-TDS integrated with metamaterial for carbendazim detection and its limit of detection achieved 5 mg/L, which is ~10^4 times enhancement compared to squash method for THz-TDS detection.

The ability of metamaterial-based nano-sensors in detecting refractive index change realises their applications in food quality control. Dielectric properties of food are related to chemical composition and physical structure (*i.e.* density, firmness, and thickness) (Tao et al., 2012). Therefore, it is suitable to use metamaterial for the detection of the variation of chemical composition and physical structure. Taking fruits as example, some of the potential applications of nanostructured metamaterial sensors are determination of skin thickness, sweetness, ripeness and nutrient content. For example, a metamaterial-based gold nanoparticle array on a flexible silk substrate is applied on food surface to monitor changes in food quality (Tao et al., 2012).

Sensors which are integrated with nanostructured metamaterials can detect various sugar molecules. Gold film with horizontal and vertical slots achieve sensitivity of 588 nm/RIU for the sensing of water and aqueous glucose solution (N. Liu et al., 2010). Gold film with cross-shaped apertures detects concentration of aqueous glucose solutions and the sensitivity achieves ~590 nm/RIU (F. Cheng et al., 2014). Aluminium cross structure is integrated in the microfluidic sensing for various analytes including ethanol and glucose with sensitivity of 3.5 THz/RIU (Hu et al., 2016). Ring and disc resonators detect glucose concentration with a sensitivity of 225 nm/ RIU (Vafapour, 2019). Sensing of sugar molecules allows the determination of sugar levels in beverages (D. K. Lee et al., 2015).

Table 9. Applications of nanostructured metamaterials in food science

Nanostructured metamaterials	Device features	Applications	Ref.
Nano-slot antenna array	• Operate based on the change of the magnitude of maximum transmittance and resonance frequency shift due to the types and concentration of sugar molecules • Resonance at 1.7 THz	• Detect the concentration of sugar molecules which are D-glucose, cellulose and sucrose. • Detect sugar levels for beverages	(D. K. Lee et al., 2015)
Split ring resonator (thickness = 60 nm, periodicity = 180 nm) on silicon substrate	• Operate based on resonance angle change due to local refractive index change • High absorption from 100 nm to 550 nm	• Detect sucrose concentration (Sensitivity = 19.58°/RIU)	(Agarwal & Prajapati, 2019)
Ring and disc resonator (thickness = 200 nm) on glass substrate	• Operate based on resonance frequency shift due to local refractive index change. • Perfect absorption (~100%) at 154.6 THz for water sample • Polarisation insensitive	• Detect glucose concentration (Sensitivity = 225 nm/ RIU)	(Vafapour, 2019)
Gold nanoparticle array on silk substrate	• Operate based on shift of resonance due to variation of dielectric properties of food • Resonance at ~0.68 THz • Flexible and can be applied to curved surfaces of food • Adhesive and edible	• Monitor changes in food quality • Detect bacterial contamination	(Tao et al., 2012)
Gold electric-field-coupled resonator (thickness = 98 nm) on silicon substrate	• Operate based on shift of resonant frequency due to change in the effective dielectric constant in the gap of the pattern • Resonance at ~0.8 THz	• Detect microorganisms such as moulds, yeasts and bacteria	(Park et al., 2014)
Gold patches (thickness = 200 nm) on polyimide substrate	• Operate based on shift of resonant frequency due to change in pesticide concentration • Resonance at ~0.8 THz	• Detect pesticide content in food (Limit of detection of Chlorpyrifos-methy = 0.204 mg/L)	(W. Xu et al., 2017)

FUTURE RESEARCH OF NANOSTRUCTURED METAMATERIALS

Nanostructured metamaterials are trending towards realising switchable, tunable or reconfigurable applications. This feature allows the flexibility of metamaterials in sensing applications to operate at another frequency or detecting other sensing parameters or substances (Ou et al., 2011). Metamaterials can be tuned or adjusted by using thermal, electrical and mechanical approaches (Sim et al., 2020). Furthermore, multi-functional metamaterials are in research interests. For example, metamaterial structures in the nano-sensors can also harvest electromagnetic energy to power up the sensing system. In addition, new materials such as superconductors, nano-carbon materials and organic polymers can be adopted in fabricating metamaterials. For example, three-layered graphene-silicon dioxide-silicon structures which are deposited on polyimide substrate are used in a tunable metamaterial design (X. He, 2015). New fabrication techniques which reduce the fabrication time and cost are also a need in future research of nanostructured metamaterials (Zheludev, 2011).

CONCLUSION

In conclusion, nanostructured metamaterials are artificial structural materials which are useful in various sensing applications. The structural designs of metamaterials allow sensitive detection of molecules and refractive index change. Therefore, metamaterial-based nano-sensors have proven to have promising sensing applications in biomedicine and food science. Advances in the field of metamaterials have led to the realisation of nano-sensors which are sensitive, real-time, small unit cell size, and large functional sensing area. The main challenges will be in developing cost-efficient, sensitive, robust, and stable nanostructured metamaterials.

ACKNOWLEDGMENT

This research received no specific grant from any funding agency in the public, commercial, or not-for-profit sectors.

REFERENCES

Agarwal, S., & Prajapati, Y. K. (2019). Multifunctional metamaterial surface for absorbing and sensing applications. *Optics Communications*, *439*, 304–307. doi:10.1016/j.optcom.2019.01.020

Brown, J. (1953). Artificial dielectrics having refractive indices less than unity. *Proceedings of the IEE - Part IV: Institution Monographs*, *100*(5), 51–62. doi:10.1049/pi-4.1953.0009

Budak, S., Smith, C., Chacha, J., Muntele, C., & Ila, D. (2012). Characterization of gold nanodots arrangements in SiO_2/SiO_2 + Au nanostructured metamaterials. *Radiation Effects and Defects in Solids*, *167*(8), 607–611. doi:10.1080/10420150.2012.668697

Cao, C., Zhang, J., Wen, X., Dodson, S. L., Dao, N. T., Wong, L. M., Wang, S., Li, S., Phan, A. T., & Xiong, Q. (2013). Metamaterials-based label-free nanosensor for conformation and affinity biosensing. *ACS Nano*, *7*(9), 7583–7591. doi:10.1021/nn401645t PMID:23952283

Carrara, S., Baj-rossi, C., Boero, C., & De Micheli, G. (2014). Do carbon nanotubes contribute to electrochemical biosensing? *Electrochimica Acta*, *128*, 102–112. doi:10.1016/j.electacta.2013.12.123

Carrara, S., Shumyantseva, V. V., Archakov, A. I., & Samor, B. (2008). Screen-printed electrodes based on carbon nanotubes and cytochrome P450scc for highly sensitive cholesterol biosensors. *Biosensors & Bioelectronics*, *24*(1), 148–150. doi:10.1016/j.bios.2008.03.008 PMID:18455917

Chao, J., Cao, W., Su, S., Weng, L., Song, S., Fan, C., & Wang, L. (2016). Nanostructure-based surface-enhanced Raman scattering biosensors for nucleic acids and proteins. *Journal of Materials Chemistry. B, Materials for Biology and Medicine*, *4*(10), 1757–1769. doi:10.1039/C5TB02135A PMID:32263053

Chen, T., Li, S., & Sun, H. (2012). Metamaterials application in sensing. *Sensors (Basel)*, *12*(3), 2742–2765. doi:10.3390120302742 PMID:22736975

Chen, Y., & Ming, H. (2012). Review of surface plasmon resonance and localized surface plasmon resonance sensor. *Photonic Sensors*, *2*(1), 37–49. doi:10.100713320-011-0051-2

Cheng, F., Yang, X., & Gao, J. (2014). Enhancing intensity and refractive index sensing capability with infrared plasmonic perfect absorbers. *Optics Letters*, *39*(11), 3185–3188. doi:10.1364/OL.39.003185 PMID:24876008

Cheng, G., Dong, X., Wang, Y., Peng, D., Wang, X., Hao, H., Xie, S., Qu, W., Liu, Z., & Yuan, Z. (2014). Development of a novel genetically modified bioluminescent-bacteria-based assay for detection of fluoroquinolones in animal-derived foods. *Analytical and Bioanalytical Chemistry*, *406*(30), 7899–7910. doi:10.100700216-014-8228-3 PMID:25354889

Chung, T., Lee, S. Y., Song, E. Y., Chun, H., & Lee, B. (2011). Plasmonic nanostructures for nano-scale bio-sensing. *Sensors (Basel)*, *11*(11), 10907–10929. doi:10.3390111110907 PMID:22346679

Danilov, A., Tselikov, G., Wu, F., Kravets, V. G., Ozerov, I., Bedu, F., Grigorenko, A. N., & Kabashin, A. V. (2018). Ultra-narrow surface lattice resonances in plasmonic metamaterial arrays for biosensing applications. *Biosensors & Bioelectronics*, *104*, 102–112. doi:10.1016/j.bios.2017.12.001 PMID:29331424

Dong, Z. G., Liu, H., Cao, J. X., Li, T., Wang, S. M., Zhu, S. N., & Zhang, X. (2010). Enhanced sensing performance by the plasmonic analog of electromagnetically induced transparency in active metamaterials. *Applied Physics Letters*, *97*(11), 10–13. doi:10.1063/1.3488020

Du, L., Zhang, X., Mei, T., & Yuan, X. (2010). Localized surface plasmons, surface plasmon polaritons, and their coupling in 2D metallic array for SERS. *Optics Express*, *18*(3), 1959–1965. doi:10.1364/OE.18.001959 PMID:20174025

El, M., Akjouj, A., & Mir, A. (2020). Design of silver nanoparticles with graphene coatings layers used for LSPR biosensor applications. *Vacuum*, *180*, 109497-1, 109497–11. doi:10.1016/j.vacuum.2020.109497

Erzinger, G. S., Schmoeller, F., Pinto, L. H., Americo, L., Hemmersbach, R., Hauslage, J., & Hader, D.-P. (2018). Bioluminescence systems in environmental biosensors. In Bioassays (pp. 242–262). doi:10.1016/B978-0-12-811861-0.00012-7

Geng, Z., Guo, X., Cao, Y., Yang, Y., & Chen, H. (2015). Flexible, low-loss and large area metamaterials with high Q value. *Microelectronic Engineering*, *135*, 23–27. doi:10.1016/j.mee.2015.02.045

Geng, Z., Zhang, X., Fan, Z., Lv, X., & Chen, H. (2017). A route to terahertz metamaterial biosensor integrated with microfluidics for liver cancer biomarker testing in early stage. *Scientific Reports, 7*(1), 16378-1-16378–11. doi:10.103841598-017-16762-y

Gu, W., Tang, G., & Tao, W. (2015). High efficiency thermophotovoltaic emitter by metamaterial-based nano-pyramid array. *Optics Express*, *23*(24), 30681–30694. doi:10.1364/OE.23.030681 PMID:26698700

Hammond, J. L., Formisano, N., Estrela, P., Carrara, S., & Tkac, J. (2016). Electrochemical biosensors and nanobiosensors. *Essays in Biochemistry*, *60*(June), 69–80. doi:10.1042/EBC20150008 PMID:27365037

He, S., Cui, Y., Ye, Y., Zhang, P., & Jin, Y. (2009). Optical nano-antennas and metamaterials. *Materials Today*, *12*(12), 16–24. doi:10.1016/S1369-7021(09)70313-X

He, X. (2015). Tunable terahertz graphene metamaterials. *Carbon*, *82*, 229–237. doi:10.1016/j.carbon.2014.10.066

He, Y., Deng, H., Jiao, X., He, S., Gao, J., & Yang, X. (2013). Infrared perfect absorber based on nanowire metamaterial cavities. *Optics Letters*, *38*(7), 1179–1181. doi:10.1364/OL.38.001179 PMID:23546283

Hedayati, M. K., Faupel, F., & Elbahri, M. (2014). Review of plasmonic nanocomposite metamaterial absorber. *Materials (Basel)*, *7*(2), 1221–1248. doi:10.3390/ma7021221 PMID:28788511

Helgert, C., Pshenay-Severin, E., Falkner, M., Menzel, C., Rockstuhl, C., Kley, E. B., Tünnermann, A., Lederer, F., & Pertsch, T. (2011). Chiral metamaterial composed of three-dimensional plasmonic nanostructures. *Nano Letters*, *11*(10), 4400–4404. doi:10.1021/nl202565e PMID:21853984

Hokari, R., Kurihara, K., Higurashi, E., & Hiroshima, H. (2019). Optical evaluation of nanocomposite metamaterials fabricated by nano-printing technique utilizing silver nanoink. *Microelectronic Engineering*, *211*, 44–49. doi:10.1016/j.mee.2019.03.024

Holzhauser, T., & Röder, M. (2015). Polymerase chain reaction (PCR) methods for detecting allergens in foods. In *Handbook of Food Allergen Detection and Control*. Woodhead Publishing Limited., doi:10.1533/9781782420217.2.245

Hossain, M. I., Faruque, M. R. I., Islam, M. T., & Ullah, M. H. (2015). A new wide-band double-negative metamaterial for C- and S-Band applications. *Materials (Basel)*, *8*(1), 57–71. doi:10.3390/ma8010057 PMID:28787924

Hu, X., Xu, G., Wen, L., Wang, H., Zhao, Y., Zhang, Y., Cumming, D. R. S., & Chen, Q. (2016). Metamaterial absorber integrated microfluidic terahertz sensors. *Laser & Photonics Reviews*, *10*(6), 962–969. doi:10.1002/lpor.201600064

Huang, J., Wang, X., Phuah, X. L., Lu, P., Qi, Z., & Wang, H. (2019). Plasmonic Cu nanostructures in ZnO as hyperbolic metamaterial thin films. *Materials Today Nano*, *8*, 100052-1, 100052–100056. doi:10.1016/j.mtnano.2019.100052

Ishikawa, A., & Tanaka, T. (2006). Negative magnetic permeability of split ring resonators in the visible light region. *Optics Communications*, *258*(2), 300–305. doi:10.1016/j.optcom.2005.07.076

Jin, Y. (2012). Engineering plasmonic gold nanostructures and metamaterials for biosensing and nanomedicine. *Advanced Materials*, *24*(38), 5153–5165. doi:10.1002/adma.201200622 PMID:22760939

Kabashin, A. V., Evans, P., Pastkovsky, S., Hendren, W., Wurtz, G. A., Atkinson, R., Pollard, R., Podolskiy, V. A., & Zayats, A. V. (2009). Plasmonic nanorod metamaterials for biosensing. *Nature Materials*, *8*(11), 867–871. doi:10.1038/nmat2546 PMID:19820701

Keshavarz, A., & Vafapour, Z. (2019). Water-based terahertz metamaterial for skin cancer detection application. *IEEE Sensors Journal*, *19*(4), 1519–1524. doi:10.1109/JSEN.2018.2882363

Khansili, N., Rattu, G., & Krishna, P. M. (2018). Label-free optical biosensors for food and biological sensor applications. *Sensors and Actuators. B, Chemical*, *265*, 35–49. doi:10.1016/j.snb.2018.03.004

Kim, M., & Rho, J. (2015). Metamaterials and imaging. *Nano Convergence, 2*(1), 22-1-22–16. doi:10.118640580-015-0053-7

Klimov, V. V., & Guzatov, D. V. (2012). Using chiral nano-meta-particles to control chiral molecule radiation. *Physics Uspekhi*, *55*(10), 1054–1058. doi:10.3367/UFNe.0182.201210k.1130

Kobljanskyj, Y., Melkov, G., Guslienko, K., Novosad, V., Bader, S. D., Kostylev, M., & Slavin, A. (2012). Nano-structured magnetic metamaterial with enhanced nonlinear properties. *Scientific Reports, 2*, 478-1-478–6. doi:10.1038rep00478

Lai, C., Wang, G., Ling, T., Wang, T., & Chiu, P. (2017). Near infrared surface-enhanced Raman scattering based on star-shaped gold/ silver nanoparticles and hyperbolic metamaterial. *Scientific Reports, 7*, 5446-1-5446–5448. doi:10.103841598-017-05939-0

Landy, N. I., Sajuyigbe, S., Mock, J. J., Smith, D. R., & Padilla, W. J. (2008). Perfect metamaterial absorber. *Physical Review Letters*, *100*(20), 1–4. doi:10.1103/PhysRevLett.100.207402 PMID:18518577

Lee, D., Kang, J., Kwon, J., Lee, J., Lee, S., Woo, D. H., Kim, J. H., Song, C., Park, Q., & Seo, M. (2017). Nano metamaterials for ultrasensitive terahertz biosensing. *Scientific Reports*, *7*(1), 1–6. doi:10.103841598-017-08508-7 PMID:28811551

Lee, D., Kim, G., Kim, C., Jhon, Y. M., Kim, J. H., Lee, T., Son, J., & Seo, M. (2016). Ultrasensitive detection of residual pesticides using THz near-field enhancement. *IEEE Transactions on Terahertz Science and Technology*, *6*(3), 389–395. doi:10.1109/TTHZ.2016.2538731

Lee, D. K., Kang, J. H., Lee, J. S., Kim, H. S., Kim, C., Hun Kim, J., Lee, T., Son, J. H., Park, Q. H., & Seo, M. (2015). Highly sensitive and selective sugar detection by terahertz nano-antennas. *Scientific Reports, 5*, 15459-1-15459–7. doi:10.1038rep15459

Lee, J. H., Wu, Q., & Park, W. (2009). Metal nanocluster metamaterial fabricated by the colloidal self-assembly. *Optics Letters*, *34*(4), 443–445. doi:10.1364/OL.34.000443 PMID:19373335

Lee, S. H., Park, C. M., Seo, Y. M., & Kim, C. K. (2010). Reversed Doppler effect in double negative metamaterials. *Physical Review B: Condensed Matter and Materials Physics*, *81*(24), 241102-1, 241102–241104. doi:10.1103/PhysRevB.81.241102

Li, Q., Lv, S., Lu, M., Lin, Z., & Tang, D. (2016). Potentiometric competitive immunoassay for determination of aflatoxin B1 in food by using antibody-labeled gold nanoparticles. *Mikrochimica Acta*, *183*(10), 2815–2822. doi:10.100700604-016-1929-x

Liu, H., Dong, H., Chen, Z., Lin, L., Chen, H., Li, S., & Deng, Y. (2017). Magnetic nanoparticles enhanced microarray detection of multiple foodborne pathogens. *Journal of Biomedical Nanotechnology*, *13*(10), 1333–1343. doi:10.1166/jbn.2017.2418

Liu, N., Weiss, T., Mesch, M., Langguth, L., Eigenthaler, U., Hirscher, M., Sönnichsen, C., & Giessen, H. (2010). Planar metamaterial analogue of electromagnetically induced transparency for plasmonic sensing. *Nano Letters*, *10*(4), 1103–1107. doi:10.1021/nl902621d PMID:20017551

Ma, F., Li, Y., Tang, B., & Zhang, C. (2016). Fluorescent biosensors based on single-molecule counting. *Accounts of Chemical Research*, *49*(9), 1722–1730. doi:10.1021/acs.accounts.6b00237 PMID:27583695

Masiá, A., Suarez-Varela, M. M., Llopis-Gonzalez, A., & Picó, Y. (2016). Determination of pesticides and veterinary drug residues in food by liquid chromatography-mass spectrometry: A review. *Analytica Chimica Acta*, *936*, 40–61. doi:10.1016/j.aca.2016.07.023 PMID:27566339

Mcgrath, T. F., Andersson, K., Campbell, K., Fodey, T. L., & Elliott, C. T. (2013). Development of a rapid low cost fluorescent biosensor for the detection of food contaminants. *Biosensors & Bioelectronics*, *41*, 96–102. doi:10.1016/j.bios.2012.07.081 PMID:22939510

Mirela, I., & Apetrei, C. (2013). Amperometric biosensor based on polypyrrole and tyrosinase for the detection of tyramine in food samples. *Sensors and Actuators. B, Chemical*, *178*, 40–46. doi:10.1016/j.snb.2012.12.064

Monticone, F., & Alu, A. (2017). Metamaterial, plasmonic and nanophotonic devices. *Reports on Progress in Physics*, *80*(3), 036401-1-036401–036437. doi:10.1088/1361-6633/aa518f

Naik, G. V., Shalaev, V. M., & Boltasseva, A. (2013). Alternative plasmonic materials: Beyond gold and silver. *Advanced Materials*, *25*(24), 3264–3294. doi:10.1002/adma.201205076 PMID:23674224

Naser-moghadasi, M., Nia, A. Z., Toolabi, M., & Heydari, S. (2017). Microwave metamaterial absorber based on Jerusalem Cross with meandered load for bandwidth enhancement. *Optik (Stuttgart)*, *140*, 515–522. doi:10.1016/j.ijleo.2017.04.007

Nasir, M. E., Dickson, W., Wurtz, G. A., Wardley, W. P., & Zayats, A. V. (2014). Hydrogen detected by the naked eye: Optical hydrogen gas sensors based on core/shell plasmonic nanorod metamaterials. *Advanced Materials*, *26*(21), 3532–3537. doi:10.1002/adma.201305958 PMID:24643991

Nisar, M. S., Kang, S., & Zhao, X. (2020). Photothermal effect in plasmonic nanotip for LSPR sensing. *Sensors*, *20*(3), 671-1-671–13. doi:10.339020030671

Ou, J. Y., Plum, E., Jiang, L., & Zheludev, N. I. (2011). Reconfigurable photonic metamaterials. *Nano Letters*, *11*(5), 2142–2144. doi:10.1021/nl200791r PMID:21480583

Ozden, K., Mert, O., & Kocer, H. (2016). Metamaterial based broadband RF absorber at X-band. *International Journal of Electronics and Communications*, *70*(8), 1062–1070. doi:10.1016/j.aeue.2016.05.002

Pander, A., Hatta, A., & Furuta, H. (2017). FIB secondary etching method for fabrication of fine CNT forest metamaterials. *Nano-Micro Letters*, *9*(4), 44-1-44–48. doi:10.100740820-017-0145-5

Park, S. J., Cha, S. H., Shin, G. A., & Ahn, Y. H. (2017). Sensing viruses using terahertz nano-gap metamaterials. *Biomedical Optics Express*, *8*(8), 3551–3558. doi:10.1364/BOE.8.003551 PMID:28856034

Park, S. J., Hong, J. T., Choi, S. J., Kim, H. S., Park, W. K., Han, S. T., Park, J. Y., Lee, S., Kim, D. S., & Ahn, Y. H. (2014). Detection of microorganisms using terahertz metamaterials. *Scientific Reports*, *4*, 4988-1-4988–7. doi:10.1038rep04988

Patskovsky, S., Kabashin, A. V., Meunier, M., & Luong, J. H. T. (2004). Near-infrared surface plasmon resonance sensing on a silicon platform. *Sensors and Actuators. B, Chemical*, *97*(2-3), 409–414. doi:10.1016/j.snb.2003.09.023

Presnova, G., Presnov, D., Krupenin, V., Grigorenko, V., Trifonov, A., Andreeva, I., Ignatenko, O., Egorov, A., & Rubtsova, M. (2017). Biosensor based on a silicon nanowire field-effect transistor functionalized by gold nanoparticles for the highly sensitive determination of prostate specific antigen. *Biosensors & Bioelectronics*, *88*, 283–289. doi:10.1016/j.bios.2016.08.054 PMID:27567265

Qin, B., Li, Z., Hu, F., Hu, C., Chen, T., Zhang, H., & Zhao, Y. (2018). Highly sensitive detection of carbendazim by using terahertz time-domain spectroscopy combined with metamaterial. *IEEE Transactions on Terahertz Science and Technology*, *8*(2), 149–154. doi:10.1109/TTHZ.2017.2787458

Ren, M., Pan, C., Li, Q., Cai, W., Zhang, X., Wu, Q., Fan, S., & Xu, J. (2013). Isotropic spiral plasmonic metamaterial for sensing large refractive index change. *Optics Letters*, *38*(16), 3133–3136. doi:10.1364/OL.38.003133 PMID:24104668

Sapozhnikova, Y., & Lehotay, S. J. (2015). Review of recent developments and applications in low-pressure (vacuum outlet) gas chromatography. *Analytica Chimica Acta*, *899*, 13–22. doi:10.1016/j.aca.2015.10.003 PMID:26547491

Schurig, D., Mock, J. J., & Smith, D. R. (2006). Electric-field-coupled resonators for negative permittivity metamaterials. *Applied Physics Letters*, *88*(4), 1–3. doi:10.1063/1.2166681

Sharp, G. J., Khan, S. I., Khokhar, A. Z., De La Rue, R. M., & Johnson, N. P. (2014). Negative index fishnet with nanopillars formed by direct nano-imprint lithography. *Materials Research Express, 1*(4), 045802-1-045802–045811. doi:10.1088/2053-1591/1/4/045802

Shelby, R. A., Smith, D. R., & Schultz, S. (2001). Experimental verification of a negative index of refraction. *Science*, *292*(April), 77–79. doi:10.1126cience.1058847 PMID:11292865

Shi, M., Lan, F., Mazumder, P., Aghadjani, M., Yang, Z., Meng, L., & Zhou, J. (2018). Enhanced quadruple-resonant terahertz metamaterial with asymmetric hybrid resonators. *Optical Materials*, *75*, 533–537. doi:10.1016/j.optmat.2017.11.011

Sim, M. S., You, K. Y., & Esa, F. (2017). Broadband metamaterial microwave absorber for X-Ku band usingplanar split ring-slot structures. *Progress in Electromagnetics Research Symposium-Fall (PIERS-FALL)*, 215–221. 10.1109/PIERS-FALL.2017.8293138

Sim, M. S., You, K. Y., & Esa, F. (2020). Electromagnetic metamaterials in microwave regime. In Handbook of Research on Recent Developments in Electrical and Mechanical Engineering (pp. 64–86). doi:10.4018/978-1-7998-0117-7.ch002

Sim, M. S., You, K. Y., Esa, F., Dimon, M. N., & Khamis, N. H. (2018). Multiband metamaterial microwave absorbers using split ring and multiwidth slot structure. *International Journal of RF and Microwave Computer-Aided Engineering*, *28*(7), 1–13. doi:10.1002/mmce.21473

Singh, S., Dhanjal, D. S., Thotapalli, S., Kumar, V., Datta, S., Kumar, V., Kumar, M., & Singh, J. (2020). An insight in bacteriophage based biosensors with focus on their detection methods and recent advancements. *Environmental Technology & Innovation*, *20*, 101081. doi:10.1016/j.eti.2020.101081

Smith, D. R., Padilla, W. J., Vier, D. C., & Schultz, S. (2000). Composite Medium with Simultaneously Negative Permeability and Permittivity. *Physical Review Letters*, *84*(18), 1–4. doi:10.1103/PhysRevLett.84.4184 PMID:10990641

Soheilifar, M. R., & Sadeghzadeh, R. A. (2015). Design, fabrication and characterisation of scaled and stacked layers planar metamaterial absorber. *IET Microwaves, Antennas & Propagation*, *9*(1), 86–93. doi:10.1049/iet-map.2014.0350

Sreekanth, K. V., Alapan, Y., Elkabbash, M., Ilker, E., Hinczewski, M., Gurkan, U. A., De Luca, A., & Strangi, G. (2016a). Extreme sensitivity biosensing platform based on hyperbolic metamaterials. *Nature Materials*, *15*(6), 621–627. doi:10.1038/nmat4609 PMID:27019384

Sreekanth, K. V., Alapan, Y., ElKabbash, M., Wen, A. M., Ilker, E., Hinczewski, M., Gurkan, U. A., Steinmetz, N. F., & Strangi, G. (2016b). Enhancing the angular sensitivity of plasmonic sensors using hyperbolic metamaterials. *Advanced Optical Materials*, *4*(11), 1767–1772. doi:10.1002/adom.201600448 PMID:28649484

Stasyuk, N., Gayda, G., Zakalskiy, A., Zakalska, O., Serkiz, R., & Gonchar, M. (2019). Amperometric biosensors based on oxidases and PtRu nanoparticles as artificial peroxidase. *Food Chemistry*, *285*(January), 213–220. doi:10.1016/j.foodchem.2019.01.117 PMID:30797337

Strangi, G., Sreekanth, K. V., & Elkabbash, M. (2017). Hyperbolic metamaterial-based ultrasensitive plasmonic biosensors for early-stage cancer detection. In Next Generation Point-of-care Biomedical Sensors Technologies for Cancer Diagnosis (pp. 155–172). doi:10.1007/978-981-10-4726-8_7

Sugumaran, S., Jamlos, M. F., Ahmad, M. N., Bellan, C. S., & Schreurs, D. (2018). Nanostructured materials with plasmonic nanobiosensors for early cancer detection: A past and future prospect. *Biosensors & Bioelectronics*, *100*, 361–373. doi:10.1016/j.bios.2017.08.044 PMID:28946108

Tanaka, T., & Ishikawa, A. (2017). Towards three-dimensional optical metamaterials. *Nano Convergence*, *4*(1), 34-1-34–39. doi:10.118640580-017-0129-7

Tang, X., Tan, L., Shi, K., Peng, J., Xiao, Y., Li, W., Chen, L., Yang, Q., & Qian, Z. (2018). Gold nanorods together with HSP inhibitor-VER-155008 micelles for colon cancer mild-temperature photothermal therapy. *Acta Pharmaceutica Sinica. B*, *8*(4), 587–601. doi:10.1016/j.apsb.2018.05.011 PMID:30109183

Tao, H., Brenckle, M. A., Yang, M., Zhang, J., Liu, M., Siebert, S. M., Averitt, R. D., Mannoor, M. S., McAlpine, M. C., Rogers, J. A., Kaplan, D. L., & Omenetto, F. G. (2012). Silk-based conformal, adhesive, edible food sensors. *Advanced Materials*, *24*(8), 1067–1072. doi:10.1002/adma.201103814 PMID:22266768

Temmerman, R., Huys, G., & Swings, J. (2004). Identification of lactic acid bacteria: Culture-dependent and culture-independent methods. *Trends in Food Science & Technology*, *15*(7–8), 348–359. doi:10.1016/j.tifs.2003.12.007

Tiwari, A., & Turner, A. P. F. (2014). *Biosensors Nanotechnology*. doi:10.1002/9781118773826

Tretyakov, S., Barois, P., Scharf, T., Kruglay, V., & Bergmair, I. (2010). Nanostructured metamaterials: exchange between experts in electromagnetics and material science. Publications Office of the European Union. doi:10.2777/54953

Vafapour, Z. (2019). Polarization-independent perfect optical metamaterial absorber as a glucose sensor in food industry applications. *IEEE Transactions on Nanobioscience, 18*(4), 622–627. doi:10.1109/TNB.2019.2929802 PMID:31329124

Walia, S., Shah, C. M., Gutruf, P., Nili, H., Chowdhury, D. R., Withayachumnankul, W., Bhaskaran, M., & Sriram, S. (2015). Flexible metasurfaces and metamaterials: A review of materials and fabrication processes at micro- and nano-scales. *Applied Physics Reviews, 2*(1), 011303. doi:10.1063/1.4913751

Wang, P., Nasir, M. E., Krasavin, A. V., Dickson, W., Jiang, Y., & Zayats, A. V. (2019). Plasmonic metamaterials for nanochemistry and sensing. *Accounts of Chemical Research, 52*(11), 3018–3028. doi:10.1021/acs.accounts.9b00325 PMID:31680511

Wang, S., Kang, L., & Werner, D. H. (2017). Hybrid resonators and highly tunable terahertz metamaterials enabled by Vanadium Dioxide (VO_2). *Scientific Reports, 7*(1), 4326-1-4326–4328. doi:10.103841598-017-04692-8

Wong, Z. J., Wang, Y., O'Brien, K., Rho, J., Yin, X., Zhang, S., Fang, N., Yen, T. J., & Zhang, X. (2017). Optical and acoustic metamaterials: superlens, negative refractive index and invisibility cloak. *Journal of Optics, 19*(8), 084007-1-084007–084013. doi:10.1088/2040-8986/aa7a1f

Wu, D., Liu, Y., Yu, Z., Chen, L., Ma, R., Li, Y., Li, R., & Ye, H. (2016). Wide-angle, polarization-insensitive and broadband absorber based on eight-fold symmetric SRRs metamaterial. *Optics Communications, 380*, 221–226. doi:10.1016/j.optcom.2016.06.023

Xie, L., Gao, W., Shu, J., Ying, Y., & Kono, J. (2015). Extraordinary sensitivity enhancement by metasurfaces in terahertz detection of antibiotics. *Scientific Reports, 5*(1), 1–4. doi:10.1038rep08671 PMID:25728144

Xie, T., Chen, Z., Ma, R., & Zhong, M. (2017). A wide-angle and polarization insensitive infrared broad band metamaterial absorber. *Optics Communications, 383*, 81–86. doi:10.1016/j.optcom.2016.08.058

Xu, W., Xie, L., Zhu, J., Wang, W., Ye, Z., Ma, Y., Tsai, C., Chen, S., & Ying, Y. (2017). Terahertz sensing of chlorpyrifos-methyl using metamaterials. *Food Chemistry, 218*, 330–334. doi:10.1016/j.foodchem.2016.09.032 PMID:27719917

Xu, X., Peng, B., Li, D., Zhang, J., Wong, L. M., Zhang, Q., Wang, S., & Xiong, Q. (2011). Flexible visible-infrared metamaterials and their applications in highly sensitive chemical and biological sensing. *Nano Letters, 11*(8), 3232–3238. doi:10.1021/nl2014982 PMID:21696183

Yang, K., Yu, W., Huang, G., Zhou, J., Yang, X., & Fu, W. (2020). Highly sensitive detection of Staphylococcus aureus by a THz metamaterial biosensor based on gold nanoparticles and rolling circle amplification. *RSC Advances, 10*(45), 26824–26833. doi:10.1039/D0RA03116J

Yang, X., Wang, Q., Wang, K., Tan, W., Yao, J., & Li, H. (2006). Electrical switching of DNA monolayers investigated by surface plasmon resonance. *Langmuir, 22*(13), 5654–5659. doi:10.1021/la052907m PMID:16768490

Yoon, G., Kim, I., & Rho, J. (2016). Challenges in fabrication towards realization of practical metamaterials. *Microelectronic Engineering, 163*, 7–20. doi:10.1016/j.mee.2016.05.005

Yoshino, M., Kubota, Y., Nakagawa, Y., & Terano, M. (2019). Efficient fabrication process of ordered metal nanodot arrays for infrared plasmonic sensor. *Micromachines, 10*(6), 27–30. doi:10.3390/mi10060385 PMID:31181766

Yu, C., Fan, S., Sun, Y., & Pickwell-Macpherson, E. (2012). The potential of terahertz imaging for cancer diagnosis: A review of investigations to date. *Quantitative Imaging in Medicine and Surgery, 2*(1), 33–45. doi:10.3978/j.issn.2223-4292.2012.01.04 PMID:23256057

Zayats, A. V., & Smolyaninov, I. I. (2003). Near-field photonics: Surface plasmon polaritons and localized surface plasmons. *Journal of Optics. A, Pure and Applied Optics, 5*(4), S16–S50. doi:10.1088/1464-4258/5/4/353

Zeng, S., Hu, S., Xia, J., Anderson, T., Dinh, X., Meng, X., Coquet, P., & Yong, K. (2014). Graphene-MoS_2 hybrid nanostructures enhanced surface plasmon resonance biosensors. *Sensors and Actuators. B, Chemical, 207*, 801–810. doi:10.1016/j.snb.2014.10.124

Zhang, X., Fan, Y., Qi, L., & Li, H. (2016). Broadband plasmonic metamaterial absorber with fish-scale structure at visible frequencies. *Optical Materials Express, 6*(7), 2448–2457. doi:10.1364/OME.6.002448

Zhang, Z., Ding, H., Yan, X., Liang, L., Wei, D., Wang, M., Yang, Q., & Yao, J. (2018). Sensitive detection of cancer cell apoptosis based on the non-bianisotropic metamaterials biosensors in terahertz frequency. *Optical Materials Express, 8*(3), 6951–6957. doi:10.1364/OME.8.000659

Zhao, Y., Chu, J., Li, S. H., Chen, Y., Sheng, G. P., Chen, Y. P., Li, W. W., Liu, G., Tian, Y. C., Xiong, Y., & Yu, H. Q. (2011). Preparation of Pt-Fe2O3 nano-electrode array on gold nano-wires and its application to the catalytic degradation of methyl orange. *Chemical Engineering Journal, 170*(2–3), 440–444. doi:10.1016/j.cej.2010.11.104

Zheludev, N. I. (2011). A roadmap for metamaterials. *Optics and Photonics News, 22*(3), 30–35. doi:10.1364/OPN.22.3.000030

Zheludev, N. I., & Kivshar, Y. S. (2012). From metamaterials to metadevices. *Nature Materials, 11*(11), 917–924. doi:10.1038/nmat3431 PMID:23089997

ADDITIONAL READING

Hedayati, M. K., Faupel, F., & Elbahri, M. (2014). Review of plasmonic nanocomposite metamaterial absorber. *Materials (Basel)*, *7*(2), 1221–1248. doi:10.3390/ma7021221 PMID:28788511

Jin, Y. (2012). Engineering plasmonic gold nanostructures and metamaterials for biosensing and nanomedicine. *Advanced Materials*, *24*(38), 5153–5165. doi:10.1002/adma.201200622 PMID:22760939

Monticone, F., & Alu, A. (2017). Metamaterial, plasmonic and nanophotonic devices. *Reports on Progress in Physics, 80*(3), 036401-1-036401–036437. doi:10.1088/1361-6633/aa518f

Sim, M. S., You, K. Y., & Esa, F. (2020). Electromagnetic metamaterials in microwave regime. In Handbook of Research on Recent Developments in Electrical and Mechanical Engineering (pp. 64–86). doi:10.4018/978-1-7998-0117-7.ch002

Strangi, G., Sreekanth, K. V., & Elkabbash, M. (2017). Hyperbolic metamaterial-based ultrasensitive plasmonic biosensors for early-stage cancer detection. In Next Generation Point-of-care Biomedical Sensors Technologies for Cancer Diagnosis (pp. 155–172). doi:10.1007/978-981-10-4726-8_7

Tanaka, T., & Ishikawa, A. (2017). Towards three-dimensional optical metamaterials. *Nano Convergence, 4*(1), 34-1-34–39. doi:10.118640580-017-0129-7

Tretyakov, S., Barois, P., Scharf, T., Kruglay, V., & Bergmair, I. (2010). Nanostructured metamaterials: exchange between experts in electromagnetics and material science. In Publications Office of the European Union. doi:10.2777/54953

Wang, P., Nasir, M. E., Krasavin, A. V., Dickson, W., Jiang, Y., & Zayats, A. V. (2019). Plasmonic metamaterials for nanochemistry and sensing. *Accounts of Chemical Research*, *52*(11), 3018–3028. doi:10.1021/acs.accounts.9b00325 PMID:31680511

Wong, Z. J., Wang, Y., O'Brien, K., Rho, J., Yin, X., Zhang, S., Fang, N., Yen, T. J., & Zhang, X. (2017). Optical and acoustic metamaterials: superlens, negative refractive index and invisibility cloak. *Journal of Optics, 19*(8), 084007-1-084007–084013. doi:10.1088/2040-8986/aa7a1f

Xu, X., Peng, B., Li, D., Zhang, J., Wong, L. M., Zhang, Q., Wang, S., & Xiong, Q. (2011). Flexible visible-infrared metamaterials and their applications in highly sensitive chemical and biological sensing. *Nano Letters*, *11*(8), 3232–3238. doi:10.1021/nl2014982 PMID:21696183

Zheludev, N. I. (2011). A roadmap for metamaterials. *Optics and Photonics News*, *22*(3), 30–35. doi:10.1364/OPN.22.3.000030

Zheludev, N. I., & Kivshar, Y. S. (2012). From metamaterials to metadevices. *Nature Materials*, *11*(11), 917–924. doi:10.1038/nmat3431 PMID:23089997

KEY TERMS AND DEFINITIONS

Biosensor: A device with a biological recognition system to detect particular biomolecules and further quantify them through signal processing.

Electromagnetic Metamaterial: An artificial engineered structure which are made of periodic arrangement of meta-atoms, exhibit unique properties not found in natural materials, and have unusual electromagnetic responses at certain frequency range.

Figure of Merit: The ratio of the sensitivity of a nano-sensor to the full width at half maximum (FWHM).

Localised Surface Plasmon Resonance (LSPR): An optical phenomenon that occurs on a material (negative permittivity material) when the electrons in the conduction band are oscillating to the incident electromagnetic wave.

Nano-Sensor: A nano-sized sensing device that detect the presence of particular substances or measure physical quantities and convert these to measurable signals.

Nanostructured Metamaterial: A repeating array of metamaterial structures with at least one nano-sized dimension.

Sensitivity: The ratio of the resonant wavelength shift (or angular shift) to the refractive index variation of the materials under test.

Surface Plasmon Resonance (SPR): An optical phenomenon that occurs at an interface between a dielectric material (positive permittivity material) and a plasmonic material (negative permittivity material) when the incident electromagnetic wave are propagating along the interface.

Chapter 10
Nano-Structured Materials for Efficient Energy Storage and Conversion

Jahangir Ahmad
Department of Chemistry, National Institute of Technology Srinagar, India

Kowsar Majid
Department of Chemistry, National Institute of Technology Srinagar, India

ABSTRACT

As the energy demand is rapidly increasing worldwide, one of the main challenges of this century is to fulfill the energy needs for the sustenance of life. There is clearly an urgent need to develop alternative renewable energy harvesting technologies. This chapter emphasizes nano-structured materials which hold the key to fundamental advances in energy storage and conversion. Nano-structured materials offer unique properties as electrodes and electrolytes in a range of energy devices. Among the fundamental technologies in energy storage and conversion influenced by nanostructured materials, photovoltaic cells, lithium ion batteries, supercapacitors, and electro catalysts for fuel cells are highlighted in this chapter. The principles involved for hydrogen generation and nanostructured materials used for photocatalytic hydrogen generation are also discussed.

INTRODUCTION

Currently our modern society is highly dependent on fossil fuels such as coal, crude oil and natural gas for the energy supply but the excessive use of natural resources will lead to the quick depletion in a near future. At the same time, when these fuels are combusted for the production of energy, large amounts of green house gases are inevitably emitted and pollute our environment. All these have urged us to explore alternative clean energy sources for sustainable human activities (Service, 2005). In this connection, renewable energy sources like solar (Crabtree and Lewis, 2007), mechanical (Wang and Song, 2006), heat energies (Cole, 1983) are being actively investigated. Among these three energy sources sunlight

DOI: 10.4018/978-1-7998-5563-7.ch010

is the most fascinating source. A number of approaches have been pursued to tackle the challenges. The storage and harvesting techniques of solar energy are attractive and promising to tackle the energy shortage. Exploring the solar energy in a low-cost and high-efficiency way is not easy as (a) the solar energy density is far lower than any of the fossil energy (b) sunlight is staggering in different areas and in different time spans (c) as compared to fossil fuel the solar energy is difficult to be stored in the form of electricity or heat, fossil fuel stores energy in chemical bonds (Crabtree and Lewis, 2007). These are the main reasons why solar energy accounts to as little as ~0.015% of the total energy used today (Crabtree and Lewis, 2007).

Basically, solar energy can be harvested in the form of biomass, heat and electricity. Sunlight can be directly converted into electricity and has the highest efficiency and flexibility as compared to the energy conversion efficiencies into biomass and heat. The ability to produce electricity and fuels such as hydrogen using sunlight, and the ability to efficiently store them, could help revolutionize our lives in the future. Therefore, the free and clean sunlight can be explored in the form of electricity by techniques such as photovoltaic, photo electrochemical cells (PECs) and in the form of electricity-storing solar hydrogen.

On the other hand, over the past decades scientists have been studying the properties of nanomaterials. Nanomaterials are matters with at least one dimension in their physical size ranging between 1 and 100 nm. Nanomaterials appear in a variety of forms such as nanoparticles, nanowire, nanorods, nanotubes, nanofibers, nanoporous framework, etc. As the size of the materials decreases, the percentage of the atoms on the surface and the surface-to-volume ratio increase. Due to the combination of bulk and surface properties the nanostructured materials showed unusual mechanical, electrical and optical properties and because of this nanostructured materials have attracted great attention in recent years. Energy conversion and storage involve physical interaction or chemical reaction at the surface or interface, so the specific surface area, surface energy, and surface chemistry play a very important role. Nanomaterials due to their smaller dimensions may also offer more favorable heat, mass, and charge transfer, as well as accommodate dimensional changes associated with some chemical reactions and phase transitions. The aim of this chapter is to offer a brief overview of the applications of nanostructured materials in the field of energy harvesting and storage.

BACKGROUND

Over the past several decades, significant efforts has been made in developing alternative technologies to harvest and use clean, sustainable energy including solar energy wind power, biofuels, and hydrogen, as well as clean energy technologies, such as fuel cells and lithium-ion batteries. In the past although these types of energy sources have played a promising role, efforts are being made in the progress of new technology s progressing impressively to make alternative energy more practical and low cost when compared with fossil fuels. It is expected that the coming decades will usher in a long expected transition away from coal and oil as our primary fuel.

Energy harvesting at nanoscale has gained much attention in the last decade with the technological advancements seen in the field of nanotechnology. On this particular field a lot of work was done by Wang et al. group at Georgia tech institute (Dong, et al, 2012). Wang and Song (Wang et al 2006) introduced the concept of nano generator in which vertically aligned zinc oxide (piezoelectric in nature) nanorods are fabricated on various substrates using a vapor-liquid-solid process. These nanorods would generate voltage which could be used to power nano devices when deflected by a gold coated AFM tip. This is explained on the basis of Schottky contact between the semiconductor ZnO and the gold coating on the AFM tip. The research group went on to build various other configurations and devices by exploring this novel concept. Researchers like Yang et al. (Yang, et al 2009) and Zhu et al (Zhu et al, 2010) enhanced the performance by designing a laterally oriented ZnO rod array on a polymer substrate and also introduced flexibility to the system. Dong et al (2012) integrated it with a graphene based supercapacitor. Stuart and Hall reported a pioneer work in the area of plasmonic enhancement of light-sensitive devices According to these researchers there is an enhancement in the photocurrent of a factor of 18 by using silver nanoparticles on the surface of the device (165 nm thick silicon-on-insulator photo-detector) (Stuart et al, 1998). Morfa et al. have reported an enhancement in efficiency by a factor of 1.7 for organic bulk heterojunction solar cells (Morfa et al, 2008).

Although using nanostructured materials researchers have made significant contributions in the field of energy harvesting, it is important to explore inexpensive, innovative, scalable technologies based on new materials wherein a single device can be used to transform multiple sources of energy

MAIN FOCUS OF THE CHAPTER

The nanostructured materials have the ability to modulate their composition in a well-controlled manner to create properties that are not possible in their bulk counterparts provide the potential to address some of the critical challenges faced by the conventional methods of energy storage and harvesting by fossil fuels. In this chapter selected topic fields are focused on the basis of relatively recent progress in those fields, and the most recent developments of nanomaterials in energy harvesting and storage applications are also highlighted. The specific topics which are discussed are as follows (1) inorganic nanomaterials for photo voltaics, (2) nanomaterials for supercapacitors, (3) nanostructured electrodes for lithium ion batteries, (4) nanomaterials for photocatalytic hydrogen generation, (5) carbon-based nanocomposites for hydrogen storage, (6) electro catalysts for fuel cells.

Inorganic Nanomaterials for Photovoltaic

Photovoltaic cells like dye-sensitized solar cells and quantum dot-sensitized solar cells are made of the nanostructured inorganic materials which have a large specific surface area so that sufficient dye molecules and quantum dots can be adsorbed onto the inorganic materials, serving as an antenna for optical absorption. The nanostructured inorganic network must possess long lifetime, excellent charge mobility and also possess some light scattering or photon trapping capability. This chapter will summarize the applications of nanostructures in solar cells, including the effect of quantum dots, large internal surface area of nanocrystals line films for dye-sensitized solar cells, and surface plasmon resonance of metal nanoparticles.

Quantum Dots

Inorganic semiconducting materials have been used in the synthesis of nano-sized particles of controllable dimensions. As the particle size becomes very small (on a nanometric scale) as compared to the bulk material, nanosized particles giving rise to the so-called quantum confinement effect. Quantum dots are nanosized particles which exhibits a fine band gap across a wide range of energy levels. Quantum dots are semiconductor nano-crystals with dimensions comparable to the Bohr radius of an exciton given by:

$$r_{exciton} = (em_0/m^*)r_o$$

Where e is the relative dielectric constant of the semiconductor material, m_0 is the mass of a free electron, m^* is the reduced effective mass which is given by

$$m^* = m_e + m_h / m_e m_h.$$

Where m_e and m_h are the electron and hole effective masses, respectively, and r_0 is the Bohr radius of the hydrogen atom which is equal to 0.529 Å (Manasreh, 2012 and Ashby et al, 2009).

The Bohr radius of the exciton is in the range of 1–10 nm for most semiconductors e.g; Si has 4.2 nm, CdS has 3.1 nm, CdSe has 6.1 nm and ZnO has 2.2 nm. However, for some semiconductors like PbS, PbSe and InSb the excitonic Bohr radii are relatively large which is 20.4 nm, 46 nm, and 67.5 nm respectively (Fahlman, 2011 and Grahn, 1999). As a result of the comparable diamensions of quantum dots with the excitonic Bohr radius of the semiconductor, the electrons in quantum dots gives rise to the quantum confinement effect. As there is the inverse relation between energy and Bohr radius:

$$(Eg \ \alpha \ 1/r^2),$$

the quantum dots may achieve easily a strong confinement effect in a semiconductor with a larger excitonic Bohr radius. Due to the quantum confinement effect the energy band gap of a quantum dot, Eg, is dependent on the particle size. So, the energy levels in the quantum dots are tunable by changing their size, which in turn defines the band gap. In bulk materials, for a particular material there is a fixed band gap. The ability to tune the band gap makes quantum dots desirable for their applications in light emitting diodes (LEDs) for full color displays (Kim et al, 2011), and in quantum dot-sensitized solar cells. For the sun's photon distribution, the materials with a band gap of 1.34 eV showed the maximum solar conversion efficiency according to Shockley-Quiesser limit. However, the materials with lower band gap will generate electricity from lower energy photons and vice versa. In some materials like CdS and CdSe the quantum dots acting as sensitizer adsorb on a porous oxide nano crystalline film to harvest light and inject electrons into the oxide and these have been most extensively studied for quantum dot-sensitized solar cells. For quantum dot-sensitized solar cells, in order to get more quantum dots adsorbed on the photo electrode film possibly smaller quantum dots are preferred. Smaller quantum dots have also demonstrated a higher electron injection rate than their larger counterparts (Kamat, 2012). However, too small quantum dots lower the optical absorption of the photo electrode film which brings negative impacts on the solar cells. This is because too small quantum dots would lead to increased blue shift in the absorption edge.

Dye-Sensitized Solar Cells

In the early nineties the evolution of dye-sensitized solar cells (DSCs) is a major breakthrough in the application of such mesoscopic films with the report of a solar cell based on the concept of dye-sensitization. The use of nanostructures in the form of films can greatly benefit the solar cells by providing significantly higher internal surface area than bulk material. DSCs are a type of photo electrochemical system for the conversion of solar-to-electricity, which typically includes a photoanode which acts as a working electrode for light harvesting and charge separation, cathode as a counter electrode to transport the electrons received from an external circuit, and an electrolyte filled between the two electrodes that provides redox couples allowing for reduction of the photoanode (Fig. 1a). Initially the photoanode of DSCs made of a narrow band-gap semiconductor with the expectation to absorb visible light. However, due to a small interface formed between the semi-conductor photoanode and the electrolyte, the cells only achieved efficiencies in the range of 0.4–1%. Also, the semiconductor was porne to corrosion due to a reaction with the electrode. The problem of corrosion was solved by the use of wide band-gap oxides for the photoanode on which a layer of dye was coated as sensitizer for light harvesting and consequently transferring the electrons to the oxide (Fig. 1b) because the oxides were much more stable for the photo electrochemical reaction. During the last two decades tremendous research efforts on dye-sensitized solar cells have led to the identification of several designs of DSC in terms of color, transparency and portability (Kalyanasundaram, 2010). In the standard design the DSC uses mesoscopic layers of TiO_2 as the key substrate and electron-acceptor and the redox electrolyte is the mixture of iodine and iodide. The solar conversion efficiency for this design with Ru-dyes as the light absorber has reached an efficiency of 11.4% (Han et al, 2012). The Zn-porphyrin dye (YD2) has good light absorption properties and consists of polypyridine complex of Co(III) as the redox mediator and has the highest solar conversion efficiency of 12.4% (Yella et al, 2011). Recently, Miyasaka, Snaith and coworkers have reported a novel meso super-structured solar cell based on a highly crystalline Peroskite light absorber and spiro-OMeTAD as the electron couple (Lee et al, 2012). The solar conversion efficiency of this solar cell is 10.9% in a single junction device and delivers 1.1 V open circuit voltage. The efficiency of DSCs depends upon the dye used and the choice of dyes has expanded significantly. With the introduction of various donors, acceptors and p-spacer units to the basic chromophoric unit absorption and redox properties can be modified (family of dyes referred to as D–p–A dyes). Palomares et al. have discussed recent progress in the design of photosensitizers using various porphyrins, phthalocyanines and organic dyes such as squarines, indolenes and perylenes as examples (Clifford et al, 2012). Also, Yang et al. described the design of a DSC with 7.7% conversion efficiency using organic dyes with quinacridone and furan moieties as planar p-spacers (Yand et al, 2012).

In addition to the electronic properties, the performance of a dye-sensitized solar cell can be influenced by the morphological properties of the oxide anode. Mesoporous films or nanocrystalline film consisting of B15 nm sized nanoparticles provides an extremely large internal surface area for dye adsorption and limited pore diffusion due to smaller pore sizes (Fig. 1d). It was demonstrated that the internal surface area for such a nanocrystalline film with 1 cm ^{2} geometric area and 10 mm thickness was as high as B780 cm^2, meaning an B780-fold increase in the adsorption area when compared to a planar film. The nanocrystalline film in addition to provide large internal surface area, anatase TiO_2 nanoparticles with exposed (101) facets, which allow the dye molecules to form highly dense monolayer adsorption and inject electrons highly efficiently, were also thought to be an important reason for this success (Gratzel, 2004).

Besides TiO_2 nanoparticles many other nanostructures including nanoparticles, nanowires/nanorods, nanotubes, and core shell structures of oxides such as SnO_2, ZnO, Nb_2O_5, etc, have also been extensively studied for DSCs from long time, with the expectations of not only providing a large internal surface area to the photoelectrode film, but also giving rise to other functions to enhance the optical absorption or electrontransport (Zhang and Cao, 2011 and Zhang et al, 2012).

Figure 1. Dye-sensitized solar cell (DSC). (a) The structure of a DSC, (b) dye adsorption on oxide and electron injection from dye to oxide, (c) schematic drawing showing the structure of a DSC photoelectrode film made of nanoparticles, and (d) SEM image of TiO2 nano crystalline film used in conventional DSCs (Gratzel, 2003).

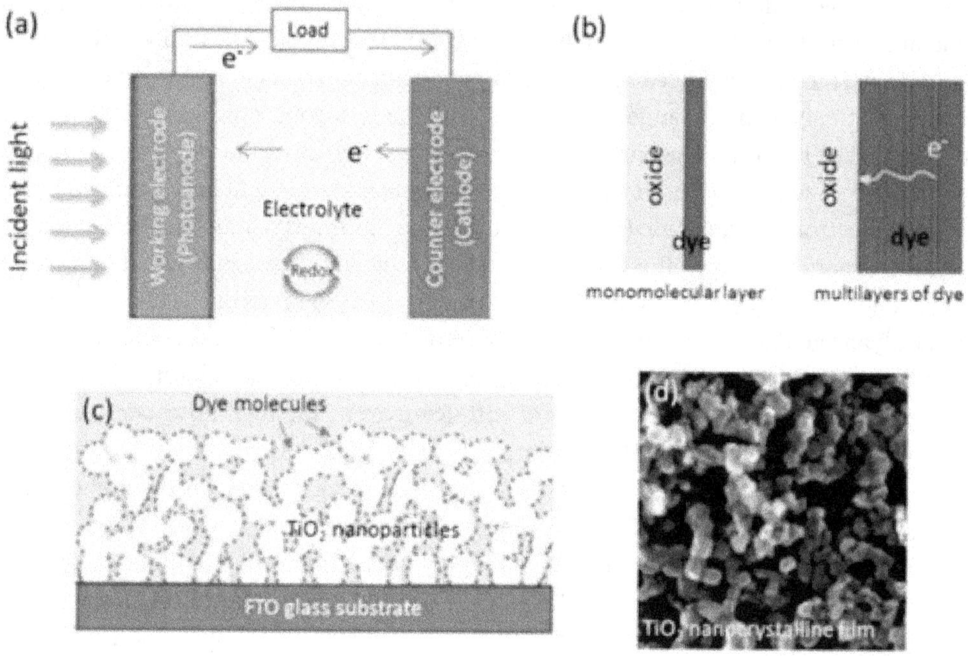

Surface Plasmon Resonance of Metal Nanoparticles

Another effective approach that can be used to enhance the optical absorption of solar cells is surface plasmon resonance (SPR) generated by metal nanoparticles is another effective approach that can be used to enhance the optical absorption of solar cell film. Surface plasmon is a process that specifically exists in metal, and it is the resonant oscillation of conduction between electrons at the interface between negative and positive permittivity material stimulated by incident light. SPR is the basis for measuring adsorption of material onto the planar metal surface or onto the surface of metal nanoparticles. In the case of metal nanoparticles due to the oscillation of electrons, the electron cloud gets deviated from the geometric center of the metal and an oscillation of the electron cloud in the metal in the direction perpendicular to that of light wave propagation, forming the so-called surface plasmon resonance.

SPR enhancement of the optical absorption of a solar cell film can be achieved through several different SPR mechanisms e.g., the far field scattering effect, the near-field localized or propagating SPR modes, and some other plasmonic modes like wave guide mode and plasmon-cavity mode (Atwater et al, 2010 and Yao et al, 2014, Feng et al 2018) (Fig. 2). In the first mechanism the enhancement of optical absorption can be achieved due to the increase of the optical path of incident photons and the decrease of the reflection at illuminated surfaces. The second mechanism is based on the fact that the number of absorption events is increased, because the metallic nanostructures can confine electromagnetic waves at the metal-dielectric interface and produce intense near field. The third mechanism involves the photoexcited carriers in the metal nanoparticles directly injecting into the semiconductor, making contributions to improve the photocurrent of the solar cell (Ferry et al, 2010).

Figure 2. Mechanisms of surface plasmon resonance enhancing optical absorption of solar cells. (a) Far field scattering leading to a prolonged optical path, (b) near field scattering causing local field enhancement, and (c) direct injection of photoexcited carriers into the semiconductor (Bharadwaj et al, 2009).

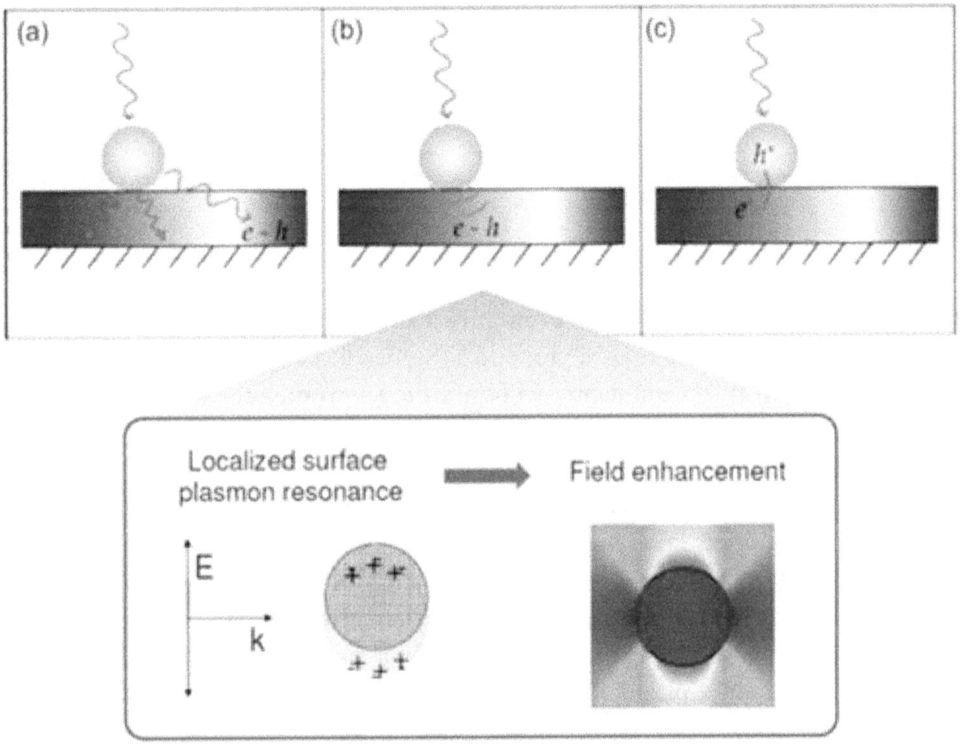

Till date, the metals like gold and silver are the most often adopted for plasmonic enhancement in solar cells because the plasmonic resonance is readily observed in Au and Ag due to their delocalized valence electrons (Kreibig and Vollmer, 1995). Catchpole et al. studied that the SPR-induced optical absorption enhancement with Ag and Au nanoparticles deposited on a Si_3N_4 under layer on silicon (Catchpole and Polman, 2008). It was described that the SPR of the metal nanoparticles gives rise to optical absorption enhancement which were originated from light scattering. The fraction of incident light scattered into the substrate (i.e., silicon) was dependent upon the shape of the nanoparticles to a large extent. Nanoparticles with different shapes like cylindrical, hemispherical, and spherical shapes were compared; it had been found that among these shapes the cylindrical nanoparticles and hemispherical nanoparticles had a much better capability of scattering light into the substrate (Fig. 3a). In the spherical nanoparticles, smaller nanoparticles gave stronger scattering than the larger ones. Among the Ag and Au nanoparticles, it was found that the Ag hemispherical nanoparticles might achieve more scattering and therefore better enhancement in the optical absorption than the Au hemispherical nanoparticles (Fig. 3b). The thickness of the Si_3N_4 under layer was also found to affect the scattering significantly (Fig. 3c).

Figure 3. Impact of (a) shape and (b) material selection of metal nanoparticles, and (c) the thickness of the underlayer on the SPR-induced optical absorption enhancement (Catchpole and Polman, 2008).

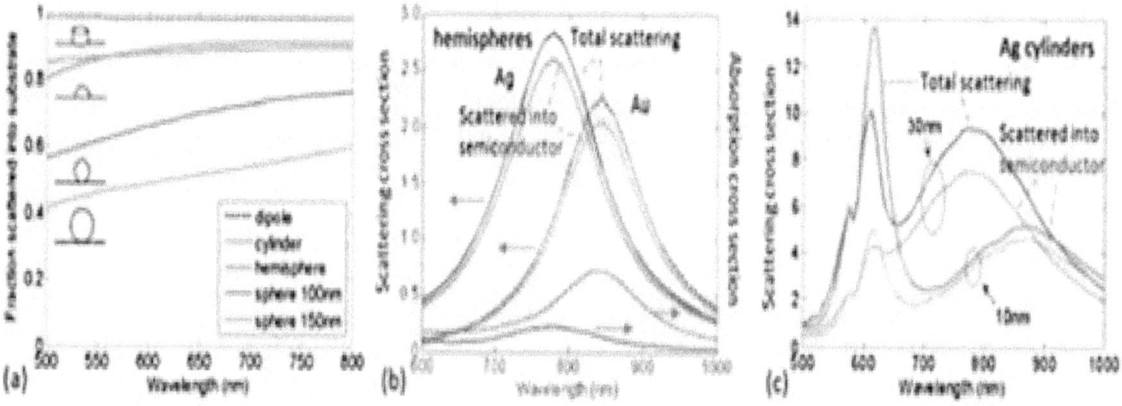

In recent years, two-dimensional (2D) atom-thick materials have attracted great attention due to their fantastic thermal, electric and optical properties (Stylianakis et al, 2017). 2D materials have been used in OPV devices to work concomitantly with metallic nanostructures to advance the stability and solar energy harvest. Lee et al. transferred graphene both on top and at the bottom of Ag NRs networks to protect them against thermal degradation. The graphene-Ag-graphene produced better transmittance than pure Ag NRs upon constructive interference of the incident light.

To know the plasmonic effect in 2D materials is of great importance. The SPR frequency of graphene resides in the range of 1012–1014 Hz. It has been reported that graphene plasmons can be excited at visible wavelength (Lange et al, 2014). However, even they were involved in the solar cells, the plasmonics from the 2D materials have scarcely been discussed. Viable approaches still need to be developed to unambiguously discriminate the plasmonics of non-metal materials from those of the metals.

Nanostructured Materials for Supercapacitors

It is the common name used electrochemical capacitors or ultra-capacitors. Supercapacitors are a class of energy storage devices which produces large energy in short intervals of time and are capable of rapid charging and discharging. They have very good storage capacities which are higher than that of conventional dielectric capacitors. They can operate in a wide range of temperatures and are also safe and environmentally friendly. In general, there are two classes of supercapacitor, each defined by the charge storage mechanism- electric double-layer capacitors (EDLC) and redox supercapacitors or pseudo-capacitors. The electrical double layer capacitors (EDLC) operates by adsorbing–desorbing charged ions from an electrolyte onto high surface area electrodes forming a double layer structure. While as the pseudo-capacitors or redox supercapacitors uses transition metal oxides or electrical conducting polymers as electrode materials, with the charge storage depending on fast faradic redox reactions.

An EDLC consists of two identical electrodes, typically carbon based, separated by an ion permeable membrane, and immersed in an ionic electrolyte. In supercapacitors energy storage occurs by the formation of an electrochemical double layer by the accumulation of charges onto active surface areas. The energy density of supercapacitors depends on the amount of active surface area available per unit mass of the electrode. Nanomaterials, very high specific surface areas, can be used as active materials in these devices. The charging and discharging of a supercapacitor can be defined by the charge separation and recombination (Conway, 1999). Figure 4 is a schematic representation of the charge discharge mechanisms in a conventional double layer supercapacitor.

Figure 4. Schematic of the mechanism of charge and discharge in an EDLC showing the charge separation and recombination during charging and discharging process leading to the formation of double layer at the electrode.

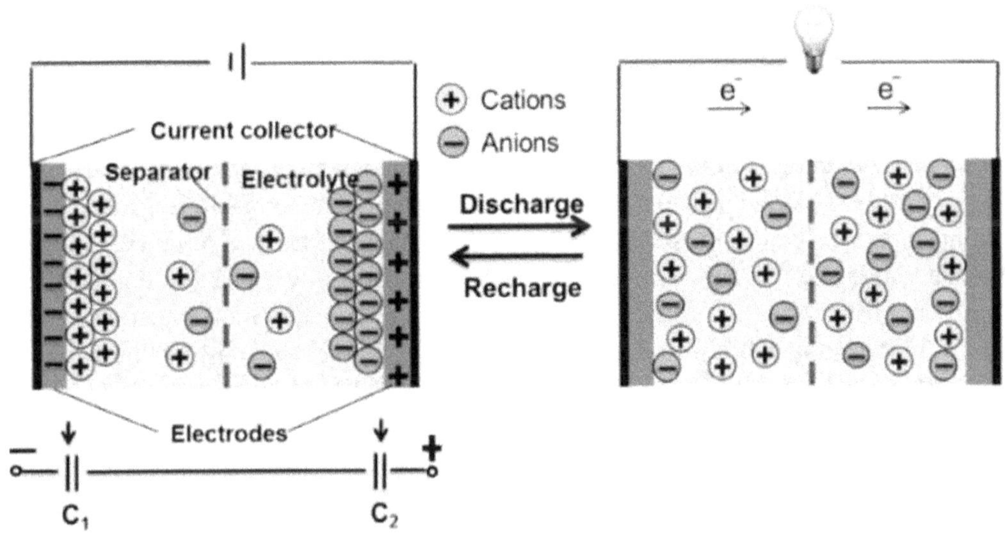

For EDLCs, the capacitance (C) is equal to C = eA/d which shows that capacitance is related to the surface area, the effective dielectric constant (e) and the double layer thickness (d). The combination of high surface area and small charge separation is necessary for high capacitance. The supercapacitor technology can be progressed by moving from conventional to nanostructured electrodes. In the case of supercapacitors, the electrode requirements are less demanding than in batteries, at least in terms of electrode compaction, because power is predominant over energy density. Thus, the nano powders with their high surface area (primary nanoparticles) are potentially more important; hence the incredible interest in nano powders and their rapid uptake for supercapacitor based storage sources. The carbon due to its high specific surface area, large specific capacitances, low material costs, etc can be used as electrodes for supercapacitors (Zhang and Zhao, 2009). The energy density of the device depends on the amount of active surface area available per unit mass of the electrode. Use of nanostructured carbons, such as aerogels (Wang et al, 2001), nanotubes (Niu et al, 1997) and nano templates (Nelson and Owen, 2003) are getting a lot of attention. The advantages of carbon aerogels lie mainly in their low ionic and electronic charging resistance and in their potential use as binderless electrodes. The carbon aerogel electrode replaces the standard carbon fibre and improves the capacitance and cyclability. The carbon nanotubes, because of their unique architecture, are now intensively studied as new electrode materials for supercapacitor structures despite of cost issue. However, it is important to keep in mind the challenges that arise by using nanostructured materials. To achieve a higher capacitance significant research effort has been made by researchers to establish correlation between specific surface area (to ensure high capacitance) and pore-size distribution (to permit easy access for the electrolyte). In general, smaller pore sizes correlate with higher energy density while larger pore sizes correlate with higher power density (Liu et al, 2010).

Graphene based electrodes show great attention due to their excellent electronic and electrical properties, good chemical stability, high surface area and easy processability. Khanra et al. reports the surface modification of graphene using 9-anthracene carboxylic acid to improve the graphene performance in supercapacitors. (Khanra et al, 2012). Fic et al. described the possible use of protic aqueous electrolytes for better control of the charge transfer processes taking place at the electrical double layer (Fic et al, 2012).

Nanostructured materials have led to the development of new supercapacitor technologies. Telcordia's researchers have introduced the so-called hybrid supercapacitors (HSCs), to obtain the benefits of nano-material electrodes, and proposed a new approach to energy storage (Amatucci et al, 2001). In HSCs is similar to that of a carbon EDLC i.e; capacitive carbon electrode and the other negative electrode consists of a nanostructured lithium titanate compound which undergoes a reversible faradic intercalation reaction (Brodd et al, 2004). The use of a nanostructured $Li_4Ti_5O_{12}$, as the negative electrode, has proved an innovation as there is no degradation in performance from charge/discharge-induced strain. The nano-material $Li_4Ti_5O_{12}$ shows excellent cyclability, rate capability and safety, thus can be explored for capacitor and battery use. The nanostructured $Li_4Ti_5O_{12}$ gives cycle life comparable to that of supercapacitors in the in the hybrid supercapacitor devices, overcomes the lifespan limitations generally associated with batteries. Besides $Li_4Ti_5O_{12}$, other nanostructured oxide materials can be engineered so as to obtain hybrid devices operating over a wide range of voltages.

For pseudo-capacitors, the capacitance involves voltage dependent reversible Faradic reactions between the electrode and the electrolyte, either in the form of surface adsorption–desorption of ions, redox reactions with the electrolyte, or doping–undoping of the electrode materials. Commonly used materials for pseudo-capacitors include conducting polymers and metal oxides or nitrides. Due to different oxidation states of the electro active material redox reactions takes place. Often, reactions do not propagate into the bulk material, and occur only at the electrode–electrolyte interface (Hall et al, 2010). Pseudo-capacitive materials includes conducting polymers, such as polyaniline, polypyrrole, and polythiophene, and metal oxides, such as RuO, MnO, CoO, etc.

Nanostructured Electrodes for Lithium Ion Batteries

Lithium-ion batteries are one of the great successes of modern science and technology (Scrosati, 1995). The development of lithium ion batteries have revolutionized the energy industry by making portable energy more efficient and robust (Nagaura and Tozawa, 1990). A typical lithium ion battery consists of three major components: anode, cathode, and electrolyte. The two electrodes are made up of a lithium-ion intercalation negative electrode (generally graphite), and a lithium-ion intercalation positive electrode (generally the lithium metal oxide, $LiCoO_2$), these being separated by a electronically insulating and ion permeable porous separator membrane, confined in an electrolyte containing lithium salt, most commonly, $LiPF_6$ in ethylene carbonate–diethyl carbonate. The device converts chemical potential into electrical energy via Faradaic reactions, which include heterogeneous charge transfer processes occurring at the surface of an electrode. In case of Li-ion battery the charging process involves an energy reversal from electrical energy to a chemical potential. Figure 5 illustrates the schematic of a typical lithium ion battery mechanism (Scrosati, 2007). On charging, lithium ions are deintercalated from the layered $LiCoO_2$

intercalation host, pass through the electrolyte, and are intercalated between the graphite layers in the anode. The process gets reversed on discharging. The battery performance is related to the intrinsic property of the materials which is the mass and charge transfer within the electrodes occurring due to Faradaic reactions and dimensional variation. The reaction rate and transfer processes for the electrode materials depends upon the composition, crystal structure, and morphology, also overall electrochemical performance can be varied accordingly (Goodenough and Kim, 2010).

Figure 5. Schematic representation of the charge and discharge mechanisms in a lithium ion battery (Jiu et al, 2006).

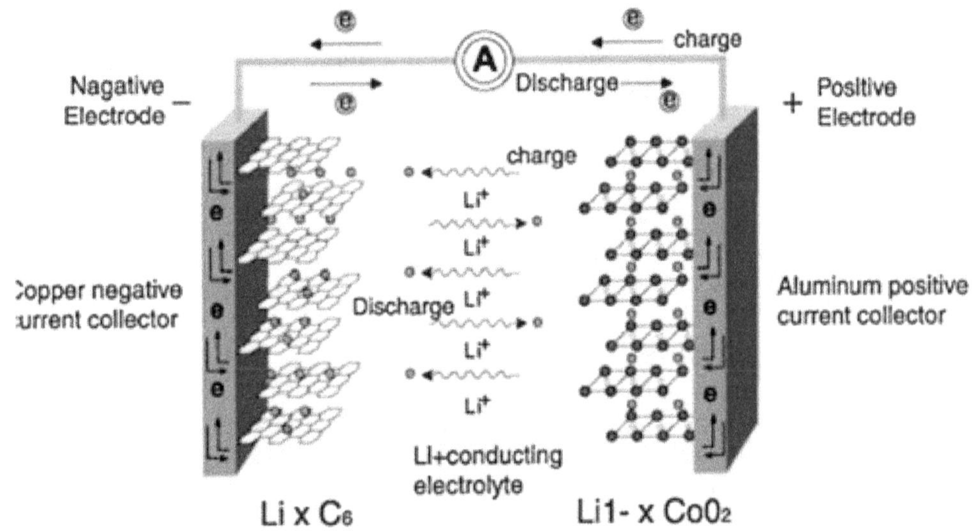

The development and implementation of nanostructured electrodes has led to great improvement in Li-ion battery performance (Guo et al, 2008).Nanostructured electrodes should offer a set of properties including large specific surface area for fast interfacial Faradaic reaction, small distance for mass and charge transport, and small dimensions to accommodate the volume change accompanied with lithium ion insertion and extraction. Nanostructured electrodes should possess more open space to accommodate more guest ions and to allow the ions to diffuse effectively in order to get high energy and power density as well as long cyclic life. Several studies have also revealed that the implementation of nanostructured electrodes has led to an increase in the specific capacity beyond the theoretical limits (Balaya et al, 2006 and Liu et al, 2011). The increased storage capacity has been attributed to the nanoscale dimensions of nanostructures that make the surface and grain interface effects more prominent. A pseudo-capacitive storage mechanism will ultimately begin to accommodate lithium ions on the surface/interface of the particles when they are below a critical particle size (Balaya et al, 2006).

Some metals acts as negative electrodes in lithium-ion batteries as it stores lithium and becomes the competitive candidates for new types of anodes. A number of metals and semiconductors, for example tin, aluminium and silicon reacts with lithium to form alloys by electrochemical processes which are partially reversible and of low voltage (relative to lithium), and provides a specific capacity much larger than that offered by conventional graphite (Huggins, 1999 and Winter and Besenhard, 1999). For example, compared with the graphite which has capacity 372 mA h g^{-1}, whereas lithium alloys such as $Li_{22}Sn_5$ and $Li_{22}Si_5$ have much higher capacity (990 mA h $g^{-1}$for $Li_{22}Sn_5$ and 4200 mA h g^{-1} for $Li_{22}Si_5$) (Jiu et al, 2006). The poor cyclic stability of the alloy electrode and the pulverization of the material occur due to large volumetric changes induced by the repeated alloying and de-alloying (Jiu et al, 2006). Attempts have been attempts to limit these side effects, among them the active/inactive nanocomposite concept represents one attractive route. Several authors have discussed the mechanism which involves mixing of two materials, one reacting with lithium whereas the other acts as an inactive confining buffer. The use of nano-size metallic clusters within this composite act as lithium hosts considerably suppresses the associated strains, and therefore improves the reversibility of the alloying reaction. By applying this concept through different systems such as SnO-based glasses (Idota et al, 1997), or composites such as Sn–Fe–C (Mao et al, 1999), Sn–Mn–C (Beaulieu et al, 2000) or Si–C (Yang et al, 2003), several authors have demonstrated that these electrodes show a considerable improvement in their cycling response in lithium cells. Recent progress on nanostructured silicon electrode is a good example (Ohara et al, 2004 and Chan et al, 2010). The Si–C nanocomposites have also attracted great interest due its capacity which is as high as 1,000 mA h g^{-1} for more than 100 cycles (Novak, 2004).

Figure 6. Schematic representation of morphological changes that occur in Si during electrochemical cycling (Chan et al, 2007).

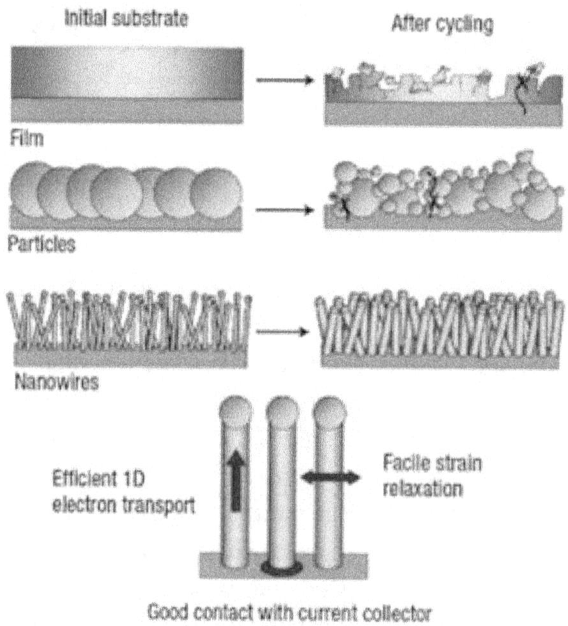

Silicon nanotubes and nanowires have shown high discharge capacities and stable cycling over tens of cycles, with reversible capacities greater than 3400 mA h g^{-1} approximately as shown in Fig. 6 (Chan et al, 2007). Nanotube and nanowire-based electrodes can accommodate material expansion during cycling, and nanowires can be grown directly onto the current collector to form a direct current pathway (Chan et al, 2007 and Song et al, 2010). The small dimensions of nanowires and nanotubes results in strain relaxation readily and was shown by partially coating Si nanowire with electrochemically inactive nickel. The ability for silicon nanowires to deform without fracture may contribute to the high reversible capacities observed (Chan et al, 2007 and Song et al, 2010).

Alternatively, for the applications of anode it has been found that the Li-insertion activities in the lithium titanites inspired interests in titanium oxide-based nanomaterials (Yang et al, 2009 and Baudrin et al, 2007). $Li_4Ti_5O_{12}$ shows a specific capacity of 175 mA h g^{-1} and serves as an excellent host for reversible Li-insertion/extraction. TiO_2 itself offers a capacity up to its value at 335 mA h g^{-1}. The redox reaction between the Li^+/Li redox couple occurs typically at 1.5–1.8 V. The TiO_2 electrodes are safer than the graphite or silicon anode due to its relative high potentials and render fewer reactions at the electrode/electrolyte interfaces. The electrochemical performance of TiO_2 electrode in its bulk form is limited because of the poor conductivity of Li+ accompanied by electrons. TiO_2 has been fabricated into various nanostructures that resulted in improved Li insertion characteristics to improve the charge/ion transport properties. With the decrease in particle size the Li-reactivity has been found to increase (Hu et al, 2006 and Guo et al, 2007). For example, 0.8 mol Li-insertion into nanostructured rutile TiO_2 (10 nm^{x}40 nm) at room temperature has been reported, while only 0.1–0.25 mol of Li into micrometer-sized rutile (Hu et al, 2006). Fig. 7 shows a comparison of the electrochemical performance of TiO rutile samples with three sizes (Baudrin et al, 2007).

Only a very amount of lithium ions (0.03Li/TiO_2) can be inserted into the bulk rutile in a galvanostatic mode (current 30 mA g^{-1}, i.e. the reaction of one lithium ion per 11 h). Nanosized TiO_2 (50 nm) could be inserted up to 0.23 Li per TiO_2 rutile. This corresponds to a specific capacity of 77 mA h g^{-1} (at 1/10 C) during the first reduction down to 1.0 V. When the size was decreased to 10 nm rutile rod particles (10 nm*200 nm), Li insertion was up to 0.85 Li during the first reduction under the same test conditions.

Figure 7. The electrochemical performance of TiO_2 rutile samples with three sizes. Nanorod: 10 nm 200 nm, commercial nano: 50 nm, bulk:1 mm. (A) Potential-capacity profiles. (B) Cycle performances. Test condition: 30 mA hg current between 3 V and 1 V in 1 M LiPF6 EC/DMC PC electrolyte at 20 1C (Baudrin et al, 2007).

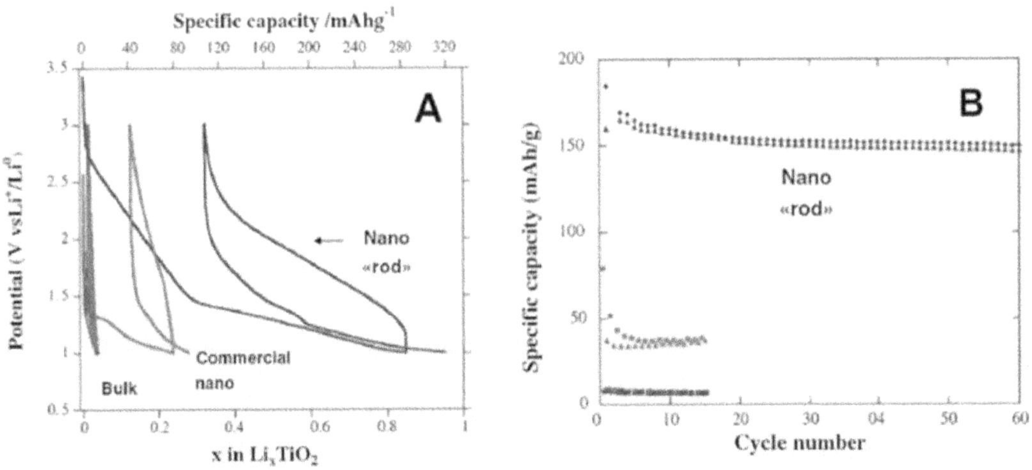

On the other hand the classical cathode materials formed by the nanomaterials such as $LiCoO_2$, $LiNiO_2$ or their solid solutions can lead to greater reaction with the electrolyte, and are safer even at high temperatures, than the use of such materials in the bulk form. Also Olivine $LiFePO_4$ has been considered a promising candidate as cathode material for large scale lithium-ion batteries used for hybrid electric vehicles (HEVs) or electric vehicles (EVs). The material has low cost, low toxicity, long cycle ability and highly safer. Earlier many researchers reported that the rate performance of $LiFePO_4$ was greatly limited by the slow diffusion of lithium ion in $LiFePO_4$, and/or the low electronic conductivity.

The poor electrochemical performance of $LiFePO_4$ is because of small diffusion coefficient (10^{-14}–$10^{-16} cm^2 s^{-1}$) of lithium ion in $LiFePO_4$. For the power performance of $LiFePO_4$ transports of lithium ions and of electrons at the interface are quite important. The carbon-coated $LiFePO_4$ nanorods with a length of up to 100 nm showed much higher rate capability of 130 mA h g^{-1} at a 10 C rate (Muraliganth et al, 2008). It was also found that the carbon-free $LiFePO_4$ with a small dimensions (100–200 nm) exhibited a similar specific capacity of 147 mA h g^{-1} at a 5 C rate and high capacity retention upon cycling to a carbon-coated $LiFePO_4$ (Delacourt et al, 2006). The improved electrochemical properties were attributed to the small size of the material, which facilitates both ionic and electronic transport within the nanostructures.

Figure 8. Schematic illustration of the photocatalytic hydrogen generation system. (A) An electrode system and (B) a photocatalytic particle system (TiO_2 is an example used here, though there are limited reports for O_2 evolution on TiO_2).

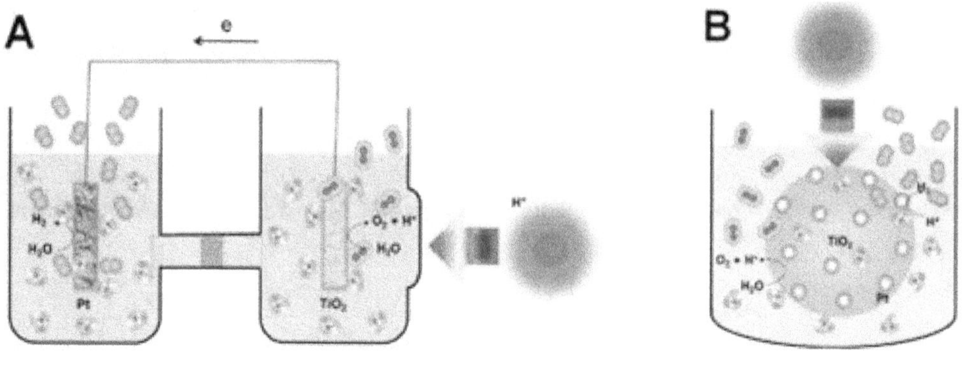

Nanomaterials for Photocatalytic Hydrogen Generation

The driving force of solar hydrogen generation is the dream of renewable clean fuels (Lewis and Crabtree, 2005 and Lewis, 2007). Hydrogen gas can be directly obtained from splitting of water using sunlight (photodecomposition of water), then this endless source of clean fuel has many applications. The key media for the photodecomposition of water into oxygen and hydrogen by the irradiation of sunlight is the semiconductor materials. There are two basic methods for the solar hydrogen generation: an electrode system and a particle system, as schematically shown in Fig. 8. Both the methods are based on the same principles in which a semiconductor acts as the light absorber by which electron–hole pairs are generated upon solar irradiation, while a metal acts as the electron trapper or a co-catalyst (Chen et al, 2010). When the semiconductor electrode or particle absorbs sunlight electrons are excited from the valence band to the conduction band photo-generated electrons and holes are produced. In the first method i.e electrode system the excited electrons can be transported to the metal electrode connected by an external circuit whereas in the second method i.e particle system the excited electrons can be directly transferred to the metal particles deposited on the surface of the semiconductor particle.

The processes in the photocatalytic generation of hydrogen by using particle system as an example are illustrated in Fig. 9. The process involves light absorption of the semiconductor photocatalyst, generation and recombination of the excited electrons and holes, separation, migration, and trap of excited charges, and transfer of excited charges to water or other molecules to produce hydrogen. The amount of hydrogen generated is largely determined by the amount of excited electrons that survived to reduce protons at the water–metal interface. Thus, the semiconductor photocatalyst should first have a sufficiently small band gap to absorb as many photons from the sun as possible. After absorbing photons, the semiconductor photocatalyst should have a high efficiency in generating excited charges, instead of producing heat.

For the photocatalytic hydrogen generation semiconductor nanomaterials are more advantageous than their bulk counterparts due to the higher surface area (Roduner, 2006), higher optical absorption (Alivisatos, 1996). As the size of nanomaterials decreases, their optical absorption may increase dramatically, Shorter charge migration length and Tunable electronic structure (Burda et al, 2005). Fujishima and Honda in 1972 reported the photocatalytic hydrogen generation on a TiO_2 single crystal under UV light irradiation (Fujishima and Honda, 1972). TiO_2 has become one of the most effective semiconductor photocatalysts (Nozik, 1975). However, the electronic band gap of TiO_2 in the ultraviolet (UV) wavelength region has largely limited the overall photocatalytic efficiency. To achiev high efficiency for solar hydrogen production the narrowing of band gap in TiO_2 is important. Various metal and nonmetal elements have been doped into the TiO_2 lattice and visible-light absorption has been obtained (et al, 1982).

Figure 9. Illustration of the processes involved in the photocatalytic hydrogen generation through water splitting (Linsebigler et al, 1995).

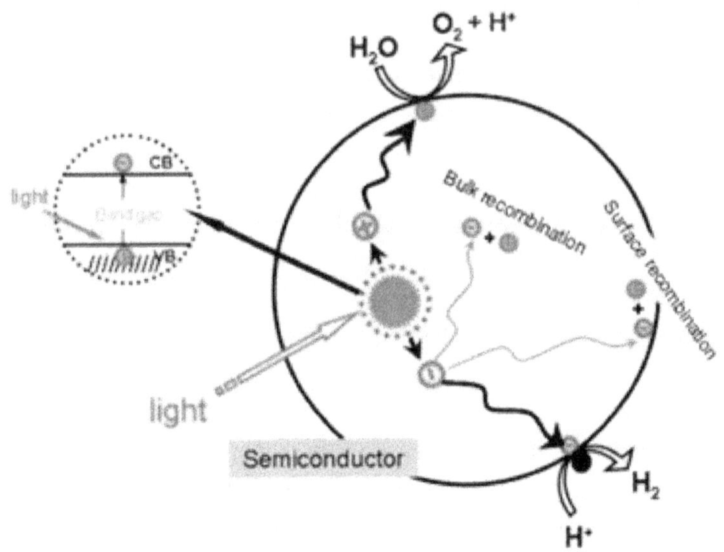

The photocatalytic activity of CdS nanorods and nanowires has also been studied for the evolution of hydrogen (Berr et al, 2010). The hydrogen evolution on non decorated CdS nanorods as well as decorated with 4.8 nm Pt nanoparticles upon exposure of UV-visible light in the presence of sodium sulfite as the hole scavenger is shown by Fig. 10 (Berr et al, 2010) The non decorated CdS system does not lead to H_2 evolution but the decorated CdS with Pt nanoparticles yields hydrogen at a rate of 5 mmol g^{-1} h^{-1}. The quantum yield of Pt-decorated samples reaches upto 3.9%, with average quantum yields in the range of 2–3%. The photocatalytic activity of Pt-decorated CdS nanorods is determined by subnanometer size Pt clusters and not by the presence of larger Pt nanoparticles (Berr et al, 2010).

Figure 10. (A) TEM images of CdS nanorods. (B) TEM images of CdS nanorods decorated with 4.8 nm large Pt nanoparticles. (C) Hydrogen evolution (in millimoles of H2 per gram of CdS; more than 99% of incoming light is absorbed by the sample) from an aqueous solution containing CdS nanorods (1) nondecorated and (2) decorated with Pt. (Berr et al, 2010).

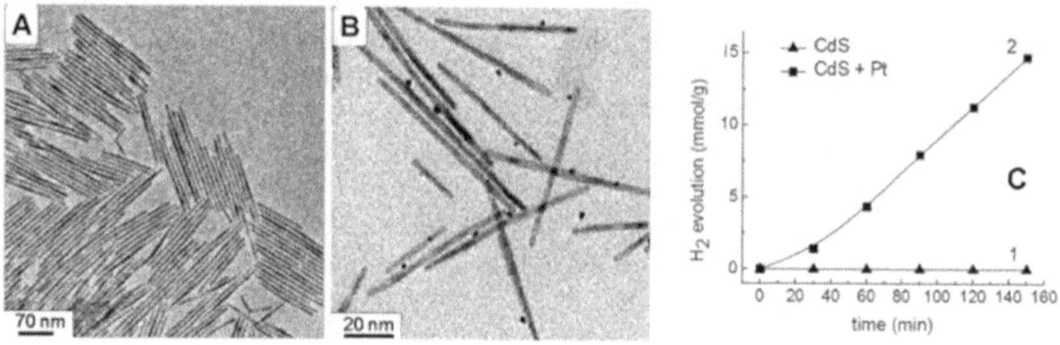

Electrocatalysts for Fuel Cells

In a polymer electrolyte membrane fuel cell, porous carbon is the most widely used electro catalyst support material and even derivatives of porous carbon can be used as electro catalyst. It is the basic material in the gas diffusion layer and it is also incorporated into composite membranes to enhance their mechanical strength. Pt (Pt alloy) nanoparticles supported on porous materials are used in most PEM fuel cell as electro catalysts. The support materials play a key role in improving Pt utilization, stability and catalytic activity. The general requirements for the electro catalyst support (Shao et al, 2009) are (1) high specific surface area and high porosity, which are necessary for improving the dispersion of catalytic metals and mass transfer; (2) high electrochemical stability under fuel cell operating conditions; (3) high electric conductivity; and (4) easy Pt recycling in the used electro catalyst.

Various nanostructured carbon materials have been developed for electro catalyst support for PEM fuel cells which includes carbon nanotubes (CNT), mesoporous carbon, the newly developed graphene, etc.

CNTs are superior to conventional carbon black for PEM fuel cell electro catalyst support in many ways (Shao et al, 2006): (1) the electrochemically durability of CNTs are high (2) CNTs provides high electric conductivity and specific interaction between Pt and CNT support resulting in a high catalytic activity (3) CNTs have few impurities (4) CNTs are free from the deep-crack structure, which is the so-called ‘‘dead zone’’ of electro catalysts because Pt nanoparticles have no catalytic activity when deposited there due to the absence of electrochemical triple-phase boundary.

Another material that has been extensively studied as catalyst supports for PEM fuel cells is Mesoporous carbon (MC) (Su, 2005). The performance of the mesoporous carbon supported electro catalysts depends upon the pore structures and sizes. The highest performance was found for the porous carbon with mesopores whose pore size is 20–25 nm as the support (Chai et al, 2004).

The newly developed carbon material which has shows enhanced activity and durability as fuel cell catalyst support is Graphene (Yoo et al, 2009 and Kou et al, 2011). Graphene has been found to enhance the electro catalytic activity of Pt cluster electro catalysts supported on it by a factor of 4 for methanol oxidation (Yoo et al, 2009). Graphene also improves the stability of Pt electro catalysts.

CONCLUSION

Nanostructured material finds extensive applications for the energy storage and conversion. In this chapter, we have summarized the recent progress of nanostructured material in various types of energy storage like photovoltaic cells, supercapacitors, lithium ion batteries, hydrogen storage and electro catalysts for PEM fuel cells. Nanostructured materials have proven to be effective in enhancing the performance of these devices in view of their novel geometrical characteristics properties. In brief, nanostructures benefit these devices by providing a large surface area to enhance the rate of electrochemical reaction, to improve the optical absorption in solar cells by generating optical effects and the quantum confinement effect which lead to nanostructured materials achieving energy conversion and storage more efficiently. This chapter also demonstrates how nanoscale materials can significantly change electrode and electrolyte properties, and consequently their performance in devices for energy storage and conversion as compared to their bulk materials. So, the need of the hour is to explore new possible cost-effective nanostructured materials for their better applications to renewable energy production and storage.

REFERENCES

Alivisatos, A. P. (1996). Perspectives on the Physical Chemistry of Semiconductor Nanocrystals. *Journal of Physical Chemistry*, *100*(31), 13226–13239. doi:10.1021/jp9535506

Amatucci, G. G., Badway, F., Du Pasquier, A., & Zheng, T. (2001). An Asymmetric Hybrid Nonaqueous Energy Storage Cell. *Journal of the Electrochemical Society*, *148*(8), A930–A939. doi:10.1149/1.1383553

Ashby, M. F., Ferreira, P. J. S. G., & Schodek, D. L. (2009). *Nanomaterials, nanotechnologies and design: an introduction for engineers and architects*. Elsevier.

Atwater, H. A., & Polman, A. (2010). Erratum: Plasmonics for improved photovoltaic devices. *Nature Materials*, *9*(10), 865. doi:10.1038/nmat2866

Balaya, P., Bhattacharyya, A. J., Jamnik, J., Zhukovskii, Y. F., Kotomin, E. A., & Maier, J. (2006). Nanoionics in the context of lithium batteries. *Journal of Power Sources*, *159*(1), 171–178. doi:10.1016/j.jpowsour.2006.04.115

Bao, N., Shen, L., Takata, T., Lu, D., & Domen, K. (2006). Highly ordered Pt loaded CdS nanowire assays for photocatalytic hydrogen production under visible light. *Chemistry Letters*, *35*(3), 318–319. doi:10.1246/cl.2006.318

Baudrin, E., Cassaignon, S., Koesch, M., Jolivet, J. P., Dupont, L., & Tarascon, J. M. (2007). J. Structural Evolution During the Reaction of Li with NanoSized Rutile Type TiO2 at Room Temperature. *Electrochemistry Communications*, *9*(2), 337–342. doi:10.1016/j.elecom.2006.09.022

Beaulieu, L. Y., & Dahn, J. R. (2000). The reaction of lithium with Sn-Mn-C intermetallics prepared by mechanical alloying. *Journal of the Electrochemical Society*, *147*(9), 3237–3241. doi:10.1149/1.1393889

Berr, M., Vaneski, A., Susha, A. S., Rodrıguez-Fernandez, J., Doblinger, M., Jackel, F., Rogach, A. L., & Feldmann, J. (2010). Colloidal CdS nanorods decorated with subnanometer sized Pt clusters for photocatalytic hydrogen generation. *Applied Physics Letters*, *97*(9), 093108. doi:10.1063/1.3480613

Bharadwaj, P., Deutsch, B., & Novotny, L. (2009). Optical Antennas. Adv. *Opt. Photonics*, *1*(3), 438–483. doi:10.1364/AOP.1.000438

Borgarello, E., Kiwi, J., Gratzel, M., Pelizzetti, E., & Visca, M. (1982). Visible light induced water cleavage in colloidal solutions of chromium-doped titanium dioxide particles. *Journal of the American Chemical Society*, *104*(11), 2996–3002. doi:10.1021/ja00375a010

Brodd, R. J., Bullock, K. R., Leising, R. A., Middaugh, R. L., Miller, J. R., & Takeuchi, E. (2004). Batteries, 1977 to 2002. *Journal of the Electrochemical Society*, *151*(3), K1–K11. doi:10.1149/1.1641042

Bruce, P. G., Scrosati, B., & Tarascon, J.-M. (2008). Nanomaterials for rechargeable lithium batteries. *Angewandte Chemie International Edition*, *47*(16), 2930–2946. doi:10.1002/anie.200702505 PMID:18338357

Burda, C., Chen, X., Narayanan, R., & El-Sayed, M. A. (2005). Chemistry and properties of nanocrystals of different shapes. *Chemical Reviews*, *105*(4), 1025–1102. doi:10.1021/cr030063a PMID:15826010

Catchpole, K., & Polman, A. (2008). Design principles for particle plasmon enhanced solar cells. *Applied Physics Letters*, *93*(19), 191113. doi:10.1063/1.3021072

Chai, G. S., Yoon, S. B., Yu, J. S., Choi, J. H., & Sung, Y. E. (2004). Ordered porous carbons with tunable pore sizes as catalyst supports in direct methanol fuel cell. *The Journal of Physical Chemistry B*, *108*(22), 7074–7079. doi:10.1021/jp0370472

Chan, C. K., Patel, R. N., O'Connell, M. J., Korgel, B. A., & Cui, Y. (2010). Solution-grown silicon nanowires for lithium-ion battery anodes. *ACS Nano*, *4*(3), 1443–1450. doi:10.1021/nn901409q PMID:20201547

Chan, C. K., Peng, H., Liu, G., McIlwrath, K., Zhang, X. F., Huggins, R. A., & Cui, Y. (2007). High-performance lithium battery anodes using silicon nanowires. *Nature Nanotechnology*, *3*(1), 31–35. doi:10.1038/nnano.2007.411 PMID:18654447

Chen, X., Shen, S., Guo, L., & Mao, S. S. (2010). Semiconductor-based Photocatalytic Hydrogen Generation. *Chemical Reviews*, *110*(11), 6503–6570. doi:10.1021/cr1001645 PMID:21062099

Choi, W. C., Woo, S. I., Jeon, M. K., Sohn, J. M., Kim, M. R., & Jeon, H. J. (2005). Platinum Nanoclusters Studded in the Microporous Nanowalls of Ordered Mesoporous Carbon. *Advanced Materials*, *17*(4), 446–451. doi:10.1002/adma.200400978

Clifford, J. N., Planells, M., & Palomares, E. (2012). Advances in high efficiency dye sensitized solar cells based on Ru(ii) free sensitizers and a liquid redox electrolyte. *Journal of Materials Chemistry*, *22*(46), 24195–24201. doi:10.1039/c2jm34289h

Cole, T. (1983). Thermoelectric energy conversion with solid electrolytes. *Science*, *221*(4614), 915–920. doi:10.1126cience.221.4614.915 PMID:17748444

Conway, B. E. (1999). *Electrochemical supercapacitors: scientific fundamentals and technological applications*. Plenum Press. doi:10.1007/978-1-4757-3058-6

Crabtree, G. W., & Lewis, N. S. (2007). Solar energy conversion. *Physics Today*, *60*(3), 37–42. doi:10.1063/1.2718755

Delacourt, C., Poizot, P., Levasseur, S., & Masquelier, C. (2006). Size effects on carbon-free LiFePO. chem. *Solid-State Lett.*, *9*(7), A352. doi:10.1149/1.2201987

Dong, X., Cao, Y., Wang, J., Chan-Park, M. B., Wang, L., Huang, W., & Chen, P. (2012). Hybrid structure of zinc oxide nanorods and three dimensional graphene foam for supercapacitor and electrochemical sensor applications. *RSC Advances*, *2*(10), 4364–4369. doi:10.1039/c2ra01295b

Feng, L., Niu, M., Wen, Z., & Hao, X. (2018). Recent Advances of Plasmonic Organic Solar Cells: Photophysical Investigations. *Polymers*, *10*(2), 123. doi:10.3390/polym10020123 PMID:30966159

Ferry, V. E., Munday, J. N., & Atwater, H. A. (2010). Design considerations for plasmonic photovoltaics. *Advanced Materials*, *22*(43), 4794–4808. doi:10.1002/adma.201000488 PMID:20814916

Fic, K., Frackowiak, E., & Beguin, F. (2012). Unusual energy enhancement in carbon-based electrochemical capacitors. *Journal of Materials Chemistry*, *22*(46), 24213–24223. doi:10.1039/c2jm35711a

Fujishima, A., & Honda, K. (1972). Electrochemical Photolysis of Water at a Semiconductor Electrode. *Nature*, *238*(5358), 37–38. doi:10.1038/238037a0 PMID:12635268

Goodenough, J. B., & Kim, Y. (2010). Challenges for Rechargeable Li Batteries. *Chemistry of Materials*, *22*(3), 587–603. doi:10.1021/cm901452z

Grahn, H. T. (1999). *Introduction to semiconductor physics*. World Scientific Pub Co Inc. doi:10.1142/3631

Gratzel, M. (2003), Dye-Sensitized Solar Cells. *J. Photochem. Photobiol., C, 4*, 145–153.

Gratzel, M. (2004). Conversion of sunlight to electric power by nanocrystalline dye-sensitized solar cells. *Journal of Photochemistry and Photobiology A Chemistry*, *164*(1-3), 3–14. doi:10.1016/j.jphotochem.2004.02.023

Guo, Y.-G., Hu, J.-S., & Wan, L.-J. (2008). Nanostructured Materials for Electrochemical Energy Conversion and Storage Devices. *Advanced Materials*, *20*(15), 2878–2887. doi:10.1002/adma.200800627

Guo, Y. G., Hu, Y. S., Sigle, W., & Maier, J. (2007). Superior Electrode Performance of Nanostructured Mesoporous TiO_2 (Anatase) through Efficient Hierarchical Mixed Conducting Networks. *Advanced Materials*, *19*(16), 2087–2091. doi:10.1002/adma.200602828

Hall, P. J., Mirzaeian, M., Fletcher, S. I., Sillars, F. B., Rennie, A. J. R., Shitta-Bey, G. O., Wilson, G., Cruden, A., & Carter, R. (2010). Energy storage in electrochemical capacitors: Designing functional materials to improve performance. *Energy & Environmental Science*, *3*(9), 1238–1251. doi:10.1039/c0ee00004c

Han, L., Islam, A., Chen, H., Malapaka, C., Chiranjeevi, B., Zhang, S., Yang, A., & Yanagida, M. (2012). High-efficiency dye-sensitized solar cell with a novel co-adsorbent. *Energy & Environmental Science*, *5*(3), 6057–6060. doi:10.1039/c2ee03418b

Hu, Y. S., Lorenz, K., Guo, Y. G., & Maier, J. (2006). High lithium electroactivity of nanometer-sized rutile TiO2. *Advanced Materials*, *18*(11), 1421–1426. doi:10.1002/adma.200502723

Idota, Y., Kabuto, T., Matsufuji, A., Maekawa, Y., & Miyasaki, T. (1997). Tin-Based Amorphous Oxide: A High-Capacity Lithium-Ion-Storage. *Materials Science*, *276*, 1395–1397.

Jiu, J., Isoda, S., Wang, F., & Adachi, M. (2006). Dye-sensitized solar cells based on a single-crystalline TiO2 nanorod film. *The Journal of Physical Chemistry B*, *110*(5), 2087–2092. doi:10.1021/jp055824n PMID:16471788

Kalyanasundaram, K. (2010). *EPFL Press*. CRC Press.

Kamat, P. V. (2012). Boosting the Efficiency of Quantum Dot Sensitized Solar Cells Through Modulation of Interfacial Charge Transfer. *Accounts of Chemical Research*, *45*(11), 1906–1915. doi:10.1021/ar200315d PMID:22493938

Khanra, P., Kuila, T., Bae, S. H., Kim, N. H., & Lee, J. H. (2012). b, Electrochemically exfoliated graphene using 9-anthracene carboxylic acid for supercapacitor application. *Journal of Materials Chemistry*, *22*(46), 24403. Advance online publication. doi:10.1039/c2jm34838a

Kim, T. H., Cho, K. S., Lee, E. K., Lee, S. J., Chae, J., Kim, J. W., Kwon, J. Y., Amaratunga, G., Lee, S. Y., & Choi, B. L. (2011). Full-colour quantum dot displays fabricated by transfer printing. *Nature Photonics*, *5*(3), 176–182. doi:10.1038/nphoton.2011.12

Kou, R., Shao, Y., Mei, D., Nie, Z., Wang, D., Wang, C., Viswanathan, V. V., Park, S., Aksay, I. A., Lin, Y., Wang, Y., & Liu, J. (2011). Stabilization of Electrocatalytic Metal Nanoparticles at Metal−Metal Oxide−Graphene Triple Junction Points. *Journal of the American Chemical Society*, *133*(8), 2541–2547. doi:10.1021/ja107719u PMID:21302925

Kreibig, U., & Vollmer, M. (1995). *Optical Properties of Metal Clusters* (Vol. 25). Springer. doi:10.1007/978-3-662-09109-8

Lange, P., Kewes, G., Severin, N., Benson, O., & Rabe, J. P. (2014), Evidence for Graphene Plasmons in the Visible Spectral Range Probed by Molecules. arXiv, arXiv:1404.

Lee, M. M., Teuscher, J., Miyasaka, T., Murakami, T. N., & Snaith, H. (in press). J. Science, (2012). *Efficient Hybrid Solar Cells Based on Meso-Superstructured Organometal Halide Perovskites*. Advance online publication. doi:10.1126cience.1228604 PMID:23042296

Lewis, N. S. (2007). Toward Cost-Effective Solar Energy Use. *Science*, *315*, 798–801.

Lewis, N. S., & Crabtree, G. (2005). *Basic research needs for solar energy utilization. Office of Science*. U. S. Department of Energy.

Linsebigler, A. L., Lu, G., & Yates, J. T. (1995). Photocatalysis on TiO2 Surfaces: Principles, Mechanisms, and Selected Results. *Chemical Reviews*, *95*(3), 735–758. doi:10.1021/cr00035a013

Liu, C., Li, F., Ma, L. P., & Cheng, H. M. (2010). Advanced Materials for Energy Storage. *Advanced Materials*, *22*(8), E28–E62. doi:10.1002/adma.200903328 PMID:20217798

Liu, Y., Liu, D., Zhang, Q., Yu, D., Liu, J., & Cao, G. (2011). Lithium iron phosphate/carbon nanocomposite film cathodes for high energy lithium ion batteries. *Electrochimica Acta*, *56*(5), 2559–2565. doi:10.1016/j.electacta.2010.11.050

Manasreh, M. O. (2012). *Introduction to Nanomaterials and Devices*. Wiley Online Library.

Mao, O., & Dahn, J. R. (1999). Mechanically alloyed Sn-Fe(-C) powders as anode materials for Li-ion batteries: I. The Sn2Fe-C system. *Journal of the Electrochemical Society*, *146*, 423–427.

Morfa, A. J., Rowlen, K. L., Reilly, T. H. III, Romero, M. J., & Lagemaatb, J. (2008). Plasmon-enhanced solar energy conversion in organic bulk heterojunction photovoltaics. *Applied Physics Letters*, *92*(1), 013504. doi:10.1063/1.2823578

Muraliganth, T., Murugan, A. V., & Manthiram, A. (2008). Nanoscale networking of $LiFePO_4$nanorods synthesized by a microwave-solvothermal route with carbon nanotubes for lithium ion batteries. *Journal of Materials Chemistry*, *18*(46), 5661–5668. doi:10.1039/b812165f

Nagaura, T., & Tozawa, K. (1990). Lithium-ion rechargeable battery. *Prog. Batter. Sol. Cells*, *9*, 209–212.

Nelson, P. A., & Owen, J. R. (2003). A high-performance supercapacitor/battery hybrid incorporating templated mesoporous electrodes. *Journal of the Electrochemical Society*, *150*(10), A1313–A1317. doi:10.1149/1.1603247

Niu, C., Sichjel, E. K., Hoch, R., Hoi, D., & Tennent, H. (1997). High power electrochemical capacitors based on carbon nanotube electrodes. *Applied Physics Letters*, *70*(11), 1480–1482. doi:10.1063/1.118568

Nozik, A. J. (1975). Photoelectrolysis of water using semiconducting TiO_2 crystals. *Nature*, *257*(5525), 383–386. doi:10.1038/257383a0

Ohara, S., Suzuki, J., Sekine, K., & Takamura, T. (2004). A thin film silicon anode for Li-ion batteries having a very large specific capacity and long cycle life. *Journal of Power Sources*, *136*(2), 303–306. doi:10.1016/j.jpowsour.2004.03.014

Prosini, P. P., Carewska, M., Scaccia, S., Wisniewski, P., & Pasquali, M. (2003). Long-term cyclability of nanostructured $LiFePO_4$. *Electrochimica Acta*, *48*(28), 4205–4211. doi:10.1016/S0013-4686(03)00606-6

Roduner, E. (2006). *Nanoscopic materials size-dependent phenomena*. The Royal Society of Chemistry.

Scrosati, B. (1995). Challenge of portable power. *Nature*, *373*, 557–558.

Scrosati, B. (2007). Nanomaterials: Paper powers battery breakthrough. *Nature Nanotechnology*, *2*(10), 598–599. doi:10.1038/nnano.2007.318 PMID:18654380

Service, R. F. (2005). Solar energy. Is it time to shoot for the sun? *Science*, *309*(5734), 548–551. doi:10.1126cience.309.5734.548 PMID:16040683

Shao, Y. Y., Liu, J., Wang, Y., & Lin, Y. H. (2009). Novel catalyst support materials for PEMfuelcells: Current status and future prospects. *Journal of Materials Chemistry*, *19*(1), 46–49. doi:10.1039/B808370C

Shao, Y. Y., Yin, G. P., Wang, J. J., Gao, Y. Z., & Shi, P. F. (2006). Multi-walled carbon nanotubes based Pt electrodes prepared with in situ ion exchange method for oxygen reduction. *Journal of Power Sources*, *161*(1), 47–53. doi:10.1016/j.jpowsour.2006.03.064

Song, T., Xia, J., Lee, J.-H., Lee, D. H., Kwon, M.-S., Choi, J.-M., Wu, J., Doo, S. K., Chang, H., Park, W. I., Zang, D. S., Kim, H., Huang, Y., Hwang, K.-C., Rogers, J. A., & Paik, U. (2010). Arrays of sealed silicon nanotubes as anodes for lithium ion batteries. *Nano Letters*, *10*(5), 1710–1716. doi:10.1021/nl100086e PMID:20369889

Stuart, H. R., & Hall, D. G. (1998). Island size effects in nanoparticle-enhanced photodetectors. *Applied Physics Letters*, *73*(26), 3815–3817. doi:10.1063/1.122903

Stylianakis, M.M., Konios, D., Petridis, C., Kakavelakis, G., Stratakis, E., Kymakis, E. (2017). Ternary solution-processed organic solar cells incorporating 2D materials. *2D Mater., 4*, 042005.

Su, F. B., Zeng, J., Bao, X., Yu, Y., Lee, J. Y., & Zhao, X. S. (2005). Preparation and characterization of highly ordered graphitic mesoporous as a Pt catalyst support for direct methanol fuel cells. *Chemistry of Materials*, *17*(15), 3960–3967. doi:10.1021/cm0502222

Wang, J., Zhang, S. Q., Guo, Y. Z., Shen, J., Attia, S. M., Zhou, B., Zheng, G. Z., & Gui, Y. S. (2001). Morphological effects on the electrical and electrochemical properties of carbon aerogels. *Journal of the Electrochemical Society*, *148*(6), D75–D77. doi:10.1149/1.1368104

Wang, Z. L., & Song, J. H. (2006). Piezoelectric Nanogenerators Based on Zinc Oxide Nanowire Arrays. *Science*, *312*(5771), 242–246. doi:10.1126cience.1124005 PMID:16614215

Winter, M., & Besenhard, J. O. (1999). Electrochemical lithiation of tin and tin-based intermetallics and composites. *J. Electrochim. Acta*, *45*(1-2), 31–50. doi:10.1016/S0013-4686(99)00191-7

Yang, J., Guo, F., Hua, J., Li, X., Wu, W., Qu, Y., & Tian, H. (2012). Efficient and stable organic DSSC sensitizers bearing quinacridone and furan moieties as a planar π-spacer. *Journal of Materials Chemistry*, *2012*(22), 24356–24365. doi:10.1039/c2jm31929b

Yang, J., Wang, B. F., Wang, K., Liu, Y., Xie, J. Y., & Wen, Z. S. (2003). Si/c composites for high capacity lithium storage materials. *Electrochemical and Solid-State Letters*, *6*(8), A154–A156. doi:10.1149/1.1585251

Yang, R., Qin, Y., Dai, L., & Wang, Z. L. (2009). Power generation with laterally packaged piezoelectric fine wires. *Nature Nanotechnology*, *4*(1), 34–39. doi:10.1038/nnano.2008.314 PMID:19119280

Yang, Z., Choi, D., Kerisit, S., Rosso, K. M., Wang, D., Zhang, J., Graff, G., & Liu, J. (2009). Nanostructures and lithium electrochemical reactivity of lithium titanites and titanium oxides: A review. *Journal of Power Sources*, *192*(2), 588–598. doi:10.1016/j.jpowsour.2009.02.038

Yao, K., Salvador, M., Chueh, C. C., Xin, X. K., Xu, Y. X., de Quilettes, D. W., Hu, T., Chen, Y. W., Ginger, D. S., & Jen, A. K. Y. (2014). General Route to Enhance Polymer Solar Cell Performance using Plasmonic Nanoprisms. *Advanced Energy Materials*, *4*(9), 1289–1295. doi:10.1002/aenm.201400206

Yella, A., Lee, H. W., Tsao, H. N., Yi, C., Chandiran, A. K., Nazeeruddin, M., Diau, E. W.-G., Yeh, C.-Y., Zakeeruddin, S. M., & Gratzel, M. (2011). Porphyrin-sensitized solar cells with cobalt (II/III)-based redox electrolyte exceed 12 percent efficiency. *Science*, *334*(6056), 629–634. doi:10.1126cience.1209688 PMID:22053043

Yoo, E., Okata, T., Akita, T., Kohyama, M., Nakamura, J., & Honma, I. (2009). Enhanced electrocatalytic activity of Pt subnanoclusters on graphene nanosheet surface. *Nano Letters*, *9*(6), 2255–2259. doi:10.1021/nl900397t PMID:19405511

Zhang, L. L., & Zhao, X. S. (2009). Carbon-based materials as supercapacitor electrodes. *Chemical Society Reviews*, *38*(9), 2520–2531. doi:10.1039/b813846j PMID:19690733

Zhang, Q. F., & Cao, G. Z. (2011). Nanostructured photoelectrodes for dye-sensitized solar cells. *Nano Today*, *6*(1), 91–109. doi:10.1016/j.nantod.2010.12.007

Zhang, Q. F., Yodyingyong, S., Xi, J. T., Myers, D., & Cao, G. Z. (2012). Oxidenanowires for solar cell applications. *Nanoscale*, *4*(5), 1436–1445. doi:10.1039/C2NR11595F PMID:22200055

Zhu, G., Yang, R., Wang, S., & Wang, Z. L. (2010). Flexible High-Output Nanogenerator Based on Lateral ZnO Nanowire Array. *Nano Letters*, *10*(8), 3151–3155. doi:10.1021/nl101973h PMID:20698630

KEY TERMS AND DEFINITIONS

Energy Harvesting: It is a process by which energy is derived from external source and stored for small autonomous devices.

Fuel Cell: It is an electrochemical cell that converts the chemical energy of fuel and oxidizing agent into electricity.

Nanostructured Material: Nanoscale particles of organic and inorganic materials whose dimensions are 1-100nm.

Supercapacitor: A supercapacitor is defined as an ultra-capacitor with a capacitance value much higher than other capacitors.

Chapter 11
Nanomaterials for Energy Harvesting and Storage:
An Overview

Arunima Nayak
Graphic Era University, Dehradun, India

Vipin Kumar Saini
https://orcid.org/0000-0002-2352-892X
Doon University, India

Brij Bhushan
https://orcid.org/0000-0002-9360-3083
Graphic Era University, Dehradun, India

ABSTRACT

The possibility of both energy and environmental crisis that may arise due to use of fossil fuels has resulted in intense research activities in the past decade on the development of technologies for harvesting and storage of energy from renewable sources. In order to meet the energy requirements for an ever-increasing population, there is a need for high performance electrochemical energy harvesting as well as storage devices. Nanomaterials and nanocomposites with diverse composition, structure, and morphologies have been applied in various energy related applications ranging from photocatalytic hydrogen generation, solar electricity generation, electric energy storage by lithium ion batteries and supercapacitors, hydrogen storage systems, etc. The aim of this chapter is to provide an overview of the recent developments in the technological advancements brought about by the use of nanotechnology in energy harvesting and storage appliances with specific focus on dye sensitized solar cells for electricity generation, lithium ion batteries, and supercapacitors for energy storage.

DOI: 10.4018/978-1-7998-5563-7.ch011

1. INTRODUCTION

Rapid increase in population vis-à-vis advancement in the economy worldwide has resulted in accelerated consumption of energy. Increased dependence and usage of appliances has also enhanced the usage of energy. It is predicted that there may be a requirement of nearly 30 TW of energy resources by the year 2050 to maintain economic growth (Doung, 2002). The excessive dependence on fossil fuel reserves to meet the increasing demand for energy has led to two significant but alarming results. Firstly fossil fuel resources are limited and there is a steady depletion of its reserves on the earth's crust; thereby the world is slowly but steadily hurtling towards a possible energy crisis. Secondly, there has been a steady increase in the green house gas emissions leading to environmental pollution, global warming and climate change. Both energy and environment crisis will threaten the sustainability and development of humans. Among the widely available renewable energy resources, solar energy is the cleanest form of energy. Converting solar energy to electrical energy via photovoltaics has been considered as the best choice and is being widely used in various consumer products (Ananthakumar et al., 2019). The first generation of solar cell technology involves the use of crystalline form of silicon as the semiconducting material. While the second generation involves the use of thin film solar cell technology, the third generation involves the use of dye or quantum sensitized and/or polymer solar cells. But a consistent supply of such harvested electrical energy to the consumer is not possible; hence highly efficient energy storage devices are desirable. Among the devices used to store electric energy are the lithium ion rechargeable batteries and the supercapacitors. The basic essence is to reinvent and restructure the traditional process streams and technologies so as to enhance the efficiency of energy generation from solar resources and improve storage performance. High cost of fabrication/maintenance, decreased efficiency as well as lower durability is some of the limitations exhibited by the traditional appliances and technologies.

Nanotechnology has provided an extensive range of nanomaterials as resources to help improve the performance of solar cells as well as storage batteries (Harris, 2001; Dai 2006; Huang et al., 2011). Some of the nanomaterials that have been extensively used as electrode materials are carbon nanomaterials, cellulose based nanomaterials, metal oxide nanomaterials, and conducting polymer based nano-composites etc (Arico et al., 2005). Nanomaterials exhibit various particle morphologies ranging from zero-dimensional nanoparticles and quantum dots; one-dimensional nanowires, nanotubes and nanobelts; two-dimensional nanoflakes and nanosheets; and three-dimensional porous nanonetworks. Some of the unique properties exhibited by such nanosized materials are greater electronic, optical, mechanical, photonic, magnetic as well as chemical reactivity as compared to their bulk counterparts. The properties that have greatly influenced the performance of solar cells, batteries and supercapacitors are the nano-sized particles of the nanomaterials as well as their higher surface area. Such properties have helped in improving the ionic transport rate and electrolyte diffusion thereby ensuring high electrochemical efficiency.

Keeping in focus the importance of the use of renewable resources like solar light for energy harvesting and the storage of the same, the present chapter will give an overview of the different nanomaterials that have been used till date for electricity generation from dye sensitized solar cells as well as for electric energy storage. The emphasis of this chapter is on the advantages of using nanomaterials for these applications. Finally challenges of utilizing nanomaterials will also be addressed. It is expected that the latest overview of such content will benefit those undergoing research on nanotechnology and renewable energy technology.

2. PHOTOVOLTAIC SOLAR CELLS

Solar Cells have the capacity to capture solar energy and convert it to electrical energy via the photovoltaic (PV) technology (Chopra et al., 2004; Goetzberger et al., 2002). The first generation PV solar cells are made from mono-crystalline and poly-crystalline silicon wafer of thickness 150-300nm (Yianoulis and Giannouli, 2008; Pelemiš and Hut, 2013). The greatest disadvantage is their high cost of manufacturing and fabrication. Also, they lose their efficiency when exposed to higher temperatures. Silicon based solar cells suffer from the difficulties in modifying its band gap. Second generation PV solar cells are made from thin films (1-2 nm) of semiconducting materials like cadmium telluride (CdTe), copper indium gallium diselenide (CIGS), amorphous silicon and nano-crystalline silicon (Chopra et al., 2004). Such solar cells have ensured lesser manufacturing cost and better efficiency under laboratory set-up. But additional complexities related to efficiency and cost is known to pick up during scale-up. Also, the second generation solar cells require greater protection than silicon based solar cells so as to ensure longer duration of outdoor operation.

Third generation solar cells include dye sensitized solar cells (DSSC) and quantum dot sensitized solar cells (QDSSC) (Ananthakumar et al., 2019). The main aim of such solar cells is to achieve high efficiency as well as to minimize the cost of fabrication. Mesoporous TiO_2 is sensitized by ruthenium complex dye in DSSC and by semiconductor quantum dots in QDSSC (Salant et al., 2010).

2.1. Use of Nanomaterials in Dye Sensitized Solar Cells (DSSC)

A DSSC device as developed by Gratzel et al., in 1991 (O'Regan and Gatzel, 1991) typically have four components: photo anode, sensitizer, electrolyte and a counter electrode (Ananthakumar et al., 2019). The photo anode is basically a nano crystalline film of mesoporous TiO_2 (1-10 μm) particles deposited on a tin-doped indium oxide (ITO) or fluorine-doped tin oxide coated transparent glass plate (FTO glass). Ruthenium based organic dye is adsorbed onto the photo anode. The counter electrode is a conducting sheet of platinum (Pt) covered with a thin layer of iodide electrolyte. The counter electrode as well as the photo anode is sealed so as to prevent leaking of the electrolyte. The power conversion efficiency of DSSC was reported to be approximately 7.12% (O'Regan and Gatzel, 1991). Enhanced power efficiency of a Gratzel DSSC over that for traditional ones is due to the large surface area and nano-crystalline form of TiO_2. The large surface area ensures greater dye adsorption which inturn causes enhanced photon absorption and greater injection of electrons from the dye to the conduction band of TiO_2. The porous nanostructure ensures efficient charge transport thereby causing minimal recombination loss of electrons. Traditional DSSC (having an efficiency of 1%) has a photo anode semi-conducting material of a narrow band gap with the aim of capturing only the visible light. More recently, 14% increase in the efficiency of DSSC has been reported (Kakiage et al., 2015). Besides the nanocrystals, effects of various other TiO_2 morphologies like nanotubes (Mor et al., 2006; Paulose et al., 2006a; Paulose et al., 2006b), nanorods (Song et al., 2005; Yang et al., 2009), as well as other one dimensional oxides of ZnO, SnO_2 (Law et al., 2005) have been investigated and have been found to enhance the power conversion efficiency of DSSC. Not only have these nano-structured morphologies enabled a higher surface area to the photo anode film but have also paved way to other properties like better photon absorption, reduced charge recombination as well as greater electron transport (Dai et al., 2012). Carbon based nanomaterials like graphene have been incorporated into the TiO_2 nanoparticles (Yella et al., 2011). Yang et al. fabricated a nano-composite material based on graphene and TiO_2 (Yang et al., 2010). The nano-composite material was used as an active photo-anode in DSSC. A 40% enhancement in the power conversion efficiency was obtained as compared to a DSSC having a standard TiO_2 based photo anode. The researchers cited that the major reason for such improvement in the device was the faster electron transport and lower recombination. In yet another study (Yang et al., 2007), a photo-anode material was fabricated using vertically aligned carbon nanotube (CNT) nanowires and TiO_2 particles. The nano-composite based photo-anode served as a support for better adsorption of dye and also helped in reducing the series resistance for the DSSC via a direct electron transport pathway from the dye coated TiO_2 to the CNT. In Quantum Dot Sensitized Solar Cells (QDSSC) quantum dots have been used as sensitizers in place of dyes (Kamat, 2013). The electrolyte used was polysulphide. The quantum dots used have been bimetallic nanoparticles (CdS, CdTe, CdSe, PbS, SnS etc) (Ellingson et al., 2005), graphene (Pan et al., 1998; Li et al., 2011) or with core shell structure of another compound (Feng et al., 2016). Advantages of using quantum dots include light absorbing capacity in the infrared region, better photo chemical stability as compared to the use of dyes as sensitizers and enhanced efficiency due to multiple electron generation. Maximum power efficiency of approximately 42% was reported from QDSSC (Hanna and Nozik, 2006; Nozik, 2008; Beard et al., 2010). Graphene quantum dots were also reported to be used as a sensitizer so as to achieve higher power conversion efficiency (Pan et al., 1998; Li et al., 2011). But the lower absorption of graphene quantum dots onto the TiO_2 surface and hence the poor charge injection was reported to result in lower efficiency.

3. LITHIUM ION BATTERIES

The high surface area and the porosity are the two inherent characteristics of several nanostructured materials. These characteristics make these materials suitable for their application in energy storage devices like Lithium ion batteries (Goodenough and Kim, 2010). The innovation in material design of these next-generation batteries are the key to the success of electric vehicles, which will solve the problem of air pollution by replacing conventional vehicles.

Like other batteries, typical Li-ion batteries also consist of a cathode and anode along with Li-ion containing electrolyte. In commercial Lithium ion batteries, the cathode and anode are made up of $LiCoO_2$ and graphite, respectively. During charging, the Lithium ions are inserted to anode from cathode, likewise these ions are extracted from the anode during discharging. This whole electrochemical insertion and extraction process is a solid-state redox reaction, which involves electrochemical charge transfer along with transfer of Li ions within a conductive solid host. The surface area of electrode and the migration distance are the critical parameters that determine battery performance (Liu and Cao, 2010). The advantages of nanostructured active electrode materials involves i) a larger electrode-electrolyte contact area; ii) short path lengths for both electronic and Lithium ion transport; iii) possibility of new reactions that are not possible with bulk materials; etc. The following section highlights some of the common nano-engineered developments for the tailoring of nanostructures and nanostructure assemblies.

3.1. Enhancement in Electrode/Electrolyte Contact Area

A higher electrode to electrolyte contact area can lead to improved high current rate charge and discharge capacities. It is because; the fine particle size of electrode offers equally short transport length which makes maximum Li diffusion possible within a very short duration (Guo et al., 2008). Similarly, the surface Li storage only depends only on the surface area rather than on diffusion time. Therefore, a higher electrode to electrolyte contact area is thus beneficial to high current rate performance. The reduction of the electrode particle size down to nanometer regime tremendously enhances the overall degree of intercalation, with improvement in the intercalation kinetics.

The Lithium ion intercalation performance of anatase TiO_2 micro and nanoparticles shows that the Li-ion solubility was increased with decreasing its particle size. For instance, it was increased from 0.55 to 0.7 Li^+ per formula unit when the micron-sized TiO_2 particles were replaced with nanoparticles smaller than 40 nm (Wagemaker et al., 2007) [4]. The Li^+ diffusion rate limiting two-phase boundary between electrode particles has an activation energy of approximately 50 kJ mol^{-1}, however, the nanomaterials <40 nm did not have the phase boundary and had an activation energy of 10–25 kJ mol^{-1} (Ganapathy et al., 2011). Another study reveals that the dissimilar diffusion along the ab-plane, and Li-ion surface storage on the nanoparticles is energetically more favorable than their bulk insertion, which is responsible for the enhanced electrochemical effects of nanostructuring TiO_2 as a Lithium ion battery electrode material (Hu et al., 2006).

The layered intercalation compounds are the popular device candidates for which nearly most of the research and commercialization of cathode materials has been focused. Some of the layered compounds involve an anion close-packed or nearly close-packed lattice where the electro-active transition metal ions occupy alternating layers, and lithium is inserted in the unoccupied layers. For instance, both $LiTiS_2$ and $LiCoO_2$ is the current commercial cathode of choice. Nanostructured $Li_{4+x}Ti_5O_{12}$ spinel has demonstrated superior electrochemical performance when compared to its bulk counterpart due to increased Li-ion occupancy (Borghols et al., 2009).

Using nanoelectrodes can greatly reduce the specific current density of the active material because of the very large surface area. The low specific current density can effectively stabilize the electrode and preserve a high capacity at high charge and discharge current densities (Zhou et al., 2005). For example, CoO nanoelectrode at a rate of 2 C (C is the current rate needed to charge or discharge the theoretical capacity in 1 hour) could sustain 85% of its total capacity. Also, besides the recently demonstrated high specific capacity, an excellent high-rate performance has been observed for rutile TiO_2 nanoelectrodes (Hu et al., 2006). The materials with surface areas between ~20-100 m2/g can be charged and discharged nearly to the nominal capacity of $Li_4Ti_5O_{12}$ (175 mAh g^{-1}) within a wide range of charge/discharge current rates (from 2 C to 250 C). The thinner films displayed similar benefits when compared to thicker films composed of the same electro-active material. For example, the layered vanadium oxides in form of uniform films of V_2O_5 were formed on FTO substrates through a combination of cathodic deposition and catalyzed gelation. The homogeneous films were composed of microflakes that ranged from 0.5 to 1.5 mm in diameter, and each flake was composed of nanoparticles measuring 20–30 nm in diameter with 10 nm gaps separating adjacent nanoparticles (Liu et al., 2011).

3.2. Reduction in Path Lengths

The commercial batteries are based on micrometer-sized electrode materials containg powders particles of a low surface area. The Li-ion diffusion in these micrometer-sized electrode materials are not beneficial particularly for high-rate charge and discharge, because of the long path length. The nanostructured materials on the other hand can provide shorter path lengths for both Li-ion and electron transport during reduction or oxidation reaction in the lithium insertion and extraction (discharge and charge) process. This suggests that nanometer-sized electrode materials are necessities for high power and high energy density energy storage and conversion.

Tarascon et al. (Tarascon et al., 2001) first reported that negative electrodes consisting of NiO, FeO, or CoO have large specific capacities of ~700 mAh g^{-1} at low charge and discharge rates. This concept has been shown to hold for nanoporous TiO_2 active materials. The nanoporous TiO_2 had a two-dimensional hexagonal mesostructure containing uniform pores with a diameter of 4 nm and 5 nm-wide pore walls of nanocrystalline anatase TiO_2. A high specific capacity (about 260 mAh g^{-1}) at high current density (10 A g^{-1}) has also been obtained for these materials.

Some chemical synthesis methods have been developed to synthesize active electrode materials directly, such as V_2O_5 (Kudo et al., 2002), TiO_2) (Hibino et al., 2004), MnO_2 (Kawaoka et al., 2004) on acetylene black carbon, for high-rate performance. The Lithium ion insertion performance of the $LiMnPO_4$ microspheres assembled with plates was far better than the other primary nanoparticle units due to the exposure of (010) facets as well as the confined thickness along the [010] direction allowing for fast Li ion diffusion and a short diffusion length (Pan et al., 2012). Synthesis of active nanostructured materials on conductive nanowires and nanotubes is one of the most promising areas of research. In shell-core micro or nanostructured active materials, the diameter of the Ni wire is too thick for practical use. Conductive nanowires or nanotubes with diameters of several nanometers to several tens of nanometers are more suitable as a core for electronic transport. Therefore, active nanocrystalline electrode materials synthesized on carbon nanotubes have been investigated for high-rate lithium ion batteries. They have clearly shown some improved charge and discharge profiles at high current densities (Moriguchi et al., 2006)

3.3. New Chemical Reactions

Advancements in the field of nanoscience open routes of reinvestigation, for the materials which were thought of as being electrochemically inactive in bulk form but that could present improved electrochemical performance at the nanoscale. One good example is the demonstration that nanoparticles of some simple transition metal oxides, sulfides, fluorides, and nitrides can provide innovative anode materials for lithium ion batteries. The reaction of such transition metal compounds with Li leads to the in situ formation of metal nanoparticles embedded in an LizX matrix (where X = O, S, F, or N).

The transition metals do not alloy with Li, that is why the mechanism of Li reactivity differs from classical Li insertion and extraction or Li-alloying processes (Jamnik et al., 2003). The mechanism for the reaction of transition metal compounds with Li during charge and discharge involves the formation and decomposition of LizX accompanying the reduction and oxidation of metal nanoparticles. It was noticed that the electrodes made of nanoparticles of transition metal oxides can deliver specific capacities of 700 mAh/g with 100% capacity retention for up to 100 charge and discharge cycles and high recharging current rates when being charged and discharged in the potential window of 3.5 V to 0.01 V (versus Li+/Li). The high Li storage capacity in nanometer-sized transition metal oxides at low potential has recently been explained by an interfacial charge storage mechanism. Here, Li ions are stored on the oxide side of the interface, while electrons are localized on the metallic side, resulting in a charge separation (Zhukovskii et al., 2006).

Therefore, the electrochemically driven size confinement of the metal particles is believed to enhance their electrochemical activity toward the formation/decomposition of Li_2O. As a result with decreasing particle size, an increasing proportion of the total number of atoms lies near or on the surface, making the electrochemical reactivity of the particles more and more important.

Nanostructured electrodes may not only introduce innovative reaction mechanisms but also improve electrochemical properties, such as specific energy storage capacity, high current charge/discharge ability, and cycle stability, over their bulk counterparts. This results from the short diffusion length and high contact area between the active materials and electrolyte. Li ion diffusion is highly dependent on the transport length and accessible sites on the surface of active materials. Those compounds exhibiting low Li ion diffusion coefficients usually show low Li ion storage capacities in bulk form, especially at high current rates. This is the case for rutile TiO_2, which can only accommodate a negligible amount of Li ions at room temperature (Ohzuku et al., 1979; Bonino et al., 1991).

3.4. Stable Cycle Performance

The use of nanomaterials can also enhance the cycling performance of the material by alleviating some of the lattice strain experienced during cycling due to the (de)intercalation of lithium. Besides their excellent high current rate charge/discharge performance, nanostructured electrode materials may also deliver good cycle stability (Liu et al., 2009). The capacity fading of lithium ion batteries upon cycling are usually caused by the large volume expansion and contraction associated with Li insertion and extraction or Li alloying/de-alloying.

For example, Si as the anode of lithium ion batteries may have the highest theoretical capacity of 4200 mAh/g (Boukamp et al., 1981; Yang et al., 1996). Though, its commercial use has been hindered due to significant drastic volume change during lithium insertion/extraction, which inevitably introduces cracking or crumbling of the anode material and thus causes loss in capacity during cycling.

Nanostructured electrodes can absorb this large volume expansion/contraction, preserving the integrity of the electrode and leading to stable cycle performance. For example, a new type of nanostructured Si/C composite electrode shows a very high reversible capacity (about 1000 mAh/g) and good capacity retention (~99.8%) from the second cycle (Holzapfel et al., 2005). It is believed that the nanosized composite electrode has accommodated the large volume change of the Si during charge and discharge processes, keeping the integrity of the electrode. Likewise, the spindle-like LFP mesocrystals demonstrated an incredibly stable cycling stability of approximately 165 mA h g 1 over the course of 50 cycles, and a moderate rate capability that terminated at 120 mA h g 1 at a rate of 5 C (Xia et al., 2011). This section has reviewed some advantages of nanostructured electrode materials for high-rate energy storage devices, especially for high-rate lithium ion batteries. Of course, there are some challenges, such as a more complex synthesis process for the nanomaterials, which will increase the cost of lithium ion batteries (Yamaki et al., 2002; Zhang, 2006; Lewandowski and Swiderska-Mocek, 2009). Therefore, the next challenge will be to develop simple synthesis methods for large-scale production of nanostructured active materials.

4. SUPERCAPACITORS

Supercapacitors are electrochemical devices that have the capacity to store energy. Such capacitors have higher electrode surface area that enables them to have higher power and energy densities as compared to the conventional capacitors and batteries. Advancement in applications on supercapacitors largely relies on research on innovativeness of the electrode materials.

4.1. Supercapacitors with Activated Carbon Based Electrodes

Supercapacitors are electrochemical devices that have been extensively researched upon and have been developed for energy storage applications. In comparison to Lithium ion batteries, supercapacitors, have exhibited improved capacitance and power deliverance capability as well as a better cycle life. The high performance of such supercapacitors is due to the physical characteristics of the electrode and electrolytic materials. The electrode materials are usually the activated carbons, transition metal oxides and conjugative polymers (Frackowiak and Beguin, 2001). It is well known that the capacitance is proportional to the specific surface area of the electrode materials (Zheng et al., 1995). Activated carbons used in commercial supercapacitors have a high surface area of 3000m^2/g (Rudge et al., 1994), but the capacitance of such devices with aqueous electrolyte was found to be 100-300F/g while the same for organic electrolytes was found to be less than 150 F/g (Burke and Arulepp, 2011; Wang et al., 2012; Lee et al., 2016). The energy storage efficiency was found to be 4-5 Wh/kg and the power density was 1-2kW/kg. Studies have demonstrated that the capacitance is also related to size of the pores of the carbon electrode and also on the size of the solvated ions. For pore sizes larger than the pore size of the solvated ion, capacitance has a direct relation to the surface area. But for lesser pore size diameter, the capacitance decreases significantly. This observation was correlated to the difficulty of access of the electrolytic ions into the porous network of the electrode thereby resulting in a decrease in the capacitance (Conway, 1999).

4.2. Supercapacitors with Carbon Nanomaterials Based Electrodes

Carbon nanotubes (CNTs) and graphene are carbon based nanomaterials exhibiting nanosized porous morphology and high surface area. Such properties are useful in enhancing the performance of energy conversion and storage. The specific surface area of graphene and CNTs is 2630 and 400 m^2/g respectively (Harris, 2000; Dai, 2006; Compton and Nguyen, 2010). While the electrical conductivity for CNTs is 5000S/cm the same for graphene is as high as 10^6 S/cm. The charge mobility of graphite is double that of CNT (10^5 cm^2/V/s). Both have a pore size of 2-50nm. Thus, because of their high surface area, high electrical conductivity and high charge transport capability as well as because of the presence of higher mesoporosity, such carbon based nanomaterials have demonstrated better electrode materials for enhancing the performance of supercapacitors. Application of CNT based electrode material in supercapacitors has demonstrated a higher capacitance as compared to that for activated carbon based electrodes; despite the lower surface area of CNTs. For e.g multiwalled carbon nanotube (MWNT) based electrodes demonstrated a capacitance of 102 F/g (Niu et al., 1997) while single walled carbon nanotube based electrodes showed a capacitance of 180 F/g (Zilli et al., 2006). CNT having a surface area of 357m^2/g recorded a theoretical capacitance of 71-178 F/g. Experimental studies showed capacitance values of 180 F/g which was in good agreement with the theoretical values. The reason as cited by An et al. (An et al., 2001) was that the mesoporosity as induced by CNT entanglement was responsible for high electrolytic penetration leading to enhanced capacitance of such device. A supercapacitor designed from single walled carbon nanotube (SWNT) and using KOH as the electrolyte demonstrated high power and energy density of 20kW/kg and 10Wh/kg respectively (An et al., 2001). Use of multiwalled carbon nanotube (MWNT) as the carbon electrode and H_2SO_4 as the electrolytic solution showed power density to the tune of 8kW/g (Niu et al., 1997). The lower performance of MWNT based supercapacitors was mainly because of its lower surface area (400 m^2/g) as compared to that for SWNT (1600 m^2/g). But, no doubt the performance of both SWNT and MWNT based supercapacitors was higher in comparison to activated carbon based device.

Graphene having a surface area of 2630m^2/g [8] has recorded a theoretical capacitance of 550F/g (Yang et al., 2015) which is the highest value as obtained from all carbon based electrode devices. Various studies have shown the use of chemically modified graphene for e.g. reduced graphene oxide in supercapacitors (Hou et al., 2011). Studies as conducted by Stoller et al. (Stroller et al., 2008) on use chemically modified graphene based devices, have demonstrated a capacitance of 99 F/g and 135 F/g in the presence of organic and aqueous electrolytic solution respectively. Graphene based composites have also been used as electrode materials like graphene-activated carbon composite, graphene-CNT hybrid films (chen et al., 2010), graphene-carbon black composite (Yu and Dai, 2010) graphene-polymer composites (Wang et al., 2010) etc. Experiments have shown that the capacitance of graphene-activated carbon composite based supercapacitors was 210 (Choi et al., 2018) and 512 F/g (Chen et al., 2018). Composites fabricated from polyaniline and graphene oxide showed a capacitance of 250 F/g (Kumarn et al., 2012). Graphene-hollow carbon nanosphere based device demonstrated a capacitance of 561 F/g (Chen et al., 2018).

Similarly, CNT based composites have been fabricated and used successfully as electrode materials so as to enhance the power and energy density of supercapacitors. Activated carbons, conjugated polymers and metal oxides have been used for development of composite materials for electrodes. Portet et al. (Portet et al., 2005) have fabricated CNT based composite with activated carbon. The developed electrode demonstrated higher capacitance as compared to that for devices using activated carbon based electrode. In another study (Liu et al., 2003), SWNT and polyacrylonitrile (PAN) dimethylformamide solution was mixed followed by CO_2 activation to develop a SWNT/activated carbon composite electrode. The device with the developed composite electrode demonstrated higher capacitance, higher power and energy density as compared to that for a pure SWNT based electrode device. Polypyrrole was used to fabricate a composite electrode material with SWNT. SWNT/polypyrrole nanocomposite electrode demonstrated a higher capacitance of 265 F/g as compared to the pure polypyrrole or the pure SWNT based electrodes (An et al., 2002). CNT-polyaniline based composite electrode, in yet another study showed a capacitance of 530 F/g (Liu et al., 2017).

Transition metal oxides for e.g RuO_2, IrO_2, V_2O_5, MnO_2, CoO_2, NiO_2, Fe_2O_3 when incorporated into carbón based electrodes have demonstrated higher capacitance due to reversible redox reactions. Studies have shown that capacitance of composite electrode fabricated from incorporation of MnO_2 onto CNT was 1250 F/g (Chen et al., 2010). Graphene oxide-MnO_2 based electrode exhibited a capacitance of 213 F/g and the capacitance was retained to a level of 98% even after 1000 charge/discharge cycles (Liu et al., 2014).

5. CONCLUSION AND FUTURE PROSPECTS

The use of nanomaterials in advancing the technology of energy harvesting and storage is evident from enormous research work that has been conducted since the last two decades in related field. The use of nano-sized inorganic conducting materials for solar devices like in dye-sensitized solar cells and in quantum dot sensitized solar cells has provided a large specific surface area for greater adsorption of dye molecules and quantum dots onto the surface of inorganic materials. Nanostructures as in quantum dots have also brought about multiple exciton generation. Maximum photon absorption, maximum charge collection, improved electron transport and minimum interface charge recombination are the reason behind improved efficiency in solar cells. In lithium ion batteries, nanomaterials as electrodes have offered significant features like fast interfacial Faradaic reaction and shorter charge migration distance. Its nano-dimensions have accommodated the volume change accompanied with lithium ion insertion and extraction. Nanomaterials with high porosity and higher surface area have accommodated easy access of electrolyte to the active material, and have provided shorter diffusion distances; thereby leading to improved energy storage and performance in supercapacitors.

Certain limitation with respect to nanomaterials is that their high surface area and high reactivity has led to significant agglomeration which in turn has resulted in decreased efficiency for their application. Fabrication of nanomaterials on a large scale has been technically not feasible due to high costs, complex processes and difficulties in controlling the homogeneity.

REFERENCES

An, K. H., Jeon, K. K., Heo, J. K., Lim, S. C., Bae, D. J., & Lee, Y. H. (2002). High-Capacitance Supercapacitor Using a Nanocomposite Electrode of Single-Walled Carbon Nanotube and Polypyrrole. *Journal of the Electrochemical Society*, *149*(8), A1058. doi:10.1149/1.1491235

An, K. H., Kim, W. S., Park, Y. S., Moon, J. M., Bae, D. J., Lim, S. C., Lee, Y. S., & Lee, Y. H. (2001). Electrochemical Properties of High-Power Supercapacitors Using Single-Walled Carbon Nanotube Electrodes. *Advanced Functional Materials*, *11*(5), 387–392. doi:10.1002/1616-3028(200110)11:5<387::AID-ADFM387>3.0.CO;2-G

Ananthakumar, S., Kumar, J. R., Babu, S. M. (2019). Third-Generation Solar Cells: Concept, Materials and Performance - An Overview. *Emerging Nanostructured Materials for Energy and Environmental Science*, 305–339.

Aricò, A. S., Bruce, P., Scrosati, B., Tarascon, J. M., & van Schalkwijk, W. (2005). Nanostructured materials for advanced energy conversion and storage devices. *Nature Materials*, *4*(5), 366–377. doi:10.1038/nmat1368 PMID:15867920

Beard, M. C., Midgett, A. G., Hanna, M. C., Luther, J. M., Hughes, B. K., & Nozik, A. J. (2010). Comparing multiple exciton generation in quantum dots to impact ionization in bulk semiconductors: Implications for enhancement of solar energy conversion. *Nano Letters*, *10*(8), 3019–3027. doi:10.1021/nl101490z PMID:20698615

Bonino, F., Busani, L., Lazzari, M., Manstretta, M., Rivolta, B., & Scrosati, B. (1981). Anatase as a cathode material in lithium—Organic electrolyte rechargeable batteries. *Journal of Power Sources*, *6*(3), 261–270. doi:10.1016/0378-7753(81)80031-6

Borghols, W. J. H., Wagemaker, M., Lafont, U., Kelder, E. M., & Mulder, F. M. (2009). Size Effects in the Li_4+xTi_5O_{12} Spinel. *Journal of the American Chemical Society*, *131*(49), 17786–17792. doi:10.1021/ja902423e PMID:19919072

Boukamp, B. A., Lesh, G. C., & Huggins, R. A. (1981). All-Solid Lithium Electrodes with Mixed-Conductor Matrix. *Journal of the Electrochemical Society*, *128*(4), 725–729. doi:10.1149/1.2127495

Burke, A., & Arulepp, M. (2001). Recent Developments in Carbon-based Electrochemcial Capacitors: Status of the Technology and Future Prospects. *Electrochem. Soc. Proc.*, *21*, 576.

Chen, J., Hong, M., Chen, J., Hu, T., & Xu, Q. (2018). Fabrication of hierarchical porous hollow carbon spheres with few-layer graphene framework and high electrochemical activity for supercapacitor. *Applied Surface Science*, *443*, 367–373. doi:10.1016/j.apsusc.2018.02.052

Chen, S., Zhu, J., Wu, X., Han, Q., & Wang, X. (2010). Graphene oxide-MnO_2 nanocomposites for supercapacitors. *ACS Nano*, *4*(5), 2822–2830. doi:10.1021/nn901311t PMID:20384318

Chen, W., Fan, Z., Gu, L., Bao, X., & Wang, C. (2010). Enhanced capacitance of manganese oxide via confinement inside carbon nanotubes. *Chemical Communications (Cambridge)*, *46*(22), 3905–3907. doi:10.1039/c000517g PMID:20411189

Choi, J.-H., Lee, C., Cho, S., Moon, G. D., kim, B., Chang, H., & Jang, H. D. (2018). High capacitance and energy density supercapacitor based on biomass-derived activated carbons with reduced graphene oxide binder. *Carbon*, *132*, 16–24. doi:10.1016/j.carbon.2018.01.105

Chopra, K. L., Paulson, P. D., & Dutta, V. (2004). Thin film solar cells: An overview. *Progress in Photovoltaics: Research and Applications*, *12*(2–3), 69–92. doi:10.1002/pip.541

Compton, O. C., & Nguyen, S. T. (2010). Graphene oxide, highly reduced graphene oxide, and graphene: Versatile building blocks for carbon-based materials. *Small*, *2010*(6), 711–723. doi:10.1002mll.200901934 PMID:20225186

Conway, B. E. (1999). *Electrochemical Supercapacitors: Scientific Fundamentals and Technological Applications*. Kluwer Academic. doi:10.1007/978-1-4757-3058-6

Dai, L. (2006). *Carbon Nanotechnology: Recent Developments in Chemistry, Physics, Materials Science and Device Applications*. Elsevier Science.

Dai, L., Chang, D. W., Baek, J-B., Lu, W. (2012). Carbon Nanomaterials for Advanced Energy Conversion and Storage. *Small*, *8*, 1130–1166.

Doung, T. G. (2003). *2002 Annual Progress Report for Energy Storage Research and Development*. Freedom Car & Vehicle Technologies Program.

Ellingson, R. J., Beard, M. C., Johnson, J. C., Yu, P., Micic, O. I., Nozik, A. J., Shabaev, A., & Efros, A. L. (2005). Highly efficient multiple exciton generation in colloidal PbSe and PbS quantum dots. *Nano Letters*, *5*(5), 865–871. doi:10.1021/nl0502672 PMID:15884885

Feng, W., Li, Y., Du, J., Wang, W., & Zhong, X. (2016). Highly efficient and stable quasi-solid-state quantum dot-sensitized solar cells based on a superabsorbent polyelectrolyte. *Journal of Materials Chemistry. A, Materials for Energy and Sustainability*, *4*(4), 1461–1468. doi:10.1039/C5TA08209A

Frackowiak, E., & Beguin, F. (2001). Carbon materials for the electrochemical storage of energy in Capacitors. *Carbon*, *39*(6), 937–950. doi:10.1016/S0008-6223(00)00183-4

Ganapathy, S., van Eck, E. R., Kentgens, A. P. M., Mulder, F. M., & Wagemaker, M. (2011). Equilibrium Lithium-Ion Transport Between Nanocrystalline Lithium- Inserted Anatase TiO2 and the Electrolyte. *Chemistry (Weinheim an der Bergstrasse, Germany)*, *17*(52), 14811–14816. doi:10.1002/chem.201101431 PMID:22120842

Goetzberger, A., Luther, J., & Willeke, G. (2002). Solar cells: Past, present, future. *Solar Energy Materials and Solar Cells*, *74*(1–4), 1–11. doi:10.1016/S0927-0248(02)00042-9

Goodenough, J. B., & Kim, Y. (2010). Challenges for Rechargeable Li Batteries. *Chemistry of Materials*, *22*(3), 587–603. doi:10.1021/cm901452z

Guo, Y.-G., Hu, J.-S., & Wan, L.-J. (2008). Nanostructured Materials for Electrochemical Energy Conversion and Storage Devices. *Advanced Materials*, *20*(15), 2878–2887. doi:10.1002/adma.200800627

Hanna, M., & Nozik, A. J. (2006). Solar conversion efficiency of photovoltaic and photoelectrolysis cells with carrier multiplication absorbers. *Journal of Applied Physics*, *100*(7), 074510. doi:10.1063/1.2356795

Harris, P. J. F. (2001). *Carbon Nanotubes and Related Structures – New Materials for the Twenty-First Century*. Cambridge University Express.

Hibino, M., Abe, K., Mochizuki, M., & Miyayama, M. (2004). Amorphous titanium oxide electrode for high-rate discharge and charge. *Journal of Power Sources*, *126*(1-2), 139–143. doi:10.1016/j.jpowsour.2003.08.025

Holzapfel, M., Buqa, H., Scheifele, W., Novák, P., & Petrat, F. M. (2005). A new type of nano-sized silicon/carbon composite electrode for reversible lithium insertion. *Chemical Communications (Cambridge)*, *28*(12), 1566–1568. doi:10.1039/B417492E PMID:15770261

Hou, J., Shao, Y., Ellis, M. W., Moore, R. B., & Yi, B. (2011). Graphene-based electrochemical energy conversion and storage, fuel cells, supercapacitors and lithium ion batteries. *Physical Chemistry Chemical Physics*, *13*(34), 15384–15402. doi:10.1039/c1cp21915d PMID:21799983

Hu, Y. S., Kienle, L., Guo, Y. G., & Maier, J. (2006). High Lithium Electroactivity of Nanometer-Sized Rutile TiO_2. *Advanced Materials*, *18*(11), 1421–1426. doi:10.1002/adma.200502723

Huang, X., Yin, Z., Wu, S., Qi, X., He, Q., Zhang, Q., Yan, Q., Boey, F., & Zhang, H. (2011). Graphene-based materials: Synthesis, characterization, properties, and applications. *Small*, *7*(14), 1876–1902. doi:10.1002mll.201002009 PMID:21630440

Jamnik, J., & Maiera, J. (2003). Nanocrystallinity effects in lithium battery materials Aspects of nano-ionics. Part IV. *Physical Chemistry Chemical Physics*, *5*(23), 5215. doi:10.1039/b309130a

Kakiage, K., Aoyama, Y., Yano, T., Oya, K., Fujisawa, J. I., & Hanaya, M. (2015). Highly-efficient dye-sensitized solar cells with collaborative sensitization by silyl-anchor and carboxy-anchor dyes. *Chemical Communications (Cambridge)*, *51*(88), 15894–15897. doi:10.1039/C5CC06759F PMID:26393334

Kamat, P. V. (2013). Quantum dot solar cells. The next big thing in photovoltaics. *The Journal of Physical Chemistry Letters*, *4*(6), 908–918. doi:10.1021/jz400052e PMID:26291355

Kawaoka, H., Hibino, M., Zhou, H., & Honma, I. (2004). Sonochemical synthesis of amorphous manganese oxide coated on carbon and application to high power battery. *Journal of Power Sources*, *125*(1), 85–89. doi:10.1016/S0378-7753(03)00823-1

Kudo, T., Ikedaa, Y., Watanabea, T., Hibinoav, M., Miyayamaa, M., Abeb, H., & Kajitab, K. (2002). Amorphous V_2O_5/carbon composites as electrochemical supercapacitor electrodes. *Solid State Ionics*, *833*, 152–153. doi:10.1016/S0167-2738(02)00383-1

Kumarn, N. A., Choi, H.-J., & Shin, Y. R. (2012). Polyaniline-grafted reduced graphene oxide for efficient electrochemical supercapacitors. *ACS Nano*, *6*(2), 1715–1723. doi:10.1021/nn204688c PMID:22276770

Law, M., Greene, L. E., Johnson, J. C., Saykally, R., & Yang, P. (2005). Nanowire dye-sensitized solar cells. *Nature Materials*, *4*(6), 455–459. doi:10.1038/nmat1387 PMID:15895100

Lee, H.-M., Kwac, L.-K., An, K.-H., Park, S.-J., & Kim, B.-J. (2016). Electrochemical behavior of pitch-based activated carbon fibers for electrochemical capacitors. *Energy Conversion and Management*, *125*, 347–352. doi:10.1016/j.enconman.2016.06.006

Lewandowski, A., & Agnieszka, S. M. (2009). Ionic liquids as electrolytes for Li-ion batteries-An overview of electrochemical studies. *Journal of Power Sources*, *194*(2), 601–609. doi:10.1016/j.jpowsour.2009.06.089

Li, Y., Hu, Y., Zhao, Y., Shi, G., Deng, L., Hou, Y., & Qu, L. (2011). An electrochemical avenue to green-luminescent graphene quantum dots as potential electron-acceptors for photovoltaics. *Advanced Materials*, *6*(6), 776–780. doi:10.1002/adma.201003819 PMID:21287641

Liu, D., & Cao, G. (2010). Engineering nanostructured electrodes and fabrication of film electrodes for efficient lithium ion intercalation. *Energy & Environmental Science*, *3*(9), 1218–1237. doi:10.1039/b922656g

Liu, D., Wang, H., Du, P., & Liu, P. (2017). Independently double-crosslinked carbon nanotubes/polyaniline composite films as flexible and robust free-standing electrodes for high-performance supercapacitors. *Carbon*, *122*, 761–774. doi:10.1016/j.carbon.2017.06.097

Liu, D., Zhang, Y., Xiao, P., Garcia, B. B., Zhang, Q., Zhou, X., Jeong, Y.-H., & Cao, G. (2009). TiO_2 nanotube arrays annealed in CO exhibiting high performance for lithium ion intercalation. *Electrochimica Acta*, *54*(27), 6816–6820. doi:10.1016/j.electacta.2009.06.090

Liu, T., Sreekumar, T. V., Kumar, S., Hauge, R. H., & Smalley, R. E. (2003). SWNT/PAN composite film-based supercapacitors. *Carbon*, *41*(12), 2440–2442. doi:10.1016/S0008-6223(03)00245-8

Liu, Y., Clark, M., Zhang, Q., Yu, D., Liu, D., Liu, J., & Cao, G. (2011). V_2O_5 Nano-Electrodes with High Power and Energy Densities for Thin Film Li-Ion Batteries. *Advanced Energy Materials*, *1*(2), 194–202. doi:10.1002/aenm.201000037

Liu, Y., Yan, D., Li, Y., Wu, Z., Zhuo, R., Li, S., Feng, J., Wang, J., Yan, P., & Geng, Z. (2014). Manganese dioxide nanosheet arrays grown on graphene oxide as an advanced electrode material for supercapacitors. *Electrochimica Acta*, *117*, 528–533. doi:10.1016/j.electacta.2013.11.121

Mor, G. K., Shankar, K., Paulose, M., Varghese, O. K., & Grimes, C. A. (2006). Use of highly-ordered TiO(2) nanotube arrays in dye-sensitized solar cells. *Nano Letters*, *6*(2), 215–218. doi:10.1021/nl052099j PMID:16464037

Moriguchi, I., Hidaka, R., Yamada, H., Kudo, T., Murakami, H., & Nakashima, N. (2006). A Mesoporous Nanocomposite of TiO_2 and Carbon Nanotubes as a High-Rate Li-Intercalation Electrode Material. *Advanced Materials*, *18*(1), 69–73. doi:10.1002/adma.200501366

Niu, C., Sichel, E. K., Hoch, R., Moy, D., & Tennent, H. (1997). High power electrochemical capacitors based on carbon nanotube electrodes. *Applied Physics Letters*, *70*(11), 1480–1482. doi:10.1063/1.118568

Nozik, A. J. (2008). Multiple exciton generation in semiconductor quantum dots. *Chemical Physics Letters*, *457*(1-3), 3–11. doi:10.1016/j.cplett.2008.03.094

O'Regan, B., & Gratzel, M. (1991). A low-cost, high-efficiency solar cell based on dye-sensitized colloidal TiO_2 films. *Nature*, *353*(6346), 737–740. doi:10.1038/353737a0

Ohzuku, T., Wakamatsu, H., Takehara, Z., & Yoshizawa, S. (1979). Nonaqueous lithium/pyromellitic dianhydride cell. *Electrochimica Acta*, *24*, 219–312. doi:10.1016/0013-4686(79)80028-6

Pan, X.-L., Xu, C.-Y., & Zhen, L. (2012). Synthesis of $LiMnPO_4$ microspheres assembled by plates, wedges and prisms with different crystallographic orientations and their electrochemical performance. *CrystEngComm*, *14*(20), 6412. doi:10.1039/c2ce25593f

Pan, Z., Xie, S., Chang, B., Wang, C., Lu, L., Liu, W., Zhou, W., Li, W., & Qian, L. (1998). Very long carbon nanotubes. *Nature*, *394*(6694), 631–632. doi:10.1038/29206

Paulose, M., Shankar, K., Varghese, O. K., Mor, G. K., & Grimes, C. A. (2006 a). Application of highly-ordered TiO2 nanotube-arrays in heterojunction dye-sensitized solar cells. *Journal of Physics. D, Applied Physics*, *39*(12), 2498–2503. doi:10.1088/0022-3727/39/12/005

Paulose, M., Shankar, K., Varghese, O. K., Mor, G. K., Hardin, B., & Grimes, C. A. (2006b). Backside illuminated dye-sensitized solar cells based on titania nanotube array electrodes. *Nanotechnology*, *17*(5), 1446–1448. doi:10.1088/0957-4484/17/5/046

Pelemiš, S., & Hut, I. (2013). Nanotechnology materials for solar energy conversion. *Contemporary Materials Renewable Energy Sources, IV*, *2*, 145–151.

Portet, C., Taberna, P., Simon, P., & Flahaut, E. (2005). Influence of carbon nanotubes addition on carbon-carbon supercapacitor performances in organic electrolyte. *Journal of Power Sources*, *139*(1-2), 371–378. doi:10.1016/j.jpowsour.2004.07.015

Rudge, A., Davey, J., Raistrick, I., Gottesfeld, S., & Ferraris, J. P. (1994). Conducting polymers as active materials in electrochemical capacitors. *Journal of Power Sources*, *47*(1-2), 89–107. doi:10.1016/0378-7753(94)80053-7

Salant, A., Shalom, M., Hod, I., Faust, A., Zaban, A., & Banin, U. (2010). Quantum dot sensitized solar cells with improved efficiency prepared using electrophoretic deposition. *ACS Nano*, *4*(10), 5962–5968. doi:10.1021/nn1018208 PMID:20866044

Song, M. Y., Ahn, Y. R., Jo, S. M., Kim, D. Y., & Ahn, J.-P. (2005). TiO_2 single-crystalline nanorod electrode for quasi-solid-state dye-sensitized solar cells. *Applied Physics Letters*, *87*(11), 113113. doi:10.1063/1.2048816

Stoller, M. D., Park, S., Zhu, Y., An, J., & Ruoff, R. S. (2008). (. Graphene-based ultracapacitors. *Nano Letters*, *8*(10), 3498–3502. doi:10.1021/nl802558y PMID:18788793

Tarascon, J.-M., & Armand, M. (2001). Issues and challenges facing rechargeable lithium batteries. *Nature*, *414*(6861), 359–367. doi:10.1038/35104644 PMID:11713543

Wagemaker, M., Borghols, W. J. H., & Mulder, F. M. (2007). Large Impact of Particle Size on Insertion Reactions. A Case for Anatase Li_xTiO_2. *Journal of the American Chemical Society*, *129*(14), 4323–4327. doi:10.1021/ja067733p PMID:17362005

Wang, D. W., Li, F., Zhao, J., Ren, W., Chen, Z. G., Tan, J., Wu, Z. S., Gentle, I., Lu, G. Q., & Cheng, H. M. (2010). Fabrication of Graphene/Polyaniline Composite Paper via In Situ Anodic Electropolymerization for High-Performance Flexible Electrode. *ACS Nano*, *3*(7), 1745–1752. doi:10.1021/nn900297m PMID:19489559

Wang, G., Zhang, L., & Zhang, J. (2012). A review of electrode materials for electrochemical supercapacitors. *Chemical Society Reviews*, *41*(2), 797–828. doi:10.1039/C1CS15060J PMID:21779609

Xia, Y., Zhang, W. K., Huang, H., Gan, Y. P., Tian, J., & Tao, X. Y. (2011). Self-assembled mesoporous LiFePO4 with hierarchical spindle-like architectures for high-performance lithium-ion batteries. *Journal of Power Sources*, *196*(13), 5651–5658. doi:10.1016/j.jpowsour.2011.02.044

Yamaki, J., Takatsuji, H., Kawamura, T., & Egashira, M. (2002). Thermal stability of graphite anode with electrolyte in lithium-ion cells. *Solid State Ionics*, *148*(3-4), 241–245. doi:10.1016/S0167-2738(02)00060-7

Yan, J., Wei, T., Shao, B., Ma, F., Fan, Z., Zhang, M., Zheng, C., Shang, Y., Quian, W., & Wei, F. (2010). Electrochemical properties of graphene nanosheet/carbon black composites as electrodes for supercapacitors. *Carbon*, *48*(6), 1731–1737. doi:10.1016/j.carbon.2010.01.014

Yang, J., Winter, M., & Besenhard, J. (1996). Small particle size multiphase Li-alloy anodes for lithium-ion-batteries. *Solid State Ionics*, *90*(1-4), 281–287. doi:10.1016/S0167-2738(96)00389-X

Yang, N., Zhai, J., Wang, D., Chen, Y., & Jiang, L. (2010). Two-dimensional graphene bridges enhanced photoinduced charge transport in dye-sensitized solar cells. *ACS Nano*, *4*(2), 887–894. doi:10.1021/nn901660v PMID:20088539

Yang, W., Ni, M., Ren, X., Tian, Y., Li, N., Su, Y., & Zhang, X. (2015). (. Graphene in supercapacitor applications. *Current Opinion in Colloid & Interface Science*, *20*(5-6), 416–428. doi:10.1016/j.cocis.2015.10.009

Yang, W., Wan, F., Wang, Y., & Jiang, C. (2009). Achievement of 6.03% conversion efficiency of dye-sensitized solar cells with single-crystalline rutile TiO2 nanorod photoanode. *Applied Physics Letters*, *95*(13), 133121. doi:10.1063/1.3240870

Yang, Y., Qu, L., Dai, L., Kang, T. S., & Durstock, M. (2007). Electrophoresis Coating of Titanium Dioxide on Aligned Carbon Nanotubes for Controlled Syntheses of Photoelectronic Nanomaterials. *Advanced Materials*, *19*(9), 1239–1243. doi:10.1002/adma.200602181

Yella, A., Lee, H.-W., Tsao, H. N., Yi, C., Chandiran, A. K., Nazeeruddin, M. K., Diau, E. W.-G., Yeh, C.-Y., Zakeeruddin, S. M., & Gratzel, M. (2011). Porphyrin-sensitized solar cells with cobalt (II/III)–based redox electrolyte exceed 12 percent efficiency. *Science*, *334*(6056), 629–634. doi:10.1126cience.1209688 PMID:22053043

Yianoulis, P., & Giannouli, M. (2008). Thin Solid Films and Nanomaterials for Solar Energy Conversion and Energy Saving Applications. *Journal of Nano Research*, *2*, 49–60. doi:10.4028/www.scientific.net/JNanoR.2.49

Yu, D., & Dai, L. (2010). Self-Assembled Graphene/Carbon Nanotube Hybrid Films for Supercapacitors. *The Journal of Physical Chemistry Letters*, *1*(2), 467–470. doi:10.1021/jz9003137

Zhang, S. S. (2006). A review on electrolyte additives for lithium-ion batteries. *Journal of Power Sources*, *162*(2), 1379–1394. doi:10.1016/j.jpowsour.2006.07.074

Zheng, J. P., Cygan, P. J., & Jow, T. R. (1995). Hydrous Ruthenium Oxide as an Electrode Material for Electrochemical Capacitors. *Journal of the Electrochemical Society*, *142*(8), 2699–2703. doi:10.1149/1.2050077

Zhou, H., Li, D., Hibino, M., & Honma, I. (2005). A self-ordered, crystalline-glass, mesoporous nanocomposite for use as a lithium-based storage device with both high power and high energy densities. *Angewandte Chemie International Edition*, *44*(5), 797–802. doi:10.1002/anie.200460937 PMID:15612076

Zhukovskii, Y. F., Balaya, P., Kotomin, E. A., & Maier, J. (2006). Evidence for Interfacial-Storage Anomaly in Nanocomposites for Lithium Batteries from First-Principles Simulations. *Physical Review Letters*, *96*(5), 058302. doi:10.1103/PhysRevLett.96.058302 PMID:16487002

Zilli, D., Bonelli, P. R., & Cukierman, A. L. (2006). Effect of alignment on adsorption of multi-walled carbon nanotube arrays. *Nanotechnology*, *17*, 5126. doi:10.1088/0957-4484/17/20/016

Chapter 12
Application of LiMn2O4 Nanostructures as Efficient Cathodes for Energy Storage Devices

Shabir Ahmad Akhoon
Department of Applied Sciences, Institute of Technology, University of Kashmir, India

Ashaq Hussain Sofi
https://orcid.org/0000-0003-4279-5481
Department of Physics, National Institute of Technology, Srinagar, India

Rayees Ahmad Khan
Department of Physics, B. S. Abdur Rahman Crescent Institute of Science and Technology, Chennai, India

Ab. Mateen Tantray
Department of Physics, National Institute of Technology, Srinagar, India

Seemin Rubab
https://orcid.org/0000-0002-0593-4449
Department of Physics, National Institute of Technology, Srinagar, India

ABSTRACT

Renewable energy resources have been investigated as alternatives to fossil fuels. Though the energy density of these renewable sources is not comparable to the fossil fuels, their abundance make them highly interesting. There are three main steps in the renewable energy utilization: harvesting, conversion, and storage. Thus, after harvesting renewable energy, storing this energy is an important aspect for its large-scale end use. Considering the fact that the energy is a basic need for life on earth, there has been a strong scientific temperament towards the renewable energy utilization. The electrical energy storage maintains the key to promote the use of renewable energy. Among the storage devices, the rechargeable lithium ion batteries (LIBs) are the most promising energy storage devices. Among various cathodes proposed for LIBs, the most promising one is the spinel lithium manganese oxide (LiMn2O4). Its non-toxicity, low cost, abundance, and ease of synthesis, besides being environmentally friendly, make it suitable for next generation green LIBs.

DOI: 10.4018/978-1-7998-5563-7.ch012

INTRODUCTION

Renewable energy resources such have been investigated as alternatives to fossil fuels. Though the energy density of these renewable sources is not comparable to the fossil fuels but their abundance make them highly interesting. Further, the renewable energy conversions are of very low efficiency and unpredictable. There are three main steps in the renewable energy utilization: harvesting, conversion and storage. Thus, after harvesting renewable energy, storing this energy is an important aspect for its large scale end use.

Considering the fact that the energy is a basic need for life on earth, there has been a strong scientific temperament towards the renewable energy utilization for its significant environmental friendly implications. Thus, a great progress has been made, in recent years both in terms of renewable energy harvesting, conversion and storage. Nanomaterials based novel designs have demonstrated very promising results in increasing the efficiency in renewable energy utilization (Akhoon, S. A., 2016; Guo, Y. G., 2007; Maier, J. 2005). The electrical energy storage maintains the key to promote the use of renewable energy and to curb the green house gas emissions. During the last twenty years, great progress has been made in the electrical storage systems, but no current system is able to meet the targets set for the demanding applications, with regards to energy and power density, price and life time (Liu, J., 2008).

Among the storage devices, the rechargeable lithium ion batteries (LIBs) are the most promising energy storage devices. These find wide applications in portable power tools, wireless communication devices and hybrid electric vehicles etc (Rajesh, Y. B. R. D., 2013; Guo, D., 2013; Tang, W.; 2012; Manjunatha, H., 2011) as demonstrated in figure 1. Lithium ion rechargeable battery is common and most popular in consumer electronics, especially in portable electronics, with low cost, high energy density, no memory effect and a slow self discharging. These are also growing in popularity for use in aerospace, military, energy storage, as a replacement to lead acid batteries and electric and hybrid electric vehicle applications. The pioneer work on lithium metal battery had begun in the year 1912 under G.N. Lewis. But due to the inherent instability of lithium metal, new research was focused towards rechargeable lithium ion battery (Buchmann, I., 2001) and in the year 1991, Sony Corporation commercialized the first lithium ion battery, with superior safety and stability.

WORKING PRINCIPLE OF A LITHIUM ION BATTERY

In a lithium ion battery, lithium ions move from positive electrode to negative electrode during charging and vice versa during the discharging process. The electrolyte and the two electrodes (anode and cathode) are the three primary functional constituent components of lithium-ion battery. Lithium ion battery consists of a lithium-ion intercalation negative electrode (generally graphite), and a lithium-ion intercalation positive electrode (generally the lithium metal oxide). The two electrodes are separated by lithium-ion conducting electrolyte (for example a solution of lithium complexes in ethylene carbonate or diethyl-carbonate), through which the movement of lithium ions takes place (Scrosati, B., 2010).

This mechanism of charging and discharging of lithium ion battery is based on the diffusion of lithium ion through the electrolyte towards the respective electrodes: delivering lithium ions to

Figure 1. Advantages of li-ion batteries in terms of size, weight and cost (http://www.cei.washington.edu; http://www.alaskareflector.org).

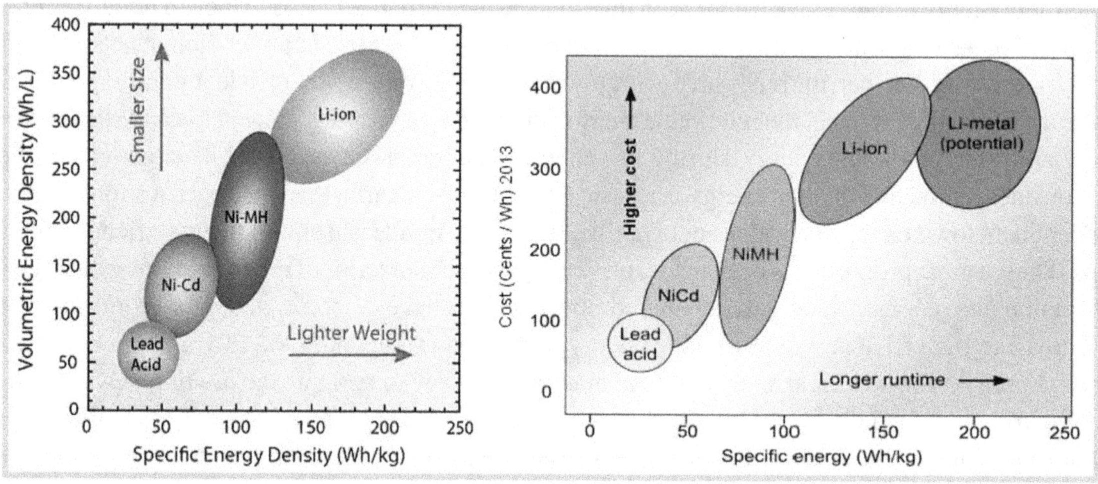

the surface of anode, transitioning to and diffusion through the electrolyte, and transitioning to and diffusion into the cathode as illustrated in figure 2. During this intercalation and deintercalation process of lithium ions, a volume change occurs in the active electrode materials, making these batteries dangerous under certain conditions. Efforts in material processing and manufacturing have been carried out from several decades to increase the performance and to manage the unavoidable volume changes in the lithium ion batteries. The active electrode materials should be both electronic and ionic conductors as both these parameters influence the current flow and hence, the power delivered. These efforts have lead to the nanostructured electrode materials. Nanostructured materials can provide a desired morphology, high surface area, and can accommodate the volume changes with minimal risk of cracking and reduced diffusion path lengths (Chan, C. K., 2008).

Figure 2. Working principal of Li-ion battery (Molenda, J., 2011).

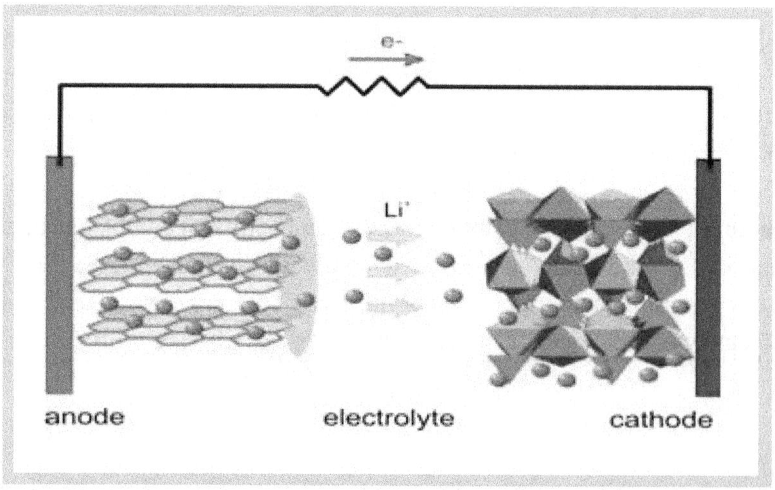

Spinel Lithium Manganese Oxide as a Cathode Electrode

The intercalation and deintercalation of lithium ion is easy because of the 3D tunnel structure of spinel lithium manganese oxide (Guo, D., 2013; Tang, W., 2012; Manjunatha, H., 2011; Guo, D., 2014) as shown in figure 3. The framework was first demonstrated by Thackeray et al. for lithium insertion host in $LiMn_2O_4$ for a rechargeable electrode in a lithium ion battery (David, W. I. F., 1987; Thackeray, M. M. 1997; Yi, T. F., 2014). It has an arrangement of fd3m space group in which lithium ion occupies a 8a tetrahedral sites, manganese at 16d sites and oxygen at 32e sites (Thirunakaran, R., 2013; Park, S. H., 2003; Yi, T., 2008). The edge-shared octahedral Mn_2O_4 host structure being highly stable and because of face-sharing of tetrahedral lithium (8a) sites and empty octahedral (16c) sites, possesses a series of tunnels which intersect each other. Lithium diffusion occurs through such tunnels. At about 4 V, the lithium intercalation/deintercalation occurs into/from the 8a tetrahedral sites while maintaining the cubic spinel symmetry (Xia, H., 2012).

Figure 3. $LiMn_2O_4$ spinel structure. (http://people.cst.cmich.edu.)

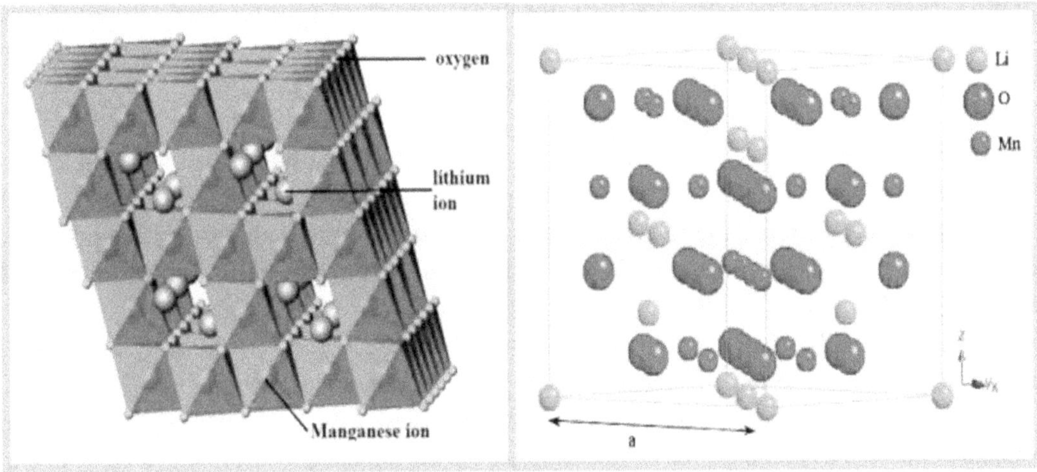

Different Synthesis Methods for $LiMn_2O_4$ Nanostructures

The usual method to produce $LiMn_2O_4$ has been the solid state reaction process (Lu, C. H., 2001; Miura, K., 1996; Tarascon, J. M., 1993; Reimers, J. N., 1992; Jones, C. D. W., 1994; Barker, J., 1996; Tarascon, J. M., 1993; Jiang, Z., 1996). But this method has several disadvantages of in-homogeneity, irregular morphology, broader particle size distribution, poor control of stoichiometry and longer periods of calcinations (Seyedahmadian, M., 2013). Spray pyrolysis has been considered as the versatile process to synthesize homogeneous $LiMn_2O_4$, but it leads to the discharge of toxic and corrosive gases (Hirose, S., 2011). Numerous other wet chemical methods, which include co-precipitation method (Thirunakaran, R., 2013; Qiu, X., 1997), emulsion drying (Lu, C. H., 2001; Park, S. B., 2006), hydrothermal method (Jiang, C. H., 2007), the sol-gel method (Seyedahmadian, M., 2013; Ikuhara, Y. H., 1999), pechini process (Liu, W., 1996) and combustion synthesis method (Zhu, C., 2014) etc have been explored to synthesize

$LiMn_2O_4$ powders to overcome the drawbacks of other methods. Among these methods, solution combustion synthesis method, solution mixture of aqueous metal salts and fuels, based on exothermic and self sustaining reaction is a promising method to synthesize $LiMn_2O_4$ powders. It is a single step method to yield nanosize particles having large specific surface area and homogeneous doping of trace amounts of various elements, besides being an environmental friendly synthesis method (Aruna, S. T., 2008).

Both the electrodes of the lithium ion batteries have been satisfactorily explored with nanostructures of transition metal oxides. These studies incorporate different nanostructures like nanorods, nanowires, nanotubes etc as the electrode materials in lithium ion batteries (Hassoun, J., 2007; Timmons, A., 2007). The nanostructuration of the cathodes with manganese oxides are suitable for both environmental and economical reasons. Wang et al demonstrated that the storage and rate capability of Li-ion batteries is greatly influenced by the electrode morphology (Wang, Y., 2006). Nanotubes and nanowires of manganese oxides have shown to enhance the performance in lithium ion batteries and thus, different morphologies have been explored as efficient electrodes and a lot of research has been devoted to it. Synthesis of ordered mesoporous, large surface area and highly crystalline cathodes has been under focus. These properties could arrange the electrolyte inside the pores with enhanced intercalation and deintercalation processes and thus, notably increase the performance of the lithium ion battery.

Among various cathodes proposed for LIBs, the most promising one is the spinel lithium manganese oxide ($LiMn_2O_4$). Its non-toxicity, low cost, abundance and ease of synthesis, besides being environmental friendly makes it suitable for next generation green LIBs (Rajesh, Y. B. R. D., 2013; Zhu, J., 2012; Chen, Z. H., 2010).

The nanostructured morphologies of $LiMn_2O_4$ could meet the requirements for enhanced LIBs for better performance from each strategic point of view (Cheng, B., 2012). Nanostructured $LiMn_2O_4$ has shown to significantly increase the intercalation/de-intercalation of Li^+ due to (a) large surface area, providing innumerable reaction sites for Li and (b) shorter diffusion lengths for Li^+ within the $LiMn_2O_4$ particles (Okubo, M., 2010; Ryu, W. H., 2011; Tang, W., 2012).

It has been very well established that the size, specific surface area, crystallinity and morphology of the nanomaterials have a great influence on their properties and applications (Ju, S. H., 2012). Thus, in this regard, several approaches have been devised to synthesize 1-D, 2-D and 3-D nanostructures of $LiMn_2O_4$ and explored as cathodes for Li-ion batteries (Wu, H. M., 2005; Liu, X., 2013; Liu, Q., 2013; Zhu, C., 2014). The results have revealed that 3D hierarchical nanostructures often produce more active sites or possess more interesting properties compared to 1D and 2D nanostructures. Among the various nanostructures, nanospheres, nanorods and nanowires have been synthesized by template methods, employing MnO_2 nanostructures as templates (Chen, Z. H., 2010; Hosono, E., 2009; Kim, D. K., 2008) and micro-cubes by sol gel method (Yi, T., 2008).

Shortcomings of $LiMn_2O_4$ as a Cathode Material

Unfortunately, during charging/discharging, $LiMn_2O_4$ suffers from serious defects of poor cycling performance and capacity fading, especially at elevated temperatures (Liu, Q., 2013). These disadvantages with $LiMn_2O_4$, as a cathode material limit its commercialization. The capacity degradation of $LiMn_2O_4$ has been reported as a result of: (a) dissolution of manganese into the electrolyte solution, (b) decomposition of electrolyte at the electrode, (c) phase transition from cubic to tetragonal upon 3V cycling and (d) micro-crack formation at the cathode surface during electrochemical cycling (Xiao, L., 2008; Liu, Q., 2013). Dissolution of Mn as Mn^{3+} and Mn^{2+} ions into the electrolyte solution has been considered to play a major part in reducing the cycling performance and capacity fading of the $LiMn_2O_4$ respectively (Park, J., 2011).

To suppress the capacity fading and improve the electrochemical properties, several attempts have been made to synthesize modified $LiMn_2O_4$ nanostructures. The partial substitution of cations for Mn and surface coating of $LiMn_2O_4$ have been proposed as the main strategies (Ouyang, C. Y., 2010; Li, C., 2006; Etacheri, V., 2011; Yi, T. F., 2009). For instance, the cation doping method shows better electrochemical performance as it weakens the Jahn-Teller effect and improves the stability of the structure (Liu, Q., 2013) and hence, improves the cycling performance.

Singhal et al. synthesized Nd doped $LiMn_2O_4$ nanopowders ($LiMn_{1.99}Nd_{0.01}O_4$) by sol-gel method (Singhal, R., 2007). The initial discharge capacity of 149 $mAhg^{-1}$ was obtained for the sample. The results of charge-dischrage characteristics in 3.4-4.3 V voltage range indicated that the small concentration doping considerably reduced the capacity fading compared to pure $LiMn_2O_4$. The capacity retention of 91% was obtained after 25 cycles. Malyovanyi et al. obtained the Fe doped ($Li_{1.2}Mn_{1.6}Fe_{0.4}O_4$) spinel structure of $LiMn_2O_4$ (Malyovanyi, S. M., 2013). The oxide showed good reversibility for the first several cycles. The initial discharge capacity of 105 mAh g^{-1} was obtained with Fe doping. The Fe doping reduced the initial discharge capacity. Also, the capacity retention of the doped samples was not so impressive after initial cycles. Thirunakaran et al. synthesized the B-doped $LiMn_2O_4$ spinel structure ($LiB_xMn_{2-x}O_4$) in which the concentration of dopant was varied (x = 0.01, 0.02, 0.05, 0.10, 0.20) (Thirunakaran, R., 2004). The sample was homogenous in size with higher degree of crystallinity. The results showed better electrochemical performance. The initial discharge capacity of 120 $mAhg^{-1}$ was obtained with the capacity retention of 75% after 30 cycles. Yang et al. synthesized $LiMn_2O_4$ nanorods with Al doping (Yang, Y., 2009). The $LiMn_{1.9}Al_{0.1}O_4$ nanorods showed more stability against the electrolyte etching than the pristine sample. The capacity retention of 96% was observed even after 100 cycles at 1C rate at room temperature. The sample also showed good capacity retention at higher current rates and also at higher temperatures.

The various other dopants used to synthesize the modified $LiMn_2O_4$ are the nonmetals like B (Chan, H. W., 2004; Thirunakaran, R., 2004; Chan, H. W., 2005), F (Chen, Y. B., 2010; Feng, C., 2010; Jayaprakash, N., 2010), S (Molenda, M., 2007), Br (Du, G., 2011), the metals like Al (Amaral, F. A., 2010), Mg (Singh, P., 2010), Cr (Peng, Z. D., 2010; Xu, W., 2011) Ti (Liu, D. Q., 2007; Lu, W., 2007), Fe (Singh, P., 2009), Ni (Wu, H. M., 2007), Co (Amaral, F. A., 2010; Luo, Q., 2009), Cu (Ein-Eli, Y., 2005), Zn (Liu, H., 2007; Tu, J., 2007; Sclar, H., 2012), Ga (Liu, D. Q., 2007), Zr (Wu, H. M., 2010), Ru (Wang, H., 2011), Ag (Son, J. T., 2004; Zhou, W. J., 2008), Sn (Wang, L., 2010), Au (Tu, J., 2006), the rear earth metals La (Sun, H., 2012), Ce (Ha, H. W., 2007), Pr (Iqbal, M. J., 2008), Nd (Suryakala, K., 2008), Sm (Balaji, S. R. K., 2010), Gd (Helan, M., 2011), and the actinide dopants: Th (Chao, L. I., 2006), U (Eftekhari, A., 2006). The modified $LiMn_2O_4$ with surface coatings (Li, X., 2008; Shi, J. Y., 2010; Qing, C., 2011; Li, C., 2006), electrolyte modification (Kamarulzaman, N., 2001), laser annealing (Pröll, J., 2011), pulsed laser deposition (Tang, S. B., 2006) and process optimization (Jeong, W. T., 2003) are the other strategies that have been reported to suppress the disadvantages associated with $LiMn_2O_4$ as cathodes for Li-ion batteries. Among these strategies, the doping method has been observed to demonstrate better electrochemical performances.

Among the various cations doped in the spinel $LiMn_2O_4$, aluminum (Al) doping has been considered as an attractive substitution as it has several advantages of being non-toxic, cheap and lighter than other transition metal elements (Ding, Y. L., 2011; Ryu, W. H., 2011). The electrochemical characteristics have also been better with Al doping than other doped samples as discussed above. Al doped $LiMn_2O_4$ as a cathode material has been observed with improved cycling performance and reduced capacity fading

(Kim, K. W., 2003; Yang, Y., 2009). The substitution of Mn^{3+} by Al^{3+} results in a strong M-O bonding in the spinel framework and increased stability against the electrolyte etching.

Thus, the morphology and the optimum cation doping of the spinel $LiMn_2O_4$, as discussed above, have an influence on its electrochemical properties. Thus, aluminum doped $LiMn_2O_4$ cathode material having a spherical or rod like morphology should be an effective way of enhancing the electrochemical performance of LIBs. While, most of the recent works have employed MnO_2 nanostructures as self-templates to synthesize nanospheres and nanorod like structures of $LiMn_2O_4$ through various synthesis techniques in a multi-step processes (Xiao, X., 2010; Xia, H., 2012; Kebede, M. A., 2015). Solution synthesis techniques have been preferred in order to obtain homogeneously cation doped compositions of $LiMn_2O_4$ and rapid synthesis of highly doped oxides in a one step process (Nkosi, F. P., 2015). Finally, it is believed that synthesis without catalysts and templates is an efficient way for large-scale production and well-dispersed nanomaterials (Zhu, C., 2014). However, it is essential to identify an ideal methodology that can solve the major shortcomings like, scalable production, ease of synthesis, low temperature synthesis, particle size distribution, and environmentally benign and single step process. All these factors do influence the overall strategy towards LIBs regarding its economies and applications.

Solution combustion synthesis provides the advantages of: scalable production, ease of synthesis, low temperature synthesis, control over particle size distribution, and environmentally benign and single step process. Owing to these advantages of solution combustion method, in this chapter, we shall discuss a facile, single step solution combustion synthesis of Al doped $LiMn_2O_4$ nanorods and nanospheres without the use of MnO_2 as self-templates. The as synthesized $LiMn_2O_4$, $LiMn_{1.6}Al_{0.4}O_4$ nanorods and $LiMn_{1.6}Al_{0.4}O_4$ nanospheres were characterized for the structural, morphological and electrochemical characteristics. The electrodes were synthesized to study their electrochemical behavior as cathodes for lithium ion battery and hence, a correlation within a short study is to be established.

Synthesis of $LiMn_2O_4$, Al Doped $LiMn_2O_4$ ($LiM_{n1.6}Al_{0.4}O$) Nanorods and Al Doped $LiMn_2O_4$ ($LiMn_{1.6}Al_{0.4}O_4$) Nanospheres

In the typical synthesis of $LiMn_2O_4$ and Al doped $LiMn_2O_4$ ($LiM_{n1.6}Al_{0.4}O$) nanorods, stoichiometric amounts analytical grade lithium acetate ($Li(C_{H3}COO).2H_2O$), manganese acetate ($Mn(CH_3COO)_2.4H_2O$), aluminum nitrate ($Al(NO_3)_3.9H_2O$) were magnetically stirred in a solution of glycine, starch and urea (5 gm each) in a 650 ml of distilled water for one hour. The solution was transferred to a furnace and heated up to 700 °C with the heat rate at 2°C per minute. The final temperature was maintained for 2 hours after which, the system was allowed to cool down under open air conditions without removal from the furnace. The foam like product was retrieved and ground to fine powder, which was characterized without any further treatment.

In the typical synthesis of $LiMn_{1.6}Al_{0.4}O_4$ nanospheres, the above mentioned procedure was repeated, with an addition of oleic acid (10 ml) during stirring of precursors. The typical synthesis is depicted in the flow chart as shown in figure 4.

Figure 4. Solution combustion synthesis of $LiMn_2O_4$ and $LiMn_{1.6}Al_{0.4}O_4$ nanorods and nanospheres.

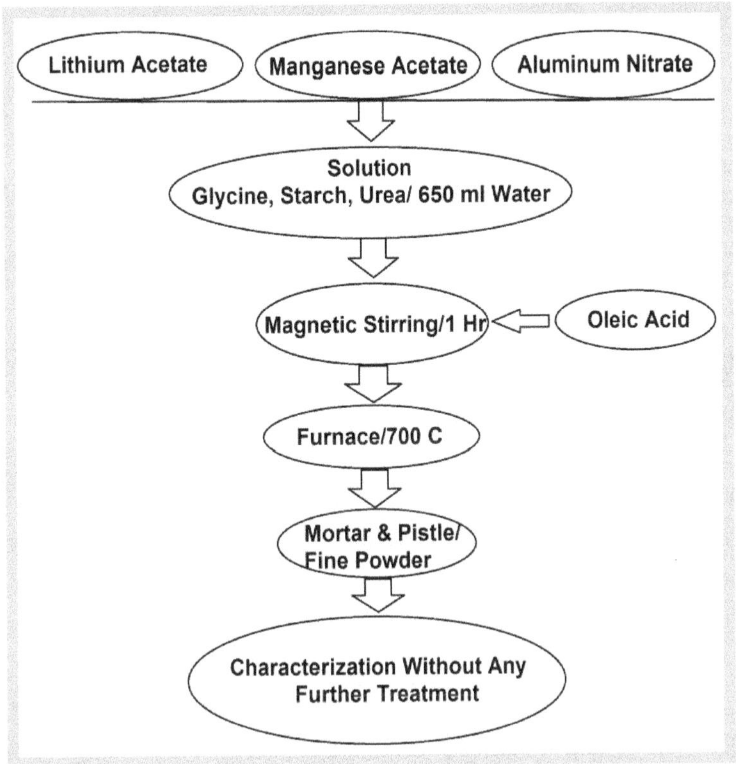

Structural Analysis

In the spinel structure of $LiMn_2O_4$, the 8a tetrahedral sites are occupied by the lithium ions. The presence of lithium at 8a tetrahedral sites gives rise to (220) reflection peaks in the XRD pattern of $LiMn_2O_4$ at around $2\theta = 30.7^{o}$ (Ra, W., 2005). As the X-ray scattering abilility of lithium atoms is very low, as evident from the figure 5, the absence of (220) reflection pleak indicate the presence of only lithium atoms at 8a tetrahedral sites in the lattice of $LiMn_2O_4$. Consiquently, the Al^{3+} ions could be considered to incorporate into the octahedral 16d sites in the lattice. Thus, the Al^{3+} ions are considered to partially substitute Mn ions in the lattice. The radius of Al^{3+} ion (0.053 nm) being smaller than that of Mn^{4+} ion (0.066 nm) and Mn^{3+} ion (0.060 nm), the partial substitution for Mn by Al in the lattice reduces the cell volume and hence, reduction in the lattice parameters. The detailed structural analysis of XRD, carried out by XRD Rietveld refinement method and the obatined parameters are determined in table 5. The crystal structure of $LiMn_2O_4$ could be stabilized because of the reduced cell volume and the stronger Al-O bond energy (502 kJ mol^{-1}) than Mn-O (362 kJ mol^{-1}) (Xiao, L., 2008; Li, Z., 2012). The substitution of Al for Mn is also evident from the XRD profile of Al doped samples.

Figure 5. XRD profile of $LiMn_2O_4$ and Al-doped $LiMn_2O_4$ samples.

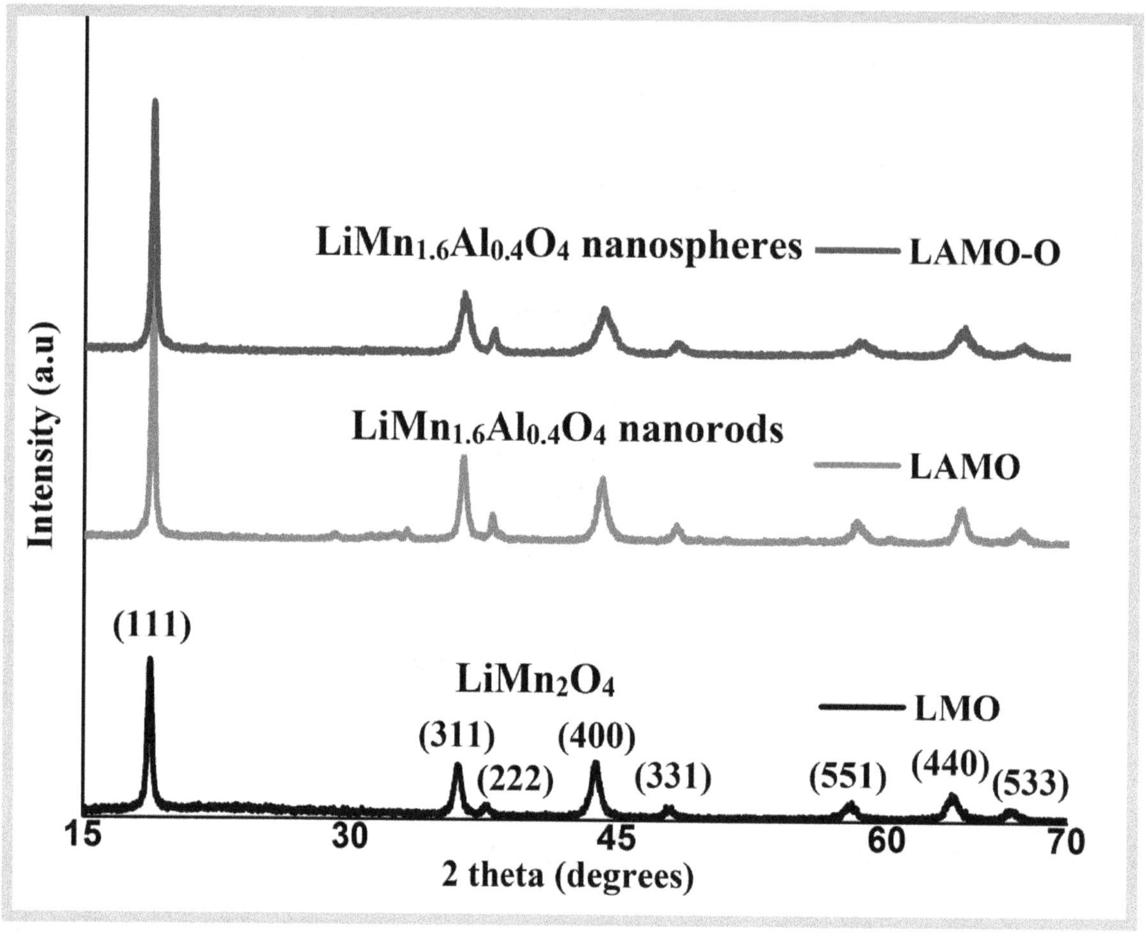

The shift in the peaks towards higher 2θ values indicate the reduction in the cell parameters due to the smaller ionic radius of Al than that of Mn as shown in figure 6 and demonstrated in table 1. Thus, the structure of LAMO-O is more strengthened, indicating the cycling performance of LAMO-O than the other samples.

Table 1. Comparison of JCPDS and observed peak positions of (111), (311) and (400) reflection peaks.

Reflection Peak	JCPDS 2θ (Degrees)	Observed 2θ (Degrees)		
		LMO	LAMO	LAMO-O
(111)	18.61	18.658	18.761	18.764
(311)	36.08	36.00	33.260	33.276
(400)	43.86	43.795	44.075	44.076

The sharp and the intense peaks in the XRD profile indicate the higher crystallinity of the sample, which is reported to influence the electrochemical properties of $LiMn_2O_4$ (Ju, S. H., 2012). The influence of Al-doping and oleic acid treatment is clearly evident from the XRD patterns of the samples as shown in figure 5 and figure 6. The intensity of the peaks and hence, crystallinity increase with Al-doping and oleic acid treatment as compared to pure $LiMn_2O_4$.

A shift towards higher 2θ values is observed in the XRD pattern of oleic acid treated Al-doped sample as shown in figure 6 and illustrated in table 1. It is reported that the precursors are influenced by the oleic acid treatment by forming a micelle structure. The micelle structure acts as a template to effectively control the crystal growth and hence, the morphology and the structure of the products (Yang, Z., 2012; Sadeghi, B., 2012). Thus, the oleic acid treatment reduces the cell volume and the lattice parameters, as calculated in table 2. This leads to the higher compactness of the structure of oleic acid treated Al-doped sample (LAMO-O) than Al-doped sample (LAMO). These properties of LAMO-O make it electrochemically more feasible as a cathode material than pristine $LiMn_2O_4$. The effect of oleic acid on the synthesis of $LiMn_2O_4$ nanostructures is studied and has been reported to effectively control the morphology of the $LiMn_2O_4$ (Akhoon, S. A., 2017).

The mixing degree of Mn atoms and the preferential lattice growth direction of the spinel $LiMn_2O_4$ have been reported to influence the stability of the structure and can be estimated by the intensity ratio of (111) and (311) reflection peaks (Guo, D., 2013). Its higher value indicates the more preferred crystal growth direction along (111) reflection plane and highly immaculate arrangement of the elements Li and Mn within the crystal structure (Yu, Z. M., 2007), leading to a stable structure. The intensity ratio (I_{111}/I_{311}) of the samples have been calculated and listed in table 2. Thus, the elements Li and Mn are arranged more orderly in the oleic acid treated sample (LAMO-O) and the (111) crystal of LAMO-O forms better. The (111) lattice growth orientation is an advantage in the intercalation and deintercalation of Li^+ ions during charging and discharging processes, which results in better electrochemical properties (Lee, Y. S., 2001; Wang, J. L., 2012; Guo, D., 2013).

It has also been reported that cycling performance and the crystallinity of $LiMn_2O_4$ is significantly related to the peak intensity ration of (311) and (400 reflection planes) (Liu, J., 2008, Wang, J. L., 2012; Lee, Y. S., 2001). As demonstrated in table 2, the Al-doped samples have higher intensity ratio (I_{311}/I_{400}) for LAMO and LAMO-O than for the pristine sample LMO.

Morphological Studies

During charging and discharging of the lithium ion battery, the Li-ions intercalate and deintercalate to and from the host electrode. Thus, the electrochemical activities and the mass-electrolyte contact are greatly influenced by the particle morphology of the host electrode (Xia, H., 2012; Fergus, J. W., 2010). Though the one dimensional nanostructures of $LiMn_2O_4$ have demonstrated an improved rate capability during the charge and discharge processes. But, these one dimensional nanostructures suffer from the disadvantages of low tap-density or volumetric-energy density. Therefore, three-dimensionally (3D) assembled nanostructured $LiMn_2O_4$ have been considered as the ideal solutions (Ryu, W. H., 2011). Such 3D nanostructures like, randomly aligned $LiMn_2O_4$ nanorods and nanospheres increase the Li^+ sites on the large surface area to improve the electrochemical properties and also, increase the volumetric energy density (Luo, J., 2007, Cho, J., 2008, Wang, J. L., 2012).

Figure 6. Comparison of peak position and intensity.

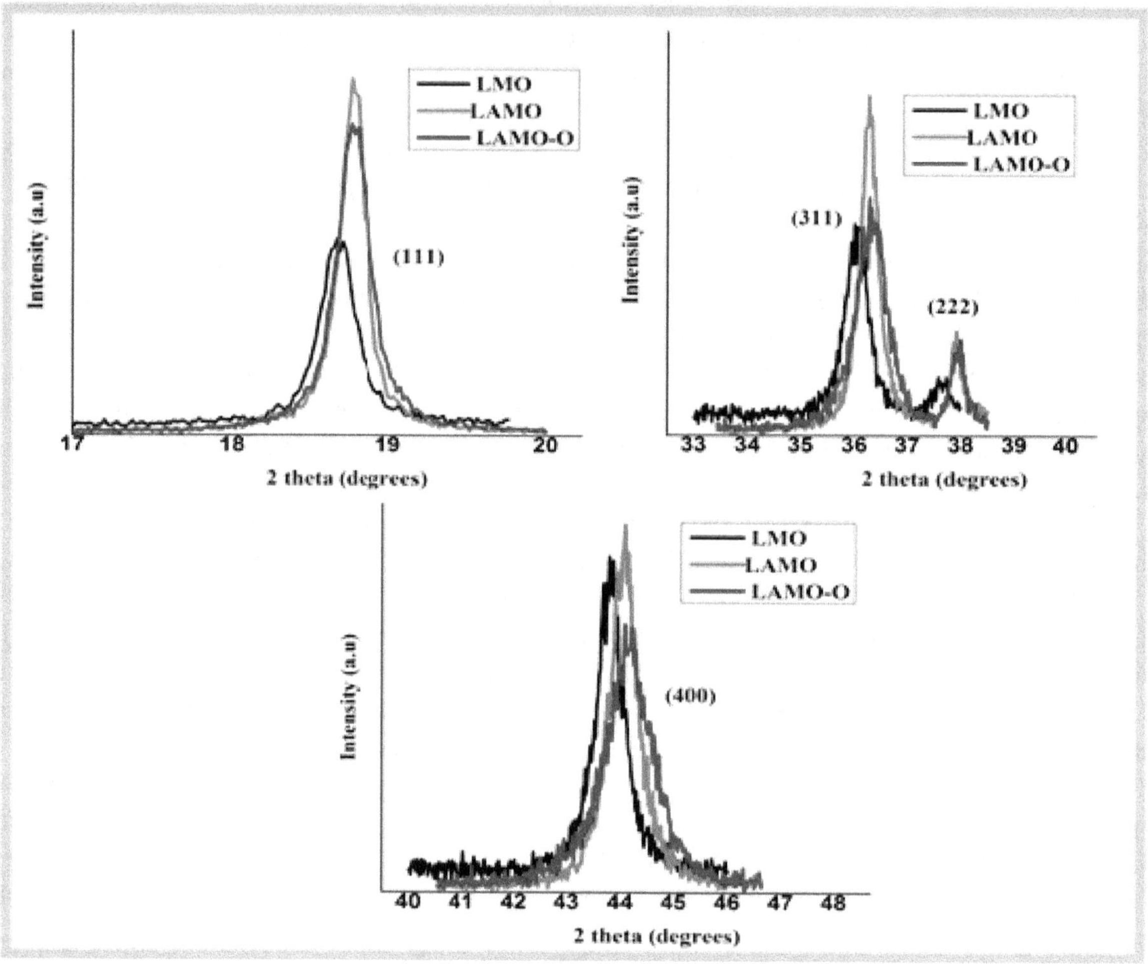

Table 2. XRD parameters of pristine and Al doped $LiMn_2O_4$ samples.

Sample	I_{111}/I_{311}	I_{311}/I_{400}	Lattice parameter 'a'	Cell Volume (nm^3)	Spacing 'd' (nm)
LMO	2.890	0.936	0.8193 nm	0.549	0.4751
LAMO	3.276	1.372	0.8127 nm	0.542	0.4725
LAMO-O	4.059	1.334	0.8109 nm	0.533	0.4721

Figure 7. FESEM images of the samples. (a) $LiMn_2O_4$ (b) $LiMn_{0.6}Al_{0.4}O_4$ nanorods and (c) $LiMn_{0.6}Al_{0.4}O_4$ nanospheres.

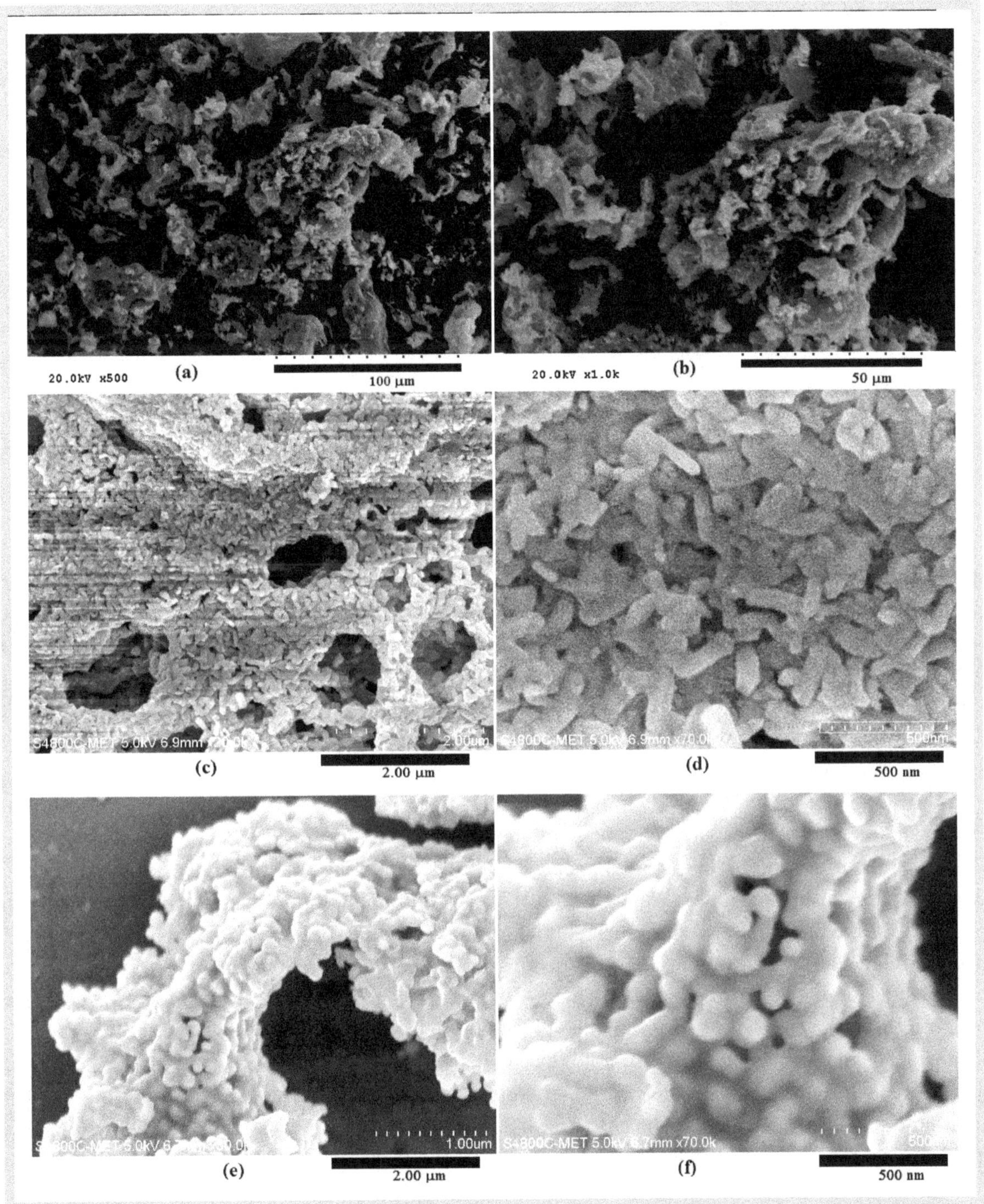

Figure 8. Charge and discharge profiles of the samples at a current rate of 100 mAg⁻¹ over 100 cycles.

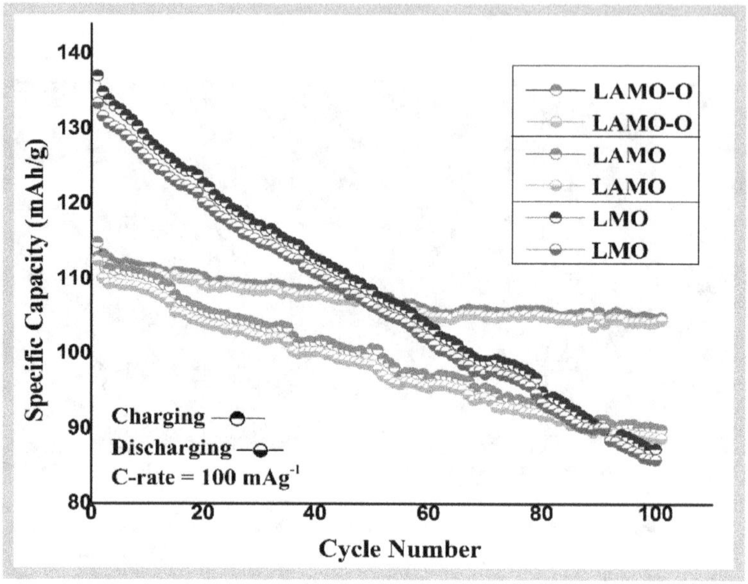

The FESEM micrographs of the $LiMn_2O_4$ samples are shown in figure 7. The images reveal the well defined structures of Al-doped and oleic acid treated $LiMn_2O_4$ samples as compared to the pristine $LiMn_2O_4$ sample. Thus, the Al-doping and oleic acid influence the morphology of the prepared $LiMn_2O_4$ samples. While, the FESEM images of pristine $LiMn_2O_4$ (figure 7a and 7b), without any Al-doping or oleic acid treatment reveal the wide distribution of micro-sized and roughly-shaped morphology, the images of 7(c) and 7(d) for Al-doped $LiMn_2O_4$ and the images of 7(e) and 7(f) for oleic acid-treated-Al-doped $LiMn_2O_4$ reveal the well defined, uniformly distributed nanorod morphology and the nano-sized-spherical morphology respectively. The

$LiMn_2O_4$ nanorods have a nearly uniform diameter of about 90 ± 10 nm, the length of about 240 ± 20 nm and the nanospheres have a diameter of about 100 nm.

The well defined morphology for Al doped samples are be defined on the basis of decomposition of the precursors during synthesis (Wang, J. L., 2012). The aluminum nitrate precursor thermally decomposed before the manganese acetate precursor to form Al_2O_3 nuclei in the Al-doped samples. These Al_2O_3 nuclei become the deposition sites for other metal salts and hence, restrain the forming of primary spinel particles (as in case of pristine sample). Thus, Al-doping acts as a self-template to synthesize $LiMn_2O_4$ nanorods, as is the case with LAMO sample. In case of oleic acid treated-Al-doped sample (LAMO-O), the influence of oleic acid on the morphology is quite evident. It is obivious that the morphology of the precursors is influenced by the oleic acid as a surafctant and hence, influences the morphology of the final products (Yang, Z., 2012). Thus, the rod-like morphology of $LiMn_{0.6}Al_{0.4}O_4$ changes to spherical morphology on the introduction of oleic acid.

Table 3. Charge capacities of the samples at different C-rates.

Sample	Capacity (mAh/g) @ 100 mAg^{-1}	Capacity retention after 100 cycles	Charge Capacity at Different C-Rates (mAh/g)					
			200 mA/g	300 mA/g	400 mA/g	500 mA/g	1000 mA/g	2000 mA/g
LMO	134	64%	126	99	85	75	40	10
LAMO	112	78%	93	76	63	56	29	10
LAMO-O	113	92%	110	102	93	83	47	16

Electrochemical Properties

The charge/discharge responses of the samples as cathodes were observed and the results are illustrated in figure 8, figure 9 and figure 10. The charge and discharge responses of the samples at a current rate of 100 mAg^{-1} over 100 cycles is shown in figure 8.

The initial discharge capacity of the pristine sample is very high as compared to Al doped samples. The initial discharge capacity for the pristine sample (LMO), Al-doped (LAMO) and oleic acid treated (LAMO-O) is found to be about 134 $mAhg^{-1}$, 112 $mAhg^{-1}$ and 113 $mAhg^{-1}$ respectively. The Al-doped samples show a low initial discharge capacity than that of the pristine sample because of the reduced electrochemically active Mn content due to the electrochemically inactive Al substitution (Kebede, M. A., 2014). Although, the Al-doped samples show a reduced initial discharge capacities, but, the capacity retention of the samples over 100 cycles is higher than that of pristine sample. The Al-doped samples show a capacity retention of about 78% for LAMO and about 92% for LAMO-O against 64% for the pristine sample at 100 mAg^{-1} (calculated in table 3).

The excellent cycling properties of the Al-doped samples may be explained on the basis of stable crystal structure and high Mn valency in the spinel due to partially substituted Al^{3+} for Mn^{3+} (Lee, Y. S., 2001). The Al^{3+} substitution may reduce the Jahn-Teller effect of the as-prepared Al-doped $LiMn_2O_4$ samples (Li, Z., 2012). Among the Al-doped samples, $LiMn_2O_4$ nanospheres show the best capacity retention of 92% after 100 cycles at a C-rate of 100 mAg^{-1} than 78% for the $LiMn_2O_4$ nanorods. The finding indicates that the cycleability is not only dependent on the Al-doping but also, on the morphology of the samples. As observed in the XRD results (table 2), the higher crystallinity and the highly ordered structure of $LiMn_2O_4$ nanospheres leads to a smooth intercalation and deintercalation of Li-ions. Thus, the highly crystalline $LiMn_2O_4$ nanospheres may absorb the stress/strain and hence, preserve the structural integrity during the Li-ion intercalation/deintercalation (Thirunakaran, R., 2009; Kebede, M. A., 2014; Kalyani, P., 2002).

Figure 9 demonstrates the capacity response of all the samples at different C-rates. The general trend of decrease in the charge capacity with the increase in the current rate from 100-2000 mAg^{-1} is observed for all the samples (Guo, D., 2013; Wang, J. L., 2012; Li, Z., 2012; Cheng, B., 2012). As discussed above, at a current rate of 100 mAg^{-1}, the initial discharge capacity of prestine sample (LMO) is higher than the Al-doped samples. At higher current rates, the discharge capacity of the pristine sample falls sharply as compared to Al-doped samples. Among the samples, $LiAl_{0.4}Mn_{1.6}O_4$ nanospheres (LAMO-O) give the best response at higher discharge rates. At 300 mAg^{-1}, the discharge capacity of $LiAl_{0.4}Mn_{1.6}O_4$ nanospheres (LAMO-O) and pristine sample becomes nearly the same (table 3.3). As the current rate is increased from 300 mAg^{-1} to 2000 mAg^{-1}, the $LiAl_{0.4}Mn_{1.6}O_4$ nanospheres (LAMO-O) show higher capacities than pristine sample (LMO).

Figure 9. Specific capacities of the samples at different current rates.

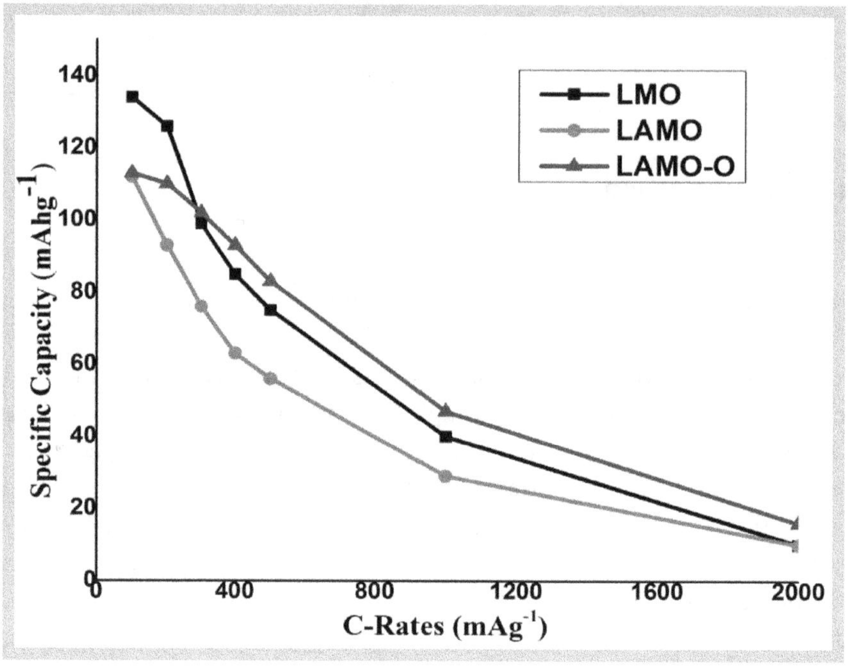

Figure 10. Cycling performance of the samples at different C-rates.

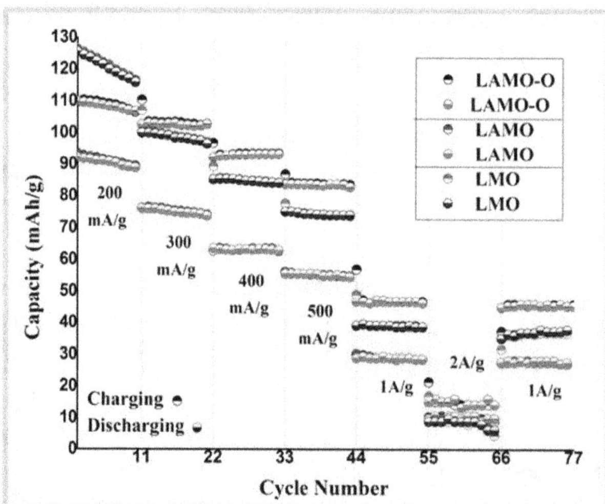

Also, the Al-doped $LiMn_2O_4$ samples are highly porous (figure 7) which could increase the mass-electrolyte contact and hence, the number of active sites increase many folds, with shorter Li^+ diffusion lengths. Thus, it would increase the rate capabilities of Al-doped $LiMn_2O_4$ (Xiao, X., 2010; Guo, X., 2010). Figure 10 shows the rate capabilities of all the samples over 10 cycles at the current-rates (C-rates) of 200 mAg^{-1}, 300 mAg^{-1}, 400 mAg^{-1}, 500 mAg^{-1}, 1000 mAg^{-1} and 2000 mAg^{-1}. As the current-rate increases, the discharge capacity (table 3) and the capacity retention (figure 11) of pritine $LiMn_2O_4$ reduces shaply as compared to the Al-doped samples. Among the Al-doped samples, Al-doped $LiMn_2O_4$ nanospheres show the best of the results even at large current densities. As the current density increases from 200 mAg^{-1} to 300 mAg^{-1}, the discharge capacity of pristine sample reduces from 126 to 99 $mAhg^{-1}$, showing a capacity retention of only 78% against 81% for $LiMn_2O_4$ nanorods and 93% for $LiMn_2O_4$ nanospheres.

Figure 11. Percentage retention of the samples at different C-rates.

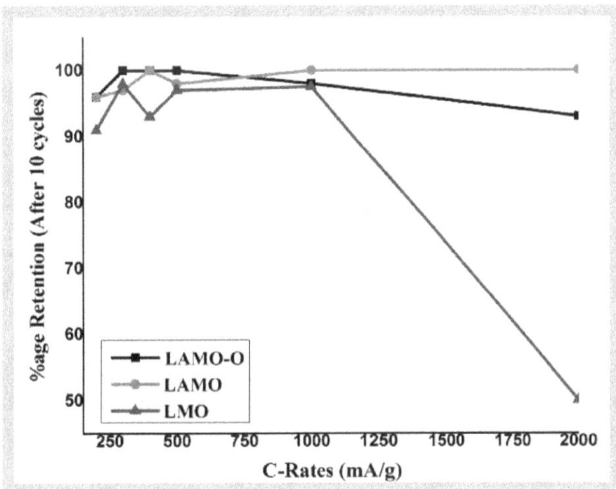

At higher C-rates, Li-ions have very short time for intercalation and deintercalation during the electrochemical process. Thus, the structural properties, which define the smooth diffusion of Li-ions influence the charge-discharge responses at higher C-rates (Xia, H., 2012). From figure 10 and table 3, it is observed that $LiMn_2O_4$ nanospheres exhibit better rate capabilities than other samples even at high current-rates of 1000 mAg^{-1} and 2000 mAg^{-1}. The time taken during intercalation and deintercalation depends on the smooth diffusion of Li-ion through the electrode structure (Das, S., 2014; Nitta, N., 2015). Hence, the best results of $LiMn_2O_4$ nanospheres at high C-rates could be explained on the basis of higher crystallinity, smaller lattice parameters, precise Li and Mn arrangements, and smaller cell volume and the results are consistent with the earlier XRD results (table 2).

CONCLUSION

The growing energy demand is adding more pressure onto the already stressed energy and environment scenario of the world. Keeping the current and future energy demands in mind, the need to explore the new ways of energy generation, utilization and storage is under the core focus of the scientific community. Given the advantages of nanotechnology and nanostructured materials, the scientific community has pinned their hopes on the nanostructured materials. Nanotechnology and nanostructured materials have been considered to reduce the energy costs and increase the efficiency of energy-conversion-devices. The research work carried out in the current study is an attempt to utilize the advantages of nanotechnology in the field of energy conversion and storage devices. The core focus has been on the synthesis of nanostructures, with modified properties to enhance their use in energy applications.

There is a tremendous challenge to store energy, especially the renewable energy and as such, lithium ion batteries have been explored as one of the promising energy storing devices. Researchers all over the world have pinned their hope on the $LiMn_2O_4$ as a promising cathode for lithium ion batteries. The particle-morphology has a great influence on the electrochemical properties of $LiMn_2O_4$ as it determines the intercalation/deintercalation of Li-ions and mass-electrolyte contact. Therefore, efforts have been focused on to control the shape, size and dimensionality of $LiMn_2O_4$ nanomaterials. In the current study, a $LiMn_2O_4$ cathode material with novel morphology has been successfully synthesized using oleic acid as a surfactant. The usual method to produce $LiMn_2O_4$ has been the solid state reaction process. But this method has several disadvantages of in-homogeneity, irregular morphology, broader particle size distribution, poor control of stoichiometry and longer periods of calcinations.

For the synthesis of spinel phase lithium manganese oxide ($LiMn_2O_4$) nanoparticles, a facile synthesis method has been presented, which is a template-free starch-glycine assisted solution combustion synthesis (SCS). The method is a simple and single step method, without using any special conditions or treatments. In this study, the Al-doped $LiMn_2O_4$ nanorods and nanospheres have been successfully synthesized through a single-step solution combustion method. The effect of oleic acid, as a surfactant has been observed to influence the morphology of the $LiMn_2O_4$. From the XRD results, it has been observed that the oleic acid treatment enhances the structural properties of Al-doped $LiMn_2O_4$. The electrochemical study reveals the better electrochemical properties for the Al-doped $LiMn_2O_4$ samples as compared to the pristine $LiMn_2O_4$ sample. Among the Al-doped $LiMn_2O_4$ samples, the oleic acid treated $LiMn_2O_4$ nanospheres demonstrate the superior results of higher cycling performance, higher capacity retention and high rate capability.

REFERENCES

Akhoon, S. A., Rubab, S., & Shah, M. A. (2016). A Review of Various Nanostructures to Enhance the Efficiency of Solar-Photon-Conversions. *Renewable and Alternative Energy: Concepts, Methodologies, Tools, and Applications: Concepts, Methodologies, Tools, and Applications, 197.*

Akhoon, S. A., Rubab, S., & Shah, M. A. (2017). Enhanced cycling properties and better rate capabilities of Al-doped $LiMn_2O_4$ nanorods and nanospheres. *Materials Research Express*, *4*(10), 105016. doi:10.1088/2053-1591/aa8e58

Amaral, F. A., Bocchi, N., Brocenschi, R. F., Biaggio, S. R., & Rocha-Filho, R. C. (2010). Structural and electrochemical properties of the doped spinels $Li_{1.05}M_{0.02}Mn_{1.98}O_{3.98}N_{0.02}$ (M= Ga^{3+}, Al^{3+}, or Co^{3+}; N= S^{2-} or F^-) for use as cathode material in lithium batteries. *Journal of Power Sources*, *195*(10), 3293–3299. doi:10.1016/j.jpowsour.2009.12.002

Balaji, S. R. K., Mutharasu, D., Shanmugan, S., Subramanian, N. S., & Ramanathan, K. (2010). Influence of Sm $^{3+}$ ion in structural, morphological, and electrochemical properties of $LiMn_2O_4$ synthesized by microwave calcination. *Ionics*, *16*(4), 351–360. doi:10.100711581-009-0400-y

Buchmann, I. (2001). *Will Lithium-Ion batteries power the new millennium*. Cadex Electronics Inc.

Chan, C. K., Peng, H., Liu, G., McIlwrath, K., Zhang, X. F., Huggins, R. A., & Cui, Y. (2008). High-performance lithium battery anodes using silicon nanowires. *Nature Nanotechnology*, *3*(1), 31–35. doi:10.1038/nnano.2007.411 PMID:18654447

Chan, H. W., Duh, J. G., & Sheen, S. R. (2004). Electrochemical performance of LBO-coated spinel lithium manganese oxide as cathode material for Li-ion battery. *Surface and Coatings Technology*, *188*, 116–119. doi:10.1016/j.surfcoat.2004.08.065

Chan, H. W., Duh, J. G., & Sheen, S. R. (2005). Surface treatment of the lithium boron oxide coated $LiMn_2O_4$ cathode material in Li-ion battery. *Key Engineering Materials*, *280*, 671–676.

Chao, L. I., Yanliang, F. A. N., Shuzhong, L. I., Bing, X. I. E., Lei, B. I., & Shuting, Y. A. N. G. (2006). Synthesis and electrochemical properties of Th-doped $LiMn_2O_4$ powders for lithium-ion batteries. *Rare Metals*, *25*(6), 58–61. doi:10.1016/S1001-0521(07)60045-X

Chen, Y. B., Hu, Y., Lian, F., & Liu, Q. G. (2010). Synthesis and characterization of spinel $Li_{1.05}Cr_{0.1}Mn_{1.9}O_{4-z}F_z$ as cathode materials for lithium-ion batteries. *International Journal of Minerals Metallurgy and Materials*, *17*(2), 220–224. doi:10.100712613-010-0217-8

Cheng, B., Chen, X., Li, X., Xu, H., Yang, J., & Qian, Y. (2012). High Rate Performance of $LiM_{0.1}Mn_{1.9}O_4$ (M= Mn, Al, Fe) as Cathodes of Lithium Ion Battery at 25 C and 55 C. *International Journal of Electrochemical Science*, *7*, 6453–6464.

Cho, J. (2008). VO_x-coated $LiMn_2O_4$ nanorod clusters for lithium battery cathode materials. *Journal of Materials Chemistry*, *18*(19), 2257–2261. doi:10.1039/b719177d

Das, S., Li, J., & Hui, R. (2014, October). Impact of Electrode Surface/Volume Ratio on Li-ion Battery Performance. *Proceedings of the COMSOL Conference*, 8-10.

Ding, Y. L., Xie, J., Cao, G. S., Zhu, T. J., Yu, H. M., & Zhao, X. B. (2011). Enhanced elevated-temperature performance of Al-doped single-crystalline $LiMn_2O_4$ nanotubes as cathodes for lithium ion batteries. *The Journal of Physical Chemistry C*, *115*(19), 9821–9825. doi:10.1021/jp201669x

Du, G., Sharma, N., Peterson, V. K., Kimpton, J. A., Jia, D., & Guo, Z. (2011). Br-Doped $Li_4Ti_5O_{12}$ and Composite TiO_2 Anodes for Li-ion Batteries: Synchrotron X-Ray and in situ Neutron Diffraction Studies. *Advanced Functional Materials*, *21*(20), 3990–3997. doi:10.1002/adfm.201100846

Eftekhari, A., Moghaddam, A. B., & Solati-Hashjin, M. (2006). Electrochemical properties of $LiMn_2O_4$ cathode material doped with an actinide. *Journal of Alloys and Compounds*, *424*(1), 225–230. doi:10.1016/j.jallcom.2005.10.088

Ein-Eli, Y., Urian, R. C., Wen, W., & Mukerjee, S. (2005). Low temperature performance of copper/nickel modified $LiMn_2O_4$ spinels. *Electrochimica Acta*, *50*(9), 1931–1937. doi:10.1016/j.electacta.2004.09.002

Etacheri, V., Marom, R., Elazari, R., Salitra, G., & Aurbach, D. (2011). Challenges in the development of advanced Li-ion batteries: A review. *Energy & Environmental Science, 4*(9), 3243–3262. doi:10.1039/c1ee01598b

Feng, C., Li, H., Zhang, P., Guo, Z., & Liu, H. (2010). Synthesis and modification of non-stoichiometric spinel ($Li_{1.02}Mn_{1.90}Y_{0.02}O_{4-y}F_{0.08}$) for lithium-ion batteries. *Materials Chemistry and Physics, 119*(1), 82–85. doi:10.1016/j.matchemphys.2009.07.049

Fergus, J. W. (2010). Recent developments in cathode materials for lithium ion batteries. *Journal of Power Sources, 195*(4), 939–954. doi:10.1016/j.jpowsour.2009.08.089

Guo, D., Chang, Z., Li, B., Tang, H., Yuan, X. Z., & Wang, H. (2013). Synthesis of high-purity $LiMn_2O_4$ with enhanced electrical properties from electrolytic manganese dioxide treated by sulfuric acid-assisted hydrothermal method. *Journal of Solid State Electrochemistry, 17*(11), 2849–2856. doi:10.100710008-013-2199-8

Guo, X., Lu, X., Fang, X., Mao, Y., Wang, Z., Chen, L., Xu, X., Yang, H., & Liu, Y. (2010). Lithium storage in hollow spherical $ZnFe_2O_4$ as anode materials for lithium ion batteries. *Electrochemistry Communications, 12*(6), 847–850. doi:10.1016/j.elecom.2010.04.003

Ha, H. W., Yun, N. J., & Kim, K. (2007). Improvement of electrochemical stability of $LiMn_2O_4$ by CeO_2 coating for lithium-ion batteries. *Electrochimica Acta, 52*(9), 3236–3241. doi:10.1016/j.electacta.2006.09.066

Helan, M., Berchmans, L. J., Syamala Kumari, V. S., RaviSankar, R., & Shanmugam, V. M. (2011). Molten salt synthesis of $LiGd_{0.01}Mn_{1.99}O_4$ using chloride–carbonate melt. *Materials Research Innovations, 15*(2), 130–134. doi:10.1179/143307511X12998222918958

Iqbal, M. J., & Ahmad, Z. (2008). Electrical and dielectric properties of lithium manganate nanomaterials doped with rare-earth elements. *Journal of Power Sources, 179*(2), 763–769. doi:10.1016/j.jpowsour.2007.12.115

Jayaprakash, N., Kalaiselvi, N., Doh, C. H., & Bhuvaneswari, D. (2010). A new class of Sol–gel derived $LiM_{1x}M_{2y}Mn_{2-x-y}O_{3.8}F_{0.2}$ (M_1= Cr, M_2= V; x= y= 0.2) cathodes for lithium batteries. *Journal of Applied Electrochemistry, 40*(12), 2193–2202. doi:10.100710800-010-0187-6

Jeong, W. T., Joo, J. H., & Lee, K. S. (2003). Improvement of electrode performances of spinel $LiMn_2O_4$ prepared by mechanical alloying and subsequent firing. *Journal of Power Sources, 119*, 690–694. doi:10.1016/S0378-7753(03)00229-5

Ju, S. H., Kang, Y. C., Sun, Y. K., & Kim, D. W. (2012). Synthesis and electrochemical properties of nanorod-shaped $LiMn_{1.5}Ni_{0.5}O_4$ cathode materials for lithium-ion batteries. *Materials Chemistry and Physics, 132*(1), 223–227. doi:10.1016/j.matchemphys.2011.11.042

Kalyani, P., Kalaiselvi, N., & Muniyandi, N. (2002). A new solution combustion route to synthesize $LiCoO_2$ and $LiMn_2O_4$. *Journal of Power Sources, 111*(2), 232–238. doi:10.1016/S0378-7753(02)00307-5

Kamarulzaman, N., Osman, Z., Muhamad, M. R., Ibrahim, Z. A., Arof, A. K., & Mohamed, N. S. (2001). Performance characteristics of $LiMn_2O_4$/polymer/carbon electrochemical cells. *Journal of Power Sources*, *97*, 722–725. doi:10.1016/S0378-7753(01)00647-4

Kebede, M. A., Phasha, M. J., Kunjuzwa, N., Le Roux, L. J., Mkhonto, D., Ozoemena, K. I., & Mathe, M. K. (2014). Structural and electrochemical properties of aluminium doped $LiMn_2O_4$ cathode materials for Li battery: Experimental and ab initio calculations. *Sustainable Energy Technologies and Assessments*, *5*, 44–49. doi:10.1016/j.seta.2013.11.005

Kebede, M. A., Phasha, M. J., Kunjuzwa, N., Mathe, M. K., & Ozoemena, K. I. (2015). Solution-combustion synthesized aluminium-doped spinel ($LiAl_xMn_{2-x}O_4$) as a high-performance lithium-ion battery cathode material. *Applied Physics. A, Materials Science & Processing*, *121*(1), 51–57. doi:10.100700339-015-9311-0

Khasanova, N. R., Drozhzhin, O. A., Fedotov, S. S., Storozhilova, D. A., Panin, R. V., & Antipov, E. V. (2013). Synthesis and electrochemical performance of $Li_2Co_{1-x}M_xPO_4F$ (M= Fe, Mn) cathode materials. *Beilstein Journal of Nanotechnology*, *4*, 860–867. doi:10.3762/bjnano.4.97 PMID:24367755

Kim, D. K., Muralidharan, P., Lee, H. W., Ruffo, R., Yang, Y., Chan, C. K., Peng, H., Huggins, R. A., & Cui, Y. (2008). Spinel $LiMn_2O_4$ nanorods as lithium ion battery cathodes. *Nano Letters*, *8*(11), 3948–3952. doi:10.1021/nl8024328 PMID:18826287

Kim, K. W., Lee, S. W., Han, K. S., Chung, H. J., & Woo, S. I. (2003). Characterization of Al-doped spinel $LiMn_2O_4$ thin film cathode electrodes prepared by liquid source misted chemical deposition (LSMCD) technique. *Electrochimica Acta*, *48*(28), 4223–4231. doi:10.1016/S0013-4686(03)00608-X

Lee, Y. S., Kumada, N., & Yoshio, M. (2001). Synthesis and characterization of lithium aluminum-doped spinel ($LiAl_xMn_{2-x}O_4$) for lithium secondary battery. *Journal of Power Sources*, *96*(2), 376–384. doi:10.1016/S0378-7753(00)00652-2

Li, C., Zhang, H. P., Fu, L. J., Liu, H., Wu, Y. P., Rahm, E., Holze, R., & Wu, H. Q. (2006). Cathode materials modified by surface coating for lithium ion batteries. *Electrochimica Acta*, *51*(19), 3872–3883. doi:10.1016/j.electacta.2005.11.015

Li, X., Cheng, F., Guo, B., & Chen, J. (2005). Template-synthesized $LiCoO_2$, $LiMn_2O_4$, and $LiNi_{0.8}Co_{0.2}O_2$ nanotubes as the cathode materials of lithium ion batteries. *The Journal of Physical Chemistry B*, *109*(29), 14017–14024. doi:10.1021/jp051900a PMID:16852760

Li, X., & Xu, Y. (2008). Enhanced cycling performance of spinel $LiMn_2O_4$ coated with $ZnMn_2O_4$ shell. *Journal of Solid State Electrochemistry*, *12*(7-8), 851–855. doi:10.100710008-007-0426-x

Li, Z., Yang, J., Wang, J., Tang, J., Lei, G., & Xiao, Q. (2012). A phase-inversion process to prepare porous $LiAl_{0.1}Mn_{1.9}O_4$ spinel for aqueous rechargeable lithium batteries. *Microporous and Mesoporous Materials*, *162*, 44–50. doi:10.1016/j.micromeso.2012.06.001

Liu, D. Q., He, Z. Z., & Liu, X. Q. (2007). Synthesis and characterization of $LiGa_xMn_{2-x}O_4$ ($0\leq x\leq 0.05$) by triethanolamine-assisted sol–gel method. *Journal of Alloys and Compounds*, *440*(1), 69–73. doi:10.1016/j.jallcom.2006.09.013

Liu, D. Q., Liu, X. Q., & He, Z. Z. (2007). The elevated temperature performance of $LiMn_2O_4$ coated with $Li_4Ti_5O_{12}$ for lithium ion battery. *Materials Chemistry and Physics*, *105*(2), 362–366. doi:10.1016/S0254-0584(03)00268-2

Liu, H., Cheng, C., & Zhang, K. (2007). The effect of ZnO coating on $LiMn_2O_4$ cycle life in high temperature for lithium secondary batteries. *Materials Chemistry and Physics*, *101*(2), 276–279. doi:10.1016/j.matchemphys.2006.05.006

Liu, J., Cao, G., Yang, Z., Wang, D., Dubois, D., Zhou, X., Graff, G. L., Pederson, L. R., & Zhang, J. G. (2008). Oriented nanostructures for energy conversion and storage. *ChemSusChem*, *1*(8-9), 676–697. doi:10.1002/cssc.200800087 PMID:18693284

Liu, Q., Wang, S., Tan, H., Yang, Z., & Zeng, J. (2013). Preparation and doping mode of doped $LiMn_2O_4$ for Li-ion batteries. *Energies*, *6*(3), 1718–1730. doi:10.3390/en6031718

Lou, X. W., Wang, Y., Yuan, C., Lee, J. Y., & Archer, L. A. (2006). Template-free synthesis of SnO_2 hollow nanostructures with high lithium storage capacity. *Advanced Materials*, *18*(17), 2325–2329. doi:10.1002/adma.200600733

Lu, W., Belharouak, I., Liu, J., & Amine, K. (2007). Thermal properties of $Li_{4/3}Ti_{5/3}O_{4/}$ $LiMn_2O_4$ cell. *Journal of Power Sources*, *174*(2), 673–677. doi:10.1016/j.jpowsour.2007.06.199

Luo, J., Cheng, L., & Xia, Y. (2007). $LiMn_2O_4$ hollow nanosphere electrode material with excellent cycling reversibility and rate capability. *Electrochemistry Communications*, *9*(6), 1404–1409. doi:10.1016/j.elecom.2007.01.058

Luo, Q., & Manthiram, A. (2009). Effect of Low-Temperature Fluorine Doping on the Properties of Spinel $LiMn_{2-2y}Li_yM_yO_{4-\eta}F_\eta$ (M= Fe, Co, and Zn) Cathodes. *Journal of the Electrochemical Society*, *156*(2), A84–A88. doi:10.1149/1.3028317

Malyovanyi, S. M., Andriiko, A. A., & Monko, A. P. (2003). Synthesis and electrochemical behavior of Fe-doped overstoichiometric $LiMn_2O_4$-based spinels. *Journal of Solid State Electrochemistry*, *8*(1), 7–10. doi:10.100710008-003-0414-8

Molenda, J., & Molenda, M. (2011). *Composite Cathode Material for Li-Ion Batteries Based on $LiFePO_4$ System*. INTECH Open Access Publisher. doi:10.5772/21635

Molenda, M., Dziembaj, R., Podstawka, E., Proniewicz, L. M., & Piwowarska, Z. (2007). An attempt to improve electrical conductivity of the pyrolysed carbon- $LiMn_2O_{4-y}S_y$ ($0\leq y\leq 0.5$) composites. *Journal of Power Sources*, *174*(2), 613–618. doi:10.1016/j.jpowsour.2007.06.117

Nitta, N., Wu, F., Lee, J. T., & Yushin, G. (2015). Li-ion battery materials: Present and future. *Materials Today*, *18*(5), 252–264. doi:10.1016/j.mattod.2014.10.040

Nkosi, F. P., Jafta, C. J., Kebede, M., le Roux, L., Mathe, M. K., & Ozoemena, K. I. (2015). Microwave-assisted optimization of the manganese redox states for enhanced capacity and capacity retention of $LiAl_xMn_{2-x}O_4$ (x= 0 and 0.3) spinel materials. *RSC Advances*, *5*(41), 32256–32262. doi:10.1039/C5RA02643A

Ouyang, C. Y., Zeng, X. M., Sljivancanin, Z., & Baldereschi, A. (2010). Oxidation states of Mn atoms at clean and Al2O3-covered LiMn2O4 (001) surfaces. *The Journal of Physical Chemistry C, 114*(10), 4756–4759. doi:10.1021/jp911746g

Park, J., Seo, J. H., Plett, G., Lu, W., & Sastry, A. M. (2011). Numerical simulation of the effect of the dissolution of LiMn2O4 particles on Li-ion battery performance. *Electrochemical and Solid-State Letters, 14*(2), A14–A18. doi:10.1149/1.3516619

Park, S. H., Lee, Y. S., & Sun, Y. K. (2003). Synthesis and electrochemical properties of sulfur doped-$Li_xMnO_{2-y}S_y$ materials for lithium secondary batteries. *Electrochemistry Communications, 5*(2), 124–128. doi:10.1016/S1388-2481(03)00005-5

Patey, T. J., Ng, S. H., Büchel, R., Tran, N., Krumeich, F., Wang, J., Liu, H. K., & Novák, P. (2008). Electrochemistry of LiV3O8 nanoparticles made by flame spray pyrolysis. *Electrochemical and Solid-State Letters, 11*(4), A46–A50. doi:10.1149/1.2836741

Peng, Z. D., Jiang, Q. L., Du, K., Wang, W. G., Hu, G. R., & Liu, Y. X. (2010). Effect of Cr-sources on performance of $Li_{1.05}Cr_{0.04}Mn_{1.96}O_4$ cathode materials prepared by slurry spray drying method. *Journal of Alloys and Compounds, 493*(1), 640–644. doi:10.1016/j.jallcom.2009.12.172

Pröll, J., Kohler, R., Torge, M., Ulrich, S., Ziebert, C., Bruns, M., Seifert, H. J., & Pfleging, W. (2011). Laser microstructuring and annealing processes for lithium manganese oxide cathodes. *Applied Surface Science, 257*(23), 9968–9976. doi:10.1016/j.apsusc.2011.06.117

Qing, C., Bai, Y., Yang, J., & Zhang, W. (2011). Enhanced cycling stability of $LiMn_2O_4$ cathode by amorphous $FePO_4$ coating. *Electrochimica Acta, 56*(19), 6612–6618. doi:10.1016/j.electacta.2011.04.131

Ra, W., Nakayama, M., Uchimoto, Y., & Wakihara, M. (2005). Experimental and computational study of the electronic structural changes in $LiTi_2O_4$ spinel compounds upon electrochemical Li insertion reactions. *The Journal of Physical Chemistry B, 109*(3), 1130–1134. doi:10.1021/jp040499+ PMID:16851071

Rajesh, Y. B. R. D., & Dubey, R. S. (2013). Sol-Gel Synthesis and Characterization of Nanocrystalline Spinel $LiMn_2O_4$ For Battery Applications. *Nanoscience and Nanoengineering, 1*(3), 139–141.

Ryu, W. H., Eom, J. Y., Yin, R. Z., Han, D. W., Kim, W. K., & Kwon, H. S. (2011). Synergistic effects of various morphologies and Al doping of spinel $LiMn_2O_4$ nanostructures on the electrochemical performance of lithium-rechargeable batteries. *Journal of Materials Chemistry, 21*(39), 15337–15342. doi:10.1039/c1jm10146c

Sadeghi, B., Sarraf-Mamoory, R., & Shahverdi, H. R. (2012). The Effect of $LiFePO_4$ Coating on Electrochemical Performance of $LiMn_2O_4$ Cathode Material. *Iranian Journal of Chemistry and Chemical Engineering, 31*(4), 29–33.

Sclar, H., Haik, O., Menachem, T., Grinblat, J., Leifer, N., Meitav, A., Luski, S., & Aurbach, D. (2012). The effect of ZnO and MgO coatings by a sono-chemical method, on the stability of $LiMn_{1.5}Ni_{0.5}O_4$ as a cathode material for 5 V Li-ion batteries. *Journal of the Electrochemical Society, 159*(3), A228–A237. doi:10.1149/2.032203jes

Scrosati, B., & Garche, J. (2010). Lithium batteries: Status, prospects and future. *Journal of Power Sources, 195*(9), 2419–2430. doi:10.1016/j.jpowsour.2009.11.048

Shi, J. Y., Yi, C. W., & Kim, K. (2010). Improved electrochemical performance of $AlPO_4$-coated $LiMn_{1.5}Ni_{0.5}O_4$ electrode for lithium-ion batteries. *Journal of Power Sources, 195*(19), 6860–6866. doi:10.1016/j.jpowsour.2010.02.063

Singh, P., Sil, A., Nath, M., & Ray, S. (2009). Preparation and Characterization of Li $(Mn_{2-x}Fe_x)$ O_4 (x= 0.0-0.6) Spinel Nanoparticles as Cathode Materials for Lithium Ion Battery. (). Trans Tech Publications.). *Advanced Materials Research, 67*, 233–238. doi:10.4028/www.scientific.net/AMR.67.233

Singh, P., Sil, A., Nath, M. A. L. A., & Ray, S. (2010). Synthesis and characterisation of Li $(Mn_{2-X}mg_x)$ o_4(x= 0. 0-0. 3) prepared by sol-gel synthesis. *Ceramics-Silikáty, 54*(1), 38–46.

Singhal, R., Das, S. R., Tomar, M. S., Ovideo, O., Nieto, S., Melgarejo, R. E., & Katiyar, R. S. (2007). Synthesis and characterization of Nd doped $LiMn_2O_4$ cathode for Li-ion rechargeable batteries. *Journal of Power Sources, 164*(2), 857–861. doi:10.1016/j.jpowsour.2006.09.098

Son, J. T., Park, K. S., Kim, H. G., & Chung, H. T. (2004). Surface-modification of $LiMn_2O_4$ with a silver-metal coating. *Journal of Power Sources, 126*(1), 182–185. doi:10.1016/j.jpowsour.2003.07.010

Sun, H., Chen, Y., Xu, C., Zhu, D., & Huang, L. (2012). Electrochemical performance of rare-earth doped $LiMn_2O_4$ spinel cathode materials for Li-ion rechargeable battery. *Journal of Solid State Electrochemistry, 16*(3), 1247–1254. doi:10.100710008-011-1514-5

Suryakala, K., Marikkannu, K. R., Kalaignan, G. P., & Vasudevan, T. (2008). Synthesis and electrochemical characterization of LiMn2O4 and LiNd0. 3Mn1. 7O4 as cathode for lithium ion battery. *International Journal of Electrochemical Science, 3*, 136–144.

Tang, S. B., Lai, M. O., & Lu, L. (2006). Properties of nano-crystalline $LiMn_2O_4$ thin films deposited by pulsed laser deposition. *Electrochimica Acta, 52*(3), 1161–1168. doi:10.1016/j.electacta.2006.07.014

Tang, W., Wang, X. J., Hou, Y. Y., Li, L. L., Sun, H., Zhu, Y. S., Bai, Y., Wu, Y. P., Zhu, K., & Van Ree, T. (2012). Nano $LiMn_2O_4$ as cathode material of high rate capability for lithium ion batteries. *Journal of Power Sources, 198*, 308–311. doi:10.1016/j.jpowsour.2011.09.106

Thackeray, M. M. (1997). Manganese oxides for lithium batteries. *Progress in Solid State Chemistry, 25*(1), 1–71. doi:10.1016/S0079-6786(97)81003-5

Thirunakaran, R., Kim, K. T., Kang, Y. M., & Lee, J. Y. (2004). Solution synthesis of boron substituted $LiMn_2O_4$ spinel oxide for use in lithium rechargeable battery. *Ionics, 10*(3), 188–192. doi:10.1007/BF02382815

Thirunakaran, R., Ravikumar, R., Gopukumar, S., & Sivashanmugam, A. (2013). Electrochemical evaluation of dual-doped $LiMn_2O_4$ spinels synthesized via co-precipitation method as cathode material for lithium rechargeable batteries. *Journal of Alloys and Compounds, 556*, 266–273. doi:10.1016/j.jallcom.2012.12.053

Thirunakaran, R., Sivashanmugam, A., Gopukumar, S., & Rajalakshmi, R. (2009). Cerium and zinc: Dual-doped $LiMn_2O_4$ spinels as cathode material for use in lithium rechargeable batteries. *Journal of Power Sources*, *187*(2), 565–574. doi:10.1016/j.jpowsour.2008.10.134

Tu, J., Zhao, X. B., Cao, G. S., Tu, J. P., & Zhu, T. J. (2006). Improved performance of $LiMn_2O_4$ cathode materials for lithium ion batteries by gold coating. *Materials Letters*, *60*(27), 3251–3254. doi:10.1016/j.matlet.2006.02.089

Tu, J., Zhao, X. B., Xie, J., Cao, G. S., Zhuang, D. G., Zhu, T. J., & Tu, J. P. (2007). Enhanced low voltage cycling stability of $LiMn_2O_4$ cathode by ZnO coating for lithium ion batteries. *Journal of Alloys and Compounds*, *432*(1), 313–317. doi:10.1016/j.jallcom.2006.06.016

Wang, H., Tan, T. A., Yang, P., Lai, M. O., & Lu, L. (2011). High-rate performances of the Ru-doped spinel $LiNi_{0.5}Mn_{1.5}O_4$: Effects of doping and particle size. *The Journal of Physical Chemistry C*, *115*(13), 6102–6110. doi:10.1021/jp110746w

Wang, H. E., Cheng, H., Liu, C., Chen, X., Jiang, Q., Lu, Z., ... Martinu, L. (2011). Facile synthesis and electrochemical characterization of porous and dense TiO_2 nanospheres for lithium-ion battery applications. *Journal of Power Sources*, *196*(15), 6394–6399. doi:10.1016/j.jpowsour.2011.03.085

Wang, J. L., Li, Z. H., Yang, J., Tang, J. J., Yu, J. J., Nie, W. B., Lei, G. T., & Xiao, Q. Z. (2012). Effect of Al-doping on the electrochemical properties of a three-dimensionally porous lithium manganese oxide for lithium-ion batteries. *Electrochimica Acta*, *75*, 115–122. doi:10.1016/j.electacta.2012.04.136

Wang, L., Zhao, J., Guo, S., He, X., Jiang, C., & Wan, C. (2010). Investigation of SnO_2-modified $LiMn_2O_4$ composite as cathode material for lithium-ion batteries. *International Journal of Electrochemical Science*, *5*, 1113–1126.

Wu, H. M., Belharouak, I., Abouimrane, A., Sun, Y. K., & Amine, K. (2010). Surface modification of $LiNi_{0.5}Mn_{1.5}O_4$ by ZrP_2O_7 and ZrO_2 for lithium-ion batteries. *Journal of Power Sources*, *195*(9), 2909–2913. doi:10.1016/j.jpowsour.2009.11.029

Wu, H. M., Tu, J. P., Chen, X. T., Li, Y., Zhao, X. B., & Cao, G. S. (2007). Effects of Ni-ion doping on electrochemical characteristics of spinel $LiMn_2O_4$ powders prepared by a spray-drying method. *Journal of Solid State Electrochemistry*, *11*(2), 173–176. doi:10.100710008-005-0082-y

Wu, H. M., Tu, J. P., Yuan, Y. F., Li, Y., Zhao, X. B., & Cao, G. S. (2005). Structural, morphological and electrochemical characteristics of spinel $LiMn_2O_4$ prepared by spray-drying method. *Scripta Materialia*, *52*(6), 513–517. doi:10.1016/j.scriptamat.2004.10.037

Xi, L. J., Wang, H. E., Lu, Z. G., Yang, S. L., Ma, R. G., Deng, J. Q., & Chung, C. Y. (2012). Facile synthesis of porous $LiMn_2O_4$ spheres as positive electrode for high-power lithium ion batteries. *Journal of Power Sources*, *198*, 251–257. doi:10.1016/j.jpowsour.2011.09.100

Xia, H., Luo, Z., & Xie, J. (2012). Nanostructured $LiMn_2O_4$ and their composites as high-performance cathodes for lithium-ion batteries. *Progress in Natural Science*, *22*(6), 572–584. doi:10.1016/j.pnsc.2012.11.014

Xiao, L., Zhao, Y., Yang, Y., Cao, Y., Ai, X., & Yang, H. (2008). Enhanced electrochemical stability of Al-doped $LiMn_2O_4$ synthesized by a polymer-pyrolysis method. *Electrochimica Acta, 54*(2), 545–550. doi:10.1016/j.electacta.2008.07.037

Xiao, X., Lu, J., & Li, Y. (2010). $LiMn_2O_4$ microspheres: Synthesis, characterization and use as a cathode in lithium ion batteries. *Nano Research, 3*(10), 733–737. doi:10.100712274-010-0037-1

Xu, W., Yuan, A., Tian, L., & Wang, Y. (2011). Improved high-rate cyclability of sol–gel derived Cr-doped spinel $LiCr_yMn_{2-y}O_4$ in an aqueous electrolyte. *Journal of Applied Electrochemistry, 41*(4), 453–460. doi:10.100710800-011-0255-6

Yang, Y., Xie, C., Ruffo, R., Peng, H., Kim, D. K., & Cui, Y. (2009). Single nanorod devices for battery diagnostics: A case study on LiMn2O4. *Nano Letters, 9*(12), 4109–4114. doi:10.1021/nl902315u PMID:19807129

Yang, Y., Xie, C., Ruffo, R., Peng, H., Kim, D. K., & Cui, Y. (2009). Single nanorod devices for battery diagnostics: A case study on $LiMn_2O_4$. *Nano Letters, 9*(12), 4109–4114. doi:10.1021/nl902315u PMID:19807129

Yang, Z., Cao, G. S., Xie, J., & Zhao, X. B. (2012). Oleic acid-assisted preparation of LiMnPO4 and its improved electrochemical performance by Co doping. *Journal of Solid State Electrochemistry, 16*(3), 1271–1277. doi:10.100710008-011-1523-4

Yi, T., Hu, X., Wang, D., & Huo, H. (2008). Effects of Al, F dual substitutions on the structure and electrochemical properties of lithium manganese oxide. Journal of University of Science and Technology Beijing, Mineral, Metallurgy. *Material, 15*(2), 182–186.

Yi, T. F., Zhu, Y. R., Zhu, X. D., Shu, J., Yue, C. B., & Zhou, A. N. (2009). A review of recent developments in the surface modification of $LiMn_2O_4$ as cathode material of power lithium-ion battery. *Ionics, 15*(6), 779–784. doi:10.100711581-009-0373-x

Ying, J., Jiang, C., & Wan, C. (2004). Preparation and characterization of high-density spherical $LiCoO_2$ cathode material for lithium ion batteries. *Journal of Power Sources, 129*(2), 264–269. doi:10.1016/j.jpowsour.2003.10.007

Yu, Z. M., & Zhao, L. C. (2007). Structure and electrochemical properties of $LiMn_2O_4$. *Transactions of Nonferrous Metals Society of China, 17*(3), 659–664. doi:10.1016/S1003-6326(07)60152-6

Zhou, W. J., He, B. L., & Li, H. L. (2008). Synthesis, structure and electrochemistry of Ag-modified $LiMn_2O_4$ cathode materials for lithium-ion batteries. *Materials Research Bulletin, 43*(8), 2285–2294. doi:10.1016/j.materresbull.2007.08.013

Zhou, Y. K., Shen, C. M., Huang, J., & Li, H. L. (2002). Synthesis of high-ordered $LiMn_2O_4$ nanowire arrays by AAO template and its structural properties. *Materials Science and Engineering B, 95*(1), 77–82. doi:10.1016/S0921-5107(02)00197-6

Chapter 13
Nanomedicine in Human Health Therapeutics and Drug Delivery:
Nanobiotechnology and Nanobiomedicine

Manzoor A. Mir
University of Kashmir, India

Basharat A. Bhat
University of Kashmir, India

Bashir A. Sheikh
University of Kashmir, India

Gulzar Ahmed Rather
https://orcid.org/0000-0001-7513-8109
Department of Biomedical Engineering, Sathyabama Institute of Science and Technology, Chennai, India

Safiya Mehraj
University of Kashmir, India

Wajahat R. Mir
University of Kashmir, India

ABSTRACT

The 21st century has seen a massive spring up in the applications of nanobiotechnology. Incorporation of functionalized and modified nanostructures in various biomedical applications has generated significant research interests such as implant and tissue engineering, diagnosis, and therapy, thereby aiding in improvement of human health. The unique properties of nanoparticles including non-toxicity and biocompatibility with a large surface area make it possible to modify their surface with different chemicals including different polymers, antibodies, and drug molecules. Therefore, they are utilized for targeted drug delivery in order to carry drugs and selectively release them in desired tissues which reduces destructive effects on healthy cells. This chapter mainly covers the basic properties of nanoparticles including nanomedicine, their preparation and focuses on their diagnosis, and therapeutic applications in disease including cancer and other challenging ailments.

DOI: 10.4018/978-1-7998-5563-7.ch013

INTRODUCTION

Nanoparticles are at the main edge of the quickly creating field of material science in nanotechnology with numerous potential applications in clinical medication and research. Nanoparticles can be portrayed as a particulate material whose dimensional range lies in the nanoscale (i.e., 1–100 nm). Nanoparticles of different shapes, for example, circles, poles, wires, planets, stars, confines, and multi case can be custom fitted utilizing distinctive nano substance methodology (Beyth et al., 2015; Huh and Kwon, 2011; Jeevanandam et al., 2018; Vimbela et al., 2017). Nanoparticles have a fewkind properties not found in their mass partners, which incorporate high surface-to-volume proportion, high surface vitality, novel mechanical, warm, electrical, attractive, and optical practices, and so forth. (Jaison et al., 2018). These properties make them appropriate for a wide scope of utilizations, going from hardware to vitality gathering and capacity, to interchanges, to science, and to medication (Beatriz et al., 2017).

Nanomaterials are considered to have an admirable potential in the field of biosensors for its capacity of effective sign catch of the organic acknowledgment occasion (transduction) at nanoscale level. Nanoparticle-based "atomic" imaging shows a field where this new innovation has made way for a transformative jump in indicative imaging. In view of the ongoing advancement in nanobiotechnology, nanoparticles can possibly become valuable apparatuses as remedial and demonstrative instruments sooner rather than later (Mir et al., 2019).

The prior utilization of nanomaterials incorporate the Lycurgus Cup from the fourth-century Promotion which was utilized as shown in the English Gallery in London, some late medieval church windows and furthermore the renowned Damascene Swords: When light sparkled from outside on the antique Roman cup, the cup looked olive green and when lit up from inside it sparkled ruby red. It was seen that the colloidal nanoparticles of silver and gold contained in the glass were liable for this marvel. A comparative impact was seen in late medieval church windows, which lit up glowing red and yellow, on the grounds that nanoparticles of gold and silver had been combined into the glass. In 2006 nanometer-size particles of carbon were found in a Damascene Sword from the seventeenth century, as a result of these, the amazing swords had versatility and opposition (Reibold et al., 2006). These surprising properties of hues and materials were at that point being created a huge number of years prior yet medieval craftsmen and counterfeiters, notwithstanding, didn't have the foggiest idea about the reason for these astonishing impacts.

NANOBIOTECHNOLOGY

Nanobiotechnology is a multi-vital method that joins nanotechnology and biotechnology to build the properties of restorative operators, e.g., target conveyance of therapeutics by nanoparticles, in a characterized way (Saji et al., 2010). Nanotechnology is one of the recent emerging sciences that employ its applications in different fields ranging from health to the agricultural sciences (Stewart 2016 and Gartland 2018). Nanotechnology is defined by keeping in view the different properties of nanomaterials used in science including physical and chemical properties of nanomaterial and their ability of metabolization(Priyaet al., 2015).

Nanobiotechnology plays an astonishing role in generating many helpful tools to study biosystems(Qamar et al., 2019). According to the recent research micro-organisms, plant extracts and even fungi generate nanomaterials through various biological pathways(Shafiq et al., 2016; and Verma et al.,

2019). These derived nanoparticles are having exceptional properties that are different from the larger molecules of the same element. Because of their greater surface area to volume ratio values nanoparticles differ in properties like electrical, optical, and chemical from those observed in bulk compounds(Roy et al., 2015). By and by, nanomaterials have been broadly investigated for business applications like analytic, treatment and for inquiring about. Another rising field in the present period of cutting-edge nanotechnology and nanorobotics is nanomedicine.

Nanotechnology is a rising field in the advancement of gadgets, materials, or different structures composites having in any event one measurement estimated from 1 to 100 nanometers. In the interim, Biotechnology manages natural subjects that incorporate metabolic and other physiological procedures. A blend of these two advancements, for example, nanobiotechnology assumes a significant job in the assembling and applying numerous valuable devices in the investigation of numerous life forms (Jaison et al., 2018).

Nanotechnology is a differing field, which ranges from augmentations of customary gadget fundamental science to totally new strategies dependent on sub-atomic self-get together, from creating novel materials having measurements on the nanoscale to examining whether we can legitimately control matters on/in the nuclear scale/level. Nanobiotechnology is an advanced field in which nanoscale tools are developed for the manufacturing of different kinds of nanomaterialsand applied to study biological sciences. Nanobiotechnology presents tremendous potential for advancing natural science subsequently encouraging social insurance benefits everywhere throughout the world (Jaison et al., 2018).

Nanomedicine

For the most part, medication is the science, building, and practice of diagnosing, treating, relieving, observing, foreseeing and forestalling ailments. Nanomedicine is a developing field of nanobiotechnologyin which knowledge and techniques of nanosciences are used in medical biology for disease treatment and remediation (Albert, 2016). Nanomedicine contrasts from different sorts of medication in that it includes the improvement and use of materials and advancements with nanometer lengths. In this manner, nanomedicine is an interdisciplinary field, where nanosciences, nanoengineering, and nanotechnology associate with the existence sciences (Beatriz et al.,2017).

In nanomedicine, nanodimensional materials are used which include nanorobots, vaccine delivery, and sensory purposes, and nanosensors for diagnosis. For example, a nanoparticle-based technique has been established which is used for the imaging modalities and treatment of cancer diagnosis(Ying-Yu Ma et al., 2017).Nanomaterial influences the boundaries of nanomedicine starting from microfluidics, biosensors, drug delivery, and microarray tests to tissue engineering (Arayne, 2007; Patra, 2014; and Joseph 2017).The field of nanomedicine which comprise of biosensors, drug delivery, and tissue engineering has been powered by nanobiotechnology by employing curative agents at the nanoscale level (Mirza and Siddiqui 2014). Nanoparticles are very small sized nanospheres which are designed at the molecular level. Similarly, nanobodies have been used for the diagnostic, drug delivery and treatment purposes and it has presently got the prominence in medical field (Mir et al., 2019).

Nanomedicine alludes to the utilization of nanoscale structures for conclusions, treatment and, avoidance of infections in this way helping in the improvement of human wellbeing (Patil et al., 2008). Nanomaterials are similar to the size of cell organelles including nanosize proteins; henceforth they can be utilized to target wanted destinations without meddling with other cell hardware (Salata, 2004).

Nanomedicine is the reconciliation of nanotechnology in medication and it has been commonly characterized as the clinical utilization of nanotechnology. Nanomedicine is the theoretical field in the region of nanotechnology as it includes building and re-designing of sub-atomic constructing agents that have the capacity of re-requesting the issue either at the nuclear level or at the sub-atomic level. It is believed that nanomedicine enhances the natural healing powers of the human body as well as increases its immunization capabilities (Jayanta et al., 2018). By and by nanomedicine is utilized in a few zones of science (1) the finding that prompts the ID of a malady through the discovery of explicit side effects of the pathology; (2) treatment and explicit treatment of an infection; (3) regenerative medication that expects to permit recovery of harmed human tissue or organs; and (4) the sensor frameworks, which is a lot of interfaces, recognizing as an electrical sign, a physical wonder to speak to it and to obtain information on it (Jayanta et al., 2018) (Table 2).

Nanomedicine along these lines permits a new beam of expectation in the field of wellbeing. As a developing order, nanomedicine is step by step being made by opening up new viewpoints on key issues: streamlining drug conveyance, explicitly focusing on tissues or cells, progressively ideal controlling the pace of arrival of the medication into the body, and giving early and precise location of sicknesses. Nanomedicine is a promising field; because of the chance offered by scaling down and ultra-scaling down to collaborate in a focused on the path with natural elements, for example, tissues, cells, and even atoms (Rachid et al., 2019).

Nanomaterials are not sifted through the blood, so they can flow in the living being until they arrive at their objective. Dynamic substances can be embodied in their empty insides and their surface can be altered so they conquer characteristic hindrances, for example, cell layers like "Trojan horses", and with the guide of biosensors (for instance antibodies) perceive specific cells and tissues, join themselves to these and discharge the dynamic substances to the objective over a generally extensive period. In nutshell, the coordination of nanotechnology and biotechnology has prompted the establishment of nanomedicine. It has given novel leaps forward in fix of different infirmities and clutters, tranquilizes conveyance frameworks, location, and analysis of various maladies (Beatriz et al., 2017).

Preparation of Nanoparticles

One of the primaries considered NP conveyance framework which includes virus-like particles (VLPs), which turns into a wellspring of fascination because of their simplicity of creation and capacity to animate solid resistant reactions (Kingsman and Kingsman, 1988; Roldao et al., 2010; Zeltins, 2012). Majority in the size scope of 20–150 nm, VLPs involves a self-gathered viral envelope, which is produced from a solitary protein to shape a multimeric complex showing a high thickness proportion of epitopes (Grgacic and Anderson, 2006; Zeltins, 2012).

Baculovirus expression system is used commonly for the generation of VLPs, and has a very satisfactorily good safety profile since baculovirus do not naturally infect humans. The most extensively studied VLP component is *Autographa california* multiple nuclear polyhedrosis virus (AcMNPV) (Hu, 2005).The vector which is responsible for encoding the modified VLP can then be used to infect insect cells BTI-TN-5B1-4 derived from *Trichoplusiani*) or (Sf9 or Sf21 derived from *Spodoptera frugiperda*) so as to produce adequate amounts of the viral protein which can then self-gather into multimeric complexes (Figure 1A).

Liposomes are also self-assembling as that of VLPs, but consist of an aqueous core with phospholipid bilayer shell (Heurtault et al., 2010; Henriksen-Lacey et al., 2011). Large number of methods has been published for the synthesis of liposomes which are beyond the scope of this chapter (Riaz, 1996; Samad et al., 2007; Shailesh et al., 2009). An enormous number of techniques have been distributed for getting ready liposomes which are past the extent of this part (Riaz, 1996; Samad et al., 2007; Shailesh et al., 2009). In any case, all among them include reverse-phase evaporation process by dissolving phospholipids, (for example, phosphatidylcholine or monophosphoryl lipid A) in an organic solvent (e.g., methanol, chloroform). Water is then included, alongside an antigen, and the solvent is dissipated bringing about huge unilamellar vesicles (Kersten and Crommelin, 1995; Zhu et al., 2005).

Different ways to encapsulate antigens in liposomes incorporate utilizing repeat freeze-defrost cycles (Zhu et al., 2005), a pH angle (Waterhouse et al., 2005), or an ammonium sulfate strategy (Haran et al., 1993) with antigen encapsulation rates changing somewhere in the range of 25 and 72% (Fries et al., 1992; Baca-Estrada et al., 2000; Zhao et al., 2007) (Figure 1B).

A Colloidal saponin which contains micelles of around 40 nm can be used as self-adjuvanting vaccine delivery systems and these are together referred as ISCOMs. Two types of ISCOMs have been described, both of which consists of saponin (most often Quil A from the tree *Quillaia saponaria*), cholesterol (typically either phosphatidylethanolamine or phosphatidylcholine) and phospholipid, (Kersten et al., 1988; Lovgren and Morein, 1988; Barr et al., 1998). Traditionally, ISCOMs have been utilized to entangle viral envelope proteins, for example, from herpes simplex virus type 1, hepatitis B, and influenza. However, proteins from a wide range of bacteria and parasites including *Escherichia coli*, *Plasmodium falciparum*, and *Brucella aborus,* have also been used to collect ISCOMs (Morein and Simons, 1985; Classen and Osterhaus, 1992; Morein et al., 1995). ISCOM matrices are the complexes without viral proteins which are also used (Barr et al., 1998)(Figure 1C).

Polymeric NPs because of their capacity to convey tranquilizes just as being biodegradable have become a source of attraction (Li et al., 2000). The most regularly utilized poly(α-hydroxy acids) for getting ready polymeric NPs that are either poly(lactic corrosive) (PLA) or poly(lactic-co-glycolic corrosive) (PLGA) which are frequently synthesized utilizing a twofold emulsion solvent evaporation strategy (O'Donnell and McGinity, 1997; Sahoo et al., 2002; Lu et al., 2009).

At first, a polymer of decision is broken down in an organic solvent like ethyl acetic acid derivation or methylene chloride followed by the expansion of the antigen which is then vortexed to get an essential emulsion. With the expansion of an emulsifying operator (e.g., polyvinyl liquor or polyvinyl pyrrolidine) a water-in-oil-in-water emulsion is shaped. This result in the precipitation of polymer around the antigen (Figure 1D). Other good candidates for vaccine delivery are Hydrophilic polysaccharide polymers with both chitosan and dextran being chosen for synthesizing NPs. More consideration has been centered around chitosan NPs in view of their biocompatibility, its biodegradability into non-lethal items in vivo and its capacity to open up tight intersections between epithelial cells (Sonaje et al., 2012). Chitosan NPs can be set up in various ways.

Rather than the previously mentioned NPs, which comprises of organic or biodegradable materials, non-degradable NPs are additionally being examined for antibody conveyance (Calvo et al., 1997; Anne Saupe et al., 2006; Bhumkar et al., 2007b; Lee et al., 2010). Among those the most usually considered are gold, silica, and carbon to produce a shell in which antigens are epitomized or, all the more generally, to give a surface to covalent connection (Figure 1E).Gold NPs are frequently used in the size range of 2–50 nm, though they considerably vary in their size. As opposed to the delivery of entire microorganisms, similarly, as with conventional vaccines, the previously mentioned NP delivery systems are centered around little sub-atomic antigens delivered by the pathogen. These parts are typically communicated on the microbial layer and may incorporate glycoproteins, polysaccharides, proteins, lipoproteins (Table 1).

Applications of Nanomedicine

With the advancement of numerous products of nanotechnology that came up with a scope of treating pathophysiological conditions and anatomical changes of diseased or inflamed tissues. This has proven to be effective in the following ways:

1. By knowing various pathophysiological features of diseased tissues, drugs can be targeted in a specific manner (Vasir and Labhasetwar, 2005). 2. Unlike different normal drugs, there is greater concentrations of various nanoproducts (Vasir, Reddy and Labhasetwar2005) 3. Effective retention and transmission of the nanosystems in the inflamed tissues or tumors with an increased vascular permeability which is in turn adhered with an impaired lymphatic drainage in tumors (Maeda et al., 2000; Matsumura and Maeda, 1986). 4. Nanosystems possess an ability of selective localization and targeting in inflammed tissues (Allen and Cullis, 2004). 5. Efficiently delivering and transporting drugs to the brain, nanoparticles overcome the presence of blood–brain barrier (meninges) (Alyautdin et al., 2004; Garcia-Garcia et al., 2005). 6. Nanoparticles loaded with drugs increase the efficacy of drugs and decreases toxicity of drugs in specific tissues and organs which in turn is responsible for selective delivery of biologically active compounds (Fenget al., 2004; de Kozak et al., 2004) (Figure 2).

In present day scenario the various applications of nanotechnology are not only confined to the production of numerous anti-cancerous drug (nanodrugs) but its applications have also implemented to the treatment of various disorders such as obesity and the disorders of central nervous system (Wang and Xue, 2018). Nanobiotechnology has wide range of clinical applications for example disease diagnosis, target-specific drug delivery, and molecular imaging which is otherwise very difficult to be carefully examined at present. New promising nanoproducts are also undergoing clinical trials. Advancement of nanotechnology to the field of biological systems will build new foundations of diagnosis, treatment, and prevention of disease in future.

Nanomedicine and Cancer Treatment

In recent years, Cancer is among one of the leading reasons of mortality all over the world. Cancer malaises which comprises of a group of disorders characterized by indefinite proliferation of growth cells accompanied by delayed or no apoptosis. Conventional treatment methods of cancer which involves radiation, chemotherapy or surgery have few side effects. However, early diagnostics and targeted drug delivery to various organs are still not well developed (Jabir et al., 2012). With respect to these drawbacks, incidences of various types of cancers (blood, lung, colon, breast, etc.) are increasing with every passing day. Therefore, there is an immediate need to search for the rational alternatives to decipher these issues.

With the advent of various nanomedicines which have been successfully practiced for detection of tumor, targeted drug delivery and treatment (Sutradhar and Amin, 2014). Biosynthesized nanoparticles owing to their inherent benefits have promised potential to facilitate molecular interactions and cross biological barriers without affecting healthy cells. Borse et al. (2015). Biosynthesis of platinum nanoparticles against A431 and MCF-7 cell lines came up with the evaluation of *in vitro* anticancerous activities of *Saccharomyces boulardii*. Breast cancer malevolence is one of the leading causes of death among women. Silver nanoparticles obtained from *Cryptococcus laurentii* were found effective for antitumor activity against cancer cell lines and normal breast cell lines.

One of the major advantage of using nanomaterials as a carrier for anticancer drugs is the possibility of targeted delivery to the tumor, their ability to enclose or bind thousands of molecules of a drug and deliver to the required site, and to overcome solubility and stability issues (Moghimi, Hunter and Murray, 2005; Wilkinson, 2003; Peer et al., 2007; Martin, 2005). In addition, nanoplatforms like dendrimers, liposomes, lipid nanoparticles, micelles, and gold nanoparticles can offer solutions to various problems in diagnosis and treatment of cancer. Multifunctional nanoparticles (MNPs) for simultaneous diagnosis, imaging, and treatment, an area referred to as "theranostics" are also being developed for personalized medicine (Fernandez, Manchanda, and McGoran, 2011; Jain, 2012; Omedi, 2011; Torchilin, 2006) (Figure 3). Among the clinically successful inorganic nanoparticles are iron oxide and gold for imaging and thermal ablation of tumors and silica for cancer imaging. Nanoparticles therapeutics is especially useful for cancer and disorders of the central nervous system because they are able to cross the blood brain barrier (BBB) (Tosi et al., 2008). 'Smart' gold nanoparticles which can react to mild acidic environments and quickly form aggregates, and shift the absorption spectra from red and near infrared. Gold nanoparticles were used for photo acoustic imaging in cancer microenvironment, and confirmed the cancer-specific growth at the cellular level and an amplified signal which is twice higher than the control in vivo (Figure 4) (Jaejunget al., 2016)

Role of theranostic nanomedicine in cancer treatmentis defined as nanomedicine that combines diagnostics with therapeutics (Janib et al., 2010) (Figure 5). Nanomedicine has applied nanotechnology in various medical fields such as imaging, diagnosis and, or therapy in human diseases. Theranostics combines the last two fields, while as theranostic nanomedicine produces "nanoparticle-based drugs" simultaneously capable of the diagnosis and treatment of a disease (Muthu et al., 2014). Important advantage of theranostic nanomedicine in the treatment of cancer is the potential for a rapid review of the outcome for a treatment in individual patients, in order to plan the next therapy or to decide to repeat the same therapeutic session (personalized medicine). We feel that the use of magnetic NPs in conjunction with MRI imaging may advance the concept of personalized nanomedical theranostic treatment in cancer for an individual patient (Choi et al., 2012a,b).As MRI scanners are currently readily available in hospitals, this seems to be the most appropriate technique for monitoring the effects of cancer nanomedicine therapies. Moreover, magnetic NPs have an enormous advantage in this type of therapy, due to their paramagnetic propriety: they can be easily used as a contrast agent.

In recent years, Nanotheranostics based cancer therapy has emerged as an appealing and minimally invasive therapeutic strategy for cancer treatment (Khlebtsov et al., 2006, Huff et al., 2007). It can deliver a specific amount of photo energy directly into the tumor site to increase treatment efficiency and also minimize the damage to the surrounding healthy tissues. Noble metal-based nanostructures, such as gold nanospheres, gold nanorods, gold nanoshells, gold nanocages, copper-based semiconductor NPs, and carbon nanotubes are the chief nanomaterials that have been well prepared and demonstrated powerfull NIR laser-induced PTT efficacy (Catarina et al., 2018). However, their promising clinical applications were largely limited, due to the innate toxicity and unknown long-term toxicity of these aforementioned PTT agents.

Nano Particle-Based Drug Delivery System

Nanoparticles can be delivered to various targeted sites, which comprises of locations that are inaccessible to be easily reached by standard drugs. For example, if a therapeutic is chemically attached to a nanoparticle, it can then be oriented to the site of the infection or disease by radio or magnetic signals (Sarwar et al., 2019). Nanodrugs can also be designed in a way that they are released only at times when some specific molecules are present with them or any external stimuli triggers (such as infrared heat).

Various harmful side effects from potent medications can be avoided by decreasing the effective dosage that is required to treat the patient. This can be achieved by encapsulating drugs in nano sized materials (such as hollow polymer capsules, organic dendrimers, and nano shells), release of nanodrugs can be controlled much more precisely than ever before (Sarwar et al., 2019). Drugs are designed to carry a therapeutic payload (radiation, gene therapy or chemotherapy) as well as for various imaging applications (Lavan, Lynn and Langer, 2002). Many agents, which cannot be administered orally due to their poor bioavailability, have now scope to be used in therapy with the help of nanotechnology (El-Shabouri, 2002; Hu, Tang and Cui, 2004).

Nano-formulations offer protection to agents who are otherwise vulnerable to denaturation or degradation when exposed to extreme pH, and also prolong half-life of a drug by expanding retention of the formulation through bioadhesion (Arangoa et al., 2001; Arbos et al., 2004). Another broad application of nanotechnology is the delivery of antigens for vaccination (Diwan, 2003; Koping-Hoggard, Sanchez and Alonso, 2005). Recent advances in development of suitable animal models and encapsulation have effectively demonstrated that nanoparticles and microparticles are capable of enhancing immunization (Lutsiak et al., 2002) (Figure 6).

Nanoparticles are found to be expedient in targeted drug delivery, drug bioavailability, bioactivity and stability. Types of drug delivery nano-vehicles include water-soluble polymer such as natural antibodies and synthetic polymers, nanosphere of natural or synthetic polymers, liposome composed of vesicle with bilayer wall, polymeric micelles and emulsions stabilized by amphipathic surface coatings (Brakmane et al., 2012; Salouti and Ahangari, 2014; Omlor et al., 2015). Surface properties and small size of nanoparticles assist pharmacologically active compounds to reach within all the cellular compartments of the human body at optimum rate. Toxicokinetics can also be controlled when drugs form conjugates with nanoparticles by encapsulation or through different linker molecules. They reduce the toxic side effects of drug carrier systems while keeping therapeutic effects to the patients.

NANOPARTICLES AS VACCINE DELIVERY VEHICLES

Vaccines are defined as killed microbes, live attenuated microbes, or altered constituents of microbes. Different types of vaccines have many applications to control vast number of infectious diseases; but some vaccines have demerits and not safe for use to meet the current challenge of various infectious diseases (Nak-Hyung Lee, 2012).

Several research studies encompassing the polysaccharide or naked DNA based vaccines development encoding a protective antigen used for extensive array of infectious diseases for which no licensed vaccines are available. To overcome these challenges a range of vaccines are being developed which are primarily based on isolated polysaccharides or naked DNA encoding a protective antigen. Compared to existing vaccines with various drawbacks, these are much safer and less reactive (polysaccharides or naked DNA). They are weak immunogens and require different adjuvants to enhance their efficacy. Aluminium based adjuvants are the commonly ones used but can also induce different local reactions and more interestingly it may fail to produce the cell mediated immunity (Guy, 2007; Harandi et al., 2010).

To tackle these drawbacks, the development of some novel adjuvants and delivery systems is the need of the time for the next generation of vaccines. Thus, much attention is being paid towards the utility of nanoparticles as delivery vehicles for vaccines (Rashmirekha, Maxim, and Avinash, 2018). In this context, the nanoparticle surface is either decorated or encapsulated within by the vaccine antigen. NPs provide a method for delivering antigens by encapsulating antigenic material, which may otherwise degrade rapidly upon injection or induce a short-lived, localized immune response. Conjugation of various antigens onto the surface of NPs can led to the presentation of the immunogen to the immune systems in similar fashion as it would be presented by the pathogen, thereby provoking a similar response. Moreover, NPs which are made from some composites not only enable site directed delivery of antigens but also the continuous release of antigens so as to maximize exposure to the immune system. The potential for NPs is also explored to deliver vaccines through various non-traditional methods which comprises of inhalation, topical, or optical delivery as well as combining several antigens to the same particle in order to protect against more than one disease. The possible outcome is that the particulate vaccines generated using various technologies will be far better at providing potent antigen-specific towards humoral and cellular immune responses and thereby provide window to next generation vaccines to be generated against a wide range of infectious diseases.

Nanotechnology in Gene therapy

Gene therapy involves the modification or the prevention of a particular diseased or any abnormal condition of a person and can be achieved by the delivery of defined genes to specific target cells (Emerich and Thanos, 2003). Presently vectors that are usually viral based are more frequently used in gene therapy and some cases involve the application of various non-viral techniques as well. At present times the replacement of defective genes of a diseased person with functional ones is practiced without the use of vectors. In addition, the activity of genes are being altered in vivo by several techniques without carrying the gene transfer.

Current gene therapy procedures encompass several drawbacks including the inherent impoverishment and hurdles of effective pharmaceutical processing and progression and potential immunogenicity of viral vectors involved in gene delivery. Moreover, gene therapy is also associated with the drawback of the chance of reversion of an engineered mutant back to the wild type (Yotsuyanagi and Hazemoto, 1998; Young, Searle, Onion and Mautner, 2006).

In order to combat and address these issues, nanotechnological tools in human gene therapy have been applied and tested. The significant role of nanoparticle-based non-viral vectors (usually 50-500 nm in size) in transportation of plasmid DNA has also been elucidated. Non-viral gene delivery system involves the usage of number of nanoparticles (nanostructures) with great deal of specificity and accuracy. Therefore, successful introduction of less immunogenic nanosized gene carriers as a substitution of the disputed viral vectors seems more beneficial in replacing and altering defected genes in humans (Davis, 1997).

Nanotechnology and Liposomes

The structure of liposome comprises of a lipid bilayer, making it a good candidate for gene therapy as it has the unique property to cross easily the targct lipid bilayer or other bio-membranes. More recently, several groups of liposomes have shown fruitful results while being applied in local gene delivery (Hart, 2005; Ewert et al., 2005). Liposomes have comprehensively made their way to targeted therapy as well. A more significant reporter expression in the brain of rhesus monkey has been reported which involved the linking of nanoparticle treated liposome to a mAb for human insulin reporter (Zhang et al.,2003).

These interesting and comprehensive trails with great deal of success witness the future of targeted therapy and the significant role of nanosized particles for the advancement of molecular medicine.

Nanotechnology in Cardiac Therapy

At present times the role of nanotechnology is established to a great extent as it offers the more promising tools to be applied in modern cardiovascular science to explore several existing dimensions and frontiers at cellular level and the effective treatment of various cardiovascular diseases presenting a substantial challenge.

These tools also find their application in imaging, diagnosis and tissue engineering (Wickline et al., 2006). Downsized nanoscale sensors comprising of quantum dots (QDs), nanobarcodes and nanocrystals possess the capability of sensing and monitoring complex immune signals that arise in response to inflammatory or cardiac events (Guccione, Li, and Bednarski, 2004). Moreover, the field of nanobiotechnology plays an important role to detect and describe some clinically significant mechanisms involved in cardiac disorders. In addition, nanotechnology helps in designing of atomic -scale machines that can be further integrated into biological systems at molecular level. The applicability of such newly designed nanomachines may significantly modify many hypothesis and ideas critical for the treatment of cardiovascular disorders. The emerging field of nanotechnology may have a quite significant impact in handling several issues including unstable plaques and clarification of valves.

Subsequently, as evident from several facts the implication of nanotechnology may prove as an important milestone by achieving success in localized and sustained arterial and cardiac drug therapy and hence in the specific and targeted management of cardiovascular diseases (Panyam and Labhasetwar, 2003).

Nanotechnology in Dental Care

Recent research indicates that nanotechnology might have a future medical application in the area of dentistry. The use and emergence of nanodentistry by the aid of nanomaterials and nanorobotics will incorporate better oral health (West and Halas, 2000; Shi, Tsai, Garrison, Ferrari and Ratner, 1999) (Sims, 1999; Slavkin, 1999). The successful application of nanotechnology in the dental science will benefit millions of people who are presently receiving poor dental care and more importantly this will be a significant breakthrough in the field of health sciences (Ure and Harris, 2003; Fartash, Tangerud, Silness and Arvidson, 1996). This may further lead to the evolution of various nano-dental based techniques important for complex tooth repair. Reconstructive dental nanorobots could be used in selective and precise occlusion of specific tubules within minutes and hence will facilitate speedy and permanent recovery. The advantage of nanodentistry in natural tooth maintenance could also be significant (Shellhart and Oesterle, 1999).

Nanobiotechnology and Parkinson's Disease

The nanobiotechnology finds its application in the diagnosis and treatment of Parkinson's disease via the use of biosensors, which have the ability to reversibly measure biological activities in real time (Mehrotra, 2016). For preventing Parkinson's disease advancement early detection of this disease is necessary and it was carried out with electrochemical nanobiosensors using a miR biomarker and the same gave fruitful results than others (Piwek and Elis, 2016).

One of the important hurdles in the treatment of this disease was the inability of drugs to cross the blood-brain barrier (Fymat, 2016) but nanobiotechnology has solved this problem as the nanoparticle enclosed with drugs provide a route for drugs to easily cross the blood-brain barrier (Rizvi and Saleh,2018). Presently the treatment of Parkinson's diseases and other diseases of central nervous system(CNS) is limited as the drug development for curing brain diseases are having slowest success rates as compared other therapeutic means (Cotterell et al.,2018).

Nanobiotechnology and Malaria

The evolution of nanotechnology in recent years has indicated the potential for new control approaches against vectors of malaria. Biosynthesized nanoparticles have lethal effects on larval as well as adult stages of malarial vectors (Kuppusamy, Yusoff, Maniam, Govindan, 2016; Santhoshkumar, 2011).

Silver and Gold nanoparticles were the most potent insecticides and Silver nanoparticles were found as the broad-spectrum nanoparticles with important properties including anti-inflammatory, anti-microbial and anti-tumor effects (Qamar., Asgher, Khalid and Sadaf,2019). Thus, nanotechnology can provide fruitful results in controlling malaria by checking the population of larval stages via the plasmodicidal activity of the nanoparticles.

FUTURE CHALLENGES OF NANOMEDICINE

Nanotechnology-based approaches can be used for efficient diagnosis, drug delivery and disease treatment.In future, nanotechnology is expected to provide devices to examine tissue in minute details. Biosensors that are smaller than a cell would give us an inside look at cellular function. Tissues could be analyzed down to the molecular level, giving a completely detail of cellular, subcellular and molecular activities. Such a detailed diagnosis will ultimately lead to appropriate treatment. Moreover, it is expected that within a short span of time, exhaustive research will lead to better understanding of how to coat or chemically alter nanoparticles to reduce their toxicity, which will ultimately broaden their use for disease diagnosis and for drug delivery.

CONCLUSION

Recent advances in the field of nanomedicine provide an opportunity and possibility in nanoparticle-based detection, diagnosis and treatment of disease. The development of nanotechnology and nanoparticle application in biomedicine at commercial level have unravel a broad spectrum of human health benefits with decreased hazards. The main objective of this chapter was to investigate the use of important nanoparticles for possible use as biomedicines. Some of these nanoparticles (Ag) exhibit high thermal and electrical conductivity, chemical stability, catalytic activity and more specifically increased Raman scattering. These unique properties of nanoparticles have been specifically employed in drug delivery, bio-imaging, biosensors and treatment of various challenging diseases including cancer, Parkinson's disease etc. However, the adverse side effects of nanostructures have been limited the widespread use of nanostructures and more investigation in this field is required.

ACKNOWLEDGMENT

This article was written by BAS, BAB, DR THD and edited and compiled by Dr MAM.Authors are thankful to Dr MAM for his supervision and mentorship.

Conflict of Interest

The authors declare no conflict of interest

REFERENCES

Akerblom, L., Nara, P., Dunlop, N., Putney, S., & Morein, B. (1993). HIV experimental vaccines based on the iscom technology using envelope and GAG gene products. *Biotechnol. Ther., 4*, 145–161.

Albert, D. (2016). *Nanomedicine*. Immune Rebalancing. The Future of Immunosuppression.

Allen, T. M., & Cullis, P. R. (2004). Drug delivery systems: Entering the mainstream. *Science, 303*(5665), 1818–1822. doi:10.1126cience.1095833 PMID:15031496

Alving, C. R., Richards, R. L., Moss, J., Alving, L. I., Clements, J. D., Shiba, T., Kotani, S., Wirtz, R. A., & Hockmeyer, W. T. (1986). Effectiveness of liposomes as potential carriers of vaccines: Applications to cholera toxin and human malaria sporozoite antigen. *Vaccine, 4*(3), 166–172. doi:10.1016/0264-410X(86)90005-8 PMID:3532603

Alyautdin, R.N., Tezikov, E.B., Ramge, P., Kharkevich, D.A., Begley, D.J., & Kreuter, J. (1998). Significant entry of tubocurarine into the brain of rats by adsorption to polysorbate 80-coated poly butyl cyanoacrylate nanoparticles: an insitu brain perfusion study. *J Micro Encapsule, 15*, 67–74.

Arangoa, M. A., Campanero, M. A., Renedo, M. J., Ponchel, G., & Irache, J. M. (2001). Gliadin nanoparticles as carriers for the oral administration of lipophilic drugs. Relationships between bioadhesion and pharmacokinetics. *Pharmaceutical Research, 18*(11), 1521–1527. doi:10.1023/A:1013018111829 PMID:11758758

Arayne, M. S., Sultana, N., & Qureshi, F. (2007). nanoparticles in delivery of cardiovascular drugs. *Pakistan Journal of Pharmaceutical Sciences, 20*, 340–348. PMID:17604260

Arbos, P., Campanero, M. A., Arangoa, M. A., & Irache, J. M. (2004). Nanoparticles with specific bioadhesive properties to circumvent the pre-systemic degradation of fluorinated pyrimidines. *Journal of Controlled Release, 96*(1), 55–65. doi:10.1016/j.jconrel.2004.01.006 PMID:15063029

Baca, E. M., Foldvari, M., Snider, M., Harding, K., Kournikakis, B., & Babiuk, L. A. (2000). Intra nasal immunization with liposome-formulated Yersinia pestis vaccine enhances mucosal immune responses. *Vaccine, 18*(21), 2203–2211. doi:10.1016/S0264-410X(00)00019-0 PMID:10717339

Baca-Estrada, M. E., Foldvari, M., Snider, M., Harding, K., Kournikakis, B., Babiuk, L. A., & Griebel, P. (2000). Intra nasal immunization with liposome-formulated Yersinia pestis vaccine enhances mucosal immune responses. *Vaccine*, *18*(21), 2203–2211. doi:10.1016/S0264-410X(00)00019-0 PMID:10717339

Barr, I. G., Sjolander, A., & Cox, J. C. (1998). ISCOMs and others aponin based adjuvants. *Advanced Drug Delivery Reviews*, *32*(3), 247–271. doi:10.1016/S0169-409X(98)00013-1 PMID:10837647

Beatriz, P. (2017). Diverse applications of nanomedicine. *ACS Nano*. DOI: doi:10.1021/acsnano.6b0604011

Beyth, N., Houri-Haddad, Y., Domb, A., Khan, W., & Hazan, R. (2015). *Alternative antimicrobial approach: nano-antimicrobial materials*. Evid Based Compl. Altern Med.

Bhumkar, D. R., Joshi, H. M., Sastry, M., & Pokharkar, V. B. (2007b). Chitosan reduced gold nanoparticles as novel carriers for transmucosal delivery of insulin. *Pharmaceutical Research*, *24*(8), 1415–1426. doi:10.100711095-007-9257-9 PMID:17380266

Borse, V., Kaler, A., & Banerjee, U.C. (2015). Microbial synthesis of platinum nanoparticles and evaluation of their anticancer activity. *Int. J. Emerg. Trends Electr. Electron., 11*.

Brakmane, G., Winslet, M., & Seifalian, A. M. (2012). Systematic review: The applications of nanotechnology in gastroenterology. *Alimentary Pharmacology & Therapeutics*, *36*(3), 213–221. doi:10.1111/j.1365-2036.2012.05179.x PMID:22686286

Calvo, P., Remuñan-López, C., Vila-Jato, J. L., & Alonso, M. J. (1997). Chitosan and chitosan/ethylene oxide-propylene oxide block copolymer nanoparticles as novel carriers for proteins and vaccines. *Pharmaceutical Research*, *14*(10), 1431–1436. doi:10.1023/A:1012128907225 PMID:9358557

Caputoa, A. (2009). Induction of humoral and enhanced cellular immune responses by novel core-shell nanosphere-and microsphere-based vaccine formulations following systemic and mucosal administration. *Vaccine*, *27*(27), 3605–3615. doi:10.1016/j.vaccine.2009.03.047 PMID:19464541

Chen, Y. S., Hung, Y. C., Lin, W. H., & Huang, G. S. (2010). Assessment of gold nanoparticles as a size-dependent vaccine carrier for enhancing the antibody response against synthetic foot and mouth disease virus peptide. *Nanotechnology*, *21*(19), 195101. doi:10.1088/0957-4484/21/19/195101 PMID:20400818

Choi, K.Y., Jeon, E.J., & Yoon, H.Y. (2012b). Theranostic nanoparticles based on PEGylated hyaluronic acid for the diagnosis, therapy and monitoring of colon cancer. *Biomaterials, 33*(26), 6186-6193.

Choi, K.Y., Liu, G., & Chen, X. (2012a). Theranostic nanoplatforms for simultaneous cancer imaging and therapy: current approaches and future perspectives. *Nanoscale, 4*(2), 330-342.

Classen, I., & Osterhaus, A. (1992). The iscom structure as an immune enhancing moiety: Experiences in viral systems. *Australian Orthodontic Journal*, *15*, 260–268.

Cotterell, P. (2018). Parkinson's disease: Symptoms, treatment options and nursing care. *Nursing Standard*, *33*(7), 53–58. doi:10.7748/ns.2018.e11207 PMID:30198239

Davis, S. S. (1997). Biomedical applications of nanotechnology—Implications for drug targeting and gene therapy. *Trends in Biotechnology*, *15*(6), 217–224. doi:10.1016/S0167-7799(97)01036-6 PMID:9183864 de Kozak, Y., Andrieux, K., Villarroya, H., Klein, C., Thillaye Goldenberg, B., Naud, M. C., Garcia, E., & Couvreur, P. (2004). Intraocular injection of tamoxifen-loaded nanoparticles: A new treatment of experimental autoimmune uveoretinitis. *European Journal of Immunology, 34*(12), 3702–3712. doi:10.1002/eji.200425022 PMID:15517615

Demento, S. L., Cui, W., Criscione, J. M., Stern, E., Tulipan, J., Kaech, S. M., & Fahmy, T. M. (2012). Role of sustained antigen release from nanoparticle vaccines in shaping the T cell memory phenotype. *Biomaterials, 33*(19), 4957–4964. doi:10.1016/j.biomaterials.2012.03.041 PMID:22484047

Dhar, S., Daniel, W. L., Giljohann, D. A., Mirkin, C. A., & Lippard, S. J. (2009). Polyvalent oligonucleotide gold nanoparticle conjugates as delivery vehicles for platinum (IV) 0000 warheads. *Journal of the American Chemical Society, 131*(41), 14652–14653. doi:10.1021/ja9071282 PMID:19778015

Diwan, M., Elamanchili, P., Lane, H., Gainer, A., & Samuel, J. (2003). Biodegradable nanoparticle mediated antigen delivery to human cord blood derived dendritic cells for induction of primary T cell responses. *Journal of Drug Targeting, 11*(8-10), 495–507. doi:10.1080/10611860410001670026 PMID:15203918

El-Shabouri, M. H. (2002). Positively charged nanoparticles for improving the oral bioavailability of cyclosporin-A. *International Journal of Pharmaceutics, 249*(1-2), 101–118. doi:10.1016/S0378-5173(02)00461-1 PMID:12433438

Emerich, D. F., & Thanos, C. G. (2003). Nanotechnology and medicine. *Expert Opinion on Biological Therapy, 3*(4), 655–663. doi:10.1517/14712598.3.4.655 PMID:12831370

Ewert, K., Evans, H. M., Ahmad, A., Slack, N. L., Lin, A. J., Martin-Herranz, A., & Safinya, C. R. (2005). Lipoplex structures and their distinct cellular pathways. *Advances in Genetics, 53*, 119–155. doi:10.1016/S0065-2660(05)53005-0 PMID:16240992

Fartash, B., Tangerud, T., Silness, J., & Arvidson, K. (1996). Rehabilitation of mandibular edentulism by single crystal sapphire implants and over dentures: 3- year results in 86 patients. A dual center international study. *Clinical Oral Implants Research, 7*(3), 220–229. doi:10.1034/j.1600-0501.1996.070304.x PMID:9151586

Feng, S. S., Mu, L., Win, K. Y., & Huang, G. (2004). Nanoparticles of biodegradable polymers for clinical administration of paclitaxel. *Current Medicinal Chemistry, 11*(4), 413–424. doi:10.2174/0929867043455909 PMID:14965222

Fernandez, A., Manchanda, R., & McGoran, A. (2011). Theranostic applications of nanomaterials in cancer therapy: drug delivery, image-guided therapy and multifunctional platforms. *Appl Biochem Biotechnol., 165*(7-8), 1628-51.

Fries, L. F., Gordon, D. M., Richards, R. L., Egan, J. E., Hollingdale, M. R., Gross, M., Silverman, C., & Alving, C. R. (1992). Liposomal malaria vaccine in humans: A safe and potent adjuvant strategy. *Proceedings of the National Academy of Sciences of the United States of America, 89*(1), 358–362. doi:10.1073/pnas.89.1.358 PMID:1729706

Fymat, A. L. (2016). Recent developments in nanomedicine research. *Journal of Nanomedicine Research, 4*(4), 12. doi:10.15406/jnmr.2016.04.00096

Fynan, E. F., Webster, R. G., Fuller, D. H., Haynes, J. R., Santoro, J. C., & Robinson, H. L. (1993). DNA vaccines: Protective immunizations by parenteral, mucosal, and gene-gun inoculations. *Proceedings of the National Academy of Sciences of the United States of America*, *90*(24), 11478–11482. doi:10.1073/pnas.90.24.11478 PMID:8265577

Garcia-Garcia, E., Gil, S., Andrieux, K., Desmaële, D., Nicolas, V., Taran, F., Georgin, D., Andreux, J. P., Roux, F., & Couvreur, P. (2005). A relevant in vitro rat model for the evaluation of blood–brain barrier translocation of nanoparticles. *Cellular and Molecular Life Sciences*, *62*(12), 1400–1408. doi:10.100700018-005-5094-3 PMID:15905957

Grgacic, E. V. L., & Anderson, D. A. (2006). Virus-likeparticles: Passporttoimmunerecognition. *Methods (San Diego, Calif.)*, *40*(1), 60–65. doi:10.1016/j.ymeth.2006.07.018 PMID:16997714

Guccione, S., Li, K. C., & Bednarski, M. D. (2004). Vascular-targeted nanoparticles for molecular imaging and therapy. *Methods in Enzymology*, *386*, 219–236. doi:10.1016/S0076-6879(04)86010-5 PMID:15120254

Guy, B. (2007). The perfect mix: Recent progress in adjuvant research. *Nature Reviews. Microbiology*, *5*(7), 505–517. doi:10.1038/nrmicro1681 PMID:17558426

Haran, G., Cohen, R., Bar, L. K., & Barenholz, Y. (1993). Transmembrane ammonium sulfate gradients in liposomes produce efficient and stable entrapment of amphipathic weak bases. *Biochimica et Biophysica Acta*, *1151*(2), 201–215. doi:10.1016/0005-2736(93)90105-9 PMID:8373796

Harandi, A. M., Medaglini, D., & Shattock, R. J. (2010). Vaccine adjuvants: Apriority for vaccine research. *Vaccine*, *28*(12), 2363–2366. doi:10.1016/j.vaccine.2009.12.084 PMID:20064476

Hart, S. L. (2005). Lipid carriers for gene therapy. *Current Drug Delivery*, *2*(4), 423–428. doi:10.2174/156720105774370230 PMID:16305445

Henriksen-Lacey, M., Korsholm, K. S., Andersen, P., Perrie, Y., & Christensen, D. (2011). Liposomal vaccine delivery systems. *Expert Opinion on Drug Delivery*, *8*(4), 505–519. doi:10.1517/17425247.2011.558081 PMID:21413904

Heurtault, B., Frisch, B., & Pons, F. (2010). Liposomes as delivery systems for nasal vaccination: Strategies and outcomes. *Expert Opinion on Drug Delivery*, *7*(7), 829–844. doi:10.1517/17425247.2010.488687 PMID:20459361

Hu, L., Tang, X., & Cui, F. (2004). Solid lipid nanoparticles (SLNs) to improve oral bioavailability of poorly soluble drugs. *The Journal of Pharmacy and Pharmacology*, *56*(12), 1527–1535. doi:10.1211/0022357044959 PMID:15563759

Hu, Y. C. (2005). Baculo virus as a highly efficient expression vector in insect and mammalian cells. Act a Pharmacol.Sin. 26, 405–416. folding in vivo by anonlytic baculovirus. *The Biochemical Journal*, *382*, 695–702.

Huff, T.B., Tong, L., Zhao, Y., Hansen, M.N., Cheng, J.X., & Wei, A. (2007). Hyperthermic effects of gold nanorods on tumor cells. *Nanomedicine, 2*(1), 125-132.

Huh, A. J., & Kwon, Y.J. (2011) Nanoantibiotics: A new paradigm for treating infectious diseases using nanomaterials in the antibiotics resistant era. *J. Control Release., 156*(2), 128–45.

Jabir, N. R., Tabrez, S., Ashraf, G. M., Shakil, S., Damanhouri, G. A., & Kamal, M. A. (2012). Nanotechnology-based approaches in anticancer research. *International Journal of Nanomedicine, 7*, 4391–4408. PMID:22927757

Jaejung, S., Jeesu, K., Sekyu, H., Mansik, J., Sanghwa, J., Chulhong, K., & Sungjee, K. (2016). "Smart" Gold Nanoparticles for Photoacoustic Imaging: Imaging Contrast Agent Responsive to Cancer Microenvironment and Signal Amplification by pH-induced Aggregation. *Chemical Communications, 52*(53), 8287–8290. Advance online publication. doi:10.1039/C6CC03100E PMID:27292365

Jain, K. K., (2012). Role of nano diagnostics in personalized cancer therapy. *Clin Lab Med., 32*, 15-31.

Jaison, J., Ahmed, B., & Yen, S. (2018). Review on nanoparticles and nanostructured materials: History, sources, toxicity and regulations. *Beilstein Journal of Nanotechnology, 9*, 1050–1074. doi:10.3762/bjnano.9.98 PMID:29719757

Janib, S.M., Moses, A.S., & MacKay, J.A. (2010). Imaging and drug delivery using theranostic nanoparticles. *Adv. Drug Deliv. Rev., 62*(11), 1052-1063.

Jayanta, K., Patra, Gitishree, D., & Fernandes, F. (2018). Nano based drugdelivery systems: recent developments and future prospects. *J. Nanobiotechnol, 16*.

Jeevanandam, J., Barhoum, A., Chan, Y. S., Dufresne, A., & Danquah, M. K. (2018). Review on nanoparticles and nanostructured materials: History, sources, toxicity and regulations. *Beilstein Journal of Nanotechnology, 9*, 1050–1074. doi:10.3762/bjnano.9.98 PMID:29719757

Joseph, R. R., & Venkatraman, S. S. (2017). Drug delivery to the eye: What benefits do nanocarriers offer? *Nanomedicine (London), 12*(6), 683–702. doi:10.2217/nnm-2016-0379 PMID:28186436

Kang, C. Y., Luo, L., Wainberg, M. A., & Li, Y. (1999). Development of HIV/AIDS vaccine using chimeric gag env virus-like particles. *Biological Chemistry, 380*(3), 353–364. doi:10.1515/BC.1999.047 PMID:10223338

Karkada, M., Weir, G. M., Quinton, T., Fuentes-Ortega, A., & Mansour, M. (2011). Aliposome-based platform, Vacci Max, and its modified water-free platform DepoVax enhance efficacy of in vivo nucleic acid delivery. *Vaccine, 28*(38), 6176–6182. doi:10.1016/j.vaccine.2010.07.025 PMID:20656034

Kazanji, M., Laurent, F., & Pery, P. (1994). Immune responses and protective effect in mice vaccinated orally with surface sporozoite protein of Eimeria falciformis in ISCOMs. *Vaccine, 12*(9), 798–804. doi:10.1016/0264-410X(94)90288-7 PMID:7975858

Kersten, G. F., & Crommelin, D. J. (1995). Liposomes and ISCOMS as vaccine formulations. *Biochimica et Biophysica Acta, 1241*(2), 117–138. doi:10.1016/0304-4157(95)00002-9 PMID:7640293

Kersten, G. F., Teerlink, T., Derks, H. J., Verkleij, A. J., van Wezel, T. L., Crommelin, D. J., & Beuvery, E. C. (1988). Incorporation of the major outer membrane protein of Neisseria gonorrhoeae in saponin-lipid complexes (iscoms): Chemical analysis, some structural features, and comparison of their immunogenicity with three other antigen delivery systems. *Infection and Immunity*, *56*(2), 432–438. doi:10.1128/IAI.56.2.432-438.1988 PMID:3123391

Khlebtsov, B., Zharov, V., Melnikov, A., Tuchin, V., & Khlebtsov, N. (2006). Optical amplification of photothermal therapy with gold nanoparticles and nanoclusters. *Nanotechnology, 17*(20), 5167-5179.

Kingsman, S. M., & Kingsman, A. J. (1988). Polyvalent recombinant antigens; a new vaccine strategy. *Vaccine*, *6*(4), 304–306. doi:10.1016/0264-410X(88)90174-0 PMID:2847436

Koping-Hoggard, M., Sanchez, A., & Alonso, M. J. (2005). Nanoparticles as carriers for nasal vaccine delivery. *Expert Review of Vaccines*, *4*(2), 185–196. doi:10.1586/14760584.4.2.185 PMID:15889992

Kuppusamy, P., Yusoff, M. M., Maniam, G. P., & Govindan, N. (2016). Biosynthesis of metallic nanoparticles using plant derivatives and their new avenues in pharmacological applications – an updated report. *Saudi Pharmaceutical Journal*, *24*(4), 473–484. doi:10.1016/j.jsps.2014.11.013 PMID:27330378

LaVan, D. A., Lynn, D. M., & Langer, R. (2002). Timeline: Moving Smaller in drug discovery and delivery. *Nature Reviews. Drug Discovery*, *1*(1), 77–84. doi:10.1038/nrd707 PMID:12119612

Lee, P.-W., Hsu, S.-H., Tsai, J.-S., Chen, F.-R., Huang, P.-J., Ke, C.-J., Liao, Z.-X., Hsiao, C.-W., Lin, H.-J., & Sung, H.-W. (2010). Multifunctional core-shell polymeric nanoparticles for transdermal DNA delivery and epidermal Langerhans cell stracking. *Biomaterials*, *31*(8), 2425–2434. doi:10.1016/j.biomaterials.2009.11.100 PMID:20034662

Li, X., Deng, X., Yuan, M., Xiong, C., Huang, Z., Zhang, Y., & Jia, W. (2000). In vitro degradation and release profiles of poly-DL-lactide- poly(ethyleneglycol) microspheres with entrapped proteins. *Journal of Applied Polymer Science*, *78*(1), 140–148. doi:10.1002/1097-4628(20001003)78:1<140::AID-APP180>3.0.CO;2-P

Lovgren, K., & Morein, B. (1988). The requirement of lipids for the formation of immuno- stimulating complexes (iscoms). *Biotechnology and Applied Biochemistry*, *10*, 161–172. PMID:2838046

Lu, J. M., Wang, X., Marin-Muller, C., Wang, H., Lin, P. H., Yao, Q., & Chen, C. (2009). Current advances in research and clinical applications of PLGA-based nanotechnology. *Expert Review of Molecular Diagnostics*, *9*(4), 325–341. doi:10.1586/erm.09.15 PMID:19435455

Lutsiak, M. E., Robinson, D. R., Coester, C., Kwon, G. S., & Samuel, J. (2002). Analysis of poly (d, l-lactic-co-glycolic acid) nanosphere uptake by human dendritic cells and macrophages in vitro. *Pharmaceutical Research*, *19*(10), 1480–1487. doi:10.1023/A:1020452531828 PMID:12425465

Maeda, H., Wu, J., Sawa, T., Matsumura, Y., & Hori, K. (2000). Tumor vascular permeability and the EPR effect in macromolecular therapeutics: A review. *Journal of Controlled Release*, *65*(1-2), 271–284. doi:10.1016/S0168-3659(99)00248-5 PMID:10699287

Manzoor, A. Mir., Umar, M., Bashir, A. S., & Syed, S. H. (2019). Nanobodies: The “magic bullets” in therapeutics, drug delivery and diagnostics. *Human Antibodies*, 1–23. doi:10.3233/HAB-190390

Martin, C. R. (2006). Welcome to nanomedicine. *Nanomedicine (London), 1*(1), 5. doi:10.2217/17435889.1.1.5

Matsumura, Y., & Maeda, H. (1986). A new concept for macromolecular therapeutics in cancer chemotherapy: Mechanism of tumoritropic accumulation of proteins and the antitumor agent smancs. *Cancer Research, 46*, 6387–6392. PMID:2946403

Md, F., Zakir, H., & Hafsa, A. (2012). Prospects and applications of nanobiotechnology: A medical perspective. *Journal of Nanobiotechnology*.

Mehrotra, P. (2016). Biosensors and their applications - A review. *Journal of Oral Biology and Craniofacial Research, 6*(2), 153–159. doi:10.1016/j.jobcr.2015.12.002 PMID:27195214

Mirza, A. Z., & Siddiqui, F. A. (2014). Nanomedicine and drug delivery: A mini review. *International Nano Letters, 4*(1), 94. doi:10.100740089-014-0094-7

Moghimi, S. M., Hunter, A.C., & Murray, J. C. (2005). Nanomedicine: current status and future prospects. *FASEB J., 19*, 311-30.

Morein, B., Lövgren, K., Rönnberg, B., Sjölander, A., & Villacrés-Eriksson, M. (1995). Immunostimulating complexes. Clinical potential in vaccine development. *Clinical Immunotherapeutics, 3*(6), 461–475. doi:10.1007/BF03259065

Morein, B., & Simons, K. (1985). Subunit vaccines against enveloped viruses: Virosomes, micelles and other protein complexes. *Vaccine, 3*(2), 83–93. doi:10.1016/0264-410X(85)90055-6 PMID:3898625

Musumeci, T., Ventura, C. A., Giannone, I., Ruozi, B., Montenegro, L., Pignatello, R., & Puglisi, G. (2006). PLA/PLGA nanoparticles for sustained release of docetaxel. *International Journal of Pharmaceutics, 325*(1-2), 172–179. doi:10.1016/j.ijpharm.2006.06.023 PMID:16887303

Muthu, M.S., Leong, D.T., Mei, L., & Feng, S.S. (2014). Nanotheranostics—application and further development of nanomedicine strategies for advanced theranostics. *Theranostics, 4*(6), 660-677.

Nak-Hyung, L., Jung-Ah, L., & Seung-Yong, P. (2012). A review of vaccine development and research for industry animals in Korea. *Clinical and Experimental Vaccine Research, 1*(1), 18–34. doi:10.7774/cevr.2012.1.1.18 PMID:23596575

O'Donnell, P. B., & McGinity, J. W. (1997). Preparation of microspheres by the solvent evaporation technique. *Advanced Drug Delivery Reviews, 28*(1), 25–42. doi:10.1016/S0169-409X(97)00049-5 PMID:10837563

Olsson, S. E., Villa, L. L., Costa, R. L. R., Petta, C. A., Andrade, R. P., Malm, C., Iversen, O.-E., Høye, J., Steinwall, M., Riis-Johannessen, G., Andersson-Ellstrom, A., Elfgren, K., von Krogh, G., Lehtinen, M., Paavonen, J., Tamms, G. M., Giacoletti, K., Lupinacci, L., Esser, M. T., ... Barr, E. (2007). Induction of immune memory following administration of a prophylactic quadrivalent human papilloma virus (HPV) types 6/11/16/18 L1 virus-like particle (VLP) vaccine. *Vaccine, 25*(26), 4931–4939. doi:10.1016/j.vaccine.2007.03.049 PMID:17499406

Omedi, Y., (2011). Smart multifunctional theranostics: simultaneous diagnosis and therapy of cancer. *Bioimpacts, 1*(3), 145-7.

Omlor, A. J., Nguyen, J., Bals, R., & Dinh, Q. T. (2015). Nanotechnology in respiratory medicine. *Respiratory Research, 16*(1), 64. doi:10.118612931-015-0223-5 PMID:26021823

Panyam, J., & Labhasetwar, V. (2003). Biodegradable nanoparticles for drug and gene delivery to cells and tissue. *Advanced Drug Delivery Reviews, 55*(3), 329–347. doi:10.1016/S0169-409X(02)00228-4 PMID:12628320

Patil, M., Mehta, D. S., & Guvva, S. S. (2008). Future impact of nanotechnology on medicine and dentistry. *Journal of Indian Society of Periodontology, 12*(2), 34. doi:10.4103/0972-124X.44088 PMID:20142942

Patra, J. K., & Baek, K. H. (2014). Green nanobiotechnology: Factors affecting synthesis and characterization techniques. *Journal of Nanomaterials, 2014*, 219. doi:10.1155/2014/417305

Peer, D., Karp, J. M., & Hong, S. (2007). Nanocarriers as an emerging platform for cancer therapy. *Nat Nanotechnol., 2*, 751-60.

Pillai, G., & Coronel, M. L. C. (2013). Science and technology of the emerging nanomedicines in cancer therapy: A primer for physicians and pharmacists. *SAGE Open Medicine, 1*. Advance online publication. doi:10.1177/2050312113513759 PMID:26770691

Piwek, L., Ellis, D. A., Andrews, S., & Joinson, A. (2016). The rise of consumer health wearables: Promises and barriers. *PLoS Medicine, 13*(2), 1001953. doi:10.1371/journal.pmed.1001953 PMID:26836780

Priya, S., & Bernice, S. (2016). Defining Nano, Nanotechnology and Nanomedicine: Why Should It Matter? *Science and Engineering Ethics, 22*(5), 1255–1276. doi:10.100711948-015-9705-6 PMID:26373718

Qamar, S. A., Asgher, M., Khalid, N., & Sadaf, M. (2019). Nanobiotechnology in health sciences: Current applications and future perspectives. *Biocatalysis and Agricultural Biotechnology, 22*, 101388. doi:10.1016/j.bcab.2019.101388

Quan, F. S., Huang, C., Compans, R. W., & Kang, S. M. (2007). Virus-like particle vaccine induces protective immunity against homologous and heterologous strains of influenza virus. *Journal of Virology, 81*(7), 3514–3524. doi:10.1128/JVI.02052-06 PMID:17251294

Rachid, S., Lee, B., David, Q., Brajesh, K., & Luis, C. (2019). Nanoparticles for Environment, Engineering, and Nanomedicine. Hindawi *Journal of Nanotechnology*.

Rashmirekha, P., Maxim, S., & Avinash, S. (2018). Nanoparticle Vaccines against Infectious Diseases. *Frontiers in Immunology*. PMID:30337923

Reibold, M., Paufler, P., Levin, A. A., Kochmann, W., Pätzke, N., & Meyer, D. C. (2006). Materials: Carbon nanotubes in an ancient Damascus sabre. *Nature, 444*(7117), 286. doi:10.1038/444286a PMID:17108950

Riaz, M. (1996). Liposomes preparation methods. *Pakistan Journal of Pharmaceutical Sciences, 19*, 65–77. PMID:16414777

Rimmelzwaan, G. F., Siebelink, K. H., Huisman, R. C., Moss, B., Francis, M. J., & Osterhaus, A. D. (1994). Removal of the cleavage site of recombinant feline immunodeficiency virus envelope protein facilitates incorporation of the surface glycoprotein in immune- stimulating complexes. *The Journal of General Virology, 75*(Pt 8), 2097–2102. doi:10.1099/0022-1317-75-8-2097 PMID:8046415

Rizvi, S. A. A., & Saleh, A. M. (2018). Applications of nanoparticle systems in drug delivery technology. *Saudi Pharmaceutical Journal, 26*(1), 64–70. doi:10.1016/j.jsps.2017.10.012 PMID:29379334

Roldao, A., Mellado, M. C., Castilho, L. R., Carrondo, M. J., & Alves, P. M. (2010). Virus-like particles in vaccine development. *Expert Review of Vaccines, 9*(10), 1149–1176. doi:10.1586/erv.10.115 PMID:20923267

Roy, R., Pal, A., & Chaudhuri, A. N. (2015). Antimicrobial Effect of Silver Nanoparticle on Pathogenic Organisms Isolated from East Kolkata Wetland. *International Journal of Applied Research, 1*, 745–752.

Sahoo, S. K., Panyam, J., Prabha, S., & Labhasetwar, V. (2002). Residual polyvinyl alcohol associated with poly (d,l-lactide-co-glycolide) nanoparticles affects their physical properties and cellular uptake. *Journal of Controlled Release, 82*(1), 105–114. doi:10.1016/S0168-3659(02)00127-X PMID:12106981

Sailaja, G., Skountzou, I., Quan, F. S., Compans, R. W., & Kang, S. M. (2007). Human immunodeficiency virus like particles activate multiple types of immune cells. *Virology, 362*(2), 331–341. doi:10.1016/j.virol.2006.12.014 PMID:17276476

Saji, V. S., Choe, H. C., & Young, K. W. K. (2010). Nanotechnology in biomedical applications—A review. *Int J Nano Biomater, 3*(2), 119–139. doi:10.1504/IJNBM.2010.037801

Salata, O. V. (2004). Applications of nanoparticles in biology and medicine. *Journal of Nanobiotechnology, 2*(1), 3. doi:10.1186/1477-3155-2-3 PMID:15119954

Salouti, Mojtaba, Ahangari, & Azam. (2014). *Nanoparticle based Drug Delivery Systems for Treatment of Infectious Diseases, Application of Nanotechnology in Drug Delivery*. Academic Press.

Samad, A., Sultana, Y., & Aqil, M. (2007). Liposomal drug delivery systems: Anul date review. *Current Drug Delivery, 4*(4), 297–305. doi:10.2174/156720107782151269 PMID:17979650

Santhoshkumar, T., Rahuman, A. A., Rajakumar, G., Marimuthu, S., Bagavan, A., Jayaseelan, C., Zahir, A. A., Elango, G., & Kamaraj, C. (2011). Synthesis of silver nanoparticles using Nelumbo nucifera leaf extract and its larvicidal activity against malaria and filariasis vectors. *Parasitology Research, 108*(3), 693–702. doi:10.100700436-010-2115-4 PMID:20978795

Sarwar, H., Khalid, H., Basher, M. K., Mia, M. N. H., Rahman, M. T., & Jalal Uddin, M. (2019). Smart nanocarrier-based drug delivery systems for cancer therapy and toxicity studies: A review. *Journal of Advanced Research, 15*, 1–18. doi:10.1016/j.jare.2018.06.005 PMID:30581608

Saupe, A., McBurney, W., Rades, T., & Hook, S. (2006). Immunostimulatory colloidal delivery systems for cancer vaccines. *Expert Opinion on Drug Delivery, 3*(3), 345–354. doi:10.1517/17425247.3.3.345 PMID:16640495

Shafiq, S. A., Al-Shammari, R. H., & Majeed, H. Z. (2016). Study of Biosynthesis silver nanoparticles by Fusarium graminaerum and test their antimicrobial activity. *International Journal of Innovation and Applied Studies, 15*, 4.

Shailesh, S., Neelam, S., Sandeep, K., & Gupta, G. D. (2009). Liposomes: A review. *Journal of Pharmacy Research, 2*, 1163–1167.

Shellhart, W. C., & Oesterle, L. J. (1999). Uprighting molars without extrusion. *The Journal of the American Dental Association, 130*(3), 381–385. doi:10.14219/jada.archive.1999.0208 PMID:10085661

Slavkin, H. C. (1999). Entering the era of molecular dentistry. *The Journal of the American Dental Association, 130*(3), 413–417. doi:10.14219/jada.archive.1999.0212 PMID:10085665

Slupetzky, K., Gambhira, R., Culp, T. D., Shafti Keramat, S., Schellenbacher, C., Christensen, N. D., Roden, R. B. S., & Kirnbauer, R. (2007). A papilloma virus like particle (VLP) vaccine displaying HPV 16 L2 epitopes induces cross neutralizing antibodies to HPV 11. *Vaccine, 25*(11), 2001–2010. doi:10.1016/j.vaccine.2006.11.049 PMID:17239496

Sonaje, K., Chuang, E.-Y., Lin, K.-J., Yen, T.-C., Su, F.-Y., Tseng, M. T., & Sung, H.-W. (2012). Opening of epithelial tight junctions and enhancement of paracellular permeation by chitosan: Microscopic, ultrastructural, and computed-tomographic observations. *Molecular Pharmaceutics, 9*(5), 1271–1279. doi:10.1021/mp200572t PMID:22462641

Sutradhar, K. B., & Amin, M. L. (2014). Nanotechnology in cancer drug delivery and selective targeting. *ISRN Nanotechnology*. doi. doi:Org /10.1155 / 2014 / 939378

Takamura, S., Niikura, M., Li, T. C., Takeda, N., Kusagawa, S., Takebe, Y., Miyamura, T., & Yasutomi, Y. (2004). DNA vaccine encapsulated virus like particles derived from an orally transmissible virus stimulate mucosal and systemic immune responses by oral administration. *Gene Therapy, 11*(7), 628–635. doi:10.1038j.gt.3302193 PMID:14973544

Theron, J., Walker, J.A., & Cloete, T.E. (2008). Nanotechnology and water treatment: applications and emerging opportunities. *Critical Reviews in Microbiology, 34*(1), 43-69.

Torchilin, V. P. (2006). Multifunctional nanocarriers. *Adv Drug Deliv Rev., 58*, 1532-55.

Tosi, G., Constantino, L., Ruozi, B., Forni, F., & Vandelli, M.A. (2008). Polymeric nanoparticles for drug delivery to central nervous system. *Exp Opin Drug Deliv., 5*(2), 155-74.

Ure, D., & Harris, J. (2003). Nanotechnology in dentistry: Reduction to practice. *Dental Update, 30*(1), 10–15. doi:10.12968/denu.2003.30.1.10 PMID:12619307

Vasir, J. K., & Labhasetwar, V. (2005). Targeted drug delivery in cancer therapy. *Technology in Cancer Research & Treatment, 4*(4), 363–374. doi:10.1177/153303460500400405 PMID:16029056

Vasir, J. K., Reddy, M. K., & Labhasetwar, V. (2005). Nanosystems in drug targeting: Opportunities and challenges. *Current Nanoscience, 1*(1), 47–64. doi:10.2174/1573413052953110

Verma, M. L., Kumar, P., Sharma, D., Verma, A. D., & Jana, A. K. (2019). Advances in Nanobiotechnology with Special Reference to Plant Systems. In *Plant Nanobionics* (pp. 371–387). Springer. doi:10.1007/978-3-030-12496-0_13

Villa, L. L., Costa, R. L. R., Petta, C. A., Andrade, R. P., Ault, K. A., Giuliano, A. R., Wheeler, C. M., Koutsky, L. A., Malm, C., Lehtinen, M., Skjeldestad, F. E., Olsson, S.-E., Steinwall, M., Brown, D. R., Kurman, R. J., Ronnett, B. M., Stoler, M. H., Ferenczy, A., Harper, D. M., ... Barr, E. (2005). Prophylactic quadrivalent human papilloma virus (types6,11,16, and 18) L1virus-like particle vaccine in young women: A randomised double blind placebo controlled multicenter phase II efficacy trial. *The Lancet. Oncology*, *6*(5), 271–278. doi:10.1016/S1470-2045(05)70101-7 PMID:15863374

Vimbela, G. V., Ngo, S. M., Fraze, C., Yang, L., & Stout, D. A. (2017). Antibacterial properties and toxicity from metallic nanomaterials. *International Journal of Nanomedicine*, *12*, 3941–3965. doi:10.2147/IJN.S134526 PMID:28579779

Wang, R., & Xue, X. (2018). Theranostical application of nanomedicine for treating central nervous system disorders. *Science China. Life Sciences*, *61*(4), 392–399. doi:10.100711427-017-9292-7 PMID:29675554

Wang, T., Zou, M., Jiang, H., Ji, Z., Gao, P., & Cheng, G. (2011). Synthesis of a novel kind of carbon nanoparticle with large mesopores and macropores and its application as an oral vaccine adjuvant. *European Journal of Pharmaceutical Sciences*, *44*(5), 653–659. doi:10.1016/j.ejps.2011.10.012 PMID:22064451

Waterhouse, D. N., Madden, T. D., Cullis, P. R., Bally, M. B., Mayer, L. D., & Webb, M. S. (2005). Preparation, characterization, and biological analysis of liposomal for mulations of vincristine. *Methods in Enzymology*, *391*, 40–57. doi:10.1016/S0076-6879(05)91002-1 PMID:15721373

West, J. L., & Halas, N. J. (2000). Applications of nanotechnology to biotechnology commentary. *Current Opinion in Biotechnology*, *11*(2), 215–217. doi:10.1016/S0958-1669(00)00082-3 PMID:10753774

Wickline, S. A., Neubauer, A. M., Winter, P., Caruthers, S., & Lanza, G. (2006). Applications ofnanotechnology to atherosclerosis, thrombosis, and vascular biology. *Arteriosclerosis, Thrombosis, and Vascular Biology*, *26*(3), 435–441. doi:10.1161/01.ATV.0000201069.47550.8b PMID:16373609

Wilkinson, J. M. (2003). Nanotechnology applications in medicine. *Med Device Technol., 14*, 29-31.

Ying-Yu, M., Ke-Tao, J., Shi-Bing, W., Hui-Ju, W., Xiang-Min, T., & Dong-Sheng, H. (2017). *Molecular Imaging of Cancer with Nanoparticle-Based Theranostic Probes*. Hindawi Contrast Media & Molecular Imaging Volume.

Yotsuyanagi, T., & Hazemoto, N. (1998). Cationic liposomes in gene delivery. *Japanese Journal of Clinical Medicine*, *56*, 705–712. PMID:9549361

Young, L. S., Searle, P. F., Onion, D., & Mautner, V. (2006). Viral gene therapy strategies:from basic science to clinical application. *The Journal of Pathology*, *208*(2), 299–318. doi:10.1002/path.1896 PMID:16362990

Zeltins, A. (2012). Construction and characterization of viruslike particles: A review. *Molecular Biotechnology*, *53*(1), 92–107. doi:10.100712033-012-9598-4 PMID:23001867

Zhang, Y., Schlachetzki, F., Li, J. Y., Boado, R. J., & Pardridge, W. M. (2003). Organ specific gene expression in the rhesus monkey eye following intravenous nonviral gene transfer. *Molecular Vision*, *9*, 465–472. PMID:14551536

Zhao, W., Wu, W., & Xu, X. (2007). Oral vaccination with liposome- encapsulated recombinant fusion peptide of urease B epitope and cholera toxin B subunit affords prophylactic and therapeutic effects against H.pylori infection in BALB/cm ice. *Vaccine*, *25*(44), 7664–7673. doi:10.1016/j.vaccine.2007.08.034 PMID:17913305

Zhu, J., Yan, F., Guo, Z., & Marchant, R. E. (2005). Surface modification of liposomes by saccharides: Vesicles and stability of lactosyl liposomes studied by photon correlation spectroscopy. *Journal of Colloid and Interface Science*, *289*(2), 542–550. doi:10.1016/j.jcis.2005.03.088 PMID:15922349

Zuhong, L., Yangjun, C., Ya, Y., Yan, Y., & Yanhong, Z. (2019). Recent Advances in Nanomaterials-Based Chemo-Photothermal Combination Therapy for Improving Cancer Treatment. Review article. *Frontiers in Bioengineering and Biotechnology*.

Chapter 14
Applications of Nano Materials in Cold Storage:
Usage of Nano Particles in Cold Storage

Kapilan N.
Nagarjuna College of Engineering and Technology, India

Vidhya P.
SRSMN Government First Grade College, India

ABSTRACT

Nano particles (NPs) have superior properties and hence can be used for various applications. The cold storage is most widely used in the preservation of agricultural and horticultural products. The cold storage maybe operated by vapour compression or vapour absorption cooling system. The operating cost of this system can be reduced by using renewable energy systems and thermal energy storage systems. The NPs are used to increase the performance of renewable energy and thermal storage systems. In recent years, phase change materials are used to increase heat transfer rate in solar cold storage units. The NPs can be used to absorb the ethylene gas produced during storage of fruits, so that the shelf life, freshness, firmness, and texture of the fruits can be maintained for longer storage duration. The NPs coatings also increases the shelf life and freshness of the fruits. This chapter discusses NPs, types of NPs, basics of cold storage systems, use of NPs in solar integrated cold storage, and effect of NPs coatings on fruits stored in cold storage.

INTRODUCTION

The function of the cold storage system is similar to the domestic refrigerator. However it is large in size and used for refrigerating large quantity of agricultural products such as fruits, vegetables, perishable items etc. The required condition in the cold storage is maintained by controlling temperature, humidity and other process variables. The most important functions of the cold storage unit are to increase the shelf life, product quality and taste of stored items and also to reduce deterioration of the perishable products.

DOI: 10.4018/978-1-7998-5563-7.ch014

The increase in ambient temperature due to climate change will increase food and agricultural spoilage. Hence the demand of the cold storage systems increase which may result in increase in CO_2 emission as power is required to drive this system. Hence it is necessary to use energy efficient technologies and utilize renewable energy resources for the reduction in energy consumption of the cold storage unit and indirectly to reduce CO_2 emission (James & James, 2010). In recent years, automatic control systems are used in cold storage systems to reduce energy consumption and also to enhance refrigeration quality (Ma & Mao, 2018).

BACKGROUND

The fruits and vegetables are sensitive to the temperature and cannot be stored in ambient condition for longer time. The higher ambient temperature increases deterioration of fruits and vegetables. This problem can be overcome by the introduction of cold storage which is maintained at lower temperature and increases the shelf life of the stored items. However, very low temperature may affect the quality of the fruits and vegetables and storage. In cold storage, low temperature is maintained with the help of cold storage equipment and precision instruments. The cold storage helps to stabilize the market prices of fruits and vegetables. The performance of the cold storage system can be increased with the use of latest technologies such as using phase change materials and nanoparticles. This book chapter discusses the basic parts of cold storage system, energy efficiency, nano particles, types of nano particles, phase change materials, solar cold storage and nano particle coatings. This book chapter will be useful to the researchers, farmers, students and different stake holders of agricultural community.

PARTS OF COLD STORAGE SYSTEM

The major parts of cold storage systems are components of vapour compression refrigeration (VCR) or vapour absorption refrigeration (VAR) systems. In VCR based system, the major components used are compressor, condenser, evaporator, wind curtain and door. The compressor supplies the driving force to the cold storage system and may be called as heart of cold storage. It increases the pressure of the refrigerant and ensures its circulation in the system. It consumes lot of energy and energy efficient compressors are used. The compressor compresses the refrigerant vapour and the compressed refrigerant vapour is condensed into liquid refrigerant using condenser. Air or water is used as the cooling medium in the condenser. The water cooled condenser is compact as compared to air cooled condenser. The liquid refrigerant is allowed to expand in the expansion device and after expansion the pressure and temperature reduces. The low temperature refrigerant flows in the evaporator or ceiling unit and absorbs the heat from the cold storage and produces the cooling effect. The anti-moisture fan provided in the cold storage circulates room air into the evaporator coils. The wind curtain is located at the top of the door and blows the air such that cold air loss is minimized. The cold storage unit door is made of low thermal conductivity materials to reduce heat loss. In VAR based system is similar to VCR system and it uses generator, pump and absorber unit instead of compressor. A typical cold storage unit is shown in Figure 1.

Figure 1. Typical Cold Storage Unit

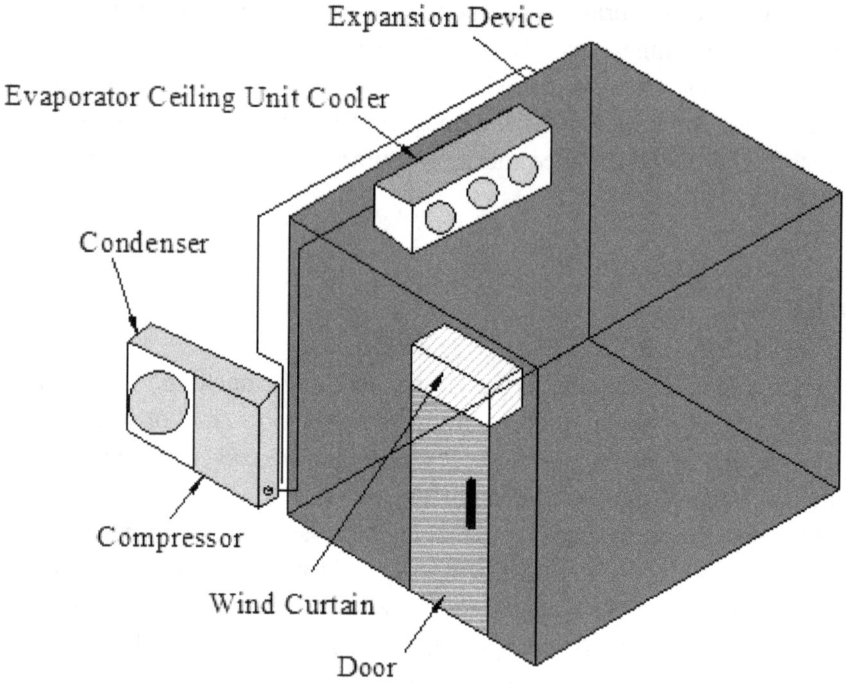

ENERGY EFFICIENCY

The use of energy efficient components and good quality insulation materials can reduce the operating cost of the cold storage units. The effective insulation reduces the heat loss and maintaining required cooling temperature in the cold storage reduces energy wastage. The temperature distribution, thermal storage system, charging and discharging rate plays a key role in optimizing the performance of the cold storage (Wang et al., 2019). It is suggested that the variety of cooling load is linear dependent on the variety of room temperature (Tian et al., 2019). It is reported that the current energy utilization with storage tank can be reduced by 72% as compared to the direct cooling mode. The initial cost of cold storage system with the partial storage of is lower than a non-storage cold storage system. The partial cold water storage system consumes less energy (Shaibani et al., 2019).

It is suggested that the best performance can be achieved with recirculated water as compared to stagnant water and stirred water when cold storage system used flooded tube (Sait, 2018).The capacity and performance of the cold storage system is reduced due to the deposition of frost on the surface of the evaporator. Hence periodic defrosting is carriedout to improve the performance. The defrosting can be achieved by electric heater and reversed cycle method. These methods reduce temperature fluctuations and increases energy utilization. Hence this new defrosting system increases operational stability of the compressor (Wang et al., 2017).

NANO PARTICLES

The size of the nano-particles is generally between 1 nm to 100 nm and properties of the NPs may or may not vary with their size. The NPs are produced in different shapes and sizes based on their applications (Cho et al., 2013). The NPs may be in spherical, flat, tubular, cylindrical, conical, hollow core and spiral shapes and few NPs are crystalline or amorphous (Machado et al., 2015). The distinctive properties of the NPs are high surface area to volume ratio, surface charge, pore size, crystalline and amorphous structures and sensitivity to heat, sunlight, air and moisture. In recent years, NPs are most widely used in various applications and research work in this area is significant. This is due to their excellent physical and chemical properties. The important properties which are enhanced by the NPs are thermal conductivity, electrical properties, wettability, light absorption, anti oxidant, anti microbial, anti fungal etc. The important physical properties of the NPs include conductivity, resistivity, hydrophilicity, suspension, diffusion, settling, elastic, ductile, tensile strengths and flexibility. The NPs are selected for particular applications based on the above said properties. Figure 2 shows the image of the NPs taken using scanning electron microscope.

Figure 2. Image of the NPs taken using scanning electron microscope.

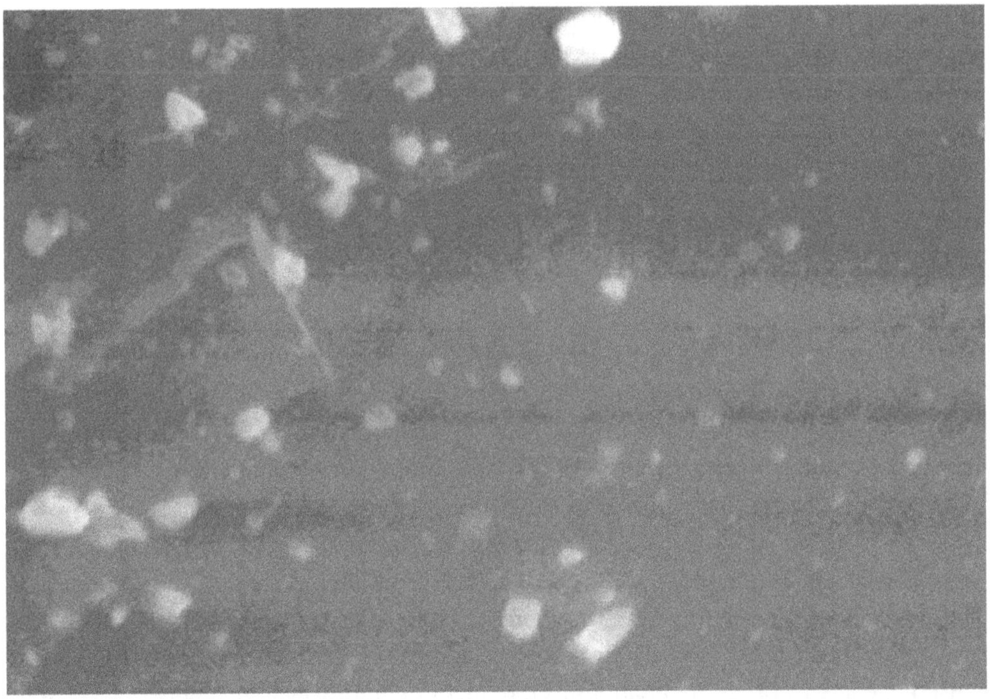

The NPs particles may be classified into four major types (Jeevanandam et al., 2018) and discussed below.

- **Organic based NPs**: This type of NPs is produced from organic materials. The required structures of this type of NPs may be obtained by utilization of non covalent interactions for the self-assembly. The required structures which can be obtained are liposomes, dendrimers, polymer NPs and micelles.

- **Inorganic based NPs**: This type of NPs is produced from inorganic materials. This includes metal and metal oxide NPs. The fanousinorganic based NPs are Ag, Au and metal oxides such as TiO_2 and ZnO NPs.
- **Carbon based NPs:** This type of NPs contain carbon and produced in different morphologies such as spheres, hollow tubes or ellipsoids. The carbon block, carbon nanotubes, graphene, carbon nanofibers and carbon onions are also included in this type. The carbon-based NPs are generally produced by chemical vapor deposition, arc discharge and laser ablation.
- **Composite based NPs**: The multiphase NPs with one phase on the nano-scale dimension that can either combine NPs with other NPs or highly complicated structures, such as a metal-organic frameworks. It is combinations of metal based or carbon based or organic-based nano-material with any form of metal or polymer or ceramic materials to get desired properties and also for the required application.

The metal-based NPs are produced from metals by either destructive or constructive methods. The NPs are produced from metals such as silver (Ag), copper (Cu), gold (Au), aluminium (Al), iron (Fe), lead (Pb), and zinc (Zn) (Salavati-niasari et al., 2008). The metal oxide based NPs are produced to modify the properties such as reactivity, efficiency etc (Tai et al., 2007). The famous NP metal oxides are Titanium oxide (TiO_2), Silicon dioxide (SiO_2), Aluminium oxide (Al_2O_3), Cerium oxide (CeO_2), Iron oxide (Fe_2O_3) and Zinc oxide (ZnO). The NPs can be produced from carbon and available in different forms such as carbon block, carbon nano-tubes (CNT), carbon nano-fibers and grapheme (Bhaviripudi et al., 2007). Table 1 shows the important properties of the NPs.

PHASE CHANGE MATERIALS

The Phase change materials (PCMs) are materials which are used store/release a large amount of energy through forming and breaking molecular bonds. The PCMs are classified into organic and inorganic PCMs. The Inorganic PCMs have large latent heat and hence this type of PCMs can be used in high temperature energy storage. Both types of PCMs have low thermal conductivity (Zalba et al., 2003). Figure 3 shows the stages of phase change of PCM from solid state to gaseous state.

The NPs can be dispersed in the PCM to increase the thermal conductivity. The PCM has higher thermal storage capacity and hence it can be used in the cold storage during power failure, frequent door openings and to maintain the temperature in the cold storage with in safe limits (Wei et al., 2019).In cold storage applications, PCM is used to increase the conventional insulation performance. The PCM is generally used in energy storage applications as it reduces operating cost during peak load demand. The use of PCM in agricultural distribution system improves the quality of agricultural products. Also lower phase transition temperature maintains the quality of agricultural products as it maintains the freshness of the agricultural products (Bai et al., 2019).

Table 1. Important properties of the NPs

Name of the NPs	Properties	Reference
Iron oxide	Higher reactivity and super paramagnetic properties	14
Titanuim oxide	large specific surface area, enhanced adsorption, higher surface area, magnetic property and photo catalytic characteristic	15
Zinc oxide	Strong UV absorption, anti corrosive, superior antibacterial, antimicrobial, and excellent UV-blocking properties	16
Cerium oxide	Antioxidant and antimicrobial activities	17, 18
Aluminum oxide	High hardness, insulation, reactivity, larger surface area, sensitivity to heat, moisture and sunlight	19, 20
Carbon block	Higher surface area, electrical conductivity and higher strength	21
Carbon nano tubes	Higher thermal conductivity, tensile strength, elastic structural, thermal, electrical characteristics, bio-sensing and high surface-to-volume ratio	22,23
Graphene	Higher thermal, electrical conductivity and light absorption, antibacterial properties and tissue regenerative capacities	24, 25
Carbon nano fiber	Higher mechanical, electrical, and thermal properties	26
Silver NPs	Higher thermal and electrical conductivity, chemical stability, antibacterial, antioxidants, nonlinear optical behavior and catalytic activity	27, 28

Figure 3. Phase change of PCM from solid to gaseous state

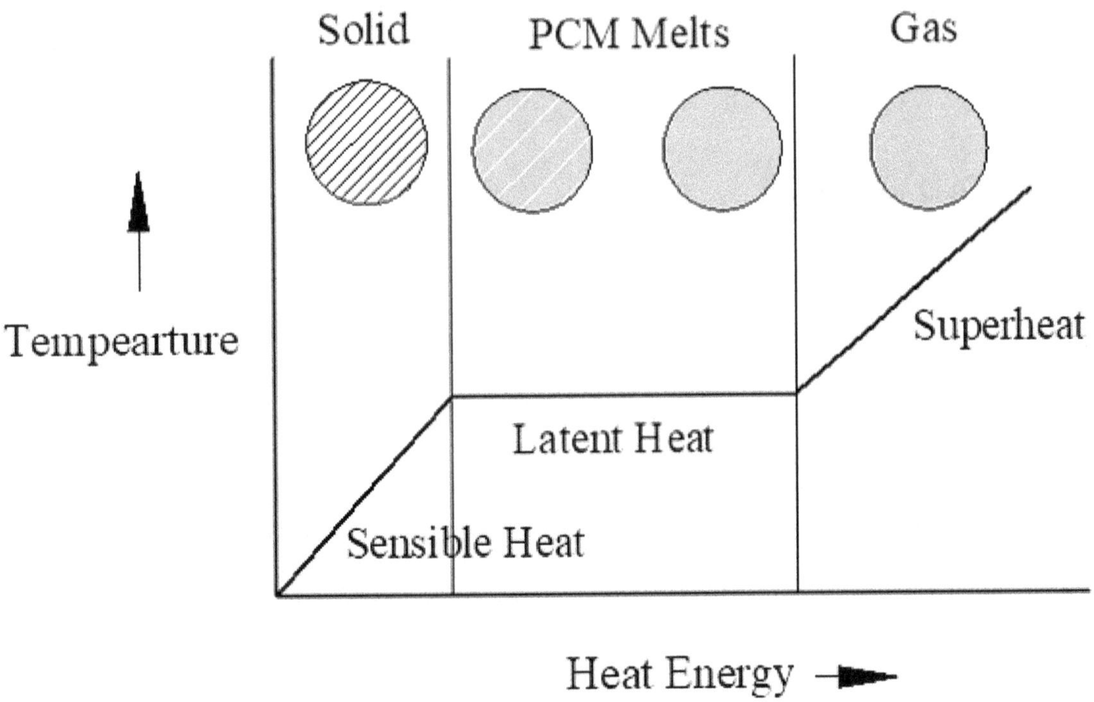

The main disadvantage of the PCMs is leakage issue and this problem can be solved by using microencapsulated PCMs. The PCM microcapsules consist of core and polymer which act as shell. This type of PCMs has higher surface per volume and can provides effective heat transfer performance. The NPs are added to the PCM to enhance heat transfer rate and efficient storage process (Li et al., 2013). The composite building material prepared by mixing composite PCM (CPCM) and the cement results in good stability, higher heat storage, higher thermal conductivity and better compression resistance (Zhang et al., 2017). The paraffin can be utilized as the PCM in summer to cool air and to store cold during daytime and nighttime respectively. The cold storage system works efficiently due to larger difference in temperature between inlet and outlet and higher cold power (Stritih & Butala, 2007). The addition of Ag NPs to PCM improves thermal conductivity and it is reported that the increase in dosage of Ag NPs increases the thermal conductivity (Zeng et al., 2007). It is also reported that the NPs embedded PCM results in higher heat extraction rate during the solidification. This is due to lower latent heat and higher thermal conductivity (Khodadadi & Hosseinizadeh, 2007).

The use of PCM in falling film type of cold energy regenerator increases heat transfer rate and enhances cold storage characteristics and reduces pumping power (Cheng & Zhai, 2018). The enhancement in PCM melting time maintains the product stored in cold storage for a longer period (Jiang et al., 2018). The solar cold storage unit which uses PCM and integrated with ejector provides a stable COP (Kozak et al., 2017). The metal foam is a solid metal, containing a large volume fraction of pores and can be used as thermal energy storage due to strong mixing capability, higher porosity and high surface-area to volume ratio (Chen, Yang, Jiang et al, 2014).

The Al_2O_3 NPs was added to paraffin PCM using surfactant which is non-ionic. The 5 and 10 wt.% of Al_2O_3 NPs were added to prepare paraffin emulsion. The density value predicted based on mixture theory agrees with theoretical values. The measured dynamic viscosity and thermal conductivity of this emulsion show a nonlinear increase with the mass fraction of the NPs as compared to paraffin (Ho & Gao, 2009).

SOLAR COLD STORAGE

The solar cold storage system is shown in the Figure 4. The solar thermal energy system is integrated with the cold storage. The vapour absorption system is used as it is a heat driven system. The solar collector absorbs the heat energy and additional heater is provided so that the required water temperature is achieved. Different types of NPs are used in solar collector to increase the heat absorption capacity. A return on investment of hybrid cold storage system which uses both solar thermal energy and solar PV system is less than four years (Chen, Worall, Omer et al, 2014). The solar cold storage unit uses PCM to manage the peak power demand or there is reduction in sun shines. The use of fins in PCM based thermal energy storage unit enhances solidification, improves capacity of thermal energy storage and provides higher heat flux during melting(Basu & Ganguly, 2016).The application of microcapsule PCM in solar powered cold storage system improves efficiency of the system and reduces the electrical energy consumption. The PCM has higher heat transfer rate as compared to water (Talukdar et al., 2019).

Figure 4. Solar powered Cold Storage System

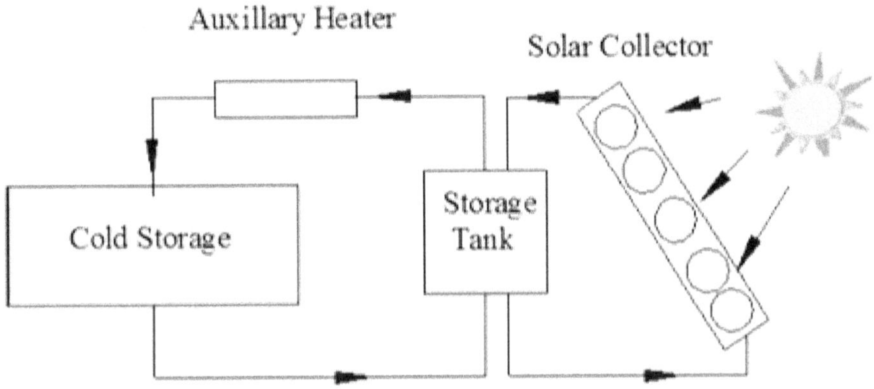

The solar powered cooling system integrated with PCM cold storage gives the maximum COP and solar thermal ratio was 0.193 and 0.097 respectively (Zheng et al., 2017). The thermal conductivities of metallic NPs made from metals like of copper, silver and iron and non-metallic materials like SiC, CuO, alumina and carbon nano-tubes are better than the liquids. These NPs can be used in solar absorption refrigeration system to increase heat transfer rate. AgO nano-fluid used in the system gives good improvement in performance due to better heat transfer rate. Hence the nano- fluids improve the performance of solar thermal system by improving the performance of the heat extraction mechanisms and can play a crucial role in the development of new technologies (Ahmed et al., 2019).

In Italy, water–lithium bromide vapour ARS was integrated with thermal solar flat-plate collectors to reduce the conventional energy required and an external heater increase the water temperature. In this system, Al_2O_3 based nano-fluid (3 vol %) was used to increase the heat transfer and it is reported that the nano-fluid increases the heating energy saving by 36%. It is suggested that the nano-fluids can be used in closed loop system to improve the renewable energy systems' efficiency (Colangelo et al., 2019). It is reported that triple effect absorption refrigeration cycle needs high temperature heat reservoir and other systems can be operated on lower temperatures than triple effect cycle (Ratlamwala & Abid, 2018).

A study was carried out to understand the impact of adding NPs such as multiwall carbon nano-tubes and carbon black on the thermal conductivity, viscosity, steam absorption, optical properties and photo-thermal conversion of aqueous lithium bromide solutions. It is reported that a low NPs concentration increased the photo-thermal conversion of the samples. It is suggested that the adding low cost commercial carbon black NPs in aqueous lithium bromide improves the performance of solar absorption system (Zeiny et al., 2019). The NPs of Al_2O_3, Ag, Cu, and CuO with different concentrations were used for the preparation of nano-fluids and used in the solar energy operated double-effect aqueous lithium bromide ARS. The results show Ag NPs gives superior performance as compared to other types. It is also reported that the COP of the system increases by 3.9% by the addition of Ag NPs with the concentration of 2.5% (Aramesh et al., 2019).

The use of binary nano-fluid in aqueous lithium bromide ARS increases the light trapping efficiency. Also the surface localized heat generation increases the evaporation rate. The addition of iron oxide NPs to the pure water increases the solar radiative energy and it is suggested that the iron oxide NPs [REMOVED HYPERLINK FIELD]can be used for the solar ARS (Nourafkan et al., 2019).

Figure 5. Coating of NPs on fruit

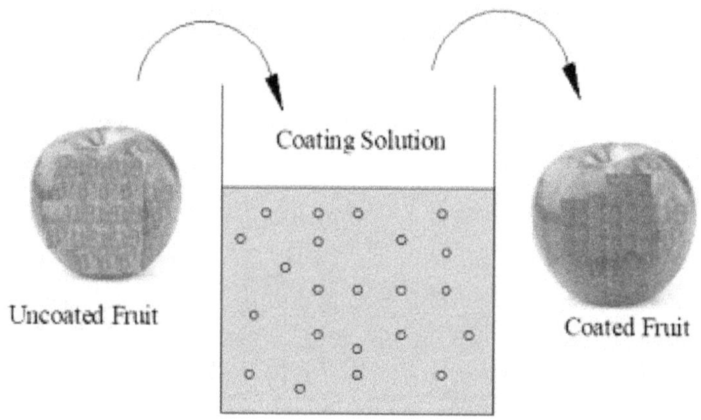

The solar absorption system can be integrated with heat pump system to enhance the performance of solar energy system. This system can be integrated with PCM heat storage to get good cooling effect and also to get higher output-input ratio depends upon various climate conditions. The PCM's phase transition temperature influences the performance of heat storage system (Wang et al., 2012). The PCM can be utilized in solar-driven ejector based cold storage system (Allouche et al., 2017).

EFFECT OF NPS COATING

The quality of the food items stored in cold storage is affected by psychrotrophic microorganisms (Wei et al., 2019). The quality of probiotic products is affected by the probiotic bacteria during longer storage period (Song et al., 2019). The campylobacter jejuni level can be reduced with the help of irradiation in chicken livers and cold storage(Gunther et al., 2019).The value of peroxide, total oxidation and thiobarbituric acid level of mussels' meat increases during cold storage (Zhou et al., 2019). The ozone treatment reduces postharvest disease in different fruits (Lv et al., 2019).The utilization of both low temperature and rice acidification reduces the growth of pathogenic aeromonas species (Hoel et al., 2018). The effect of cold storage on protein properties of stored food items can be reduced with the help of ultrasound (Chen et al., 2019). During cold storage, the galacturonic acid value changes (Fishman et al., 2019). During cold storage, firmness of fruit treated with atmosphere packaging is higher than the aminoethoxy vinyl glycine (Zheng et al., 2019). The genus pseudomonas affects the food products (Ozturk et al., 2019). The MicroRNAs reduces the pear' aroma when it is stored in cold storage (Zhang et al., 2019).The campylobacter jejuniis inactivated during cold storage due to heat stress (Shi et al., 2018).

The properties and qualities of the fruits, vegetable and other perishable items stored in the cold storage may change during storage. Hence NPs may be used to overcome these issues. The shelf life of loquat fruit can be increased by coating of chitosannanosilica. However, it affects the external and internal quality (Sun et al., 2019). During cold storage the growth of yeast and mold on pomegranate arils can be reduced by applying coating of combination of nano-ZnO and carboxymethyl cellulose. This coating reduces weight and soluble solids content during cold storage. It is also reported that total anthocyanin, vitamin C and antioxidant content was higher with the coated arils (Song et al., 2016). Figure 5 shows the process of NPs coating on the fruit. Figure 6 shows the NPs coated apple.

Figure 6. NPs Coated Apple

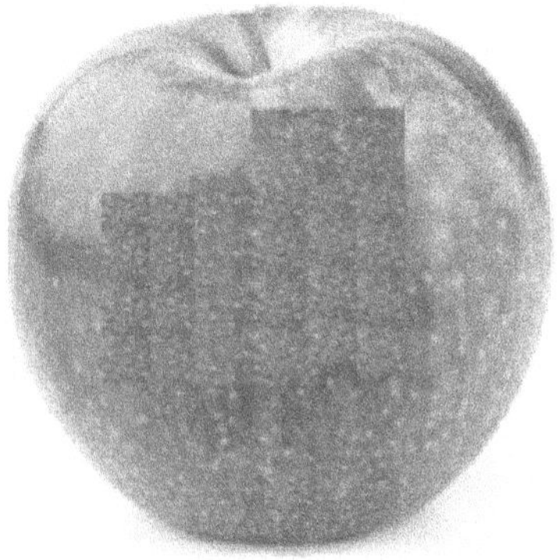

The ethylene produced by the fruits during storage increases the respiration rate and lowers shelf-life of fruits stored in cold storage. The increase in respiration of the fruits results in texture and appearance. Hence ethylene absorbents are used in cold storage to overcome these problems and also to maintain firmness and to reduce weight loss. This increases the storage period of the fruits. The use of zeolite NPs coated with potassium permanganate in the cold storage unit reduces weight loss, increases the shelf life and enhances freshness of stored nectarine and peach (Emadpour et al., 2015). The small sachets containing potassium permanganate coated zeolite NPs can be placed inside fruit boxes to remove ethylene and to increase the shelf life of the Cabbage and Iceberg Lettuce (Rezaii Kalaj et al., 2009). The TiO_2 NPs increases photo-catalytic degradation of ethylene and hence it can be used cold storage units to increase shelf life of fruits (Hussain et al., 2011). The shelf life of fruits can be increased when the fruits are treated with silver NPs as compared to chemical or other types of treatment (Ijaz et al., 2020). The guargum based coatings containing Ag NPs increases anti oxidant activity with reduction in bacteria, mold and yeast levels. Hence improvement in shelf life of the fruits was observed when the fruits were stored at 4°C in cold storage (Shah et al., 2015). The shelf life and quality of strawberry can be increased with the use of nano-silver or nano-silicate based polyethylene and polypropylene packing materials as compared to conventional packaging materials (Zandi et al., 2013). Silver NPs treated tomato fruits has highest firmness as compared untreated samples during forty days of storage in cold storage and this due to the characteristics of the silver NPs (Salem et al., 2019). The coating of silver and ZnO NPs on the packaging materials increases shelf life of orange juice due to reduction in microbial growth. These NPs enhances the shelf life of fresh orange juice for 28 days (Emamifar et al., 2011).

The addition of 4% concentration of nano-ZnO to polybutylene succinate packaging material improve shelf life of fresh-cut apples during cold storage (Naknaen, 2014). The chitosan can be used as a food preservative due to its non-toxicity, biodegradability, versatility and biocompatibility. The chitosan polycationic structure interacts with negatively charged bacterial cell envelope and reduces the microbial activities (Hu & Gänzle, 2019). The coating of nano-chitosan emulsion on fresh apple reduces ethylene production, respiration rate, peroxide activity and weight loss during storage period as compared to uncoated apples. These trails show the potential advantages of using nano-chitosan coatings (Sahraei

Khosh Gardesh et al., 2016). It is reported that the chitosan is bio fungicide to control anthracnose of fresh fruits can be used as nano-emulsions instead of conventional form as it is cost effective and also reduces the amount of chemical used (Zahid et al., 2012). The coating of chitosan on bananas inhibits conversion of starch to sugar as the coating act as a barrier (Maqbool et al., 2011). The quality of Fuji apple fruit can be increased with nano-SiOx/chitosan added packing materials and hence the storage period may be increased and are longer (Li et al., 2009).

The Chitosan NPs coated on full mature peach fruits with the concentrations of 0.2, 0.4 and 0.8%. The fruit weight loss, decay etc increases during the cold storage. However chitosan NPs with 0.4% concentration results in best qualities of peach fruits as compared to other concentrations (Gad et al., 2016). It is reported that the chitosan may be used as edible coating to increase shelf life of strawberry fruits (Vargas et al., 2006). It is reported that spraying Florida Prince Peach with Chitosan and Calcium Chloride increases shelf life and firmness of this fruit during cold storage period. Also, lowest fruit titratable acidity percentage was observed (El-Badawy, 2012). The combined use of nano-chitosan and copper improves the shelf life and freshness of the strawberry fruit (Eshghi et al., 2014). The chitosan has good film-forming capacity and increases shelf life of fresh foods (Fan et al., 2009). It is reported that chitosan coating was safe and effective method for increasing shelf life of strawberry fruits in cold storage (Vargas et al., 2006).

FUTURE RESEARCH DIRECTIONS

From the literature survey, we found that the research work can be continued in the following areas

1. The renewable energy sources can be integrated with cold storage system to reduce the operating cost.
2. The low-cost renewable energy system can be developed, to reduce the initial cost of the cold storage system.
3. The studies on the effect of nano particle coating on the environment is not explored and hence research work can be carried out in this area.
4. The nanoparticles can enter into the food chain and can affect the human being. The research work in this area is limited and there is a good scope for the research work
5. The low-cost nano particles which is suitable for various types of fruits can be developed
6. The environmentally friendly nanoparticles can be developed and can be used in cold storage system.

CONCLUSION

Most of the countries are facing food crops wastage due to poor cold storage facilities. The cold storage can preserve the vegetables, fruits, etc for longer duration and the stored items can be used in off season. Hence cold storage is getting popularity and used in various applications and installed based on the need at different locations. The energy efficient solar powered cold storage units are developed to reduce the operating cost. Different types of cold storage systems with various capacities are available commercially and selection is depends upon the applications. The cold storage temperature and storage duration affects the quality of the food stored in the cold storage. Different techniques were used to increase the shelf life of the stored items. The use of PCM with NPs increase the performance of solar powered cold storage units. The NPs coatings are used to enhance the shelf life of the fruits. The selection of NPs is based on the type of fruits, demand and cost. From this work we conclude that the NPs can be utilized n agriculture sector to improve the shelf life of agricultural products and fruits and to minimize environmental pollution by reducing the use of conventional chemical used in cold storage. However, a life cycle analysis can be carried out before recommending any type of NPs in agriculture activities and cold storage.

REFERENCES

Ahmed, A., Baig, H., Sundaram, S., & Mallick, T. K. (2019). Use of Nanofluids in Solar PV/Thermal Systems. *International Journal of Photoenergy. Article ID, 8039129*, 1–17.

Allouche, Y., Varga, S., Bouden, C., & Oliveira, A. C. (2017). Dynamic simulation of an integrated solar-driven ejector based air conditioning system with PCM cold storage. *Applied Energy*, *190*, 600–611. doi:10.1016/j.apenergy.2017.01.001

Aramesh, M., Pourfayaz, F., Haghir, M., Kasaeian, A., & Ahmadi, M. H. (2019). Investigating the effect of using nanofluids on the performance of a double-effect absorption refrigeration cycle combined with a solar collector. *Proceedings of the Institution of Mechanical Engineers, Part A: Journal of Power and Energy*. 10.1177/0957650919889811

Bai, B., Zhao, K., & Li, X. (2019). Application research of nano-storage materials in cold chain logistics of e-commerce fresh agricultural products. *Results in Physics*, *13*, 102049. doi:10.1016/j.rinp.2019.01.083

Basu, D. N., & Ganguly, A. (2016). Solar thermal–photovoltaic powered potato cold storage – Conceptual design and performance analyses. *Applied Energy*, *165*, 308–317. doi:10.1016/j.apenergy.2015.12.070

Bhaviripudi, S., Mile, E., Iii, S A S., Zare, A. T., Dresselhaus, M. S., Belcher, A. M., & Kong, J. (2007). CVD Synthesis of Single-Walled Carbon Nanotubes from Gold Nanoparticle. *Catalysts*, *129*(6), 1516–1517. PMID:17283991

Chen, J., Yang, D., Jiang, J., Ma, A., & Song, D. (2014). Research Progress of Phase Change Materials (PCMs) Embedded with Metal Foam (a Review). *Procedia Materials Science*, *4*, 389–394. doi:10.1016/j.mspro.2014.07.579

Chen, X., Worall, M., Omer, S., Su, Y., & Riffat, S. (2014). Experimental investigation on PCM cold storage integrated with ejector cooling system. *Applied Thermal Engineering*, *63*(1), 419–427. doi:10.1016/j.applthermaleng.2013.11.029

Chen, Y., Sheng, L., Gouda, M., & Ma, M. (2019). Impact of ultrasound treatment on the foaming and physicochemical properties of egg white during cold storage. *Lebensmittel-Wissenschaft + Technologie*, *13*, 108303. doi:10.1016/j.lwt.2019.108303

Cheng, X., & Zhai, X. (2018). Thermal performance analysis of a cascaded cold storage unit using multiple PCMs. *Energy*, *143*, 448–457. doi:10.1016/j.energy.2017.11.009

Cho, E. J., Holback, H., Liu, K. C., Abouelmagd, S. A., Park, J., & Yeo, Y. (2013). Nanoparticle characterization : State of the art, challenges and emerging technologies. *Molecular Pharmaceutics, 10*(6), 2093–2110. doi:10.1021/mp300697h PMID:23461379

Colangelo, G., Milanese, M., & Risi, A. D. (2019). Energy simulation of a nanofluid solar cooling system in Italy. *Proceedings of the Institution of Civil Engineers. Engineering Sustainability, 172*(1), 32–39. doi:10.1680/jensu.16.00027

El-Badawy, H. (2012). Effect of Chitosan and Calcium Chloride Spraying on Fruits Quality of Florida Prince Peach Under Cold Storage. *Research Journal of Agriculture and Biological Sciences, 8*, 272-281.

Emadpour, M., Ghareyazie, B., & Kalaj, Y.REntesari, MBouzari, N. (2015). Effect of the potassium permanganate coated zeolite nanoparticles on the quality characteristic and shelf life of peach and nectarine. *Agricultural Technology (Thailand), 11*(5), 1263–1273.

Emamifar, A., Kadivar, M., Shahedi, M., & Soleimanian-Zad, S. (2011). Effect of nanocomposite packaging containing Ag and ZnO on inactivation of Lactobacillus plantarum in orange juice. *Food Control, 22*(3–4), 408–413. doi:10.1016/j.foodcont.2010.09.011

Eshghi, S., Hashemi, M., Mohammadi, A., Badii, F., Mohammadhoseini, Z., & Ahmadi, K. (2014). Effect of nano-chitosan-based coating with and without copper loaded on physicochemical and bioactive components of fresh strawberry fruit (Fragaria x ananassa Duchesne) during storage. *Food and Bioprocess Technology, 7*(8), 2397–2409. doi:10.100711947-014-1281-2

Fan, W., Sun, J., Chen, Y., Qiu, J., Zhang, Y., & Chi, Y. (2009). Effects of chitosan coating on quality and shelf life of silver carp during frozen storage. *Food Chemistry, 115*(1), 66–70. doi:10.1016/j.foodchem.2008.11.060

Farias, I. A. P. (2018). Antimicrobial Activity of Cerium Oxide Nanoparticles on Opportunistic Microorganisms: A Systematic Review. *BioMedical Research International. Article ID, 1923606*, 1–14.

Fawole, O. G., Cai, X., & Mackenzie, A. R. (2016). Gas flaring and resultant air pollution: A review focusing on black Environ. *Pollution, 216*, 182–197. doi:10.1016/j.envpol.2016.05.075 PMID:27262132

Fishman, M. L., Chau, H. K., Hotchkiss, A. T. Jr, White, A., Garcia, R. A., & Cooke, P. H. (2019). Effect of long term cold storage and microwave extraction time on the physical and chemical properties of citrus pectin. *Food Hydrocolloids, 92*, 104–116. doi:10.1016/j.foodhyd.2018.12.047

Gad, M. M., Zagzog, O. A., & Hemeda, O. M. (2016). Development of Nano-Chitosan Edible Coating for Peach Fruits Cv. Desert Red. *International Journal of Environment, 05*(04), 43–55.

Ge, Z. (2018). Graphene Family Nanomaterials: Properties and Potential Applications in Dentistry. *International Journal of Biomaterials. Article ID, 1539678*, 1–12.

Gunther, N. W. IV, Abdul-Wakeel, A., Scullen, O. J., & Sommers, C. (2019). The evaluation of gamma irradiation and cold storage for the reduction of Campylobacter jejuni in chicken livers. *Food Microbiology, 82*, 249–253. doi:10.1016/j.fm.2019.02.014 PMID:31027780

Haider, A., & Kang, I.-K. (2015). Preparation of Silver Nanoparticles and Their Industrial and Biomedical Applications: A Comprehensive Review. *Advances in Materials Science and Engineering*, 1–16.

Ho, C. J., & Gao, J. Y. (2009). Preparation and Thermophysical Properties of Nanoparticle-in-Paraffin Emulsion as Phase Change Material. *International Communications in Heat and Mass Transfer*, *36*(5), 467–470. doi:10.1016/j.icheatmasstransfer.2009.01.015

Hoel, S., Vadstein, O., & Jakobsen, A. N. (2018). Growth of mesophilic Aeromonas salmonicida in an experimental model of nigiri sushi during cold storage. *International Journal of Food Microbiology*, *285*, 1–6. doi:10.1016/j.ijfoodmicro.2018.07.008 PMID:30005315

Hu, Z., & Gänzle, M. G. (2019). Challenges and opportunities related to the use of chitosan as a food preservative. *Journal of Applied Microbiology*, *1269*(5), 1318–1331. doi:10.1111/jam.14131 PMID:30325559

Huang, X., Boey, F., & Zhang, H. U. A. (2010). Graphene-nanoparticle. *Composites*, *6*, 159–166.

Hussain, M., Bensaid, S., Geobaldo, F., Saracco, G., & Russo, N. (2011). Photocatalytic Degradation of Ethylene Emitted by Fruits with TiO_2 Nanoparticles. *Industrial & Engineering Chemistry Research*, *50*(5), 2536–2543. doi:10.1021/ie1005756

Ijaz, M., Zafar, M., Afsheen, S., & Iqbal, T. (2020). A Review on Ag-Nanostructures for Enhancement in Shelf Time of Fruits. *Journal of Inorganic and Organometallic Polymers*, *30*(5), 1475–1482. doi:10.100710904-020-01504-x

James, S. J., & James, C. (2010). The Food Cold-Chain and Climate Change. *Food Research International*, *43*(7), 1944–1956. doi:10.1016/j.foodres.2010.02.001

Jeevanandam, J., Barhoum, A., Chan, Y. S., Dufresne, A., & Danquah, M. K. (2018). Review on nanoparticles and nanostructured materials: History, sources, toxicity and regulations. *Beilstein Journal of Nanotechnology*, *9*, 1050–1074. doi:10.3762/bjnano.9.98 PMID:29719757

Jiang, J. (2018). The Advancing of Zinc Oxide Nanoparticles for Biomedical Applications. Bioinorganic Chemistry and Applications. *Article ID*, *1062562*, 1–18.

Jiang, J.-F., Li, S.-F., & Liu, Z.-H. (2018). Study on heat transfer and cold storage characteristics of a falling film type of cold energy regenerator with PCM. *Applied Thermal Engineering*, *143*, 676–687. doi:10.1016/j.applthermaleng.2018.07.127

Khodadadi, J. M., & Hosseinizadeh, S. F. (2007). Nanoparticle-enhanced phase change materials (NEPCM) with great potential for improved thermal energy storage. *International Communications in Heat and Mass Transfer*, *34*(5), 534–543. doi:10.1016/j.icheatmasstransfer.2007.02.005

Kim, S., & Chung, B. H. (2016). Antioxidant activity of levan coated cerium oxide nanoparticles. *Carbohydrate Polymers*, *150*, 400–407. doi:10.1016/j.carbpol.2016.05.021 PMID:27312651

Kozak, Y., Farid, M., & Ziskind, G. (2017). Experimental and comprehensive theoretical study of cold storage packages containing PCM. *Applied Thermal Engineering*, *115*, 899–912. doi:10.1016/j.applthermaleng.2016.12.127

Li, G., Hwang, Y., Radermacher, R., & Chun, H.-H. (2013). Review of cold storage materials for subzero applications. *Energy*, *51*, 1–17. doi:10.1016/j.energy.2012.12.002

Li, H., Li, F., Wang, L., Sheng, J., Xin, Z., Zhao, L., Xiao, H., Zheng, Y., & Hu, Q. (2009). Effect of nano-packing on preservation quality of Chinese jujube. *Food Chemistry, 114*(2), 547–562. doi:10.1016/j.foodchem.2008.09.085

Lv, Y., Tahir, I. I., & Olsson, M. E. (2019). Effect of ozone application on bioactive compounds of apple fruit during short-term cold storage. *Scientia Horticulturae, 253*, 49–60. doi:10.1016/j.scienta.2019.04.021

Ma, X., & Mao, R. (2018). Fuzzy Control of Cold Storage Refrigeration System with Dynamic Coupling Compensation. *Journal of Control Science and Engineering, 18*, 1–7. doi:10.1155/2018/6836129

Machado, S., Pacheco, J. G., Nouws, H. P. A., Albergaria, J. T., & Delerue-Matos, C. (2015). Characterization of green zero-valent iron nanoparticles produced with tree leaf extracts. *The Science of the Total Environment, 53*, 76–81. doi:10.1016/j.scitotenv.2015.06.091 PMID:26151651

Maqbool, M., Ali, A., Alderson, P. G., Zahid, N., & Siddiqui, Y. (2011). Effect of a Novel Edible Composite Coating Based on Gum Arabic and Chitosan on Biochemical and Physiological Responses of Banana Fruits during Cold Storage. *Journal of Agricultural and Food Chemistry, 59*(10), 5474–5482. doi:10.1021/jf200623m PMID:21476593

Munuswamy, D. B., Madhavan, V. R., & Mohan, M. (2015). Synthesis and Surface Area Determination of Alumina Nanoparticles by Chemical Combustion Method. *International Journal of Chemtech Research, 8*(11), 413–419.

Naknaen, P. (2014). Utilization possibilities of antimicrobial biodegradable packaging produced by poly (butylene succinate) modified with zinc oxide nanoparticles in fresh-cut apple slices. *International Food Research Journal, 21*(6), 2413–2420.

Nourafkan, E., Asachi, M., Jin, H., Wen, D., & Ahmed, W. (2019). Stability and photo-thermal conversion performance of binary nanofluids for solar absorption refrigeration systems. *Renewable Energy, 140*, 264–273. doi:10.1016/j.renene.2019.01.081

Ozturk, B., Uzun, S., & Karakaya, O. (2019). Combined effects of aminoethoxyvinylglycine and MAP on the fruit quality of kiwifruit during cold storage and shelf life. *Scientia Horticulturae, 251*, 209–214. doi:10.1016/j.scienta.2019.03.034

Parveen, S., Rana, S., & Fangueiro, R. (2013). A Review on Nanomaterial Dispersion, Microstructure, and Mechanical Properties of Carbon Nanotube and Nanofiber Reinforced Cementitious Composites. *Journal of Nanomaterials. Article ID, 710175*, 1–19. doi:10.1155/2013/710175

Piriyawong, V. (2012). Preparation and Characterization of Alumina Nanoparticles in Deionized Water Using Laser Ablation Technique. *Journal of Nanomaterials. Article ID, 819403*, 1–6.

Ratlamwala, T. A., & Abid, M. (2018). Performance analysis of solar assisted multi-effect absorption cooling systems using nanofluids: A comparative analysis. *International Journal of Energy Research, 42*(9), 2901–2915. doi:10.1002/er.3980

Rezaii Kalaj, Y., Ghareyazie, B., Emadpour, M., & Omrani, A. (2009). Effect of the Removal of Ethylen Hormone by Potassium Permangenate Coated Zeolite Nanoparticles on the Increased Quality and Quantity of Storage of Iceberg Lettuce (Lactuca sativa L.) and Chinese Cabbage (Brassica pekinensis). *Journal of Agricultural Sciences and Natural Resources*, *15*, 1–11.

Ruales-lonfat, C., Barona, J. F., Sienkiewicz, A., Bensimon, M., & Vélez-colmenares, J. (2015). Applied Catalysis B : Environmental Iron oxides semiconductors are efficients for solar water disinfection : A comparison with photo-Fenton processes at neutral pH, *Applied Catalyst. B. Environment*, *166-167*, 497–508.

Sahraei Khosh Gardesh, A., Badii, F., Hashemi, M., & Ardakani, A. YMaftoonazad, NGorji, A. M. (2016). Effect of nano-chitosan based coating on climacteric behavior and postharvest shelf-life extension of apple cv. *Golab Kohanz. Lebensmittel-Wissenschaft + Technologie*, *70*, 33–40.

Saifuddin, N. (2013). Carbon Nanotubes: A Review on Structure and Their Interaction with Proteins. *Journal of Chemistry. Article ID*, *676815*, 1–18.

Sait, H. H. (2018). Design and analysis of a flooded tube for cold energy storage. *International Journal of Refrigeration*, *94*, 151–160. doi:10.1016/j.ijrefrig.2018.07.018

Salavati-niasari, M., Davar, F., & Mir, N. (2008). Synthesis and characterization of metallic copper nanoparticles via thermal decomposition. *Polyhedron*, *27*(17), 3514–3518. doi:10.1016/j.poly.2008.08.020

Salem, E. H., Nawito, M A S., & El-Raouf Ahmed, A. E. A. (2019). Effect of Silver Nano-Particles on Gray Mold of Tomato Fruits. *Journal of Nanotechnology Research*, *1*, 108–118.

Shah, S. W. A., Jahangir, M., Qaisar, M., Khan, S. A., Mahmood, T., Saeed, M., Farid, A., & Liaquat, M. (2015). Storage Stability of Kinnow Fruit (Citrus reticulata) as Affected by CMC and Guar Gum-Based Silver Nanoparticle Coatings. *Molecules (Basel, Switzerland)*, *2015*(20), 22645–22661. doi:10.3390/molecules201219870 PMID:26694344

Shaibani, A. R., Keshtkar, M. M., & Sardari, P. T. (2019). Thermo-economic analysis of a cold storage system in full and partial modes with two different scenarios: A case study. *Journal of Energy Storage*, *24*, 100783. doi:10.1016/j.est.2019.100783

Shi, F., Zhou, X., Yao, M.-M., Tan, Z., Zhou, Q., Zhang, L., & Ji, S.-J. (2018). miRNAs play important roles in aroma weakening during the shelf life of 'Nanguo' pear after cold storage. *Energy Research*, *116*, 942–952. PMID:30717027

Siddiqi, K. S., Husen, A., & Rao, R. A. K. (2018). A Review on Biosynthesis of Silver Nanoparticles and Their Biocidal Properties. *Journal of Nanobiotechnology*, *16*(1), 14. doi:10.118612951-018-0334-5 PMID:29452593

Song, A.-X., Mao, Y.-H., Siu, K.-C., Tai, W. C. S., & Wu, J.-Y. (2019). Protective effects of exopolysaccharide of a medicinal fungus on probiotic bacteria during cold storage and simulated gastrointestinal conditions. *International Journal of Biological Macromolecules*, *133*, 957–963. doi:10.1016/j.ijbiomac.2019.04.108 PMID:31028812

Song, H., Yuan, W., Jin, P., Wang, W., Wang, X., Yang, L., & Zhang, Y. (2016). Effects of chitosan/nano-silica on postharvest quality and antioxidant capacity of loquat fruit during cold storage. *Postharvest Biology and Technology*, *119*, 41–48. doi:10.1016/j.postharvbio.2016.04.015

Stritih, U., & Butala, V. (2007). Energy saving in building with PCM cold storage. *International Journal of Energy Research*, *31*(15), 1532–1544. doi:10.1002/er.1318

Sun, Y., Singh, Z., Tokala, V. Y., & Heather, B. (2019). Harvest maturity stage and cold storage period influence lemon fruit quality. *Scientia Horticulturae*, *249*, 322–328. doi:10.1016/j.scienta.2019.01.056

Tai, C. Y., Tai, C., Chang, M., & Liu, H. (2007). *Synthesis of Magnesium Hydroxide and Oxide Nanoparticles Using a Spinning Disk Reactor.* Academic Press.

Talukdar, S., Afroz, H. M. M., Hossain, M. A., Aziz, M., & Hossain, M. M. (2019). Heat transfer enhancement of charging and discharging of phase change materials and size optimization of a latent thermal energy storage system for solar cold storage application. *Journal of Energy Storage*, *24*, 100797. doi:10.1016/j.est.2019.100797

Tian, S., Shao, S., & Liu, B. (2019). Investigation on transient energy consumption of cold storages: Modeling and a case study. *Energy*, *180*, 1–9. doi:10.1016/j.energy.2019.04.217

Uekawa, N. (2012). Characterization of Titanium Oxide Nanoparticles Obtained by Hydrolysis Reaction of Ethylene Glycol Solution of Alkoxide. *Journal of Nanotechnology*. *Article ID*, *102361*, 1–8.

Vargas, M., Albors, A., Chiralt, A., & González-Martínez, C. (2006). Quality of cold-stored strawberries as affected by chitosan–oleic acid edible coatings. Post. *Bio/Technology*, *41*, 164–171.

Wang, D., Jiang, J., Tao, L., Kou, Z., & Yao, L. (2017). Experimental investigation on a novel cold storage defrosting device based on electric heater and reverse cycle. *Applied Thermal Engineering*, *127*, 1267–1273. doi:10.1016/j.applthermaleng.2017.08.122

Wang, L., Ma, A., Tan, Y., Cui, X., & Cui, H. (2012). Study on Solar-Assisted Cascade Refrigeration System. *Energy Procedia*, *16*, 1503–1509. doi:10.1016/j.egypro.2012.01.236

Wang, X., Dennis, M., Jiang, J., Zhou, L., Zhai, X., & Lipiński, W. (2019). Performance of a novel cold thermal storage material in an emulated air conditioning system using different storage strategies. *International Journal of Refrigeration*, *104*, 259–269. doi:10.1016/j.ijrefrig.2019.05.038

Wei, Q., Wang, X., Sun, D.-W., & Pu, H. (2019). Rapid detection and control of psychrotrophic microorganisms in cold storage foods: A review. *Trends in Food Science & Technology*, *86*, 453–464. doi:10.1016/j.tifs.2019.02.009

Yusof, Y. (2016). Enhanced Structural, Thermal, and Electrical Properties of Multiwalled Carbon Nanotubes Hybridized with Silver Nanoparticles. Journal of Nanomaterials. *Article ID*, *6141496*, 1–9.

Zahid, N., Ali, A., Manickam, S., Siddiqui, Y., & Maqbool, M. (2012). Potential of chitosan-loaded nano-emulsions to control different Colletotrichum spp. And maintain quality of tropical fruits during cold storage. *Journal of Applied Microbiology*, *113*(4), 225–239. doi:10.1111/j.1365-2672.2012.05398.x PMID:22805053

Zalba, B., Marin, J. M., Cabeza, L. F., & Mehling, H. (2003). Review on thermal energy storage with phase change: Materials, heat transfer analysis and applications. *Applied Thermal Engineering*, *23*(3), 251–283. doi:10.1016/S1359-4311(02)00192-8

Zandi, K., Weisany, W., Ahmadi, H., Bazargan, I., & Naseri, L. (2013). Effect of Nanocomposite-Based Packaging on Postharvest Quality of Strawberry during Storage. *Bulletin of Environment. Pharmacology and Life Sciences*, *2*(5), 28–36.

Zeiny, A., Haruna, M. A., & Wen, D. (2019). Aqueous lithium bromide nano-solution for solar absorption refrigeration systems. *AIP Conference Proceedings*, *2123*, 020083. doi:10.1063/1.5117010

Zeng, J. L., Sun, L. X., Xu, F., Tan, Z. C., Zhang, Z. H., Zhang, J., & Zhang, T. (2007). Study of a PCM based energy storage system containing Ag nanoparticles. *Journal of Thermal Analysis and Calorimetry*, *87*(2), 369–373. doi:10.100710973-006-7783-z

Zhang, Q., Rao, Y., Jiao, Y., Li, L., Li, Y., & Jin, L. (2017). preparation and performance of composite building materials with phase change material for thermal storage. *Energy Procedia*, *143*, 125–130. doi:10.1016/j.egypro.2017.12.659

Zhang, Y., Wei, J., Yuan, Y., & Yue, T. (2019). Diversity and characterization of spoilage-associated psychrotrophs in food in cold chain. *International Journal of Food Microbiology*, *290*, 86–95. doi:10.1016/j.ijfoodmicro.2018.09.026 PMID:30317110

Zheng, J., Li, S., Xu, Y., & Zheng, X. (2019). Effect of oxalic acid on edible quality of bamboo shoots (Phyllostachys prominens) without sheaths during cold storage. *Lebensmittel-Wissenschaft + Technologie*, *109*, 194–200. doi:10.1016/j.lwt.2019.04.014

Zheng, L., Zhang, W., & Liang, F. (2017). Experiment Study on Thermal Conductivity of Microcapsule Phase Change Suspension Applied to Solar Powered Air Conditioning Cold Storage System. *Procedia Engineering*, *205*, 1237–1244. doi:10.1016/j.proeng.2017.10.364

Zhou, X., Zhou, D.-Y., Liu, Z.-Y., Yin, F.-W., Liu, Z.-Q., Li, D.-Y., & Shahidi, F. (2019). Hydrolysis and oxidation of lipids in mussel Mytilus edulis during cold storage. *Food Chemistry*, *272*, 109–116. doi:10.1016/j.foodchem.2018.08.019 PMID:30309519

Chapter 15
Nanomaterials in Food Packaging

Nairah Noor
University of Kashmir, India

Asima Shah
University of Kashmir, India

Adil Gani
University of Kashmir, India

Zanoor Ul Ashraf
University of Kashmir, India

F. A. Masoodi
University of Kashmir, India

ABSTRACT

Nano-materials hold great promise regarding their application in the food industry due to their size-dependent properties, high surface area, longer retention, easy absorption, and unique optical properties. The role of nanomaterials have been extended for increasing the stability and bioavailability of nutrients, encapsulation of flavors, bioactives, enhancing the physical and mechanical properties of food packaging (nanocomposites), pesticide and growth hormone delivery, antimicrobial agents to boost preservation of foodstuffs, detection of foodborne pathogens, biodegradable nano-sensors for monitoring of temperature and moisture, etc. There are various types of nanomaterials like nanoparticles, nano-emulsions, and nano-clays which are synthesized by several methods to be used in the food industry. However, there is some food safety concerns associated with these nanomaterials when used in food systems. It is, therefore, very necessary to formulate and develop some method for the detection of nanomaterials, in particular when used in-vivo.

DOI: 10.4018/978-1-7998-5563-7.ch015

1. INTRODUCTION

The evolution of food packaging in the global economy is driven by the demand posed by consumers as well as the advancement in technology. In the current scenario, packaging not only enables the easy distribution of food to consumers but is also being designed to facilitate the preservation and communication to consumers. It is the third-largest industry in the world and in developed nations, it represents 2% of Gross National Product (GNP) (Han, 2005).The main functions of packaging include containment, protection of food against unfavourable external and internal conditions including gases, microbes, water vapour and physical damage. Also, the introduction of convenience foods for busy lifestyle consumers has triggered a rapid growth in designing the packaging materials that offer convenience features. Talking about the advances in the packaging, the concept of intelligent packaging and active packaging has changed the whole idea of packaging. In an intelligent packaging system, the package provides a feedback to the consumers with respect to the deterioration or the unfavourable time/temperature to which the package has been subjected to. In case of active packaging systems, the preservatory and protective function of the package is initiated by an intrinsic and or/extrinsic factors .However there are major challenges in the packaging technology that needs to be addressed. These include low mechanical strength, insufficient barrier properties, non-sustainability and waste generation. Many of these properties are fulfilled by the glass and metal but plastics are still the first choice of the manufacturers owing to their easy formability, light weight and low cost. So the consumption of plastics by the packaging industry accounts to 40% with food packaging industry consuming half of it (Rhim, Park, & Ha, 2013). However the major drawback of these is that the raw material for manufacturing of most of the plastics comes from petroleum products which are is not sustainable and produces environmental hazards. Another concern of the existing packaging system is to enhance the shelf life of the product without any detrimental effect on the quality and safety of the food. There may be loss of the nutritive quality due to the migration of moisture, oxygen and other gases. Also an increase in the microbial population due to contamination or temperature abuse may cause a public health hazard. In case of respiring products, O_2 permeability of a packaging material is a major criterion for the effective functioning. To get the barrier properties of the packaging material in line with the specific characteristics of the food, many polymer blends have been studied and designed but the formation of these composites is still a major issue due to the limitation of high costs and non-biodegradable nature of these materials. So in an attempt to address these concerns, nanotechnology has been exploited to make the necessary interventions in the food packaging sector. Nanotechnology comprises of the fabrication and application of the particles (having at least one of the dimension) ranging from approximately 1-100nm in length. Nanotechnology has evolved as novel tool in various industries like food processing, textile industries, medicine, cosmetics, electronics and computing (Maynard & Michelson, 2014). The use of materials having the particles of nano - dimensions may serve to improve the barrier, mechanical and anti- microbial properties. The addition of nanoparticles to the polymers results in the formation of nano-composites with improved thermal and mechanical strength. Further nanosensors may be employed to provide the feedback to the consumers with respect to the food quality and food safety. The major systems of the packaging where nanotechnology has a potential to provide enhancements are active packaging, intelligent packaging and composite manufacturing. The following sections provide an insight into the nanomaterials, their properties, applications, potential (eco) toxicological effects, public perception and global legislation of nanoparticles in various packaging systems.

2. NANOPARTICLES IN FOOD PACKAGING

The nanoparticles used in the food packaging system can have different sources based upon the end use, food matrix to be packed, processing storage conditions and. The following section deals with the nanoparticles derived from metals, non –metals and food grade polymers and their incorporation and binding to the food packaging materials.

2.1. Nanoparticles From Metals And Non-Metals

Metals form a broad category of substances from which the nanoparticles can be derived in abundance. In fact all the metals exist in the form of nanoparticles. However a small proportion of these including gold (Au), iron (Fe), silver (Ag), zinc oxide (ZnO), titanium dioxide (TiO2), iron oxide (Fe3O4, Fe2O3) (Chaudhry et al., 2008), copper oxide (CuO), copper (Cu) and palladium (Pd) (Llorens et al., 2012) have been used on commercial scale to enhance the properties of the food packaging materials. The most striking feature that allows metal nanoparticles to be used in food packaging applications is the anti-microbial property. Ag (Silver) nanoparticles are the widely used for its anti microbial activity. It is a shelf stable, broad spectrum anti –microbial and has been used to target a wide range of microbes including bacteria, yeasts, fungi and algae. The anti-microbial activity of the Ag may be attributed to any one of the following reasons; (a) it might interfere with the binding of sulfhydrl or disulfide groups on the active sites of the membrane proteins thereby hampering various vital cellular processes. (b) It may develop an oxidative stress and (c) It might damage the replication mechanism of DNA (Luoma, 2008). However the exact reason for its working as an anti microbial is still under study. Likewise Gallium has also been found as a potent anti-microbial against various pathogenic bacteria and fungi (Kelson, Carnevali, & Truong-Le, 2013).The similar analogy of gallium with respect to Fe makes it a good choice to deprive bacteria of Fe by destroying the mechanism of Fe uptake. However its use at commercial scale is limited owing to its toxicity. Apart from metals, non metallic sources have also been exploited for designing of nanoparticles and these include mostly organic materials such as polymers and proteins, clays, chitosan and poly-lactic acid. Chitosan nanoparticles have been recently exploited for their anti-bacterial properties. (Hajipour et al., 2012). It is extracted from fungi and insects in the form of deacetylated chitin. In food packaging operations, macromolecular chitosan has been used as a wall material for various antimicrobials (Ouattara et al., 2000), as a coating materials on surfaces (Coma, Deschamps, & Martial-Gros, 2003) and as an antimicrobial deposit in polymer packaging (Park, Marsh, & Dawson, 2010). Nanoclays including nano scale montmorillinite (MMT), also called as bentonite has been used as depositions in various polymers which has the added benefits of increasing the polymer strength, thermal stability and increased gas barrier properties (Majeed et al., 2013)

2.2. Food Grade Nanoparticles

This category of nanoparticles includes the particles of nano dimensions that are derived from food compatible sources (Cruz-Romero, Murphy, Morris, Cummins, & Kerry, 2013).The toxicity of these nanoparticles is negligible as compared to metallic and metal oxide nanoparticles. But the apprehensions regarding the accumulation and increased bioavailability of these nanoparticles in the human body is still persistent. As a matter of fact, the in-depth study of the effects on human exposure needs to be undertaken to establish the toxicity. Various food grade derived substances like curcumin and ascorbyl-di-palmitate having source as turmeric and Vitamin C respectively have been reduced to nano level and are used as an anti-microbial additives when incorporated in cellulosic packaging films (Sonkaew, Sane, & Suppakul, 2012). Similarly food grade nanocapsules based on chitosan have also been formulated by incorporating alcoholic lecithin and sodium caseinate on chitson matrix (Sato, Quintas, Vincente, & Cunha, 2011).

2.3. Incorporation And Attachment In Food Packaging

There are two main techniques of incorporating nanoparticles in food packaging: (1) Immobilization of nanoparticles at the surface or within the packaging material and 2) By using independent pads of nanoparticles in the existing package (De Azeredo, 2013). The latter method serves the advantage in a sense that a close contact can be established between the nanoparticles and the food. However, there are chances of migration and additional manufacturing costs. So food industries are now focussing on the methods that incorporate nanoparticles within polymers or using nanoparticle surface coatings. The use of polymers in food packaging has been carried successfully over years, so these can be the first choice to allow for the incorporation of nanoparticles. These provide a good matrix for immobilization of nanoparticles and have numerous advantages including low cost, prevention of aggregation, ease of manufacture and uncontrollable release (Guo, Yuan, Lu, & Li, 2013). Both inorganic and biodegradable polymers have been exploited for these purpose including polyolefins (polyvinyl chloride (PVC), polystyrene (PS), polyethylene terephthalate (PET), polypropylene (PP), polyethylene (PE) and polylactic acid. Due to the environmental concerns, biodegradable polymers are mostly sorted for incorporation of nanoparticles but polyolefins also make a good choice for the carriers of nanoparticles owing to their ability to reduce the material required for packaging and improved thermal properties and strength (Silvestre, Duraccio, & Cimmino, 2011). Nanoparticles can be immobilized within the polymers either by in situ methods (casting and coating methods) wherein the nanoparticles are incorporated into liquid polymers or by adherhing the nanoparticles with polymers in the final stage of processing. In another case, if a polymer exists in solid form, reduction of polymer atoms into ions can form nanoparticles. A number of methods of forming nancomposites have been reported including casting, diffusion and in situ synthesis of forming nanoparticles and polymers. The distribution of the nanoparticles in the polymer is dependent upon the method employed for the formation of nanoparticles. A study carried out by Nobile et al. (2004) a novel technique of plasma coating was used to deposit nanoparticles on a polyethylene based packaging. Another novel technique of incorporating nanoparticles on the polymer matrix having improved immobilization is Self-Assembling Block Copolymer. It consists of a forming a uniform assembly of nanostructure by using an anionic polymerization process. This is followed by the attachment of the nanoparticles to polymer and the process is called as templating. The result of such process is a copolymer which is then exposed to the chemical reaction form a nanoscale pattern. This process has been projected as a way of delivering drugs for various pharmaceutical industries but limited knowledge is available for its use in packaging systems.

3. PROPERTIES OF NANOPARTICLES USED IN FOOD PACKAGING

For the successful marketing of food products, certain characteristics of the packaging material like moisture barrier, gas barrier, structural integrity, transparency and anti- bacterial properties are important. So for nanoparticle packaging, all these properties have to been taken into consideration, which will make it acceptable to both industries and consumers. The important desirable characteristic of a packaging material i.e. transparency enables consumers to have a view of the contents before purchasing. A study carried out by Nazarov et al. (2013) revealed that more finely the nanoparticles were distributed throughout the polymer, more transparent the polymers were in appearance. However the presence of large sized particles demonstrated loss in the transparency. The food constituents also have a pronounced effect on transparency of the packaging materials for example, Kanmani & Rhim (2014) reported that with the increase in EAgNP content, the transparency of the gelatin films decreased. In another study carried out by Martinez-Abad, Lagaron, & Ocio (2012), two food sources i.e. apple and chicken were observed for the relative change in transparency after contact nano particle packaging. The workers reported that the loss of transparency was more in chicken owing to high protein content. This can form an important basis for selection of the packaging material for high protein foods as the reduction of transparency can diminish the marketability of the high protein foods. Apart from these properties, the nanopackages should also fulfil the other dimensions including strength, oxygen barrier/scavenging, antimicrobial and biosensing properties.

3.1. Gas And Moisture Barrier Properties

For the effective maintenance of the sensorial properties of food, the food package must provide the necessary barrier to the moisture and gases (Simon, Chaudhry, & Bakos, 2008).Owing to their high aspect ratios, nanomaterials can serve to improve the gas barrier properties by creating an obstacle to the gas and moisture, as the path through which gas/moisture has to travel increases. These are generally applied as filler in the walls of the packaging materials. A classic example of nanomaterial in this regard is nanoclay. Commercially, Nanocor in collaboration with a company named Voridan has developed Imperm – a nanocomposite comprising of nanoclay particles. Imperm in turn has been employed by a number of companies to create their own nanocomposite material with enhanced gas barrier property.

3.2. Antibacterial Properties

The packaging materials that contain nanoparticles have also been exploited to provide anti-microbial activity. This can be attributed to the ability of the nanoparticles to release the ions which prevents the growth of microbes and the ability to prevent the binding and growth of bacteria at the surface of the packaging material (Lichter, VanVliet, & Rubner, 2009). Various sources of nanoparticles including Ag, TiO_2, MMT and ZnO have shown to possess anti-microbial activities (Cushen, Kerry, Morris, Cruz-Romero, & Cummins, 2012). The most important characteristics that influences the anti-microbial activity of the nanoparticle is the size of the particle and it has been reported that the particles in the range of 1 and 10 nm displayed enhanced anti-microbial properties (Fernandez et al., 2009). But in a recent study carried out by Xiu et al. (2012), size of Ag nanoparticles was shown to have an indirect effect on the anti-microbial activity. It was reported that Ag nanoparticles have increased surface area for oxidation of Ag into Ag ions which in turn increases the anti-microbial activity. Conversely the aggregation of the nanoparticles lowers the reactive surface area thereby reducing the anti-microbial activity (Zook, Halter, Cleveland, & Long, 2012).Ag nanoparticles have been studied on extensive scale owing to their high anti –microbial properties. The ions released from the Ag nanoparticles are effective against *Escherichia coli* (*E. coli*) and *Staphylococcus aureus* (*S. aureus*) (Fernandez et al., 2009). In another study carried out by Rhim et al. (2006) Ag- Chitosan nanocomposites have shown to possess improved antimicrobial properties. Many such combinations have been studied for their anti-microbial properties like Ag-Zeolite nanoparticles and Ag – Agar nanoparticle. The production of these polymers incorporated with nanoparticles can provide a synergistic approach for improving both the anti-microbial as well as the strength properties.

4. FOOD PACKAGING BASED ON POLYMER NANOMATERIALS

The added features of nanoparticles when incorporated in food packaging can uplift the domain of food packaging with respect to the following three areas viz; "Improved", "Active" and "Intelligent" packaging (Silvestre, Duraccio & Cimmino, 2011). These three categories specify the applications of nanotechnology in food packaging industry. The use of polymer nanomaterials can upgrade the conventional packaging systems in terms of safety, economy and biodegradability, mechanical strength, moisture and barrier properties, less requirement of energy, reduction in emission of CO_2. The benefits of the polymers in packaging industry have been exploited from decades but the research in the polymer nanotechnology is still in infancy. The important factors like safety, standardization, trained manpower and technology transfer need due consideration for the successful implementation of nanotechnology in polymers. The whole idea should synchronize with various level of packaging like selection of raw materials, production, scrutinizing the food and polymer interaction, applications and waste elimination. Apart from these factors cost, impacts on health and environment also needs to be analyzed. The applications of the nanobased polymers for food packaging can be studied under the following categories.

1) Active -nano packaging
2) Improved Polymer nanomaterials for packaging/Nanostructured coating
3) Intelligent- nano packaging.

In case of "Improved" polymer nanomaterials, the use of nanoparticles improves the gas barrier, moisture/temperature stable, flexibility properties of the polymer materials. The first reported category of the nanoparticles was that of clay. These comprise of the nanostructured layers which are separated by interlayer galleries. A homogenous dispersion of the polymer matrix and clay is necessary for exploiting the potential of nanoparticles incorporated into the polymer matrix. This can only take place when the clay –polymer interaction is possible i.e. when there are positive enthalpy conditions. As a matter of fact both enthalpy as well as entropic factors has direct bearing on the morphology of the nanoparticles in the polymer structure (Paiva, Morales & Diaz, 2008). In order to form continuous nanocomposites from polar polymers, alkyl-ammonium is used as a surfactant as it offers maximum enthalpy. In active nano packaging, the use of nanoparticles enables the food, environment and package interaction which ultimately extends the shelf life of the food. The third category, i.e. "Intelligent nano packaging" involves the use of nano-devices in the polymer matrix which detect any breach in the temperature/time of environment around the food or communicates the actual condition of the food package to the consumers.

4.1. Active Nano Packaging

This system employs the deliberate incorporation of the substances into the polymer matrix that have the ability to release or absorb components in and out of the food package or the environment surrounding the food. These include carbon dioxide absorbers/emitters, ethylene absorbers and oxygen scavengers. Currently, only anti-microbial active systems have been developed using nano materials. These systems have exploited metal oxides, metal nanoparticles and carbon nanotubes. The metal nanoparticles derived from zinc, silver and gold have been mostly studied for their anti-microbial properties. Silver nanoparticles have shown to be more applicable and have been commercialized. Various studies have shown that silver nanoparticles are anti-fungal and show anti-bacterial action against 150 different types of bacteria (Kumar & Munstedt, 2005). The anti-microbial action of the silver nanoparticles can be attributed to any one of the mechanisms i) these adhere to the surface of the cell and degrade the lipopolysaccharides, thereby forming pits or holes in the membrane. ii) These penetrate inside the cytoplasm of the bacterial cell and damage the DNA iii) release Ag^+ ions that bind to the electro donor groups. The silver nanoparticles have been used in the form of nanocomposites and have shown higher anti- microbial activity as compared to the micro-composites. Damm, Munstedt, & Rosch (2008) reported that polyamide 6/silver-nanocomposites were more effective against *Escherichia coli* as compared to micro composites and the anti-bacterial activity of the silver nanocomposites was more persistent for longer time as compared to micro composites. When used in combination with other metals, enhancement in the anti-bacterial properties have been observed. The examples of these combinations are siver/zeolite and silver/gold composites. Apart from silver nanoparticles, metal oxides like zinc oxide (ZnO), magnesium oxide (MgO), silicon oxide (SiO_2) and Titanium dioxide (TiO_2) have also shown the potential to be used as the anti-microbials owing to their ability to block UV. ZnO nanoparticles when incorporated in polymers like polypropylene have shown to absorb UV light besides improving the polymer stability. Likewise carbon nanotubes have displayed the anti –bacterial properties against *E. coli.* This can be attributed to the fact that thin and long carbon nanotubes cause an irreversible damage to the microbial cells by puncturing them (Kang, Pinault, Pfefferle, & Elimelech, 2007.) However due to cytotoxic nature, their application in food industry has been halted.

The deteriorative reactions in most of the foods are accelerated by the inclusion of oxygen in the package. So many nano-active food packaging systems have been developed which scavenge the oxygen. The food deterioration reactions may be direct or indirect with indirect reaction involving the spoilage of food by the growth of aerobes in the package, whereas direct oxidation is a common phenomenon that causes the browning and rancidity reactions in foods. Both of these result in deterioration of food quality and produces off-colors, off-flavours, off-odours and loss of nutrients. Oxygen scavengers work by removing the Oxygen which may either enter the package from outside or may be residual. An example of such type is the one made from TiO_2 nanoparticles. Similarly ethylene nano scavengers derived from silver have been shown to absorb ethylene with its simultaneous decomposition (Li et al., 2009). Since ethylene hastens the ripening process in fruits and vegetables, removing it can extend the shelf life of such perishable commodities.

4.2. Nanostructured Coating Or Improved Polymer Nanomaterials

The use of nano-materials in the form of nano-coatings on the food packaging material has been gaining much response due to the enhanced properties of moisture barrier and anti-microbial activity. These nano-materials can be either incorporated in the form of a laminate thereby forming a nano-composite layer or can be simply applied on to the package polymer. Metal oxide based nanoparticles have been used for their anti-microbial and barrier properties. These have been coated successfully on biodegradable and non-biodegradable polymers, reduce the use of materials and have simple film conversion process.

The food packaging industry has exploited the use of paper/paperboard material to the fullest but owing to its hydrophilic nature, its use is restricted in various foods. To improve the moisture barrier properties of paper/paperboard, various hydrophobic thermoplastics and metal oxides have been successfully coated in the form of additional barrier layer. In a study carried out by Hirvikorpi, Vaha-Nissi, Harlin, & Karppinen (2010), a coating of 25nm thick layer of aluminium oxide on PLA displayed an increase in the moisture and oxygen barrier properties. In another study carried out by Johnston et al. (2008) the anti-microbial properties of the package were enhanced by using calcium silicate nanoparticles as the coating material. Also, TiO_2 nanoparticles when used in a coating, were found to be effective against *E. coli* (Fu, Vary, & Lin, 2005). Similarly, ZnO nanoparticles were used to improve the anti-microbial and water barrier properties of PVC (Li, et al., 2010).

4.3. Intelligent Nano-Packaging

The most striking feature of the intelligent packaging is to communicate the quality conditions of the food package to the consumers. It overtakes the static technique of analysing the quality of food by the use of "Best Before" and "Use By" approach employed by the manufacturers. The packaging materials used by these systems must possess the properties that help them to monitor the environment present inside and outside the package (Yam, Takhistov, & Miltz, 2005). These intelligent packs usually come up with the indicators which help in detection and identification of any breach in the storage conditions that may result in deterioration reactions in food package. Initial developments in this aspect of packaging were the use of devices that would provide the time-temperature history, expiry date and integrity of the food package. More recently, different type of indicators have been developed using nanotechnology including freshness indicators, oxygen indicators, and pathogen sensors. The use of silicate nanoparticles in pH indicators is the latest entry in these intelligent systems. (Jurmanovic et al., 2006).The governing factors for their widespread use include robustness, cost, interaction with foods and packaging materials. Some of them are discussed below:

4.3.1. Oxygen Indicators

The presence of oxygen in some food packages is detrimental to the quality of the product as it can cause the growth of aerobes during the course of storage. So one of the aspects in development of intelligent packaging has been the designing of the oxygen indicators .The use of such non-toxic and irreversible oxygen sensors is to ensure that the package is free from oxygen. The application of nanotechnology in monitoring the oxygen conditions can be seen with the development of colorimetric oxygen indicator activated by ultra-violet radiations (Lee Mao, Flynn, & Belcher, 2002).This type of an indicator comprises of TiO_2 nanoparticles, an electron donor (Sacrificial donor) and a redox dye. The whole assembly is encapsulated into a polymer matrix of coating and film (Mills & Hazafy, 2008, 2009). When the sensor is exposed to UV radiation, the valence electrons become excited and jump to conduction band. This creates an electron-hole pairs on the surface of the TiO_2 semi-conductor. The photo generated holes in the valence band are quickly filled with the electrons donated by the sacrificial electron donor, like glycerol in this case. This inhibits the re-filling of holes by electrons and consequently the conduction band gets accumulated with excited electrons. These electrons then reduce the methylene blue dye (MBOx) to a leuko state (MDRd; colorless).This step marks the activation of the indicator and upon ingression of oxygen, MBRd is oxidized and the colourless sensor becomes blue again. The extent of the color change in the indicator depends on the amount of oxygen that reacts with the dye.

4.3.2. Detection Of Spoilage And Pathogenic Microorganisms

For detecting various food borne pathogens, a number of sensors have been developed and these consists of a polymer matrix into which nanoparticles are embedded. When these sensors detect any food borne pathogen, a response or a change which is particular for each pathogen is produced. At present there are three kinds of bacteria including *Vibrio parahemolyticus, Salmonella spp.* and *Bacillus cereus* that can be detected using these sensors. Another method that has been employed to detect bacteria is the use of nanomaterials (quantum dots) to which the antibodies are conjugated. Quantum dots possess the property of high fluorescence that is resistant to delayed decay life-time, higher sensitivity and photobleaching. In a study carried out by Yang and Li (2006), quantum dots were used to detect *E. coli* O157:H7 and *Salmonella Typhimurium*. The workers conjugated the anti-E. coli O157 and anti- Salmonella antibodies to CdSe/ZnS quantum dots having the wavelength of 525 and 705 nm using a light source at 395 nm for excitation. The two emission peaks made it possible to detect the two different pathogen simultaneously, with no cross-talk between the emission peaks. The use of DNA-based biochips as a tool of nano-packaging has been used to identify the pathogenic bacteria in fish or meat, fungi in fruits. Owing to their ability of identifying the microbes and various compounds in foods with greater precision, these budding technologies may find a way to be used as an intelligent label. So their in-depth studies and research is expected to increase in coming times.

4.3.3. Time, Temperature, And Humidity Indicators

The loss in the shelf life of a food product can be attributed to the temperature abuses production, packaging, distribution or storage. The increase in the temperature can increase the deteriorative reactions (physical, chemical and biological) and lead to loss of quality and finally make the product unfit for consumption. In other cases, a relative decrease in temperature can cause chill injury and other changes which again have a pronounced effect on the quality of the food. The overall effect of temperature on the shelf stability of the food is accumulative and depends on the degree to which the food has been subjected to the temperature abuse. To observe the changes occurring during handling, distribution and storage of the food, time-temperature indicators (TTIs) are a good choice. Their use in food packaging system began in late 20th century and provides information about the temperatures to which the food has been subjected to. At the consumer level, it assures them about the quality and safety of their purchase and for manufacturers it helps them to trace the chain of supply in case of any temperature abuse. These can be differentiated into two classes: one that provides a colour change which is associated with a chemical reaction (starts immediately after the package is applied with label) and the other which is dependent upon the transfer or migration of a dye via porous material and is time and temperature dependent. In this regard, nanosensors have been developed which respond to the time, temperature, humidity and oxygen changes, microbial contamination changes and provide a visible effect. These can be applied in the food packaging materials as "reactive particles". The application of nanotechnology in this aspect of packaging can be understood in case of triangle shaped Ag nanoplates which have been developed to monitor the time-temperature changes. (Zeng, Roberts, & Xia, 2010). The built up of the nano-plates is such that it has sharp corners and in visible spectrum of radiation and exhibits a strong in-plane dipole resonance. But with increase in the storage time, the sharp corners of the nano-plates become somewhat round in appearance and there is a shift of resonance position from cyan to blue. So if the food pack has been subjected to a storage condition in excess of the stipulated time and temperature, the device will help us to detect the same. The key to the success of these TTI 's is that the kinetics of the deteriorative reactions must match with the kinetics of the TTI's response. This is a major challenge in using such devices as the reactions cannot be programmed easily. Similarly humidity indicators have also been developed as a component of intelligent packaging as ingress of moisture is the main factor responsible for the deteriorative reactions in foods particularly the dried and intermediate moisture foods. The monitoring of moisture transfer in and out of the package can provide an outlook on the quality, safety and integrity of the package. An example of this category includes the humidity indicator developed by (Zhou, 2013). The indicator consists of a nanocrystalline cellulose film which was developed by iridescent technology. The rigid rods of crystallites form self assembly as a result of casting and develop a chiral nematic structure. The colour of the dry films is blue-green .Upon the ingress of moisture, the colour becomes red. These films are structured such that when they interact with electromagnetic field a simultaneous change is seen in colour.

4.3.4. Freshness Indicators

These provide the real information of the product quality to the consumers, producers or retailers. The principle of their action is that they display the significant changes in any one of constituents or display the accumulation of any metabolite or marker spoilage compound (amines and sulphides).The accumulation of these marker compounds is due to the time/temperature abuse or any microbial activity. In order to detect their presence a number of techniques have been employed. In a study carried out by (Smolander et al., 2004), a coating of 1-10nm thickness of transition metal (silver and copper) was deposited on the paper or plastic packages and used for packaging of fresh meats. Upon spoilage, the coated metals of nano-range react with the sulphide volatiles produced as a result of spoilage and undergo a change in color which can be used as a tool to monitor the freshness. In raw sea foods, trimethylamine is accumulated on spoilage and this can be detected by using bioelectronic nose which has a peptide receptor. The sensors are made up of the carbon-nanotubes transistors which have sensitivity as low as 10 fM. Carbon nanotubes have also been employed to detect the changes volatile compounds, ethylene and CO_2 in case of ripening of fruits.

5. EFFECTS OF NANOPACKAGING ON FOODS

The overall properties of the nano-materials are a result of its constituents i.e. the polymer and the substance in the nanoform. The type of the polymer used has a controlling action on the release of the nano-particles from the matrix. The use of nano-materials on commercial level has been successful to some extent only after thorough studies. A study carried out by Brayner et al. (2006) reports that nano-materials can inhibit the growth of prokaryotic cells whereas in eukaryotic cells these can cause death. These features of the nano-materials can be exploited in controlling the growth of the spoilage organisms. The most accepted mechanism for this is believed to be the large surface area of the nano-materials which absorbs the nutrients and deprives the pathogenic and spoilage cells of the nutrients which ultimately leads to cell death (Geys, Nemery, & Hoet, 2010). As explained before the use of Ag nanoparticles has been commercialized owing to their anti-microbial properties. Also these nanoparticles have the ability to absorb and decompose ethylene. Thus when Ag nanoparticles are incorporated into the food packaging films, they can absorb and decompose ethylene (Hu & Fu, 2003) which in turn can increase the shelf life of the fruits and vegetables. An, Zhang Wang, & Tang (2008) reported an increase in the shelf life of asparagus when a coating of Ag nanomaterials was applied on it. Li, et al. (2009) also reported that there was a delay in the senescence in case of the Chinese fruit jujube when polyethylene nanocomposite incorporated with Ag nanoparticles was used for its packaging. Another application of the Ag nanoparticles is seen in case of modified atmospheric packaging for the preservation of poultry. In this, Ag nanoparticles are embedded in absorbant pads and have shown to retard the growth of *Escherichia coli* and *Staphylococcus aureus*. (Fernandez et al. 2009).Similarly packaging films incorporated with TiO_2 powder have shown to anti-microbial activity against *Escherichia coli* (Chawengkijwanich & Hayata, 2008).

6. ASSESSMENT OF RISK

The application of nanotechnology in the food packaging system may pose various risks to humans and the environment. So a preliminary risk assessment is an essential factor to be taken into consideration which helps to isolate and measure these risks. The Directorate General of Health and Consumer Protection in EU has established a Scientific Committee on Emerging and Newly Identified Health Risks (SCENIHR).The main functions of the committee are to discuss and present the overall facts on the matters related to consumer safety or public health when any new potential hazard is identified (SCENIHR, 2010).Thus nanotechnology can also be included as a matter of discussion in this committee. There is a need to analyze the effects of this developing technology on human health and to look for the ways to reduce or eliminate the implications of this emerging technology. In this regard an integrated system is the need of the hour that can compile the massive research going in the area to establish the recognised terminology and also enable the risk analysis on immediate basis. In this system, the workers from various fields like food technology, toxicology and risk assessment will be required to analyze the whole situation. Also a well established communication regarding the advantages of the nanotechnogies in the food packaging system between the producers and consumers is a must.

7. TOXICOLOGICAL EFFECTS

The lack of safety tests for nanotechnologies in the food systems is a limiting factor for its application on commercial scale. Also there are major differences among the legislations in the entire world regarding the standardization safety of these novel technologies. According to Tiede et al. (2008), toxicological and risk assessment studies are practically unavailable particulary in the food industry. To start with, the toxicity testing used for the conventional packaging systems can be employed as an initial step to analyze the hazards associated with the nanomaterials. This can be followed with some modifications in the aforementioned methodology owing to the differences between nano-materials and conventional materials. In order to establish the toxicity, certain properties of the nano-materials (polymer matrix as well as the substance in nano-form) including shape, reactivity, solubility, size and various physico-chemical parameters needs to be analyzed. According to Handy and Shaw (2007), when a new nanomaterial is to be studied for toxicological effects, the first step is to examine the physical and chemical properties in order to establish safety in handling of the raw materials, its application and disposal. Next, the materials are examined by subjecting them to various acute, chronic, oral, skin irritation, dermal and mutagenicity tests. It has been shown that that some of the materials at nanoscale possess significant toxicity as compared to the same materials at macro level. In a study carried out by Cui et al. (2005) there was an inhibition of human kidney cell proliferation when carbon tubes having single walls were tested. Further the nanotubes had negative effect on the growth of cells. Since different nanomaterials have different properties, so studying the toxicological effects should be carried separately basis (Munro et al., 2009). Also some nanoparticles have been reported to induce oxidative stress, inflammation, and symptoms of early tumour formation (Carlson et al., 2008). The toxicological effects observed in such studies can help in screening the nanomaterials to be used in packaging systems. Further the migration tests employed for conventional packaging can form the basis for assessing the nanomaterials for migration. These tests are well established, reliable and reproducible and can help to assess the applications of these nanomaterials for food.

8. GLOBAL LEGISLATION

The regulatory aspects of the nanotechnology are covered under both the vertical and horizontal legislation. Vertical legislation has developed recently and takes into consideration the industrial domain where the nanotechnology is likely to be applied and therefore is more practical to the users of nanotechnology. In case of horizontal legislation, there is no particular regulation regarding nanotechnology as it is much broader. The risks associated with the nanotechnology have forced the global agencies to take extra precautions while applying this novel technology to food systems. However the perception varies from region to region, like in Australia and Europe, these regulations are bound by horizontal legislation (Lyons & Whelan, 2010) whereas in Taiwan, the legislation has introduced Nano Mark System: which is the symbol of quality for consumers and signifies that the product had been manufactured using a genuine nanotechnology (Chau, Wu, & Yen, 2007). However, this system excludes food but includes the nano-ingredients. In U.S.A, there are a number of regulatory agencies associated with the use of products based on nanotechnology. However there are no strict guidelines or framework which can provide the necessary protection and assessment to the consumers regarding the usage of the products based on nanotechnologies (Corley, Scheufele, & Hu, 2009). Similarly NICNAS is a regulatory authority in Australia which governs the legislation concerning chemicals and has included various administrative procedures to address the issue of nanotechnology (NICNAS, 2010).It determines the data handling, type and volumes of the nanomaterials used and is in charge of the legislation necessary to protect the people from the risks posed by the use of nanotechnology.

9. PUBLIC PERCEPTION

The public understanding of nanotechnology is a crucial factor that will determine its future development. The benefits offered by this promising technology are sometimes over shadowed by the apprehensions and risks associated with it. Any development or innovation in food science is a sensitive issue from the consumer's point of view. In a study carried out by Cobb & Macoubrie (2004), it was reported that the perception of nanotechnology among the participants in U.S.A. was optimistic, however the knowledge regarding the same was limited. Among the participants from Europe, it was observed that the perceptions regarding the nanotechnology were overall positive (Gaskell et al., 2005). In a study carried out by Siegrist et al. (2007): the workers presented a comprehensive nanosystems along with proper explanation among 153 consumers regarding the nanocoatings as a barrier against moisture and O_2 on tomatoes, anti-bacterial food materials, juice fortified with encapsulated vitamin A in wall materials such as starch and bread fortified with nanoencapsulated omega-3 fatty acids. They observed that nano-engineered foods had less buyers in comparison to that of the nanopackaging and it was deduced that foods where the nanomaterials formed a part within the system has less acceptability that the nano materials which were not present within the foods.

10. CONCLUSION

The demand to meet the requirements of the food industry has pushed the researchers to apply nanotechnology at various levels of production, packaging, storage and distribution. It has a potential of eliminating the loopholes present in the conventional packaging systems. The application of nanotechnology will definitely fulfil the domains of quality, safety, shelf life extensibility and security of the food products. The positive perception of nanotechnogy among the consumers can be maximized only when the toxicological, risk &exposure assessment and risk management studies are available worldwide. The lack of knowledge on the toxicology, bioaccumulation, risk assessment and management has created uncertainty among consumers towards the acceptability of nanopacked foods. Once the facts are established, nanotechnology in packaging industry can revolutionize the whole idea of global marketing and can help the producers to break the geographic barriers with their wide range of products.

ACKNOWLEDGMENT

Authors are thankful to the Department of Science & Technology, GOI (INSPIRE fellowship scheme) for financial support.

REFERENCES

An, J., Zhang, M., Wang, S., & Tang, J. (2008). Physical, chemical and microbiological changes in stored green asparagus spears as affected by coating of silver nanoparticles-PVP. *Lebensmittel-Wissenschaft + Technologie*, *41*(6), 1100–1107. doi:10.1016/j.lwt.2007.06.019

Brayner, R., Ferrari-Iliou, R., Brivois, N., Djediat, S., Benedetti, M. F., & Fievet, F. (2006). Toxicological impact studies based on *Escherichia coli* bacteria in ultrafine ZnO nanoparticles colloidal medium. *Nano Letters*, *6*(4), 866–870. doi:10.1021/nl052326h PMID:16608300

Carlson, C., Hussain, S. M., Schrand, A. M., Braydich-Stolle, K., Hess, K. L., & ... . (2008). Unique cellular interaction of silver nanoparticles: Size-dependent generation of reactive oxygen species. *The Journal of Physical Chemistry B*, *112*(43), 13608–13619. doi:10.1021/jp712087m PMID:18831567

Chau, C. F., Wu, S. H., & Yen, G. C. (2007). The development of regulations for food nanotechnology. *Trends in Food Science & Technology*, *18*(5), 269–280. doi:10.1016/j.tifs.2007.01.007

Chaudhry, Q., Scotter, M., Blackburn, J., Ross, B., Boxall, A., Castle, L., Aitken, R., & Watkins, R. (2008). Applications and implications of nanotechnologies for the food sector. *Food Additives and Contaminants*, *25*(3), 241–258. doi:10.1080/02652030701744538 PMID:18311618

Chawengkijwanich, C., & Hayata, Y. (2008). Development of TiO_2 powder-coated food packaging film and its ability to inactivate *Escherichia coli in vitro* and in actual tests. *International Journal of Food Microbiology*, *123*(3), 288–292. doi:10.1016/j.ijfoodmicro.2007.12.017 PMID:18262298

Cobb, M. D., & Macoubrie, J. (2004). Public perceptions about nanotechnology: Risks, benefits and trust. *Journal of Nanoparticle Research*, *6*(4), 395–405. doi:10.100711051-004-3394-4

Coma, V., Deschamps, A., & Martial-Gros, A. (2003). Bioactive packaging materials from edible chitosan polymer-antimicrobial activity assessment on dairy-related contaminants. *Journal of Food Science*, *68*(9), 2788–2792. doi:10.1111/j.1365-2621.2003.tb05806.x

Corley, E., Scheufele, D., & Hu, Q. (2009). Of risks and regulations: How leading U.S. nanoscientists form policy stances about nanotechnology. *Journal of Nanoparticle Research*, *11*(7), 1573–1585. doi:10.100711051-009-9671-5 PMID:21170136

Cruz-Romero, M. C., Murphy, T., Morris, M., Cummins, E., & Kerry, J. P. (2013). Antimicrobial activity of chitosan, organic acids and nano-sized solubilisates for potential use in smart antimicrobially-active packaging for potential food applications. *Food Control*, *34*(2), 393–397. doi:10.1016/j.foodcont.2013.04.042

Cui, D., Tian, F., Ozkan, C. S., Wang, M., & Gao, H. (2005). Effect of single wall carbon nanotubes on human HEK293 cells. *Toxicology Letters*, *155*(1), 73–85. doi:10.1016/j.toxlet.2004.08.015 PMID:15585362

Cushen, M., Kerry, J., Morris, M., Cruz-Romero, M., & Cummins, E. (2012). Nanotechnologies in the food industry e recent developments, risks and regulation. *Trends in Food Science & Technology*, *24*(1), 30–46. doi:10.1016/j.tifs.2011.10.006

Damm, C., Munstedt, H., & Rosch, A. (2008). The antimicrobial efficacy of polyamide6/silver-nano and microcomposites. *Materials Chemistry and Physics*, *108*(1), 61–66. doi:10.1016/j.matchemphys.2007.09.002

De-Azeredo, H. M. C. (2013). Antimicrobial nanostructures in food packaging. *Trends in Food Science & Technology*, *30*(1), 56–69. doi:10.1016/j.tifs.2012.11.006

Ferdnandez, A., Soriano, E., Lopez-Carballo, G., Picouet, P., Lloret, E., Gavara, R., & … . (2009). Preservation of aseptic conditions in absorbent pads by using silver nanotechnology. *Food Research International*, *42*(8), 1105–1112. doi:10.1016/j.foodres.2009.05.009

Fu, G., Vary, P. S., & Lin, C. T. (2005). Anatase TiO_2 nanocomposites for antimicrobial coatings. *The Journal of Physical Chemistry B*, *109*(18), 8889–8898. doi:10.1021/jp0502196 PMID:16852057

Gaskell, G., Eyck, T. T., Jackson, J., & Veltri, G. (2005). Imagining nanotechnology: Cultural support for technological innovation in Europe and the United States. *Public Understanding of Science (Bristol, England)*, *14*(1), 81–90. doi:10.1177/0963662505048949

Geys, J., Nemery, B., & Hoet, P. H. M. (2010). Assay conditions can influence the outcome of cytotoxicity tests of nanomaterials: Better assay characterization is needed to compare studies. *Toxicology In Vitro*, *24*(2), 620–629. doi:10.1016/j.tiv.2009.10.007 PMID:19850119

Guo, L., Yuan, W., Lu, Z., & Li, C. M. (2013). Polymer/nanosilver composite coatings for antibacterial applications. *Colloids and Surfaces. A, Physicochemical and Engineering Aspects*, *439*(0), 69–83. doi:10.1016/j.colsurfa.2012.12.029

Hajipour, M. J., Fromm, K. M., Akbar Ashkarran, A., Jimenez de Aberasturi, D., Larramendi, I. R., Rojo, T., Serpooshan, V., Parak, W. J., & Mahmoudi, M. (2012). Antibacterial properties of nanoparticles. *Trends in Biotechnology*, *30*(10), 499–511. doi:10.1016/j.tibtech.2012.06.004 PMID:22884769

Han, J. H. (2005). *Innovations in food packaging* (2nd ed.). Academic Press.

Handy, R. D., & Shaw, B. J. (2007). Toxic effects of nanoparticles and nanomaterials: Implications for public health, risk assessment and the public perception of nanotechnology. *Health Risk & Society*, *9*(2), 125–144. doi:10.1080/13698570701306807

Hirvikorpi, T., Vaha-Nissi, M., Harlin, A., & Karppinen, M. (2010). Comparison of some coating techniques to fabricate barrier layers on packaging materials. *Thin Solid Films*, *518*(19), 5463–5466. doi:10.1016/j.tsf.2010.04.018

Hu, A. W., & Fu, Z. H. (2003). Nanotechnology and its applications in packaging and packaging machinery. *Packaging Engineering*, *24*, 22–24.

Johnston, J. H., Borrmann, T., Rankin, D., Cairns, M., Grindrod, J. E., & McFarlane, A. (2008). Nanostructured composite calcium silicate and some novel applications. *Current Applied Physics*, *8*(3-4), 504–507. doi:10.1016/j.cap.2007.10.060

Jurmanovic, S., Kordi, S., & Steinberg, M. D. (2010). Organically modified silicate thin films doped with colourimetric pH indicators methyl red and bromocresol green as pH responsive sol–gel hybrid materials. *Thin Solid Films*, *518*(8), 2234–2240. doi:10.1016/j.tsf.2009.07.158

Kang, S., Pinault, M., Pfefferle, L. D., & Elimelech, M. (2007). Single-walled carbon nanotubes exhibit strong antimicrobial activity. *Langmuir*, *23*(17), 8670–8673. doi:10.1021/la701067r PMID:17658863

Kanmani, P., & Rhim, J. W. (2014). Physicochemical properties of gelatin/silver nanoparticle antimicrobial composite films. *Food Chemistry*, *148*, 162–169. doi:10.1016/j.foodchem.2013.10.047 PMID:24262541

Kelson, A. B., Carnevali, M., & Truong-Le, V. (2013). Gallium-based anti-infectives: Targeting microbial iron-uptake mechanisms. *Current Opinion in Pharmacology*, *13*(5), 707–716. doi:10.1016/j.coph.2013.07.001 PMID:23876838

Kumar, R., & Munstedt, H. (2005). Silver ion release from antimicrobial polyamide/silver composites. *Biomaterials*, *26*(14), 2081–2088. doi:10.1016/j.biomaterials.2004.05.030 PMID:15576182

Lee, S. W., Mao, C., Flynn, C. E., & Belcher, A. M. (2002). Ordering of quantum dots using genetically engineered viruses. *Science*, *296*(5569), 892–895. doi:10.1126cience.1068054 PMID:11988570

Li, H., Li, F., Wang, L., Sheng, J., Xin, Z., Zhao, L., Xiao, H., Zheng, Y., & Hu, Q. (2009). Effect of nano-packing on preservation quality of Chinese jujube. *Food Chemistry, 114*(2), 547–552. doi:10.1016/j.foodchem.2008.09.085

Li, X. H., Xing, Y. G., Li, W. L., Jiang, Y. H., & Ding, Y. L. (2010). Antibacterial and physical properties of poly (vinyl chloride)-based film coated with ZnO nanoparticles. *Food Science & Technology International, 16*(3), 225–232. doi:10.1177/1082013209353986 PMID:21339138

Lichter, J. A., Van Vliet, K. J., & Rubner, M. F. (2009). Design of antibacterial surfaces and interfaces: Polyelectrolyte multilayers as a multifunctional platform. *Macromolecules, 42*(22), 8573–8586. doi:10.1021/ma901356s

Llorens, A., Lloret, E., Picouet, P. A., Trbojevich, R., & Fernandez, A. (2012). Metallic-based micro and nanocomposites in food contact materials and active food packaging. *Trends in Food Science & Technology, 24*(1), 19–29. doi:10.1016/j.tifs.2011.10.001

Lyons, K., & Whelan, J. (2010). Community engagement to facilitate, legitimize and accelerate the advancement of nanotechnologies in Australia. *NanoEthics, 4*(1), 53–66. doi:10.100711569-009-0070-2

Majeed, K., Jawaid, M., Hassan, A., Abu Bakar, A., Abdul Khalil, H. P. S., Salema, A. A., & Inuwa, I. (2013). Potential materials for food packaging from nanoclay/natural fibres filled hybrid composites. *Materials & Design, 46*(0), 391–410. doi:10.1016/j.matdes.2012.10.044

Martinez-Abad, A., Lagaron, J. M., & Ocio, M. J. (2012). Development and characterization of silver-based antimicrobial ethylene-vinyl alcohol copolymer (EVOH) films for food-packaging applications. *Agricultural and Food Chemistry, 60*(21), 5350–5359. doi:10.1021/jf300334z PMID:22577863

Maynard, A., & Michelson, E. (2014). *The nanotechnology consumer products Inventory*. Retrieved 26/06/2014, from http://www. nanotechproject.org/cpi/

Mills, A., & Hazafy, D. (2008). A solvent-based intelligence ink for oxygen. *Analyst (London), 133*(2), 213–218. doi:10.1039/B713450A PMID:18227944

Mills, A., & Hazafy, D. (2009). Nanocrystalline SnO_2-based, UVB-activated, colourimetric oxygen indicator. *Sensors and Actuators. B, Chemical, 136*(2), 344–349. doi:10.1016/j.snb.2008.12.048

Munro, I. C., Haighton, L. A., Lynch, B. S., & Tafazoli, S. (2009). Technological challenges of addressing new and more complex migrating products from novel food packaging materials. *Food Additives and Contaminants, 26*(12), 1534–1546. doi:10.1080/02652030902995277 PMID:19938328

Nazarov, M. M., Khaydukov, E. V., Sokolov, V. I., Panchenko, V. Y., & Shkurinov, A. P. (2013, september). *Polymer matrix with nanoparticles as a high refraction material for the waveguides*. Paper presented at the Infrared, Millimeter, and Terahertz Waves (IRMMW-THz), 2013 38th International Conference. 10.1109/IRMMW-THz.2013.6665809

NICNAS. (2010). National industrial chemicals notification and assessment scheme. Australian Government. *Gazette*.

Nobile, M. A., Cannarsi, M., Altieri, C., Sinigaglia, M., Favia, P., Iacoviello, G., & D'Agostino, R. (2004). Effect of Ag-containing nanocomposite active packaging system on Survival of Alicyclobacillus acidoterrestris. *Journal of Food Science*, *69*(8), E379–E383. doi:10.1111/j.1365-2621.2004.tb09899.x

Ouattara, B., Simard, R. E., Piette, G., Begin, A., & Holley, R. A. (2000). Diffusion of Acetic and Propionic Acids from Chitosanbased Antimicrobial Packaging Films. *Journal of Food Science*, *65*(5), 768–773. doi:10.1111/j.1365-2621.2000.tb13584.x

Paiva, L. B., Morales, A. R., & Diaz, F. R. V. (2008). Organoclays: Properties preparation and applications. *Applied Clay Science*, *42*(1-2), 8–24. doi:10.1016/j.clay.2008.02.006

Park, S., Marsh, K. S., & Dawson, P. (2010). Application of chitosanincorporated LDPE film to sliced fresh red meats for shelf life extension. *Meat Science*, *85*(3), 493–499. doi:10.1016/j.meatsci.2010.02.022 PMID:20416821

Rhim, J. W., Hong, S. I., Park, H. M., & Ng, P. K. W. (2006). Preparation and characterization of chitosan-based nanocomposite films with antimicrobial activity. *Journal of Agricultural and Food Chemistry*, *54*(16), 5814–5822. doi:10.1021/jf060658h PMID:16881682

Rhim, J. W., Park, H. M., & Ha, C.-S. (2013). Bio-nanocomposites for food packaging applications. *Progress in Polymer Science*, *38*(10-11), 1629–1652. doi:10.1016/j.progpolymsci.2013.05.008

Luoma, S. N. (2008). Silver Nanotechnologies and the Environment: Old Problems or New Challenges? Project on emerging Nanotechnologies, Woodrow Wilson International Center for Scholars.

Sato, A. C. K., Quintas, M. A., Vincente, A. A., & Cunha, R. L. (2011). *Food Grade nanoparticles obtained from natural source ingredients.* Paper presented at the ICEF 11th International Congress on Engineering and Food.

Siegrist, M., Cousin, M.-E., Kastenholz, H., & Wiek, A. (2007). Public acceptance of nanotechnology foods and food packaging: The influence of affect and trust. *Appetite*, *49*(2), 459–466.

Silvestre, C., Duraccio, D., & Cimmino, S. (2011). Food packaging based on polymer nanomaterials. *Progress in Polymer Science*, *36*(12), 1766–1782.

Simon, P., Chaudhry, Q., & Bakos, D. (2008). Migration of engineered nanoparticles from polymer packaging to food - a physicochemical view. *Journal of Food and Nutrition Research*, *47*(3), 105–113.

Smolander, M., Hurme, E., Koivisto, M., & Kivinen, S. (2004). *Indicator.* International Patent WO2004/102185 A1.

Sonkaew, P., Sane, A., & Suppakul, P. (2012). Antioxidant activities of curcumin and ascorbyl dipalmitate nanoparticles and their activities after incorporation into cellulose-based packaging films. *Journal of Agricultural and Food Chemistry*, *60*(21), 5388–5399.

Tiede, K., Boxall, A. B. A., Tear, S. P., Lewis, J., David, H., & Hassellov, M. (2008). Detection and characterization of engineered nanoparticles in food and the environment. *Food Additives and Contaminants*, *25*, 795–821.

Xiu, Z., Zhang, Q., Puppala, H. L., Colvin, V. L., & Alvarez, P. J. J. (2012). Negligible particle specific antibacterial activity of silver nanoparticles. *Nano Letters*, *12*(8), 4271–4275.

Yam, K. L., Takhistov, P. T., & Miltz, J. (2005). Intelligent packaging: Concepts and applications. *Journal of Food Science*, *70*, R1–R10.

Yang, L., & Li, Y. (2006). Simultaneous detection of *Escherichia coli* O157:H7 and *Salmonella Typhimurium* using quantum dots as fluorescence labels. *Analyst (London)*, *131*, 394–401.

Zeng, J., Roberts, S., & Xia, Y. (2010). Nanocrystal-based time-temperature indicators. *Chemistry (Weinheim an der Bergstrasse, Germany)*, *16*, 12559–12563.

Zhou, C. (2013). Theoretical analysis of double-microfluidic-channels photonic crystal fiber sensor based on silver nanowires. *Optics Communications*, *288*, 42–46.

Zook, J., Halter, M., Cleveland, D., & Long, S. (2012). Disentangling the effects of polymer coatings on silver nanoparticle agglomeration, dissolution, and toxicity to determine mechanisms of nanotoxicity. *Journal of Nanoparticle Research*, *14*(10), 1–9.

Chapter 16
Routes of Synthesis and Characterizations of Nanoparticles

Gulzar Ahmed Rather
https://orcid.org/0000-0001-7513-8109
Sathyabama Institute of Science and Technology, India

Arghya Chakravorty
https://orcid.org/0000-0002-7522-8304
Vellore Institute of Technology, Vellore, India

Basharat Ahmad Bhat
University of Kashmir, India

Ishfaq Majeed Malik
University of Kashmir, India

Fayaz Hussain Mir
University of Kashmir, India

Siva Sankar Sana
North University of China, China

Vimala Raghavan
https://orcid.org/0000-0001-9351-9407
Vellore Institute of Technology, Vellore, India

Anima Nanda
Sathyabama Institute of Science and Technology, India

Moharana Choudhury
Voice of Environment (VoE), India

ABSTRACT

An interesting aspect of nanotechnology is the remarkable size-dependent physico-chemical properties of nanomaterials that have led to the rise of synthesis procedures for nanomaterials across a range of sizes, shapes, and chemical compositions. This chapter will concentrate on the different methods such as electron irradiation, laser ablation, and chemical reduction, biological methods, photochemical methods; microwave processing, chemical vapour condensation (CVC), arc discharge, hydrogen plasma-metal reaction, and laser pyrolysis in the vapour phase. This chapter will also include the various characterization techniques for the conformation of nanomaterials such as UV-visible spectroscopy, x-ray diffraction, and electron microscopy (e.g., transmission electron microscopy [TEM], scanning electron microscopy [SEM], and atomic force microscopy [AFM]).

DOI: 10.4018/978-1-7998-5563-7.ch016

INTRODUCTION

Over the time, nanotechnology has gained a great attention. The nanoparticles are the fundamental and essential component of nanotechnology. Nanoparticles are particles in sizes between 1 and 100 nanometers and consist of carbon, silicon, metal oxides or organic matter (Hasan et al., 2015; Chakravorty et al., 2020a). Compared to their respective particles at higher scales, nanoparticles exhibit unique physical, chemical, and biological properties at nanoscales, this phenomenon is due to the volume of a relatively larger surface, increased reactivity or stability in a chemical process, increased mechanical strength etc. (Ealias et al., 2017). Nanomaterials are particles of nanoscale size with improved thermal conductivity, catalytic reactivity, nonlinear optical performance and chemical stability because of their large area-to-volume ratio (Agarwalk et al., 2017).

Based on synthesis, nanoparticles can be of different sizes and shapes like spherical, cylindrical, tetrahedral and hexagonal. The surface can be irregular or uniform with surface variations. Some nanoparticles are amorphous or crystalline with single or multi crystal solids either loose or agglomerated (Machado et al., 2015). Over time, specific metallic and metal oxide nanoparticles are developed using copper, zinc, gold, silver, etc., and used for various applications in fields such as agriculture, drug delivery for medicine farming, etc. Nanoparticles can be synthesized through different approaches such as physical, chemical or biological method. Different synthesis methods and characterization techniques have been used for obtaining nanoparticles depending on the material. This chapter elaborates the different methods of nanomaterial synthesis and different methods for their characterization.

PHYSICAL SYNTHESIS METHODS

The physical methods for the synthesis of nanoparticles come under the top-down approaches or the destructive methods where the bulk materials are reduced to nanometer sized particles (Chakravorty et al., 2019). Physical techniques utilize properties like mechanical pressure, high energy radiations, thermal energy or electrical energy for the generation of nanoparticles. Inert gas condensation, Laser pyrolysis, Sputtering, Laser ablation, Vacuum arc, High energy ball milling are some of the important physical synthesis techniques of nanoparticles and are briefly discussed as under:

Inert Gas Condensation

The Inert gas condensation is the oldest technique synthesizing nanoparticles in the gas phase (Du et al., 2005). It is the technique where the ultrafine metal particles/nanoparticles are generated under the vacuum conditions via the evaporation of a metallic source in an inert gas. Though the technology is old, its applications in the production of nanosized powders/ particles are relatively recent.

The Inert gas condensation (IGC) technique for the synthesis of silver and platinum nanoparticles was found to be the most productive method (Maicu et al., 2014). In its basic design, the method involves evaporation of the metallic source using radiofrequency heating or electron or laser beam as the heating source inside the vacuum chamber. The vapors of the metallic source move from hot source towards the cooler inert gas via the combination of diffusion and convective flow losing energy with each collision, leading to nucleation subsequently the particle formation. The particles thus formed migrate towards cold finger, where they are collected for the subsequent consolidation. Ward *et al.* used this technique for the formation of Mn nanoparticles (Ward et al., 2006).

Pulse Vapor Deposition

The Pulse-vapor deposition (PVD) technique is the frequently used method for the production of nanomaterials, typically in the range of few nanometers to several micrometers (Mark,T. et al., 2003). It is an eco-friendly vacuum deposition technique consisting of the following three steps:

I. Vaporization of the solid state precursor/source material
II. Transportation of the vaporized material
III. Nucleation and generation of thin-films and nanomaterials (Okuyama,K. et al., 2003)

The commonly used PVD methods for the generation of nanoparticles are as:

Sputtering

Among the various physical synthesis methods, the sputter deposition has the capability to generate metallic and intermetallic compounds (Gonzalez, G. et at., 2001). It is the PVD technique in which particles are ejected from the target material in the gaseous phase via the bombardment of energetic ions onto the target material (Shah, P. et al., 2006). Sputtering is usually the accumulation of thin layer of nanoparticles and the properties like thickness of the layer, temperature, substrate type, etc. determine the shape and the size of synthesized nanoparticles (Lugscheider, E. et al., 1998).

Based on the same principle of sputtering, several parameters such as gas species, target- substrate distance, chamber pressure, sputtering time, etc. can be modified to produce metal nanoparticles (Bapat, A. et al., 2003; Kruis,F. et al., 1998; Wu, W.Y. et al., 2002) e.g. Mo nanoparticles were generated by Kath et al. via the sputtering method keeping the target-substrate distance of about nine centimeters (Kaatz, F. H. et al., 1993).

Vacuum Arc

Vacuum arc is another vacuum-based PVD technique in which the arc is used to cause evaporation of the target material. This method proves fruitful in the generation of metallic, ceramic and composite nanomaterials and films. Mg-Al NPs were produced by Akbari *et al.* by varying Mg and Al concentrations using the same technique (Akbari, M. K. et al., 2015). Inter-metallic Fe-Sn NPs were generated by Lein *et al.* using vacuum arc discharge process (Lei, J. P. et al., 2007).

Laser Ablation

In laser ablation technique, the precursor material is targeted by the high energy laser pulses to cause the vaporization of the precursor target (Chen, Y. et al., 2002). The target either metallic or non-metallic material is heated locally to high temperatures to cause its vaporization &during the pulse, a supersonic jet of evaporated material i.e., plume is ejected. As the temperature decreases due to the adiabatic expansion of plume, the particles formed are transported by the carrier gas to the powder collector. In order to obtain different products, the carrier gas may also contain reactive gas components e.g. to obtain oxides oxygen is added, for nitrides ammonia is added & for carbides methane is added (Dieter, V. 2013). In a normal laser ablation process the laser can be either pulsed or continuous. Using the laser ablation technique Gopal et al. synthesized colloidal zinc metallic NPs (Singh, S. C. and Gopal, R. 2007).

In order to synthesize NPs from various solvents, laser ablation synthesis in solution (LASis) technique is commonly used. Here the target metal submerged in a liquid solution is irradiated by a high energy laser beam and causes the plume to condense ultimately resulting in the production of nanoparticles (Amendola, V. and Meneghetti, M. 2009).

Pulse laser deposition (PLD) is the vacuum-based PVD process that utilizes the laser energy to eject the nanomaterials from their target substrates. PLD utilizes the pulsed laser beams usually coming from either excimer laser or NdLYAG laser, for the ablation of the target material. A variety of materials viz., polymers, metallic systems, fullerenes, oxides, nitrides, carbides, etc. can be generated by PLD technique (Bhardwaj et al., 2020). Lee *et al.* reported the production of FeCo NPs in an inert gas atmosphere using PLD technique (Happy et al., 2004). Using the same technique Quintana et al. reported the synthesis of selenium nanoparticles on the three different substrates (I) metallic Au film (II) glass (III) Si wafers (Quintana, M.et al., 2002).

Pulsed Wire Discharge Method

This method is used in synthesizing nanoparticles via a distinct mechanism as compared to other physical methods. In this technique the precursor material usually a metallic wire is vaporized by a pulsed current, which is then cooled by ambient gas to produce nanomaterials. Synthesis of a wide variety of nanomaterials has been recorded by this method (Satyanarayana, T. et al., 2018). The technique being expensive in nature is not used for common industrial purposes and moreover this technique is beneficial for the synthesis of those metal nanoparticles whose precursors are having high electrical conductivity and are available in thin wire forms (Tanaka et al., 2020).

Laser Pyrolysis

The carbon dioxide laser pyrolysis technique was developed during early 1980s by Haggerty *et al.* It is a vapor- phase synthesis process (Daraio, C. et al., 2012; Swihart, M. T. 2003) used to generate a wide variety of nanoparticles such as oxide nanoparticles (TiO_2, SiO_2, Al_2O_3), non-metal NPs (Si, SiC) as well as ternary composites like Si/C/N &Si/Ti/C. In this top-down synthesis strategy, the NP synthesis occurs quickly as soon as the degree of super saturation of condensable product reaches the vapor phase (Swihart, M. T. 2003). Ammonia, sulphur-hexafluoride, ethylene gas are added with reactant precursors as additional chemicals as inert photo-sensitizers to carry out the energy transfer process between precursor material and the laser light (Chetna, D. et al., 2015). The particle growth occurs via coagulation/ coalescence once the nucleation occurs. It has been observed that spherical particle synthesis occurs at higher temperatures while non-spherical/or loose agglomerates of particles are formed at lower temperatures (Swihart, M. T. 2003). In this technique the condensable products are formed at the bridge point of laser beam & the molecular flow of vapor phase precursor reactants. Several nanoparticles have been generated by this method e.g. ceramic nanoparticles (SiC, SiO_2, TiO_2) (Amato, R. et al., 2013), carbon coated TiO_2 nanoparticles, SiC nanoparticles (Scarisoreanu, M. et al., 2013), MoS_2 nanoparticles (Swihart, M. T. 2003).

High Energy Ball Milling

High energy ball milling (HEBM) also called as mechanical alloying method/technique was first used by Benjamin in 1970 to synthesize fine, uniform dispersion of different nanoparticles with varying shapes & dimensionalities (Xing, T. et al., 2013). In HEBM the moving balls transfer their energy to the milled material resulting in rupturing of their chemical bonds & milled material into smaller particles. The physical and morphological qualities of the nanoparticles formed by this method are determined by several factors like the type of mill, milling temperature, ball to powder weight ratio, milling media, etc. (Satyanarayana, T. et al., 2018). Carvahlo *et al.* produced supermagnetic magnetite nanoparticles by HEBM using metallic iron powder as the precursor material (de Carvalho et al., 2013). One of the demerits of this technique is the contamination with the iron but the application of tungsten carbide and the inert atmosphere &/or high vacuum processes reduced the impurity levels within acceptable limits (Namita, R. 2015).

Chemical Methods

There are various chemical methods (Figure 1) which are used to synthesize nanoparticles. Chemical methods are able to produce large quantity of nanoparticles with proper size and shape. However these methods use toxic chemicals for the preparation of nanoparticles, which can be hazardous to humans and environment (Agarwal, H.et al. 2017).

Figure 1. Chemical methods of nanoparticle synthesis

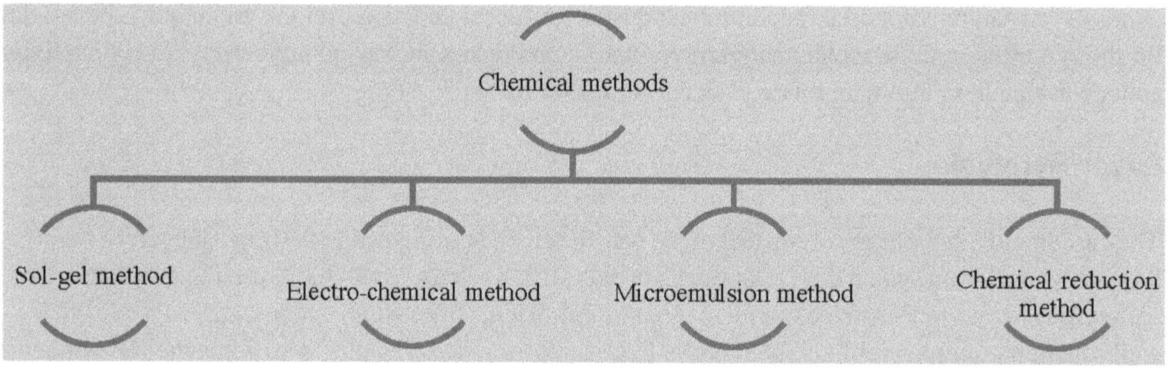

Sol-Gel Method

In the sol–gel processing technique, there are two types of components namely 'sol' which is a colloidal suspension of solid particles in a liquid and 'gel' which are polymers containing liquid. Thus, this process includes the formation of 'sols' in the liquid that lead to the creation of a network of polymers by the connection of sol particles. Condensation and Hydrolysis are the main steps of sol–gel process, in which the hydrolysis use water to disintegrate the bonds of the precursor that is also the first step in formation of the gel phase and then this process is followed by condensation that leads to the production of nanoparticles.

The sol-gel method is relatively rapid and a simple method and is widely used in the design of nanoparticles (Jayaprakash, J.et al., 2014). This method is often applied for the synthesis of nanoparticles as it ensures the control of the size of nanoparticles. Synthesis of CdSe NPs using sol–gel method and realized quantum size effect in fabricated NPs, which is important for developing advanced optoelectronic devices (Goncalves, L.F. et al., 2014); Sol-gel technique is also a promising method for the synthesis of variety of NPs such as metal aluminate NPs, magnetic Fe–Co NPs, ZnO and Fe_2O_3 NPs, ZrB_2 NPs, $GdVO_4$ NPs, Ta_2O_5 NPs (Bayal,N. et al., 2012; Nautiyal,P. et al., 2015; Reda, S.M., 2010; Zhang,Y.et al., 2011; Chumba,N.et al.,2014; Sreethawong, T. et al., 2013). Moreover, in the sol-gel method, the size of nanoparticles is proportionally related with the temperature, physical conditions are very important for the design of functional nanoparticles using this approach (Nithya, K. et al., 2014). Karthik,K.et al., 2011) synthesized CuO NPs with dimensions of 25 nm by a sol-gel method.

Electrochemical Method

This method is used for the synthesis of important nanoparticles which are used in the present research field. In this method, nanoparticles are synthesized by passing electric current between two electrodes which are separated by an electrolyte. Nanoparticle synthesis occurs at the electrolyte-electrode interface. One of the most important advantages of this technique is the ability to control the size and morphology of the resulting CuO NPs by changing current density, time, temperature, composition or voltage (Jadhav, S. et al., 2011).Platinum nanocrystals with high catalytic activity were obtained by electro deposition from a solution containing a metal precursor mixed with urea as a growth directing agent (Zhang, M. et al., 2014).

Microemulsion

The microemulsion method is one of the ideal techniques for the preparation of inorganic nanoparticles, yet the mechanism of nanoparticle formation in the microemulsion has not yet been understood well. However, some researchers have suggested a mechanism for nanoparticle synthesis within microemulsions. When the microemulsion material, including reactants, is mixed together, reactant exchange takes place during the collision of water droplets in the microemulsion. The reactant exchange is too fast and a precipitation reaction occurs in the nanodroplets, which is followed by nucleation growth and coagulation of primary particles, resulting in the final nanoparticles surrounded by water and/or stabilized by surfactants used. Microemulsion method is also used to synthesize nanoparticles of copper with size of 3-13 nm (Salzemann, C. et al., 2004). Microemulsions are thermodynamically stable, and consist of small droplets which possess large interfacial area. These characteristics facilitate their use in nanoparticle synthesis.

Chemical Reduction Method

Michael Faraday, in 1857, reported a systematic study of the synthesis and colors of colloidal gold using chemical reduction technique. The chemical reduction of copper salts is the easiest, simplest and the most commonly used synthetic method for copper nanoparticles. In fact, the production of nano sized metal copper particles with good control of morphologies and sizes using chemical reduction of copper salts can be achieved (Park,B.et al.,2007). One of the most important methods for the synthesis of copper nanoparticles is the reduction chemical method. In this technique a copper salt is reduced by a reducing agent such as polyols, sodium borohydride, hydrazine, ascorbic acid, hypophosphite (Song, X.Y et al., 2004; Su, X.D. et al., 2007; Wu, C. et al., 2006; Zhu, H.T. et al., 2004; Dang, T. et al., 2011; Park, B. et al., 2007).

Biological Methods

The usage of nanoparticles (NPs) in medical sciences, agriculture, cosmetics, electronics and drug delivery is increasing day-by-day leading to a genuine concern about the issues related to their environment and biological safety. The nanoparticles can be produced by different methods including physical, chemical and biological methods. However, the physical and chemical methods are expensive and hazardous to health in addition to being toxic to environment. The biological methods use biological entities such as microorganisms and plants to synthesize nanoparticles (NPs) and these methods are ecofriendly and cost effective. Various biological methods used for the synthesis of nanoparticles are given in figure 1.

Figure 2. Schematic presentation of various biological methods used in the synthesis of NPs.

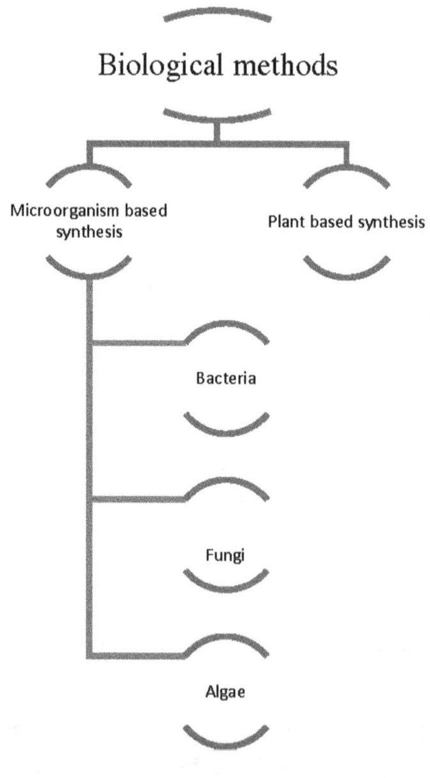

Microbial-Mediated Synthesis Of Nanoparticles

The biological synthesis of nanoparticle is bottom-up approach because formation of nanoparticle occurs due to the reduction of metallic ions by the biomolecules such as enzymes, proteins, and sugars secreted by the microorganism (Prabhu, S. et al., 2012).

Nanoparticle formation by the microorganisms can be either extracellular or intracellular depending upon the type of microorganism. However extracellular synthesis of nanoparticles is more advantageous because the product is easily recovered by simple down streaming without lysis of host cell (Kuppusamy, P. et al., 2014). Microorganisms such as bacteria, fungi, algae and yeasts have been extensively employed for the production of nanoparticles because of their rapid growth and easy cultivation. Table (1) shows some micro organisms that have been used to synthesize a variety of nanoparticles.

Biosynthesis Of Nanoparticles From Bacteria

The major bacterial species used for the synthesis of metallic nanoparticles include *Actinobacter sp., Escherichia coli, Klebsiella pneumonia, Lactobacillus spp., Bacillus cereus, Corynebacterium sp., and Pseudomonas spp.* (Tollamadugu, K.V. et al., 2011; Iravani, S., 2014; Sunkar, S. et al., 2012). Bacteria are known to synthesise metallic nanoparticles by either intracellular or extracellular mechanisms. For example, silver nanoparticles have been synthesized using *Pseudomonas stutzeri*AG259 bacterium via a mechanism involving the NADH-dependent reductase enzyme that provides an electron and oxidizes to NAD^+. The biological reduction of Ag ions to Ag nanoparticles occurs as a result of electron transfer (Ahmad, A. et al., 2003). In a similar study, Husseiny et al. were able to reduce Au ions using *Pseudomonas aeruginosa* that resulted in the extracellular synthesis of Au nanoparticles (Husseiny, M. I. et al., 2011).

Biosynthesis Of Nanoparticles From Fungi

Biosynthesis of nanoparticles using fungi has been extensively studied globally and the synthesis occurs at both extracellular and intracellular locations. Various fungal species like *Verticillium luteoalbum, Fusarium oxysporum, Trichothecium spp., Asperigillus oryzae, Trichoderma viride*, etc., have been reported to synthesize nanoparticles with different shapes and sizes. For example Ag NPs in the size range of 25±12 nm have been prepared by exposing fungal biomass (*Verticillium*) to the aqueous solution of Ag^+ ions, where the NPswere not toxic since the biomass (fungal cells) continues to grow. The NPs were found to grow on the surface of mycelia as a result of electrostatic interaction between the Ag+ ions and negatively charged carboxylate groups of enzymes present in the cell wall of the fungus (Mukherjee, P. et al., 2001).

Fungi possess some additional attributes when compared to their bacterial counterparts for the synthesis of metallic nanoparticles. For instance, fungi secrete large amounts of proteins and enzymes per unit of biomass, which results in larger amounts of biomass, which results in larger amounts of nanoparticles being, manufactured (Jeevanandam, J. et al., 2016). However, few limitations in production of nanoparticles from fungi include time-consuming production process and cost-intensive down streaming processing which need to be addressed in order to develop economical method for commercial scale nanoparticles production (Narayanan, K.B. et al., 2010).

Biosynthesis of nanoparticles from algae

The biosynthesis of nanoparticles using algae is an emerging area of current research. These are competent in the production of different metal and metal oxide nanoparticle **(Patel, V. et al., 2015)**. There are various species of algae which are employed for the synthesis of nanoparticles. For example, *Chlorella vulgaris* was used to synthesize gold (Au) nanoparticles. Extracellular synthesis of gold (Au) and silver (Ag) was also reported from a marine alga (*Sargassum wightii)* (Govindaraju, K. et al., 2009).

Table 1. Biosynthesis of different nanoparticles from microbial sources.

Microbial source	Type of nanoparticles	Shape	References
Bacillus mycoides	Titanium-dioxide	Spherical	**Aenishanslins, N.A.O. et al.,(2014).**
Pencillium fellutanum	Silver	Spherical	**Kathiresan, K. et al.,(2009).**
Lactobacillus sporogens	Zinc oxide	Hxagonal	**Prasad, K.et al., (2009).**
Aeromonas hydrophila	Zinc oxide	Hexagonal	**Jayaseelana,C.et al., (2012).**
Cladosporium	Silver	Spherical	**Balaji, D.S.et al., (2009).**
Rhodobacter sphaeroides	Cadium sulphide	Spherical	**Bai, H.et al.,(2009).**
Lactobacillus crispatus	Titanium dioxide	Spherical, oval	**Salman, J.A.S.et al.,(2014).**
Bacillus sps	Silver	Spherical	**Das, V.L.et al.,(2014).**
Aspergillus flavus	Titanium dioxide	Oval	**Rajakumar, G.et al.,(2012).**
Humicola sps	Cerium oxide	Spherical	**Khan, S.A.et al.,(2013).**

Plant Mediated Synthesis Of Nanoparticles

Plants have the potential to hyper-accumulate and biologically reduce metallic ions (Kulkarni, N.et al., 2014;Kale, A.et al., 2013). As a result of these peculiar properties, plants have been considered eco-friendly route for biologically synthesizing metallic nanoparticles and for detoxification applications (Khan, A.A.et al 2013; Kale, A. et al., 2013). The synthesis of nanoparticles is initiated by addition of extracts obtained from plant parts such as leaves, roots and fruits into the aqueous solution of metal ions. With the materials present in the plant extract, such as sugar, flavonoid, protein, enzyme, polymer and organic acid, acting as a reducing agent, takes part in bioreduction of metal ions into nanoparticles (Iravani, S., 2011; Makarov, V.V. et al., 2014; Nadaroglu, H. et al., 2017; Siddiqi, KS. et al., 2016; Park, S.et al., 2016). The leaf extracts of *Jasminum sambac* were employed to prepare stable Au, Ag, Au–Ag alloy NPs (Yallappa, S. et al., 2015).

The variation in composition and concentration of these active biomolecules between different plants and their subsequent interaction with aqueous metal ions is believed to be the main contributing factors to the diversity of nanoparticle sizes and shapes produced (Li, X. et al., 2011). Properties of the plants extract such as its concentration, metal salt concentration, reaction time, reaction solution pH, and temperature significantly influence the quality, size, and morphology of the synthesized nanoparticles

(Mittal, A.K.et al., 2013; Dwivedi, A.D.et al., 2010). Table (2) shows some plant species that have been used to synthesize nanoparticles.

Table 2. Biosynthesis of different nanoparticles from plant sources.

Plant source	Type of nanoparticle	References
Zingiber officinale extract	Copper	**Subhankari, I.et al., (2013).**
Aloe vera leaf extract	Silver	**Medda, S. et al.,(2014).**
Terminalia catappa leaf extract	Gold	**Ankamwar, B., (2010).**
Cassia auriculata	Zinc oxide	**Ramesh, P. et al., (2014).**
Gloriosa superb	Copper oxide	**Naikaa, H.R. et al., (2015).**
Camellia sinensis	Zinc oxide	**Senthilkumar,.et al.,(2014).**

Figure 3. Different techniques used for nanoparticle analysis.

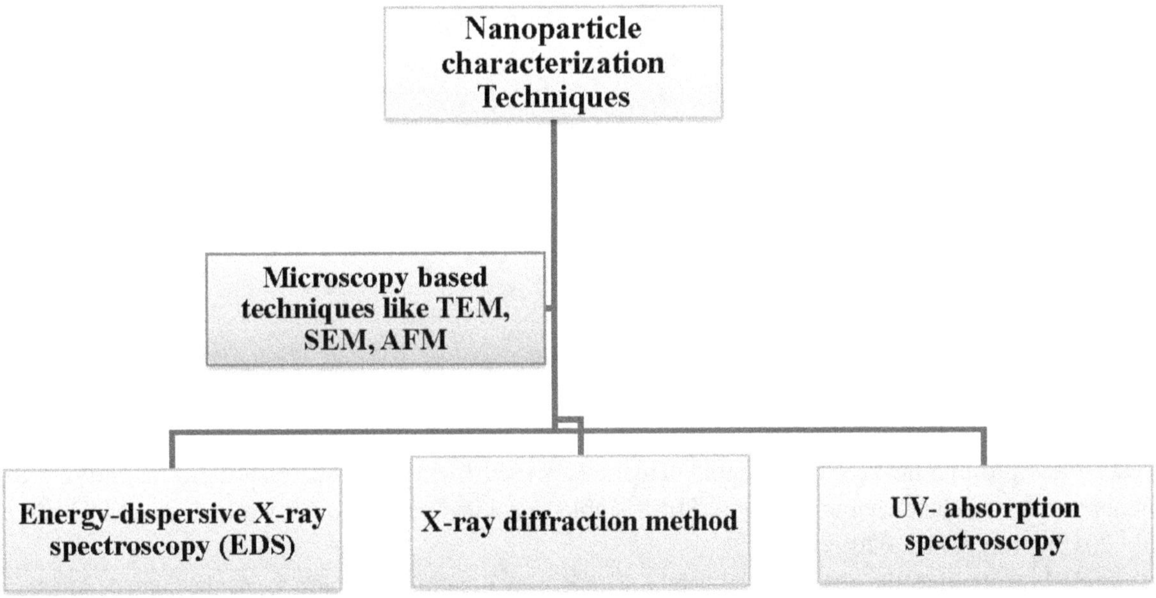

CHARACTERIZATION OF NANOPARTICLES

Nanoparticle possesses various important properties due to which they gained huge interest in the research field. Such properties include optical, high surface to volume ratio, and other physical and chemical properties. They have many applications in biological sciences such as in the treatment of various life threatening diseases. A range of several analytical techniques have been developed for nanoparticle characterization which include (UV, TEM, SEM, FTIR, XRD, DLS and AFM). These techniques are being used to characterize the elemental composition, size, shape, crystal structure, morphology, and various physical and chemical properties of nanoparticles. Till now, there is no single technique that fulfills all the requirements to characterize the nanoparticles completely (Vimala et al., 2011).

Morphological characteristics of nanoparticles can be studied by these techniques namely SEM and TEM. In research these techniques are being used to display that the synthesized nanoparticles were more or less constant in size and shape (Hasan et al., 2015; Nivetha et al., 2020).

Transmission Electron Microscopy (TEM)

TEM is the furthermost technique to characterize nanoparticle morphology and homogeneity. This technique provides the true nanoparticle size and captures accurate image of the sample.

The procedure transmission electron microscopy is that a beam of electrons is transmitted through an ultra-thin specimen and diffuses, interacting with the specimen as it passes through. The image which is formed from the interaction of the electrons diffused through the specimen; the image is magnified and focused onto an imaging device, such as a fluorescent screen which can be detected by a sensor such as a CCD camera. The interaction between electrons and sample depends upon the size, morphology and elemental composition of the sample (Velappan et al., 2020).

TEMs have huge application in cancer research, diagnostics, virology, therapeutic carriers and imaging, materials science as well as nanotechnology research (Ealias et al., 2017; Sitaaraman et al., 2020). TEMs also provide the information about the interparticle distance between two metal NPs when they brought together.

Furthermore, TEM has been also used to assess degree of penetration of NPs, location of NPs within a cell and also helped to understand the cell death pathways in melanoma cells (Agarwal et al., 2017; Raghavan et al., 2020).

Scanning Electron Microscopy (SEM)

SEM is themost widely employed technique to determine the morphologies of nanoscale materials. SEM provides high resolution images of desired nanoparticles. The mechanism of SEM technique is same as an optical microscope, but it quantifies the scattering of electrons rather than photons as electrons are accelerated through the electric potential. This makes the SEM technique versatile in magnifying the nanoparticles size and characterization. SEM is able to achieve resolution down to 1 nm (Machodo et al., 2015; Arun et al., 2020).

In SEM technique, the electrons are used for imaging which interacts and scans the surface of specimen to produce various signals that gives information about the nature of interaction, samples structure and composition. Furthermore, SEM has been used to copy both intact samples as well as partitioned samples (Du et al., 2005; Rajeev et al., 2019).

X-Ray Diffraction (XRD)

X-ray diffraction is the most comprehensive and non-destructive technique to depict NPs. This technique gives data regarding the crystalline phase, crystalline structure, texture as well as strain of nanoparticles. X-ray diffraction technique is achieved after desiccating of the sample of powdered form. The composition of the particles can be examined by comparing the position and intensity of the peaks obtained by using monochromatic beam of x-rays to obtain different peaks. These peaks help in identifying the periodic arrangements of small constituents in the sample. This technique is applicable only analyze crystalline materials but not to amorphous materials (Paul et al., 2020).

Energy-Dispersive X-Ray Spectroscopy (EDS)

This technique is used for elemental composition and chemical characterization of a sample. The procedure of this technique is that an electronic beam is applied in to the specimen. Which focuses and electrons excite in to the inner shell and some to eject from the shell, therefore, generating an electron hole. The difference of energy between the inner shell and the outer shell release in the form of X-rays and the electron in the outer shell having higher energy fills the hole [6].We can obtain information about the elemental composition of specimen by obtaining the distinctive number of peaks as determined by atomic structure (Maicu et al., 2014; Thakur et al., 2015). The electromagnetic emission spectrum of each element is unique. Therefore, EDS microanalysis facilitate for giving information about the structure and composition of such core shell of NPs (Ward et al., 2006; Deb et al.., 2017).

Fourier Transforms Infrared Spectroscopy (FTIR)

This is used to measure the surface composition, molecular structure, nature of the bonds, specific functional groups, interaction and ligand binding of NPs. Absorption electromagnetic spectrum with wavelengths ranging from (4000–400 cm^{-1}) is necessary to characterize the nanoparticles (Mark et al., 2003; Srinivasan et al., 2019). Measures infrared intensity *vs.* wavelength of light, this technique is used to determine the structural features of biological extracts and nature of linked functional group with nanoparticles. The optical properties of nanoparticles can be calculated using spectra which clearly reflect the well-known dependence of nanoparticles. The biological synthesis of silver nanoparticle from various leaf extract was examined by using Fourier Transform Infrared [FTIR] Spectroscopy which revealed distinguishing peaks (Okuyama et al., 2003; Krupa et al., 2019).

Atomic Force Microscopy (AFM)

Atomic force microscopy (AFM) is a microscopy technique generates three dimensional images with high resolution. The forces of attraction between a fine probe and the specimen is the main principle of this technique. When AFM scans the sample due to attractive or repulsive forces between the tipand the sample surface, the information obtained from the laser variation and the final results are calculated by combining forces. AFM can image in three different ways i.e. contact, non-contact and tapping approach (also known as intermediate or oscillating mode) (Gonzalez et al., 2001; Kavitha et al., 2018). The latter is the utmost common when characterizing NPs. The topological characterization of small NPs ($\leq$6 nm), such as ion-doped Y_2O_3, has been achieved by AFM without any special treatment (Shah et al., 2006; Krupa et al., 2017).

UV-Visible Absorption Spectroscopy

This technique is used to determine the optical properties of a solution. A beam of light is driven in the sample solution and the amount of absorbed light is measured. When the wavelength is wide-ranging and the absorbance is measured at each wavelength. The absorbance can be used to at the molecular level and maintain in gprecise control of molecular structure (Lugscheider et al., 1998; Chakravorty et al., 2020b).

REFERENCES

Aenishanslins, N. A. O., Saona, L. A., Dura'n-Toro, V. M., Monra's, J. P., Bravo, D. M., & Donoso, J. M. P. (2014). Use of titanium dioxide nanoparticles biosynthesized by Bacillus mycoides in quantum dot sensitized solar cells. *Microbial Cell Factories*, *13*, 90. PMID:25027643

Agarwal, H., Kumar, S. V., & Rajeshkumar, S. (2017). A review on green synthesis of zinc oxide nanoparticles–An eco-friendly approach. *Resource-Efficient Technologies*, *3*(4), 406–413. doi:10.1016/j.reffit.2017.03.002

Agarwal, H., Kumar, S. V., & Rajeshkumar, S. (2017). A review on green synthesis of zinc oxide nanoparticles–An eco-friendly approach. *Resource-Efficient Technologies*, *3*(4), 406–413. doi:10.1016/j.reffit.2017.03.002

Ahmad, A., Senapati, S., Khan, M. I., Kumar, R., Ramani, R., Srinivas, V., & Sastry, M. (2003). Intracellular synthesis of gold nanoparticles by a novel alkalotolerant actinomycete, Rhodococcus species. *Nanotechnology*, *14*(7), 824–828. doi:10.1088/0957-4484/14/7/323

Akbari, M. K., Derakhshan, R., & Mirzaee, O. (2015). Article. *Chemical Engineering Journal*, *259*, 918–926. doi:10.1016/j.cej.2014.08.053

Amendola, V., & Meneghetti, M. (2009). *Laser ablation synthesis in solution and size manipulation of noble metal nanoparticles*. Academic Press.

Ankamwar, B. (2010). Biosynthesis of gold nanoparticles (green-gold) using leaf extract of Terminalia catappa. *Journal of Chemistry*, *7*, 1334–1339.

Arun, D., Vimala, R., & Ramkumar, K. D. (2020). Investigating the microbial-influenced corrosion of UNS S32750 stainless-steel base alloy and weld seams by biofilm-forming marine bacterium Macrococcus equipercicus. *Bioelectrochemistry (Amsterdam, Netherlands)*, *135*, 107546. doi:10.1016/j.bioelechem.2020.107546 PMID:32413811

Bai, H., Zhang, Z., Guo, Y., & Jia, W. (2009). Biological Synthesis of Size-Controlled Cadmium Sulfide Nanoparticles Using ImmobilizedRhodobacter sphaeroides. *Nanoscale Research Letters*, *4*(7), 717–723. doi:10.100711671-009-9303-0 PMID:20596372

Balaji, D. S., Basavaraja, S., Deshpande, R., Mahesh, D. B., Prabhakar, B. K., & Venkataraman, A. (2009). Extracellular biosynthesis of functionalized silver nanoparticles by strains of Cladosporium cladosporioides fungus. *Colloids and Surfaces. B, Biointerfaces*, *68*(1), 88–92. doi:10.1016/j.colsurfb.2008.09.022 PMID:18995994

Bapat, A., Perrey, C. R., Campbell, S. A., Barry Carter, C., & Kortshagen, U. (2003). Synthesis of highly oriented, single-crystal silicon nanoparticles in a low-pressure, inductively coupled plasma. *Journal of Applied Physics*, *94*(3), 1969–1974. doi:10.1063/1.1586957

Bayal, N., & Jeevanandam, P. (2012). Synthesis of metal aluminate nanoparticles by sol–gel method and studies on their reactivity. *Journal of Alloys and Compounds*, *516*, 27–32. doi:10.1016/j.jallcom.2011.11.080

Bhardwaj, P., Singh, S., Kharangarh, P. R., & Grace, A. N. (2020). Surfactant decorated polypyrrole-carbon materials composites electrodes for supercapacitor. *Diamond and Related Materials*, *108*, 107989. doi:10.1016/j.diamond.2020.107989

BlancoAndujar. C. (2014). *Sodium Carbonate Mediated Synthesis of Iron Oxide NPs to Improve Magnetic Hyperthermia Efficiency and Induce Apoptosis*. University College London.

Chakravorty, A., & Abhishek, N. (2019). Processed Exudate of Pathogen Can Kill Wild Pathogens: Successful In Vitro Application of Newly Synthesized Novel Antimicrobial Therapeutic against Multiple Human Pathogens & Plant Pathogens. *Think India Journal, 22*.

Chakravorty, A., Biswas, B., Sana, S. S., Rayan, R. A., Lala, N. L., & Ramakrishna, S. (2020). A review on toxicity of turmeric derived Nano-Formulates against bacterial and fungal cells with special emphasis on electrospun nanofibers. *Materials Today: Proceedings*. Advance online publication. doi:10.1016/j.matpr.2020.05.820

Chakravorty, A., Rather, G. A., Ali, A., Bhat, B. A., Sana, S. S., Abhishek, N., & Nanda, A. (2020). *Nano Approach: Indian Spices as Antimicrobial Agents. In Ethnopharmacological Investigation of Indian Spices*. IGI Global.

Chen, Y. H., & Yeh, C. S. (2002). Laser ablation method: Use of surfactants to form the dispersed Ag nanoparticles. *Colloids and Surfaces. A, Physicochemical and Engineering Aspects*, *197*(1-3), 133–139. doi:10.1016/S0927-7757(01)00854-8

Chumha, N., Kittiwachana, S., Thongtem, T., Thongtem, S., & Kaowphong, S. (2014). Synthesis and characterization of GdVO4 nanoparticles by a malic acid-assisted sol–gel method. *Materials Letters*, *136*, 18–21. doi:10.1016/j.matlet.2014.07.175

D'Amato, R., Falconieri, M., Gagliardi, S., Popovici, E., Serra, E., Terranova, G., & Borsella, E. (2013). Synthesis of ceramic nanoparticles by laser pyrolysis: From research to applications. *Journal of Analytical and Applied Pyrolysis*, *104*, 461–469. doi:10.1016/j.jaap.2013.05.026

Dang, T. M. D., Le, T. T. T., Fribourg-Blanc, E., & Dang, M. C. (2011). The influence of solvents and surfactants on the preparation of copper nanoparticles by a chemical reduction method. *Advances in Natural Sciences: Nanoscience and Nanotechnology*, *2*(2), 025004. doi:10.1088/2043-6262/2/2/025004

Daraio, C., & Jin, S. (2012). Synthesis and patterning methods for nanostructures useful for biological applications. In *Nanotechnology for biology and medicine* (pp. 27–44). Springer. doi:10.1007/978-0-387-31296-5_2

Das, V. L., Thomas, R., Varghese, R. T., Soniya, E. V., Mathew, J., & Radhakrishnan, E. K. (2014). Extracellular synthesis of silver nanoparticles by the Bacillus strain CS 11 isolated from industrialized area. *3 Biotech, 4*(2), 121-126.

De Carvalho, J. F., De Medeiros, S. N., Morales, M. A., Dantas, A. L., & Carriço, A. S. (2013). Synthesis of magnetite nanoparticles by high energy ball milling. *Applied Surface Science*, *275*, 84–87. doi:10.1016/j.apsusc.2013.01.118

Deb, A., & Vimala, R. (2017). Graphene Mediated Drug Delivery-A Boon to Cancer Therapy. *Research Journal of Pharmacy and Technology*, *10*(5), 1571–1576. doi:10.5958/0974-360X.2017.00276.1

Dhand, C., Dwivedi, N., Loh, X. J., Ying, A. N. J., Verma, N. K., Beuerman, R. W., ... Ramakrishna, S. (2015). Methods and strategies for the synthesis of diverse nanoparticles and their applications: A comprehensive overview. *RSC Advances*, *5*(127), 105003–105037. doi:10.1039/C5RA19388E

Du, J., Liu, Z., Wu, W., Li, Z., Han, B., & Huang, Y. (2005). Preparation of single-crystal copper ferrite nanorods and nanodisks. *Materials Research Bulletin*, *40*(6), 928–935. doi:10.1016/j.materresbull.2005.03.002

Dwivedi, A. D., & Gopal, K. (2010). Biosynthesis of silver and gold nanoparticles using Chenopodium album leafextract. *Colloids and Surfaces. A, Physicochemical and Engineering Aspects*, *369*(1-3), 27–33. doi:10.1016/j.colsurfa.2010.07.020

Ealias, A. M., & Saravanakumar, M. P. (2017, November). A review on the classification, characterization, synthesis of nanoparticles and their application. In IOP Conf. *Ser. Mater. Sci. Eng*, *263*, 032019.

Goldstein, J. I., Newbury, D. E., Michael, J. R., Ritchie, N. W., Scott, J. H. J., & .... (2017). *Scanning Electron Microscopy and X-Ray Microanalysis*. Springer.

Goncalves, L. F., Kanodarwala, F. K., Stride, J. A., Silva, C. J., Pereira, M. R., & Gomes, M. J. (2014). One-pot synthesis of CdSe nanoparticles exhibiting quantum size effect within a sol–gel derived urea-silicate matrix. *Journal of Photochemistry and Photobiology A Chemistry*, *285*, 21–29. doi:10.1016/j.jphotochem.2014.04.005

Gonzalez, G., Freites, J. A., & Rojas, C. E. (2001). Synthesis and characterization of nanophase particles obtained by DC sputtering. *Scripta Materialia*, *44*(8-9), 1883–1887. doi:10.1016/S1359-6462(01)00805-3

Govindaraju, K., Kiruthiga, V., Kumar, V. G., & Singaravelu, G. (2009). Extracellular synthesis of silver nanoparticles by a marine alga, Sargassum wightii Grevilli and their antibacterial effects. *Journal of Nanoscience and Nanotechnology*, *9*(9), 5497–5501. doi:10.1166/jnn.2009.1199 PMID:19928252

Hasan, S. (2015). A review on nanoparticles: Their synthesis and types. *Research Journal of Recent Sciences ISSN*, *2277*, 2502.

Husseiny, M. I., El-Aziz, M. A., Badr, Y., & Mahmoud, M. A. (2007). Biosynthesis of gold nanoparticles using Pseudomonas aeruginosa. *Spectrochimica Acta. Part A: Molecular Spectroscopy*, *67*(3-4), 1003–1006. doi:10.1016/j.saa.2006.09.028 PMID:17084659

Iravani, S. (2011). Green synthesis of metal nanoparticles using plants. *Green Chemistry*, *13*(10), 2638–2650. doi:10.1039/c1gc15386b

Iravani, S. (2014). Bacteria in nanoparticle synthesis: Current status and future prospects. *Int. Sch. Res. Not., 359316.*

Jadhav, S., Gaikwad, S., Nimse, M., & Rajbhoj, A. (2011). Copper oxide nanoparticles: Synthesis, characterization and their antibacterial activity. *Journal of Cluster Science*, *22*(2), 121–129. doi:10.100710876-011-0349-7

Jayaprakash, J., Srinivasan, N., & Chandrasekaran, P. (2014). Surface modifications of CuO nanoparticles using Ethylenediamine tetra acetic acid as a capping agent by sol–gel routine. *Spectrochimica Acta. Part A: Molecular and Biomolecular Spectroscopy*, *123*, 363–368. doi:10.1016/j.saa.2013.12.080 PMID:24412789

Jayaseelana, C., Rahumana, A. A., Kirthi, A. V., Marimuthua, S., Santhoshkumara, T., & Bagavana, A. (2012). Novel microbial route to synthesize ZnO nanoparticles using Aeromonas hydrophila and their activity against pathogenic bacteria and fungi. *Spectrochimica Acta Part A*, *90*, 78–84. doi:10.1016/j.saa.2012.01.006 PMID:22321514

Jeevanandam, J., Chan, Y. S., & Danquah, M. K. (2016). *Biosynthesis of Metal and Metal Oxide Nanoparticles. Chem. Bio. Eng. Rev.*, *3*(2), 55–67.

Kaatz, F. H., Chow, G. M., & Edelstein, A. S. (1993). Narrowing sputtered nanoparticle size distributions. *Journal of Materials Research*, *8*(5), 995–1000. doi:10.1557/JMR.1993.0995

Kale, A., Bao, Y., Zhou, Z., Prevelige, P. E., & Gupta, A. (2013). Directed self-assembly of CdS quantum dots on bacteriophage P22 coat protein templates. *Nanotechnology*, *24*(4), 045603. doi:10.1088/0957-4484/24/4/045603 PMID:23296127

Kale, A., Bao, Y., Zhou, Z., Prevelige, P. E., & Gupta, A. (2013). Prevelige, P.E.; Gupta, A. Directed self-assembly of CdS quantum dots on bacteriophage P22 coat protein templates. *Nanotechnology*, *24*(4), 045603. doi:10.1088/0957-4484/24/4/045603 PMID:23296127

Karthik, K., Jaya, N. V., & Kanagaraj, M. (2011). Arumugam, S. Temperature-dependent magnetic anomalies of CuO nanoparticles. *Solid State Communications*, *151*(7), 564–568. doi:10.1016/j.ssc.2011.01.008

Kathiresan, K., Manivannan, S., Nabeel, M. A., & Dhivya, B. (2009). Studies on silver nanoparticles synthesized by a marine fungus, Penicillium fellutanum isolated from coastal mangrove sediment. *Colloids and Surfaces. B, Biointerfaces*, *71*(1), 133–137. doi:10.1016/j.colsurfb.2009.01.016 PMID:19269142

Kavitha, S., & Raghavan, V. (2018). Isolation and characterization of marine biofilm forming bacteria from a ship's hull. *Frontiers in Biology*, *13*(3), 208–214. doi:10.100711515-018-1496-0

Khan, A.A., Fox, E.K., Gorzny, M.L., Nikulina, E., Brougham, D.F., Wege, C., & Bittner, A.M. (2013). pH control of the electrostatic binding of gold and iron oxide nanoparticles to tobacco mosaic virus. *Langmuir, 29*, 2094–2098.

Khan, S. A., & Ahmad, A. (2013). Fungus mediated synthesis of biomedically important cerium oxide nanoparticles. *Materials Research Bulletin*, *48*(10), 4134–4138. doi:10.1016/j.materresbull.2013.06.038

Kruis, F. E., Fissan, H., & Peled, A. (1998). Synthesis of nanoparticles in the gas phase for electronic, optical and magnetic applications—A review. *Journal of Aerosol Science*, *29*(5-6), 511–535. doi:10.1016/S0021-8502(97)10032-5

Krupa, A. N. D., & Vimala, R. (2017). AgNPs doped TEOS sol–gel coatings to prevent the adhesion of marine fouling organisms. *IET Nanobiotechnology / IET, 12*(2), 99–105. doi:10.1049/iet-nbt.2017.0047

Krupa, N. D., Grace, A. N., & Raghavan, V. (2019). Process optimisation for green synthesis of ZnO nanoparticles and evaluation of its antimacrofouling activity. *IET Nanobiotechnology / IET, 13*(5), 510–514. doi:10.1049/iet-nbt.2018.5396

Kulkarni, N., & Muddapur, U. (2014). Biosynthesis of metal nanoparticles: A review. *Journal of Nanotechnology, 2014*, 510246. doi:10.1155/2014/510246

Kuppusamy, P., Yusoff, M. M., Maniam, G. P., & Govindan, N. (2016). Biosynthesis of metallic nanoparticles using plant derivatives and their new avenues in pharmacological applications–An updated report. *Saudi Pharmaceutical Journal, 24*(4), 473–484. doi:10.1016/j.jsps.2014.11.013 PMID:27330378

Lei, J. P., Dong, X. L., Zhu, X., Lei, G. M., Huang, K. H., Zhang, X. F., Lu, B., Park, W. J., & Chung, H. S. (2007). Formation and characterization of intermetallic Fe–Sn nanoparticles synthesized by an arc discharge method. *Intermetallics, 15*(12), 1589–1594. doi:10.1016/j.intermet.2007.06.010

Li, J., Zeng, H. S., Sun, S., Liu, J. P., & Wang, Z. L. (2004). Analyzing the Structure of CoFe–Fe_3O_4 Core–Shell Nanoparticles by Electron Imaging and Diffraction. *The Journal of Physical Chemistry B, 108*(37), 14005–14008. doi:10.1021/jp047602f

Li, X., Xu, H., Chen, Z. S., & Chen, G. (2011). Biosynthesis of nanoparticles by microorganisms and their applications. *Journal of Nanomaterials, 2011*, 270974. doi:10.1155/2011/270974

Lugscheider, E., Bärwulf, S., Barimani, C., Riester, M., & Hilgers, H. (1998). Magnetron-sputtered hard material coatings on thermoplastic polymers for clean room applications Surf. *CoatingsTechnol., 108-109*, 398–402.

Machado, S., Pacheco, J. G., Nouws, H. P. A., Albergaria, J. T., & Delerue-Matos, C. (2015). Characterization of green zero-valent iron nanoparticles produced with tree leaf extracts. *The Science of the Total Environment, 533*, 76–81. doi:10.1016/j.scitotenv.2015.06.091 PMID:26151651

Maicu, M., Schmittgens, R., Hecker, D., Glöß, D., Frach, P., & Gerlach, G. (2014). Synthesis and deposition of metal nanoparticles by gas condensation process. *Journal of Vacuum Science & Technology A: Vacuum, Surfaces, and Films, 32*(2), 02B113.

Makarov, V. V., Love, A. J., Sinitsyna, O. V., Makarova, S. S., Yaminsky, I. V., Taliansky, M. E., & Kalinina, N. O. (2014). "Green" nanotechnologies: Synthesis of metal nanoparticles using plants. *Acta Naturae, 6*(1 (20)), 35–44. doi:10.32607/20758251-2014-6-1-35-44 PMID:24772325

Mark, T. (2003). Vapor-phase synthesis of nanoparticles. *Current Opinion in Colloid & Interface Science, 8*(1), 127–133. doi:10.1016/S1359-0294(03)00007-4

Medda, S., Hajra, A., Dey, U., Bose, P., & Mondal, N. K. (2014). Biosynthesis of silver nanoparticles from Aloe vera leaf extract and antifungal activity against Rhizopus sp. and Aspergillus sp. *Appl. Nanosci., 5*, 875–880. doi:10.100713204-014-0387-139

Mittal, A. K., Chisti, Y., & Banerjee, U. C. (2013). Synthesis of metallic nanoparticles using plant extracts. *BiotechnologyAdvances, 31*(2), 346–356. doi:10.1016/j.biotechadv.2013.01.003 PMID:23318667

Montes, A., Bisson, M. A., Gardella, J. A. Jr, & Aga, D. S. (2017). Uptake and transformations of engineered nanomaterials: Critical responses observed in terrestrial plants and the model plant Arabidopsis thaliana. *The Science of the Total Environment*, *607-608*, 1497–1516. doi:10.1016/j.scitotenv.2017.06.190 PMID:28793406

Mukherjee, P., Ahmad, A., Mandal, D., Senapati, S., Sainkar, S. R., Khan, M. I., Parishcha, R., Ajaykumar, P. V., Alam, M., Kumar, R., & Sastry, M. (2001). Fungus-mediated synthesis of silver nanoparticles and their immobilization in the mycelial matrix: A novel biological approach to nanoparticle synthesis. *Nano Letters*, *1*(10), 515–519. doi:10.1021/nl0155274

Murugan, A., & Kumara, K., & Shanmugasundaram. (2014). Biosynthesis and characterization of silver nanoparticles using the aqueous extract of vitexnegundo.linn. *World Journal of Pharmacy and Pharmaceutical Sciences*, *3*(8), 1385–1393.

Nadaroglu, H., Gungor, A.A., Ince, S., Babagil, A., (2017). Green synthesis and characterisation of platinum nanoparticles using quail egg yolk. *Spectrochimica Acta Part a-Molecular and Biomolecular Spectros-copy, 172*, 43–7. . doi:10.1016/j.saa.2016.05.023

Naikaa, H. R., Lingarajua, K., Manjunathb, K., Kumar, D., Nagarajuc, G., Sureshd, D., & Nagabhushanae, H. (2015). Green synthesis of CuO nanoparticles using Gloriosa superba L. extract andtheir antibacterial activity. *Journal of Taibah University for Science: JTUSCI*, *9*(1), 7–12. doi:10.1016/j.jtusci.2014.04.006

Narayanan, K. B., & Sakthivel, N. (2010). Biological synthesis of metal nanoparticles by microbes. *Advances in Colloid and Interface Science*, *156*(1-2), 1–13. doi:10.1016/j.cis.2010.02.001 PMID:20181326

Nautiyal, P., Seikh, M. M., Lebedev, O. I., & Kundu, A. K. (2015). Sol–gel synthesis of Fe–Co nanoparticles and magnetization study. *Journal of Magnetism and Magnetic Materials*, *377*, 402–405. doi:10.1016/j.jmmm.2014.10.157

Nithya, K., Yuvasree, P., Neelakandeswari, N., Rajasekaran, N., Uthayarani, K., Chitra, M., & Kumar, S. S. (2014). Preparation and characterization of copper oxide nanoparticles. *International Journal of Chemtech Research*, *6*, 2220–2222.

Nivetha, R., Gothandapani, K., Raghavan, V., Jacob, G., Sellappan, R., Bhardwaj, P., ... Grace, A. N. (2020). Highly Porous MIL-100 (Fe) for the Hydrogen Evolution Reaction (HER) in Acidic and Basic Media. *ACS Omega*.

Okuyama, K., & Lenggoro, I. W. (2003). Preparation of nanoparticles via spray route. *Chemical Engineering Science*, *58*(3-6), 537–547. doi:10.1016/S0009-2509(02)00578-X

Park, B. K., Jeong, S., Kim, D., Moon, J., Lim, S., & Kim, J. S. (2007). Synthesis and size control of monodisperse copper nanoparticles by polyol method. *Journal of Colloid and Interface Science*, *311*(2), 417–424. doi:10.1016/j.jcis.2007.03.039 PMID:17448490

Park, S., Sung, H. K., & Kim, Y. (2016). Green Synthesis of Metal Nanoparticles Using Sprout Plants: Pros and Cons. *Journal of Nanoscience and Nanotechnology*, *16*(5), 4444–4449. doi:10.1166/jnn.2016.10970 PMID:27483771

Patel, V., Berthold, D., Puranik, P., & Gantar, M. (2015). Screening of cyanobacteria and micro algae for their ability to synthesize silver nanoparticles with antibacterial activity. *Biotechnology Reports (Amsterdam, Netherlands)*, *5*, 112–119. doi:10.1016/j.btre.2014.12.001 PMID:28626689

Paul, A. M., Sajeev, A., Nivetha, R., Gothandapani, K., Bhardwaj, P., Govardhan, K., ... Grace, A. N. (2020). Cuprous oxide (Cu2O)/graphitic carbon nitride (g-C3N4) nanocomposites for electrocatalytic hydrogen evolution reaction. *Diamond and Related Materials*, *107*, 107899. doi:10.1016/j.diamond.2020.107899

Perrault, S. D., & Chan, W. C. (2010). In vivo assembly of nanoparticle components to improve targeted cancer imaging. *Proceedings of the National Academy of Sciences of the United States of America*, *107*(25), 11194–11199. doi:10.1073/pnas.1001367107 PMID:20534561

Prabhu, S., & Poulose, E. K. (2012). Silver nanoparticles: Mechanism of anti-microbial action, synthesis, medica lapplications, and toxicity effects. *International Nano Letters*, *2*(1), 1–10. doi:10.1186/2228-5326-2-32

Prasad, K., & Jha, A. K. (2009). ZnO nanoparticles: Synthesis and adsorption study. *Nature and Science*, *1*(02), 129.

Prathna, T. C., & Lazar Mathew, N. (2010). Biomimetic synthesis of nanoparticles: science, technology & applicability. In Biomimetics, learning from nature. InTechOpen.

Quintana, M., Haro-Poniatowski, E., Morales, J., & Batina, N. (2002). Synthesis of selenium nanoparticles by pulsed laser ablation. *Applied Surface Science*, *195*(1-4), 175–186. doi:10.1016/S0169-4332(02)00549-4

Raghavan, V., Deb, A., & Grace, A. N. (2020). *Honokiol-Camptothecin loaded graphene oxide nanoparticle towards combinatorial anti-cancer drug delivery*. IET Nanobiotechnology.

Rajakumar, G., Rahumana, A. A., Roopan, S. M., Khannac, V. G., Elangoa, G., Kamaraja, C., & ... . (2012). Fungus-mediated biosynthesis and characterization of TiO2 nanoparticles and their activity against pathogenic bacteria. *Spectrochimica Acta Part A*, *9*, 123–129. doi:10.1016/j.saa.2012.01.011

Rajeev, P. V., Gnanasekar, S., Sellappan, R., & Grace, A. N. (2019). Synthesis and analysis of Mo2N as efficient counter electrodes for dye sensitized solar cells. *Materials Today: Proceedings*. Advance online publication. doi:10.1016/j.matpr.2019.05.438

Rajput, N. (2015). Methods of preparation of nanoparticles-a review. *International Journal of Advances in Engineering and Technology*, *7*(6), 1806.

Ramesh, P., Rajendran, A., & Shisundaram, M. M. (2014). Green synthesisof zinc oxide nanoparticles using flower extract cassia. *Journal of Nanoscience and Nanotechnology*, *2*, 41–45.

Reda, S. M. (2010). Synthesis of ZnO and Fe2O3 nanoparticles by sol–gel method and their application in dye-sensitized solar cells. *Materials Science in Semiconductor Processing*, *13*(5-6), 417–425. doi:10.1016/j.mssp.2011.09.007

Salman, J. A. S., Ibrahem, K. H., & Ali, F. A. (2014). Effect of culture media on biosynthesis of titanium dioxide nanoparticles using Lactobacillus crispatus. *International Journal of Advanced Research*, *2*, 1014–1021.

Salzemann, C., Lisiecki, I., Brioude, A., Urban, J., & Pileni, M. P. (2004). Collections of copper nanocrystals characterized by different sizes and shapes: Optical response of these nanoobjects. *The Journal of Physical Chemistry B*, *108*(35), 13242–13248. doi:10.1021/jp048491n

Satyanarayana, T., & Sudhakar Reddy, S. (2018). A Review on Chemical and Physical Synthesis Methods of Nanomaterials. *International Journal for Research in Applied Science & Engineering Technology, 6*(1).

Scarisoreanu, M., Morjan, I., Alexandrescu, R., Fleaca, C. T., Badoi, A., Dutu, E., ... Bouhadoun, S. (2014). Enhancing the visible light absorption of titania nanoparticles by S and C doping in a single-step process. *Applied Surface Science*, *302*, 11–18. doi:10.1016/j.apsusc.2014.01.135

Senthilkumar, S. R., & Sivakumar, T. (2014). Green tea (Camelli sinensis) mediated synthesis of zinc oxide (ZnO) nanoparticles and studies on their antimicrobial activities. *International Journal of Pharmacy and Pharmaceutical Sciences*, *6*, 461–465.

Shah, P., & Gavrin, A. (2006). Synthesis of nanoparticles using high-pressure sputtering for magnetic domain imaging. *Journal of Magnetism and Magnetic Materials*, *301*(1), 118–123. doi:10.1016/j.jmmm.2005.06.023

Shobha, G., Moses, V., & Ananda, S. (2014). Biological synthesis of copper nanoparticles and its impact. *International Journal of Pharmaceutical Science Invention*, *3*(8), 6–28.

Siddiqi, K. S., & Husen, A. (2016). Fabrication of metal and metal oxide nanoparticles by algae and their toxic effects. *Nanoscale Research Letters*, *11*(1), 363. doi:10.118611671-016-1580-9 PMID:27530743

Singh, S. C., & Gopal, R. (2007). Zinc nanoparticles in solution by laser ablation technique. *Bulletin of Materials Science*, *30*(3), 291–293. doi:10.100712034-007-0048-z

Sitaaraman, S. R., Santhosh, R., Kollu, P., Jeong, S. K., Sellappan, R., Raghavan, V., ... Grace, A. N. (2020). Role of graphene in NiSe2/graphene composites-Synthesis and testing for electrochemical supercapacitors. *Diamond and Related Materials*.

Song, X., Sun, S., Zhang, W., & Yin, Z. (2004). A method for the synthesis of spherical copper nanoparticles in the organic phase. *Journal of Colloid and Interface Science*, *273*(2), 463–469. doi:10.1016/j.jcis.2004.01.019 PMID:15082381

Sreethawong, T., Ngamsinlapasathian, S., & Yoshikawa, S. (2013). Facile surfactant-aided sol–gel synthesis of mesoporous-assembled Ta2O5 nanoparticles with enhanced photocatalytic H2 production. *Journal of Molecular Catalysis A Chemical*, *374*, 94–101. doi:10.1016/j.molcata.2013.04.003

Srinivasan, K., Samuel, E. J. J., Poopathi, V., & Grace, A. N. (2019). Investigation on energy dependency of dose enhancement factor produced by gold nanoparticle. *Materials Today: Proceedings*, *9*, 446–449. doi:10.1016/j.matpr.2019.02.174

Su, X. D., Zhao, J. Z., Bala, H., Zhu, Y. C., Gao, Y., Ma, S. S., & Wang, Z. C. J. (2007). Article. *PhysChemComm*, *111*(40), 14689–1469.

Subhankari, I., & Nayak, P. L. (2013). Antimicrobial activity of copper nanoparticles synthesised by ginger (Zingiber officinale) extract. *World J. Nano Sci. Technol.*, *2*, 10–13.

Sunkar, S., & Nachiyar, C. V. (2012). Biogenesis of antibacterial silver nanoparticles using the endophytic bacterium Bacillus cereus isolated from Garcinia xanthochymu. *Asian Pacific Journal of Tropical Biomedicine*, *12*(12), 953–959. doi:10.1016/S2221-1691(13)60006-4 PMID:23593575

Swihart, M. T. (2003). Vapor-phase synthesis of nanoparticles. *Current Opinion in Colloid & Interface Science*, *8*(1), 127–133. doi:10.1016/S1359-0294(03)00007-4

Tanaka, S., Nishi, M., Yamaguchi, M., Bataev, I., & Hokamoto, K. (2020). Simultaneous Initiation of Nitromethane in Two Holes by Pulsed Wire Discharge for Crack Control of a Concrete Block. *Journal of Dynamic Behavior of Materials*, *6*(1), 53–63. doi:10.100740870-019-00227-6

Thakur, H., Nirmala Grace, A., & Vimala, R. (2015). Biosorption of di-butyl phthalate from aqueous solutions using Pleurotus ostreatus: Isotherm and Kinetic study. *Journal of Chemical and Pharmaceutical Research*, *7*(4), 697–706.

Tollamadugu, K. V., Prasad, T., Kambala, V. S., & Naidu, R. (2011). A critical review on biogenic silver nanoparticles and their antimicrobial activity. *Current Nanoscience*, *7*, 531–544. doi:10.2174/157341311796196736

Umer, Naveed, & Naveedramzan. (2012). Selection of a suitable method for the synthesis of copper nanoparticles. *World Sci. Publ.Company*, *7*(5), 18.

Velappan, S., Nivedhita, P., Vimala, R., & Raja, S. (2020). Role of nano titania on the thermomechanical properties of silicon carbide refractories. *Ceramics International*, *46*(16), 25921–25926. doi:10.1016/j.ceramint.2020.07.077

Vilalta-Clemente, A., & Gloystein, K. (2008). Principles of Atomic Force Microscopy (AFM). *Proceedings of Physics of Advanced Materials Winter School.*

Vimala, R., Charumathi, D., & Das, N. (2011). Packed bed column studies on Cd (II) removal from industrial wastewater by macrofungus Pleurotus platypus. *Desalination*, *275*(1-3), 291–296. doi:10.1016/j.desal.2011.03.014

Vimala, R., Charumathi, D., & Das, N. (2011). Packed bed column studies on Cd (II) removal from industrial wastewater by macrofungus Pleurotus platypus. *Desalination*, *275*(1-3), 291–296. doi:10.1016/j.desal.2011.03.014

Vollath, D. (2013). *Nanoparticles-Nanocomposites–Nanomaterials: An Introduction for Beginners.* John Wiley & Sons.

Ward, M. B., Brydson, R., & Cochrane, R. F. (2006). Mn nanoparticles produced by inert gas condensation. *Journal of Physics: Conference Series*, *26*(1), 296–299. doi:10.1088/1742-6596/26/1/071

Wu, C., Mosher, B. P., & Zeng, T. (2006). One-step green route to narrowly dispersed copper nanocrystals. *Journal of Nanoparticle Research*, *8*(6), 965–969. doi:10.100711051-005-9065-2

Wu, W. Y., & Ting, J. M. (2002). Growth and characteristics of carbon films with nano-sized metal particles. *Thin Solid Films*, *420*, 166–171. doi:10.1016/S0040-6090(02)00804-0

Xing, T., Sunarso, J., Yang, W., Yin, Y., Glushenkov, A. M., Li, L. H., Howlett, P. C., & Chen, Y. (2013). Ball milling: A green mechanochemical approach for synthesis of nitrogen doped carbon nanoparticles. *Nanoscale*, *5*(17), 7970–7976. doi:10.1039/c3nr02328a PMID:23864038

Yallappa, S., Manjanna, J., & Dhananjaya, B. L. (2015). Phytosynthesis of stable Au, Ag and Au–Ag alloy nanoparticles using J. sambac leaves extract, and their enhanced antimicrobial activity in presence of organic antimicrobials. *Spectrochimica Acta. Part A: Molecular and Biomolecular Spectroscopy*, *137*, 236–243. doi:10.1016/j.saa.2014.08.030 PMID:25222319

Yue, J., Feliciano, T. J., Li, W., Lee, A., & Odom, T. W. (2017). Gold nanoparticle size and shape effects on cellular uptake and intracellular distribution of siRNA nanoconstructs. *Bioconjugate Chemistry*, *28*(6), 1791–1800. doi:10.1021/acs.bioconjchem.7b00252 PMID:28574255

Zhang, M., Lv, J., Li, F.-F., Bao, N., Wang, A.-J., Feng, J.-J., & Zhou, D.-L. (2014). Urea assisted electro_chemical synthesis of flower_like platinum arrays with high electrocatalytic activity. *Electrochimica Acta*, *123*, 227–232. doi:10.1016/j.electacta.2014.01.054

Zhang, Y., Li, R., Jiang, Y., Zhao, B., Duan, H., Li, J., & Feng, Z. (2011). Morphology evolution of ZrB2 nanoparticles synthesized by sol–gel method. *Journal of Solid State Chemistry*, *184*(8), 2047–2052. doi:10.1016/j.jssc.2011.05.040

Zhu, H. T., Lin, Y. S., & Yin, Y. S. (2004). A novel one-step chemical method for preparation of copper nanofluids. *Journal of Colloid and Interface Science*, *277*(1), 100–103. doi:10.1016/j.jcis.2004.04.026 PMID:15276044

Chapter 17
Role of Nanostructured Materials in Health and Medicine

Rafia Bashir
S. P. College, Cluster University, Srinagar, India

Hamida Tun-Nisa Chisti
National Institute of Technology, Srinagar, India

Tauseef Ahmad Rangreez
National Institute of Technology, Srinagar, India

Rizwana Mobin
Government College for Women, Cluster University, Srinagar, India

ABSTRACT

In the recent times, nanotechnology has been the most explored and extensively studied area. With the application of nanotechnology, many devices were devised at a lightning speed, which were earlier impossible to imagine. Nanotechnology offers multiple benefits in treating chronic human diseases by site-specific and target-oriented delivery of precise medicines. This chapter describes the importance of nanoparticle-based devices like nanotubes, quantum dots, carbon nanotubes, dendrimers, etc. and their applications for the treatment of several diseases. Applications of nanoparticles in drug delivery, tuberculosis treatment, and cancer therapy are also explained in this chapter. Nanomedicines can also be used to detect diseases at much earlier stages.

INTRODUCTION

Nanotechnology is concerned with the design, synthesis, and characterization of materials and devices that have a functional organization in at least one dimension on the nanometer (i.e., one billionth of a meter) scale. Nanotechnology has opened a new era of technology which has impact on all sectors of

DOI: 10.4018/978-1-7998-5563-7.ch017

human life: Electronics and computers, mobile phones, cosmetics, paints, food and agriculture industry, and of course healthcare. The potential impact of nanotechnology on health care is immense and pervades many aspects of a new era aptly labeled as 'Nanomedicine'. Nanomedicine is the medical use of engineered nanodevices and nanostructures to deliver drugs, heat, light or other substances to specific cells in the human body and for the detection and treatment of diseases or injuries within the targeted cells, thereby minimizing the damage to healthy cells in the body. In the field of medical science and diagnostics nanomedicine can also be regarded as another implementation of nanotechnology.

Nanomedicine is an interdisciplinary field, where nanoengineering, nanoscience, and nanotechnology interact with the life sciences. Given the broad scope of nanomedicine, we expect it eventually to involve all aspects of medicine. It is expected that nanomedicine will lead to the development of better devices, drugs, and other applications for early diagnoses and treatment of diseases with highefficacy, specificity, and personalization, with the objective being to enhance patient's quality of life. This chapter provides an overview of recent achievements, materials, and technologies belonging to nanomedicines.

Nanoparticles (NPs) are the key components of nanomedicine, however, there is no well defined nomenclature for nanoparticles; therefore, terms such as engineered nanomaterials, nonbiological complex drugs (NBCDs), nanomedicals/nanomedicines, etc. are used freely. Some functions ofglobular biological macromolecules can be replicated with the use of nanomaterials.For example lipid micelles, different polymeric nanostructures, protein constructs, ribonucleic acid (RNA) NPs (RNPs),carbon dots (C-dots), nanodiamonds (NDs), carbon nanotubes (CNTs), graphene, as well as inorganic materials such as mesoporous silica NPs (MSNP), superparamagnetic iron oxide NPs (SPIONs), quantum dots (QDs), gold nanoclusters (GNCS), plasmonic NPs, upconverting NPs (UCNPs), etc. Many of these nanoscale materials have unique size and shape dependent optical, electronic, and magnetic properties, and these properties are dependent upon the methods to synthesize, to purify, and to characterize them. These nanoparticles are size dependent so a small change in their size or shape can significantly change the properties of NPs.

Nanoparticles are used as delivery vehicles for bioactive materials, pharmaceutical agents, and also being developed for the treatment of disease.NP-based carrier systems have a unique ability to cross biological barriers in case of delivery effect. In addition to using nanomedicine to diagnose and to treat diseases, this chapter also focusses the importance of NPs' efficacy and safety in biological systems.

BACKGROUND

Since ancient times, plant-based natural products were widely used as medicines against various diseases by humans. On the basis of traditional knowledge and practices herbs are mainly used for the preparation of modern medicines. Nearly 25% of the major pharmaceutical compounds and their derivatives available today are derived from natural resources (Swamy, 2016). Natural products showed remarkable characteristics which include extraordinary chemical diversity, chemical and biological properties with macromolecular specificity and less toxicity. Despite several advantages, pharmaceutical companies are hesitant to invest more in natural product based drug discovery and drug delivery systems (Beutler et al, 2009) and instead explore the available chemical compounds libraries to discover novel drugs. In drug delivery process the use of large sized materials poses major challenges, including in vivo instability, poor solubility, poor bioavailability, poor absorption, problems with target-specific delivery, and probable adverse effects of drugs. Therefore, to solve these critical issues new drug delivery systems for targeting drugs to specific body parts could be used (Martinho et al, 2011 and Jahangirian et al, 2017).

The field of "Nanomedicine" is the science and technology of diagnosing, treating, and preventing disease and traumatic injury, of relieving pain, and of preserving and improving human health, using nanoscale structured materials, genetic engineering and nonorobots (European Science Foundation, 2005). Hence, nanotechnology plays a signifcant role in advanced medicine/drug formulations, targeting arena and their controlled drug release and delivery with immense success.

In the advanced medical research nanotechnology plays an important role particularly in the development of potential site specific delivery systems with greater efficiencies and lower drug toxicities (Ramachandran and Shanmughavel, 2010). The era of nanotechnology has allowed researchers to design drug delivery systems which have been seen to be suitable for treating chronic intracellular infections (Putheti et al, 2008). The development of nanomedicines, by the use of nanotechnology, is now part of our research and in the European Union (EU) it has been recognized as a Key Enabling Technology, capable of providing new and innovative medical solution to address unmet medical needs (Bleeker et al., 2013; Ossa, 2014; Tinkle et al., 2014; Pita et al., 2016). The application of nanotechnology for medical purposes has been termed nanomedicine and is defined as the use of nanomaterials for diagnosis, monitoring, control, prevention and treatment of diseases (Tinkle et al., 2014). Recent progress in cancer nanotechnology gives rise to exciting opportunities in which diagnosis and treatment are based on the molecular profiles of individual patients (Nie et al, 2007).The word Nanotechnology was first defined by Norio Taniguchi, Tokyo Science University in 1974 (Taniguchi, 1974). Although the application of nanotechnology to medicine seems to be a recent trend, the basic nanotechnology approaches for medical application dates back to many decades (Farokhzad and Langer, 2006). Liposomes are the lipid vesicles which were described in 1965 (Bangham, 2006), and in 1976 the description about the first controlled release polymer system of macromolecules was given (Langer and Folkman, 1976), the first long circulating stealth polymeric nanoparticle was described in 1994 (Gref et al, 1994), the first quantum dot bioconjugate was described in 1998 (Chan and Nie, 1998), and the first nanowire nanosenser was described in 2001 (Cui et al, 2001).

MAIN FOCUS OF THE CHAPTER

Recent developments in nanomedicines involve many diagnostic and therapeutic applications involving nanomaterials and nanodevices. The main aim of any novel therapeutic application is to reduce its toxicity and more target specific. Nanotechnology also finds its usein bacterial and toxin detection. The chapter will discuss about the applications of nanotechnology in targeting various systems for treating different diseases and disorders efficiently. Nanotechnology tools are used in process development and product development. Process development refers to both synthesis of drugs, drug intermediates, and to the development of analytical tools for diagnostics. One of the most important tool is miniaturization and automation in organic synthesis and biological screening on a nanoscale. Specific nanosized receptors present on the surface of the cell can recognize the drug and elicit appropriate response by delivering and releasing the therapy exactly wherever needed. Because of their small size and large surface area relative to their volume, nanoscale devices can readily interact with biomolecules. Nanoscale devices include: nanoparticles [Figure 1], nanotubes, cantilevers, semiconductor nanocrystals, and liposomes.

Figure 1. Multifunctional nanoparticle (Ferrari, 2005)

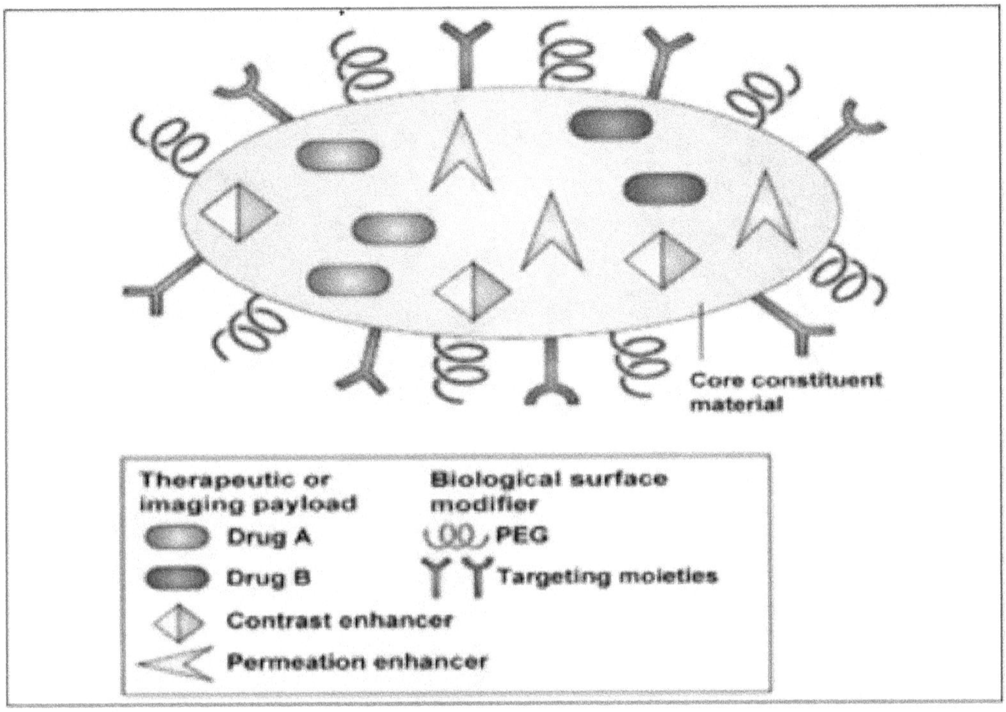

Carbon Nanotubes (CNTs)

CNTs are usually produced by catalytic chemical vapour deposition. CNTs contain metals in it and due to the presence of metals CNTs are paramagnetic in nature.Because of the paramagnetic property these are useful for certain biomedical applications. CNTs vary in diameter and in length. CNTs show unique properties like high tensile strength, heat resistance,high electrical conductivity and efficient thermal conduction and relative chemical inactivity. CNTs are smaller in size than nanopores [Figure 2]. Single walled CNTs and Multiwalled CNTs can be used to transport therapeutic and diagnostic small molecules and macromolecules to cells intracellularly (Ferreira et al, 2008 and Rathod et al, 2011). It has been reported in the literature that different uptake mechanisms like phagocytosis, diffusion and endocytosis are followed. CNTs help to identify Dioxyribonucleic acid (DNA) changes associated with cancer cells. Their diameter is about half the diameter of a DNA molecule. It helps to find out the exact location of the changes. With the help of the nano tube tip the physical shape of the DNA can be traced (Drabu et al, 2010).

Figure 2. Nanotubes (https://trickledown.wordpress.com/2008/05/27/nanotubes-and-asbestos-nutrition-and-the nintendo-wii/)

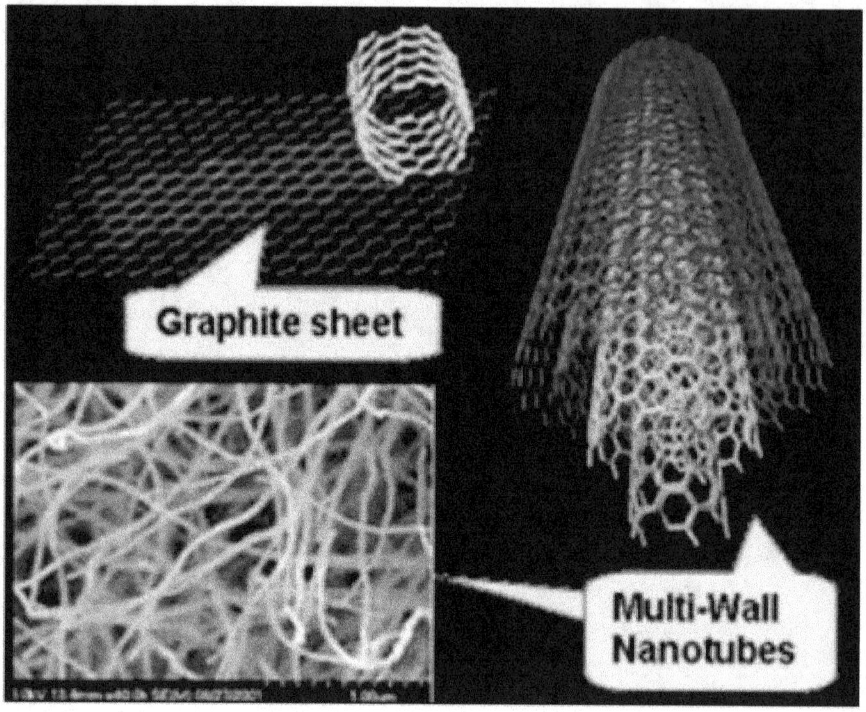

Quantum Dot's

Quantum dots are discovered by Louis E Brus whichconstitute an important class of nanomaterials (Ashoori et al, 1992). They are semiconductor nanocrystals whose excitons i.e, electrons bound to electron holes are confined in three dimensions. The nanocrystals consists elements of groups II-VI, III-V, or IV-VI of periodic tablesurrounded by a metallic shell (ZnS) and they have properties different those of their bulk semiconductors. These are tiny crystals that glow when these are stimulated by ultraviolet light [Figure 3]. The latex beads filled with these crystals when stimulated by light, emit the color that lights up the sequence of interest. Quantum dots can also be used as drug carriers or fluorescent labels for other drug carriers. These are also widely used in biological research (Stroh et al, 2005 and Michalet et al, 2005). For example, iron oxide and gold nanoparticles are the most frequently studied nanoparticles (Li et al, 2006).

Quantum dots are used in medicine for contrasting of blood and lymph vessels (including microvessels) (Lim et al, 2003), but first of all for multiplex molecular diagnostics and visualization in vivo (Gao et al, 2004). Earlier studies revealed that the conjugation of peptides with QDs leads to their selective accumulation in vessels of tumors and other tissues (Gao et al, 2004) whenthe QDs are usedfor molecular diagnostics. Later the studies showing a possibility of "QDs-peptide" conjugates use for specific visualization of tissues in vivo were performed (Pleskova et al, 2018).

The unique optical properties of quantum dots makes them potential candidates for luminescent nano-probes and carriers for biological applications. The QD nano-carriers can be loaded for drugs by the means of dissolving, dispersing, adsorption and coupling, etc (Peer et al, 2007 and Abbaspourrad et al 2013). Then, the physical and chemical properties (like dissolution rate, saturation solubility, crystal form, particle surface hydrophobicity, and hydrophilicity), physical response, and biological characteristics of drugs are changed due to the role of the carriers; thus, the absorption, distribution, metabolism, and excretion of drugs are affected (Oluwole and Nyokong, 2015). Ultimately, the efficacy of drugs can be enhanced by QD nano-carriers and also reduces the side effects of drug reactions to improve the therapeutic index of the drugs (Brigger et al 2002). Moreover, the absorption of small molecule drugs can be effectively promoted by nano-carriers for drugs. At the same time, the research about macromolecular drug delivery has also demonstrated good prospects (Bartosova et al 2012).

Figure 3. Antibody conjugated quantum dotes (Cai et al, 2007)

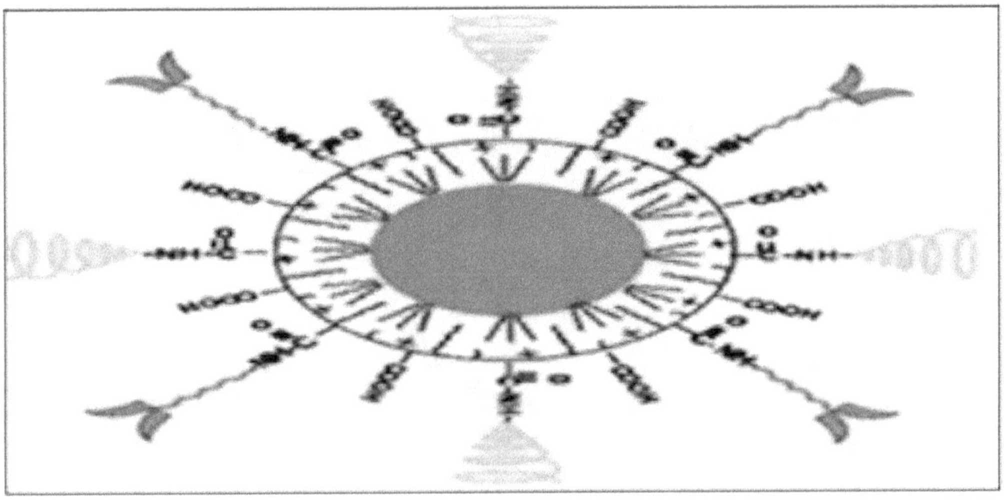

Liposomal Nanoparticles

These are the spherical nanoparticles produced by the use of lipid bilayers [Figure 4]. These nanoparticles are formed within no time when an amphiphilic lipid is added to water or other hydrophilic liquids, yielding 50 to 500 nm sized spheres. By this method hydrophilic drugs can be encapsulated by dissolving the in the liquid used for formation of the nanoparticles. Encapsulation of hydrophobic and amphiphilic drugs can be done by direct addition to the lipid solution before formation of the nanoparticles, thus a layer of drug molecules gets trapped between the lipid bilayer (Sun et al, 2014). The methods which are commonly used for the formation of liposomal nanoparticles include sonication, extrusion, reverse phase evaporation, and solvent injection (Puri et al, 2009).The drug delivery efficiency can be enhanced by liposomes and use of liposomes allows targeted drug delivery to the areas where high frequency electromagnetic radiations such as ultrasound, microwaves and radiofrequency are used (Frenkel, 2008). Hydrophobic and amphiphilic drugs can difuse easily while the hydrophilic drug molecules do not difuse easily through the lipid bilayer which leads to toxicity in normal tissues. Liposomes may ease the issue of hydrophilic drug delivery. The liposomal nanoparticle releases the drug inside the cell by fusing with the cell membrance as the lipid bilayer is similar in structure to the cell membrane. During the past 30 years liposomes have received considerable attention as pharmaceutical carriers with various applications: adjuvants in vaccination, drug delivery vehicles, signal enhancers/carriers in medical diagnostics and analytical biochemistry, solubilizers for various materials as well as support matrix for chemical ingredients.

Figure 4. Basic composition of a liposome – the hydrophobic hydrocarbon tails of the lipid molecules face away from aqueous solutions.

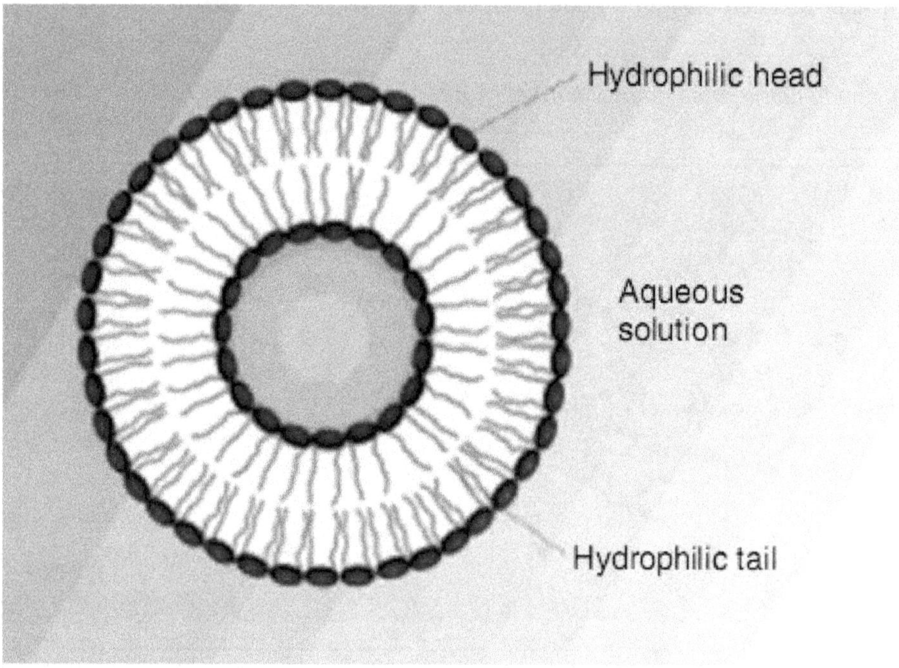

Polymeric Nanoparticles

Polymeric nanoparticles consisting of synthetic polymers in which many key properties are altered such as molecular weight, biodegradability, and hydrophobicity. Polymeric nanoparticles include nanospheres and nanocapsules which can be amorphous or crystalline. Polymeric nanoparticles are typically comprised of dense matrices with well known degradation curves which makes the release of drug easier in these nanoparticles to manipulate in comparison to many other nanoparticle drug delivery systems. These nanoparticles are able to adsorb or encapsulate a drug thereby protecting it against chemical and enzymatic degradation. The drug is confined to a cavity which is surrounded by a polymer membrane in case of nanocapsules [Figure 5], while in case of nanospheres which is matrix systemsthe drug is physically and uniformly dispersed within it.In recent years, biodegradable polymeric nanoparticles have attracted considerable attention in the controlled release of drugs targeting particularly in organs and tissues, as carriers of DNA in gene therapy and in their ability to deliver proteins, peptides and genes by the oral route (Kumaria et al, 2010).

Figure 5. Schematic representation of a nanocapsule drug carrier.

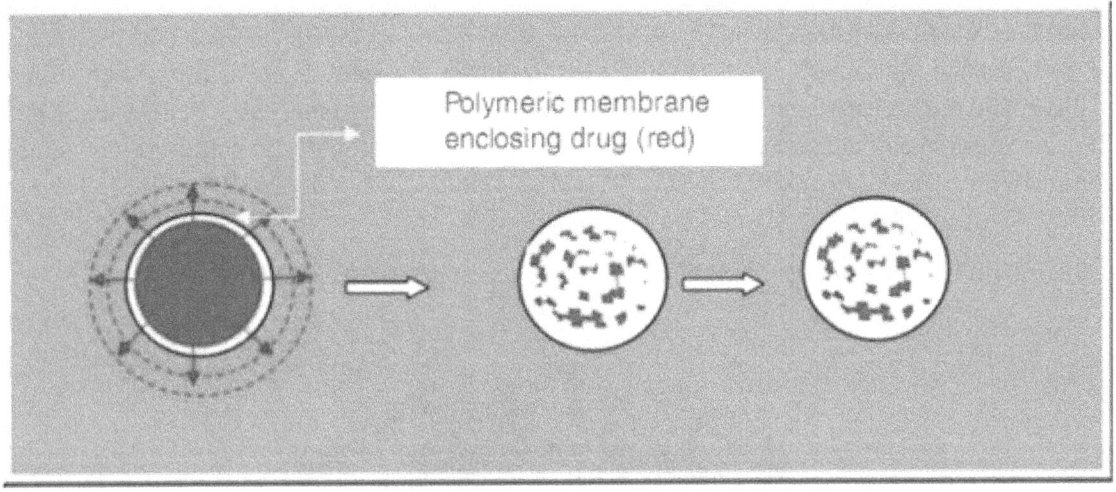

In environmentally sensitive controlled drug delivery systems the release of the drug at the intended site is triggered by the application of an external stimulus such as ultrasound which heats and opens the polymer, thereby releasing the drug.

Dendrimeric Nanoparticles

Dendrimeric nanoparticles consist of dendrimers, which are nanometre-sized, spherical macromolecules with central core, many branching units and terminal functional groups. These nanoparticles are formed layer by layer [Figure 6]. The initial core of the dendrimer is incorporated onto the previous layer before branches are allowed to form. The solubilizing properties of the cavity are determined by core chemistry, whereas the solubility and chemical behaviour of the dendrimer is determined by the external chemical groups. The specific ligands gets attached to the external surface of the dendrimer thereby targets the disease by enabling its binding to disease sites (Kukoswka-Latallo et al, 2005), while by 'decorating' the dendrimers with polyethylene glycol chains the stability and protection from phagocytes is achieved. (Kaminskas et al).

Nanotechnology for the Management of Various Diseases

Management of tuberculosis: Around the world, tuberculosis (TB) still remains the most fatal infectious disease and has socioeconomic disaster for millions of people despite the remarkable advancement in medical science and therapeutics. The treatment of tuberculosis (TB) either depends upon vaccines (i.e., preventive) or on chemotherapy (i.e., therapeutic). With the current tuberculosis chemotherapy the critical problem is that when the drug is administered intravenously or orally, it is distributed throughout the body via the systemic blood circulation and most of the molecules do not reach their targets and, consequently, stay in the body causing adverse side effects. The current anti-TB drugs are although effective, but the need of the hour is to develop urgent strategies so as to accomplish delivery of these drugs. In this connection it is worthwhile to develop a more decisive and more effective drug delivery systems for treatment of TB. Thus, nanotechnology is one of the most promising passages for the treatment of TB along with the potent strategy for the development and delivery of next-generation TB vaccines. For the long-term therapy and also improved pharmacokinetic profile of the drug the lipid nanoparticles and liposomes are successfully used to deliver the antituberclosis drugs with sustained and controlled drug release, and eventually increased bioavailability (Fine, 1995, Pandey and Khuller, 2006). The desired particle size which is required for drug localization upon administration by inhalation is between 50 and 200 nm.

Figure 6. Dendrimer (Available from: https://www.trynano.org/Dendrimers.html.)

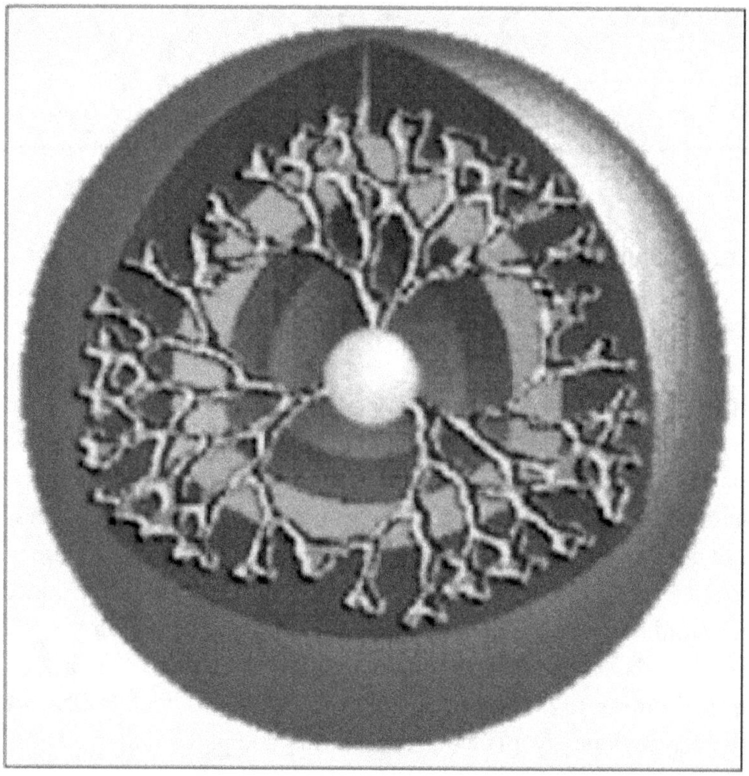

Phagocytic escape by slow release from lungs and mucociliary clearance without inducing any immune responses are promising key factors of nanosized particles. The therapeutic concentration and the lowering of drug doses were maintained by the rapid drug absorption through the pulmonary epithelia and high lung bioavailability. Also, the systemic side effects were reduced by combination of smaller dose with absence of first pass metabolism and prevention of gastrointestinal tract and with increased tolerability. In this context, nanotechnology has emerged as a promising area to rise above the limitations of some of the following factors: (a) increased patient conformity and devotion to regimes, (b) main technological margins, and (c) targeting bacterial reservoirs (e.g., alveolar macrophages) (Sosnik et al, 2010).

Nanotechnology in Pharmaceutical Aerosols

For many years pharmaceutical inhalation aerosols have been playing a crucial role in the health and well being of millions of people throughout the world. The continuous advancement in technology, the easy use and the more desirable pulmonary rather than needle delivery for systemic drugs has increased the attraction for the pharmaceutical aerosol in recent years. But the drug taken by the pulmonary route is technically challenging as oral deposition can be high and changes in inhalation technique can affect the quantity of drug delivered to the lungs. Rapid advances in nanotechnology and nanoscience have showed that bringing nanotechnology to the pharmaceutical aerosol field can help to overcome the drawbacks of conventional aerosol drug delivery system with more efficient mode of drug presentation to the lungs (Sugan and Dutta, 2004 and Buxton, 2006).

To prepare nanosuspensions for drugs which are insoluble in aqueous medium as well as in oily medium new nanotechnological principles are applied, thus gave improved pharmacokinetics which subsequently improved the bioavailability of drugs administrated as aerosols as most of the drugs are not suitable for developing aerosols. Furthermore, development of bioadhesive nanoparticles results in increase in the absorption of the drugs and enhances its bioavailabilty with the increase in mucosal residence time of the drugs(Fadi et al, 2004, Takeuchi et al, 2001 and Patel and Vavia, 2007).

Cancer Detection, Anticancer Drugs and Targeting

Nanomedicines promises a new horizon in diagnosis and treatment of cancer through targeted delivery of drugs, genes and proteins. Cancerous tissues or cells being self becomes very difficult to target the specific cells or organs; as a result, many normal cells are being killed in the process but nanomedicines specifically target to the cancerous cells with minimally induced healthy cells injuries through the use of polymeric nanoparticles, liposomes, dendrimers and nano-shells. Many devices based on nanotechnology have come to the rescue of the formulators, wherein, using biomarkers, the anticancer agents can be targeted only to specific cells or organse.g Photodynamic Therapy (PDT) using 5-aminolaevulinic acid. Quantum dots can produce exceptional images of tumor sites when used in combination with magnetic resonance imaging (Walling and Novak, 2009). These nanoparticles are much brighter than organic dyes and the use of fluorescent quantum dots could produce a higher contrast image and at a lower cost than today's organic dyes as quantum dots absorb only one light source for excitation. But the drawback is quantum dots are usually made up of quite toxic elements. Due to the high surface area to volume ratio nanoparticles allows many functional groups to be attached with it which can bind to certain tumor cells.

The anticancer drug delivery process to a solid tumor consists of five important steps which are: circulation in blood, accumulation and penetration into the tumor, cellular internalization, and intracellular drug release. Thus, the efficiency in each step gives the overall therapeutic efficiency of a nanomedicine [Figure 7] (Sun et al, 2014).These five critical steps are termed as the CAPIR cascade. A nanomedicine which efficiently finish sucessfully the whole CAPIR cascade should have a high therapeutic index. Correspondingly, such a nanomedicine should have 2R2SP properties, 2R stands for drug retention vs release, 2S stands for surface stealthy vs sticky and P stands for tumor penetration (Sun et al, 2012). The drug loaded properties of nanomedicines was given by 2R i.e., during the transport of drug in blood and tumor tissues it must tightly retain the drug without burst release, and the drug is efficiently released at the intracellular target to exert its pharmaceutical action.Similarly, the 2S gives the needed properties in terms of the NP surface, which should be stealthy while in blood circulation for passive tumor accumulation, whereas it should become sticky once nearby the tumor cells to interact with them for efficient cellular uptake. Besides the 2R2S properties, the nanomedicine should be able to penetrate in tumor tissues to reach remote tumor cells from blood vessels (Sun et al, 2014 and Sun et al, 2012).

Figure 7. (A) Five-step CAPIR cascade in targeted cancer drug delivery (Sun et al, 2014). (B) Needed properties of a nanomedicine capable of accomplishing the cascade.

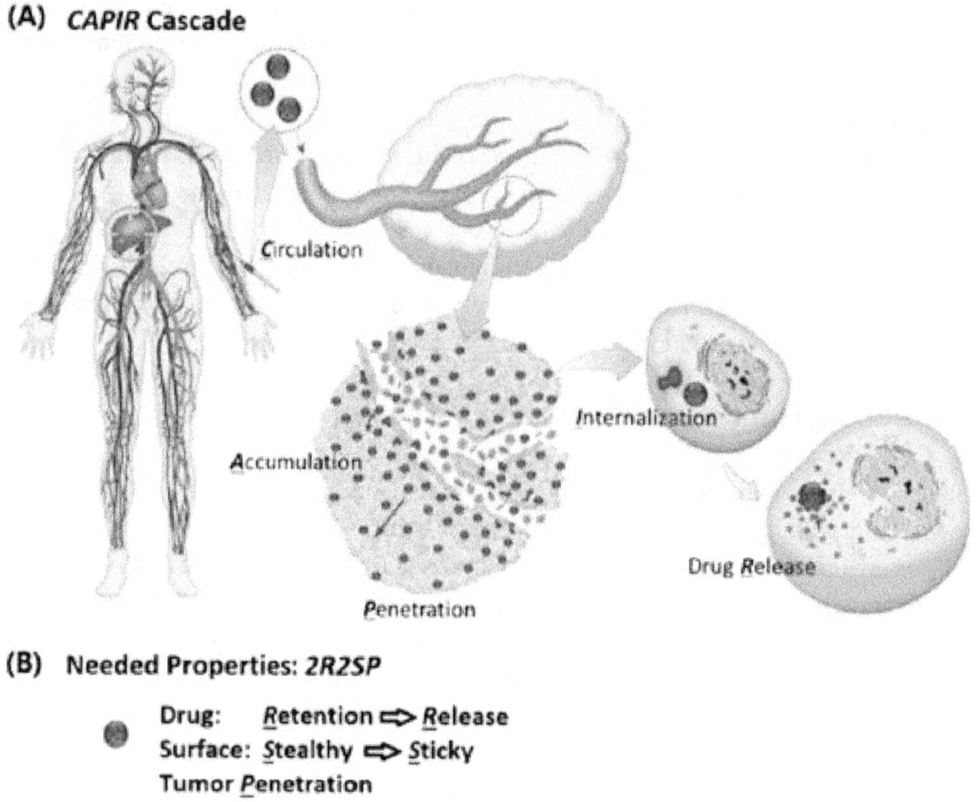

Nucleic Acid Delivery

The major barrier for the delivery of nucleic acids such as small interfering RNA or plasmid DNA is the lipid bilayer of the cell membrane. Nanomedicines have overcome this issue and several nanomedicines have been synthesized that can actively cross the lipid membrane and deliver nucleic acids with ease and reduced toxicity in vitro. Some of the nanomedicines which cross the barrier are viral and polymeric nanocapsules, cationic liposomes, and non-viral vectors like lipoplexes, polyplexes, and inorganic nanoparticles (Hart, 2010 and Patel et al, 2011).

Biochemical Sensors

Another important function of nanoparticles, especially noble metal nanoparticles, is the high catalytic activity for many chemical reactions. As the nanomaterials also have good biocompatibility, they are used to immobilize biomolecules for the fabrication of biosensors. For example Glucose nanosensors are being used for the detection of glucose levels in diabetics. Nanosensors of triglycerides are extremely useful in detecting hyperlipidemia (El-Ansary and Faddah, 2010). For the qualitative and quantitative determination of biomolecular interactions gold colloid-based optical biosensors are used. The synthesis of gold colloid-based localized surface plasmon resonance (LSPR) biosensors and their applications in immunosensing, nucleic acid detection, and quantification of toxins has added much value to this technology in recent years (Mirkin et al, 1996 and Satija et al 2010). Researchers have reported that Oligonucleotide-capped gold nanoparticles are used for the detection of polynucleotide or protein using various detection or characterization methods such as atomic force microscopy, gel electrophoresis, Raman spectroscopy, and surface plasmon resonance imaging (Han et al, 2000 and Cai et al, 2008).

Nanotechnologies in Drug Delivery

The most promising application of nanomaterials is the promise of targeted, site-specific drug delivery. The therapeutic index of nearly all drugs currently being used would be improved if they were more efficiently delivered to their biological targets through appropriate application of nanotechnologies (Sahoo and Labhasetwar, 2003 and Vasir et al, 2005). The nanomaterial based drug delivery has found significant effect to eliminate the tumorous outgrowth without any collateral damage (Wang, 2008) and the functionalized nanoparticles form the basis in designing drug delivery systems (Yokoyama et al, 1990 and Yokoyama et al, 1991). Nanomaterials were initially designed as carriers for vaccines and anticancer drugs (Couvreur et al, 1982) and then by affecting the bio-distribution and toxicodynamics of drugs these may significantly enhance the drug delivery (Thrall, 2004 and Moghimi et al, 2001). By this many types of drugs can be delivered easily which were initially difficult to deliver (Vauthier et al, 2007). A brilliant outcome of this technology is the modification of nanoparticles to deliver drugs through the blood brain barrier for targeting brain tumors (Nazarov et al, 2009). For example, doxorubicin does not cross the blood–brain barrier when it is combined with polysorbate 80 modified polybutylcyanoacrylate nanoparticles can increase its delivery to the brain.

In the recent times a number of drug delivery systems are successfully employed, however there are still certain challenges that need to be addresses. The need of the hour is to develop an advanced technology for successful delivery of drugs to its target sites. Hence the nano based drug delivery systems are currently been studied that will facilitate the advanced system of drug delivery.

Fundamentals of Nanotechnology Based Techniques in Designing of Drug

Nanomedicine is the branch of medicine that utilizes the science of nanotechnology in the prevention and cure of various diseases using the nanoscale materials, such as biocompatible nanoparticles (McNamara et al, 2015) and nanorobots (Saadeh and Vyas, 2014), for various applications including, diagnosis (Oliveira et al, 2014), delivery (De Jong and Borm, 2008), sensory (Holzinger et al, 2014). Drugs with very low solubility possess various biopharmaceutical delivery issues including limited bioaccessibility after intake through mouth, less diffusion capacity into the outer membrane, require more quantity for intravenous intake and unwanted after effects preceding traditional formulated vaccination process. However all these limitations could be overcome by the application of nanotechnology approaches in the drug delivery mechanism.

The most advanced and extensively studied technology in the area of nanoparticle applications is the drug designing because of its potential advantages such as the possibility to modify properties like solubility, difusivity, drug release profles, bioavailability and immunogenicity. This can consequently lead to the improvement and development of convenient administration routes, fewer side effects, lower toxicity, improved biodistribution and extended drug life cycle (Mirza and Siddiqui, 2014). The engineered drug delivery systems are either targeted to a specific location or are intended for the controlled release of therapeutic agents at a specific site. Their formation involves self-assembly where-in well defined structures or patterns spontaneously are formed from building blocks (Lu et al, 2016). Nanostructures can deliver the drugs by two ways which are: passive and self-delivery. In the passive method the drugs are incorporated in the inner cavity of the structure mainly via the hydrophobic effect. The intended amount of the drug is released when the nanostructure materials are targeted to the specific sites, because of the low content of the drugs which is encapsulated in a hydrophobic environment (Lu et al, 2016). Conversely, in the latter, for the easy delivery of drugs, the drugs are released directly conjugated to the carrier nanostructure material. In this method, the timing of release is important as the drug will not reach the target site and it dissociates from the carrier very quickly. The bioactivity and efficacy of the drug will be decreased if it is released from its nano-carrier system at the right time (Lu et al, 2016). Another significant aspect is the targeting of drugs that uses nanomaterials or nano formulations as the drug delivery systems and, is classified into active and passive. In active targeting, the antibodies and peptides are coupled with drug delivery system to adhere them to the receptor structures expressed at the specific site. In passive targeting, the synthesised drug carrier complex circulates through the bloodstream and is taken to the target site by affinity or binding influenced by properties like pH, temperature, molecular site and shape. The main targets in the body are the receptors on cell membranes, lipid components of the cell membrane and antigens or proteins on the cell surfaces (Kumari et al, 2012).

Biopolymeric Nanoparticles in Diagnosis, Detection and Imaging

The integration of therapy and diagnosis is defined as theranostic and is being extensively utilized for cancer treatment (Chen et al, 2014 and Swierczewska et al, 2016). Theranostic nanoparticles can be used to diagnose the disease, location of disease, identify the stage of the disease, and gives information about the treatment response. Theranostic nanoparticles can also carry a therapeutic agent for the tumor, which provides the necessary concentrations of the therapeutic agent via molecular or external stimuli (Chen et al, 2014 and Swierczewska et al, 2016). Chitosan is a biopolymer which possesses good biocompatibility due to the presence of functional groups (Swierczewska et al, 2016 and Yhee et al, 2014). It is used in the nanoparticle encapsulation or coating which thus produces nanoparticles with different functions for their potential uses in the detection and diagnosis of different types of diseases (Swierczewska et al, 2016 and Yhee et al, 2014).

Lee et al (Lee et al, 2011) examined the effect of oleic acid-conjugated chitosan (oleyl-chitosan) FeO nanoparticles in the tumour cells through the penetrability and holding (EPR) consequences under the in vivo state for the analytical uses by the magnetic resonance imaging mechanisms. The analytical techniques showed noticeable signal strength and improvement in the tumor tissues through a higher

EPR consequence after the injection of cyanine-5-attached oleyl-chitosan nanoparticles intravenously (Cyanine 5).

Alginate is a natural polymer which is derived from the brown seaweed and has been extensively studied for its potential uses in the biomedical field because of its characteristics properties like low cost of manufacture, less harmfulness, harmonious nature, and easy gelling in response to the addition of divalent cations (Gombotz and Wee, 1998 and Lee and Mooney, 2012).Baghbani et alsynthesized perfluorohexane (PFH) nanodroplets which are stabilized with alginate to drive doxorubicin and then their sensitivity towards ultrasound and imaging as well as their therapeutic properties was evaluated. Further it has been found that in the breast cancer rat models the ultrasound-facilitated treatment with PFH nanodroplets loaded with doxorubicin showed promising positive responses. The efficacy was characterized by the deterioration of the tumor (Baghbani et al, 2016).

CONCLUSION

The emerging scientific field of nanotechnology due to its outstanding features promises to revolutionize all scientific fields. Nanotechnology has been successful in overcoming the hurdles offered by conventional therapy from the very beginning. The introduction of nanomedicines represents significant advances in the field of drug delivery. Nanoparticles are rapidly becoming the focus of most efforts aiming at targets and site-specific drug delivery. The targeting ability of nanoparticles depends on certain factors such as particle size, surface charge, surface modification and hydrophobicity. Still there are many problems which need to be addressedand are related to selective binding, targeted delivery and toxicity. The options for nanoparticle design and function are extremely varied and the list of potential applications continues to grow, to the point where the drug delivery system can be tailor-made to best suit the selected drug.

REFERENCES

Abbaspourrad, A., Datta, S. S., & Weitz, D. A. (2013). Controlling release from pH-responsive microcapsules. *Langmuir, 29*(41), 12697–12702. doi:10.1021/la403064f PMID:24041287

Ashoori, R. C., Stormer, H. L., Weiner, J. S., Pfeiffer, N. L., Baldwin, K. W., & West, K. W. (1992). N-electron ground state energies of a quantum dot in magnetic field. *Physical Review Letters, 71*(4), 613–616. doi:10.1103/PhysRevLett.71.613 PMID:10055320

Baghbani, F., Moztarzadeh, F., Mohandesi, J. A., Yazdian, F., & MokhtariDizaji, M. (2016), Novel alginate-stabilized doxorubicin-loaded nanodroplets for ultrasounic theranosis of breast cancer. *Int J Biol Macromol, 93*, 512–9.

Bangham, A. D., Standish, M. M., & Watkins, J. C. (1965). Diffusion of univalent ions across the lamellae of swollen phospholipids. *Journal of Molecular Biology, 13*(1), 238–252. doi:10.1016/S0022-2836(65)80093-6 PMID:5859039

Bartosova, L., & Bajgar, J. (2012). Transdermal drug delivery in vitro using diffusion cells. *Current Medicinal Chemistry, 19*(27), 4671–4677. doi:10.2174/092986712803306358 PMID:22934776

Beutler, J. A. (2009). Natural products as a foundation for drug discovery. *Current Protocols in Pharmacology, 46*(1), 9–11. doi:10.1002/0471141755.ph0911s46 PMID:20161632

Bleeker, E. A., de Jong, W. H., Geertsma, R. E., Groenewold, M., Heugens, E. H., Koers-Jacquemijns, M., van de Meent, D., Popma, J. R., Rietveld, A. G., Wijnhoven, S. W. P., Cassee, F. R., & Oomen, A. G. (2013). Considerations on the EU definition of a nanomaterial: Science to support policy making. *Regulatory Toxicology and Pharmacology, 65*(1), 119–125. doi:10.1016/j.yrtph.2012.11.007 PMID:23200793

Brigger, I., Dubernet, C., & Couveur, P. (2002). Nanoparticles in cancer therapy and diagnosis. *Advanced Drug Delivery Reviews, 54*(5), 631–651. doi:10.1016/S0169-409X(02)00044-3 PMID:12204596

Buxton, D. (2006). The Promise of nanotechnology for heart, lung and blood diseases. *Expert Opinion of Drug Deliver*, 173.

Cai, W., Gao, T., & Hong, H. (2008). Applications of gold nanoparticles in cancer nanotechnology, J. Nanotechnology. *Science and Applications, 1*, 17–32. PMID:24198458

Cai, W., Hsu, A. R., Li, Z. B., & Chen, X. (2007). Are quantum dots ready for in vivo imaging in human subjects. *Nanoscale Research Letters, 2*(6), 265–281. doi:10.100711671-007-9061-9 PMID:21394238

Chan, W. C., & Nie, S. (1998). Quantum dot bioconjugates for ultrasensitive nonisotopic detection. *Science, 281*(5385), 2016–2018. doi:10.1126cience.281.5385.2016 PMID:9748158

Chen, F., Ehlerding, E. B., & Cai, W. (2014). Theranostic nanoparticles. *Journal of Nuclear Medicine, 55*(12), 1919–1922. doi:10.2967/jnumed.114.146019 PMID:25413134

Couvreur, P., Kante, B., Grislain, L., Roland, M., & Speiser, P. (1982). Toxicity of polyalkylcyanoacrylate nanoparticles II: Doxorubicin-loaded nanoparticles. *Journal of Pharmaceutical Sciences, 71*(7), 790–792. doi:10.1002/jps.2600710717 PMID:7120064

Cui, Y., Wei, Q., Park, H., & Lieber, C. M. (2001). Nanowire nanosensors for highly sensitive and selective detection of biological and chemical species. *Science, 293*(5533), 1289–1292. doi:10.1126cience.1062711 PMID:11509722

De Jong, W. H., & Borm, P. J. (2008). Drug delivery and nanoparticles: Applications and hazards. *International Journal of Nanomedicine, 3*, 133. doi:10.2147/IJN.S596 PMID:18686775

Drabu, S., Khatri, S., Babu, S., & Verma, D. (2010). Nanotechnology: An introduction to future drug delivery system. *Journal of Chemical and Pharmaceutical Research, 2*, 171–179.

El-Ansary, A., & Faddah, L. M. (2010). Nanoparticles as biochemical sensors. *Nanotechnology, Science and Applications, 3*, 65–76. doi:10.2147/NSA.S8199 PMID:24198472

European Science Foundation. (2005). *Nanomedicine. Forward look on Nanomedicine*. Academic Press.

Fadi, E., Hartwig, S., & Muller, B. W. (2004). In vitro evaluation of Cyclosporin A (CsA) inhalation nanosuspension. *Respir Drug Deliv, 9*(2), 433-6.

Farokhzad, O. C., & Langer, R. (2006). Nanomedicine: Developing smarter therapeutic and diagnostic modalities. *Advanced Drug Delivery Reviews, 58*(14), 1456–1459. doi:10.1016/j.addr.2006.09.011 PMID:17070960

Ferrari, M. (2005). Cancer Nanotechnology: Opportunities and Challenges. *Cancer*, *5*, 161–171. PMID:15738981

Ferreira, L., Karp, J. M., Nobre, L., & Langer, R. (2008). New Opportunities: The Use of Nanotechnologies to Manipulate and Track Stem Cells. *Cell Stem Cell*, *3*(2), 136–146. doi:10.1016/j.stem.2008.07.020 PMID:18682237

Fine, P. E. (1995). Variation in protection by BCG: Implications of and for heterologous immunity. *Lancet*, *346*(8986), 1339–1345. doi:10.1016/S0140-6736(95)92348-9 PMID:7475776

Frenkel, V. (2008). Ultrasound mediated delivery of drugs and genes to solid tumors. *Advanced Drug Delivery Reviews*, *60*(10), 1193–1208. doi:10.1016/j.addr.2008.03.007 PMID:18474406

Gao, X., Cui, Y., Levenson, R. M., Chung, L. W. K., & Nie, S. (2004). In vivo cancer targeting and imaging with semiconductor quantum dots. *Nature Biotechnology*, *22*(8), 969–976. doi:10.1038/nbt994 PMID:15258594

Gombotz, W. R., & Wee, S. (1998). Protein release from alginate matrices. *Advanced Drug Delivery Reviews*, *31*(3), 267–285. doi:10.1016/S0169-409X(97)00124-5 PMID:10837629

Gref, R., Minamitake, Y., Peracchia, M. T., Trubetskoy, V., Torchilin, V., & Langer, R. (1994). Biodegradable long-circulating polymeric nanospheres. *Science*, *263*(5153), 1600–1603. doi:10.1126cience.8128245 PMID:8128245

Han, S., Lin, J., Zhou, F., & Vellanoweth, R. L. (2000). Oligonucleotide-capped gold nanoparticles for improved atomic force microscopic imaging and enhanced selectivity in polynucleotide detection. *Biochemical and Biophysical Research Communications*, *279*(1), 265–269. doi:10.1006/bbrc.2000.3943 PMID:11112450

Hart, S. L. (2010). Multifunctional nanocomplexes for gene transfer and gene therapy. *Cell Biology and Toxicology*, *26*(1), 69–81. doi:10.100710565-009-9141-y PMID:20127400

Holzinger, M., Le Gof, A., & Cosnier, S. (2014). Nanomaterials for biosensing applications: A review. *Frontiers in Chemistry*, *2*, 63. doi:10.3389/fchem.2014.00063 PMID:25221775

Jahangirian, H., Lemraski, E. G., Webster, T. J., Rafee-Moghaddam, R., & Abdollahi, Y. (2017). A review of drug delivery systems based on nanotechnology and green chemistry: Green nanomedicine. *International Journal of Nanomedicine*, *12*, 2957–2978. doi:10.2147/IJN.S127683 PMID:28442906

Kaminskas, L. M., Kelly, B. D., McLeod, V. M., Boyd, B. J., Krippner, G. A., Williams, E. D., & Porter, C. J. H. (2009). Pharmacokinetics and tumor disposition of PEGylated, Methotrexate conjugated Poly-l-lysine Dendrimers. *Molecular Pharmaceutics*, *6*(4), 1190–1204. doi:10.1021/mp900049a PMID:19453158

Kukoswka-Latallo, J. F., Candido, K. A., Cao, Z., Nigavekar, S. S., Majoros, I. J., Thomas, T. P., & ... . (2005). Nanoparticle targeting of anticancer drug improves therapeutic response in animal model of human epithelial cancer. *Cancer Research*, *65*(12), 5317–5324. doi:10.1158/0008-5472.CAN-04-3921 PMID:15958579

Kumari, A., Kumar, V., & Yadav, S. (2012). Nanotechnology: A tool to enhance therapeutic values of natural plant products. *Trends Med Res*, *7*(2), 34–42. doi:10.3923/tmr.2012.34.42

Kumaria, A., Yadava, S. K., & Yadav, S. C. (2010). Biodegradable polymeric nanoparticles based drug delivery systems. *Colloids and Surfaces. B, Biointerfaces*, *75*(1), 1–18. doi:10.1016/j.colsurfb.2009.09.001 PMID:19782542

Langer, R., & Folkman, J. (1976). Polymers for the sustained release of proteins and other macromolecules. *Nature*, *263*(5580), 797–800. doi:10.1038/263797a0 PMID:995197

Lee, C. M., Jang, D., Kim, J., Cheong, S. J., Kim, E. M., Jeong, M. H., Kim, S. H., Kim, D. W., Lim, S. T., Sohn, M. H., Jeong, Y. Y., & Jeong, H.-J. (2011). Oleyl-Chitosan nanoparticles based on a dual probe for Optical/MR imaging in vivo. *Bioconjugate Chemistry*, *22*(2), 186–192. doi:10.1021/bc100241a PMID:21243999

Lee, K. Y., & Mooney, D. J. (2012). Alginate: Properties and biomedical applications. *Progress in Polymer Science*, *37*(1), 106–126. doi:10.1016/j.progpolymsci.2011.06.003 PMID:22125349

Li, L., Fan, M., Brown, R., Van, L. J., Wang, J., Wang, W., Song, Y., & Zhang, P. (2006). Synthesis, properties, and environmental applications of nanoscale iron-based materials: A review. *Critical Reviews in Environmental Science and Technology*, *36*(5), 405–431. doi:10.1080/10643380600620387

Lim, Y. T., Kim, S., Nakayama, A., Stott, N. E., Bawendi, M. G., & Frangioni, J. V. (2003). Selection of quantum dot wavelengths for biomedical assays and imaging. *Molecular Imaging*, *2*(1), 50–64. doi:10.1162/15353500200303100 PMID:12926237

Lu, H., Wang, J., Wang, T., Zhong, J., Bao, Y., & Hao, H. (2016). Recent progress on nanostructures for drug delivery applications. *Journal of Nanomaterials*, *2016*, 2016–2020. doi:10.1155/2016/5762431

Martinho, N., Damgé, C., & Reis, C. P. (2011). Recent advances in drug delivery systems. *Journal of Biomaterials and Nanobiotechnology*, *2*(05), 510–526. doi:10.4236/jbnb.2011.225062

McNamara, K., & Tofail, S. A. (2015). Nanosystems: The use of nanoalloys, metallic, bimetallic, and magnetic nanoparticles in biomedical applications. *Physical Chemistry Chemical Physics*, *17*(42), 27981–27995. doi:10.1039/C5CP00831J PMID:26024211

Michalet, X., Pinaud, F. F., Bentolila, L. A., Tsay, J. M., Doose, S., Li, J. J., Sundaresan, G., Wu, A. M., Gambhir, S. S., & Weiss, S. (2005). Quantum dots for live cells, in vivo imaging, and diagnostics. Science. *Science*, *307*(5709), 538–544. doi:10.1126cience.1104274 PMID:15681376

Mirkin, C. A., Letsinger, R. L., Mucic, R. C., & Storhoff, J. J. (1996). A DNA-based method for rationally assembling nanoparticles into macroscopic materials. *Nature*, *382*(6592), 607–609. doi:10.1038/382607a0 PMID:8757129

Mirza, A. Z., & Siddiqui, F. A. (2014). Nanomedicine and drug delivery: A mini review. *International Nano Letters*, *4*(1), 94. doi:10.100740089-014-0094-7

Moghimi, S. M., Hunter, A. C., & Murray, J. C. (2001). Long-circulating and target-specific nanoparticles: Theory to practice. *Pharmacological Reviews*, *53*, 283. PMID:11356986

Nanotubes and Asbestos. (n.d.). *Nutrition and the Nintendo Wii*. Available from: https://trickledown.wordpress.com/2008/05/27/nanotubes-and-asbestos-nutrition-and-the nintendo-wii/

Nazarov, G. V., Galan, S. E., Nazarova, E. V., Karkishchenko, N. N., Muradov, M. M., & Stepanov, V. A. (2009). Nanosized forms of drugs (a review). *Pharmaceutical Chemistry Journal*, *43*(3), 163–170. doi:10.100711094-009-0259-2

Nie, S., Xing, Y., Kim, G. J., & Simons, J. W. (2007). Nanotechnology applications in cancer. *Annual Review of Biomedical Engineering*, *9*(1), 257–288. doi:10.1146/annurev.bioeng.9.060906.152025 PMID:17439359

Oliveira, O. N. Jr, Iost, R. M., Siqueira, J. R. Jr, Crespilho, F. N., & Caseli, L. (2014). Nanomaterials for diagnosis: Challenges and applications in smart devices based on molecular recognition. *ACS Applied Materials & Interfaces*, *6*(17), 14745–14766. doi:10.1021/am5015056 PMID:24968359

Oluwole, D. O., & Nyokong, T. (2015). Physicochemical behavior of nanohybrids of mono and tetra substituted carboxyphenoxy phthalocyanine covalently linked to GSH-CdTe/CdS/ZnS quantum dots. *Polyhedron*, *87*, 8–16. doi:10.1016/j.poly.2014.10.024

Ossa, D. (2014). *Quality Aspects of Nano-Based Medicines*. SME Workshop: Focus on Quality for Medicines Containing Chemical Entities, London.

Pandey, R., & Khuller, G. K. (2006). Nanotechnology Based Drug Delivery System(s) for the Management of Tuberculosis. *Indian Journal of Experimental Biology*, *44*, 357–366. PMID:16708887

Patel, A. R., & Vavia, P. R. (2007). Nanotechnology and pharmaceutical inhalation aerosols. *Indian Journal of Experimental Biology*, *45*, 166–174. PMID:17375556

Patel, S., Bhirde, A. A., Rusling, J. F., Chen, X., Gutkind, J. S., & Patel, V. (2011). Nano Delivers Big: Designing Molecular Missiles for Cancer Therapeutics. *Pharmaceutics*, *3*(1), 34–52. doi:10.3390/pharmaceutics3010034 PMID:21949900

Peer, D., Karp, J. M., Hong, S., Farokhzad, Q. C., Margalit, R., & Langer, R. (2007). Nanocarriers as an emerging platform for cancer therapy. *Nature Nanotechnology*, *2*(12), 751–760. doi:10.1038/nnano.2007.387 PMID:18654426

Pita, R., Ehmann, F., & Papaluca, M. (2016). Nanomedicines in the EU—Regulatory overview. *The AAPS Journal*, *18*(6), 1576–1582. doi:10.120812248-016-9967-1 PMID:27527889

Pleskova, S., Mikheeva, E., & Gornostaeva, E. (2018). Using of Quantum Dots in Biology and Medicine. *Advances in Experimental Medicine and Biology*, *1048*, 323–334. Advance online publication. doi:10.1007/978-3-319-72041-8_19 PMID:29453547

Puri, A., Loomis, K., Smith, B., Lee, J. H., Yavlovich, A., Heldman, E., & Blumenthal, R. (2009). Lipid-based nanoparticles as pharmaceutical drug carriers: From concepts to clinic. *Critical Reviews in Therapeutic Drug Carrier Systems*, *26*(6), 523–580. doi:10.1615/CritRevTherDrugCarrierSyst.v26.i6.10 PMID:20402623

Putheti, R. R., & Okigbo, R. N., Sai Advanapu, M., & Chavanpatil, S. (2008). Nanotechnology importance in the pharmaceutical industry. *Afr J Pure Applied Chem*, *2*, 27–31.

Ramachandran, R., & Shanmughavel, P. (2010). Preparation and characterization of biopolymeric nanoparticles used in drug delivery. *Indian Journal of Biochemistry & Biophysics*, *47*, 56–59. PMID:21086757

Rathod, K. B., Patel, M. B., Parmar, P. K., Kharadi, S. R., Patel, P. V., & Patel, K. S. (2011). Glimpses of Current Advances of Nanotechnology in Therapeutics. *International Journal of Pharmacy and Pharmaceutical Sciences*, *3*, 8–12.

Saadeh, Y., & Vyas, D. (2014). Nanorobotic applications in medicine: Current proposals and designs. *American Journal of Robotic Surgery*, *1*(1), 4–11. doi:10.1166/ajrs.2014.1010 PMID:26361635

Sahoo, S. K., & Labhasetwar, V. (2003). Nanotech approaches to drug delivery and imaging. *Drug Discovery Today*, *8*(24), 1112–1120. doi:10.1016/S1359-6446(03)02903-9 PMID:14678737

Satija, J., Bharadwaj, R., Sai, V., & Mukherji, S. (2010). Emerging use of nanostructure films containing capped gold nanoparticles in biosensors. *Nanotechnology, Science and Applications, 3*, 171-88.

Sosnik, A., Carcaboso, A. M., Glisoni, R. J., Moretton, M. A., & Chiappetta, D. A. (2010). New old challenges in tuberculosis: Potentially effective nanotechnologies in drug delivery. *Advanced Drug Delivery Reviews*, *62*(4-5), 547–559. doi:10.1016/j.addr.2009.11.023 PMID:19914315

Stroh, M., Zimmer, J. P., Duda, D. G., Levchenko, T. S., Cohen, K. S., Brown, E. B., Scadden, D. T., Torchilin, V. P., Bawendi, M. G., Fukumura, D., & Jain, R. K. (2005). Quantum dots spectrally distinguish multiple species within the tumor milieu in vivo. *Nature Medicine*, *11*(6), 678–682. doi:10.1038/nm1247 PMID:15880117

Sugan, A., & Dutta, J. (2004). Nanoparticles for nanotechnology. *PSI Jilid, 50*.

Sun, Q. H., Radosz, M., & Shen, Y. Q. (2012). Challenges in Design of Translational Nanocarriers. *Journal of Controlled Release*, *164*(2), 156–169. doi:10.1016/j.jconrel.2012.05.042 PMID:22664472

Sun, Q. H., Sun, X. R., Ma, X. P., Zhou, Z. X., Jin, E. L., Zhang, B., Shen, Y. Q., Van Kirk, E. A., Murdoch, W. J., Lott, J. R., Lodge, T. P., Radosz, M., & Zhao, Y. L. (2014). Integration of Nanoassembly Functions for an Effective Delivery Cascade for Cancer Drugs. *Advanced Materials*, *26*(45), 7615–7621. doi:10.1002/adma.201401554 PMID:25328159

Sun, T., Zhang, Y. S., Pang, B., Hyun, D. C., Yang, M., & Xia, Y. (2014). Engineered nanoparticles for drug delivery in cancer therapy. *Angewandte Chemie International Edition*, *53*(46), 12320–12364. doi:10.1002/anie.201403036 PMID:25294565

Swamy, M. K., & Sinniah, U. R. (2016). Patchouli (Pogostemon Cablin Benth.): Botany, agrotechnology, and biotechnological aspects. *Industrial Crops and Products*, *87*, 161–176. doi:10.1016/j.indcrop.2016.04.032

Swierczewska, M., Han, H., Kim, K., Park, J., & Lee, S. (2016). Polysaccharide-based nanoparticles for theranostic nanomedicine. *Advanced Drug Delivery Reviews*, *99*, 70–84. doi:10.1016/j.addr.2015.11.015 PMID:26639578

Takeuchi, H., Yamamoto, H., & Kawashima, Y. (2001). Mucoadhesive nanoparticulate systems for peptide drug delivery. *Advanced Drug Delivery Reviews*, *47*(1), 39–54. doi:10.1016/S0169-409X(00)00120-4 PMID:11251244

Taniguchi, N. (1974). On the basic concept of nano-technology. *Proc. Intl. Conf. Prod. Eng. Tokyo, Part II, 10*, 5-10.

Thrall, J.H. (2004). Nanotechnology and medicine. *Radiology, 230*, 315–318.

Tinkle, S., McNeil, S. E., Mühlebach, S., Bawa, R., Borchard, G., Barenholz, Y. C., Tamarkin, L., & Desai, N. (2014). Nanomedicines: Addressing the scientific and regulatory gap. *Annals of the New York Academy of Sciences, 1313*(1), 35–56. doi:10.1111/nyas.12403 PMID:24673240

Vasir, J. K., Reddy, M. K., & Labhasetwar, V. (2005). Nanosystems in drug targeting:opportunities and challenges. *Current Nanoscience, 1*(1), 47–64. doi:10.2174/1573413052953110

Vauthier, C., Labarre, D., & Ponchel, G. (2007). Design aspects of poly(alkylcyanoacrylate) nanoparticles for drug delivery. *J. Drug Target., 15*, 641.

Walling, M. A., Novak, J., & Shepard, J. R. E. (2009). Quantum Dots for live cell & in vivo imaging. *International Journal of Molecular Sciences, 10*(2), 441–491. doi:10.3390/ijms10020441 PMID:19333416

Wang, L., Zhao, W., & Tan, W. (2008). Bioconjugated silica nanoparticles: development and applications, Bioconjugated silica nanoparticles: development and applications. *Nano Research, 1*(2), 99–115. doi:10.100712274-008-8018-3

Yhee, J. Y., Son, S., Kim, S. H., Park, K., Choi, K., & Kwon, I. C. (2014). Self-assembled glycol chitosan nanoparticles for disease-specifc theranostics. *Journal of Controlled Release, 193*, 202–213. doi:10.1016/j.jconrel.2014.05.009 PMID:24845129

Yokoyama, M., Miyauchi, M., Yamada, N., Okano, T., Sakurai, Y., Kataoka, K., & Inoue, S. (1990). Polymer micelles as novel drug carrier: Adriamycin-conjugated poly(ethylene glycol)-poly(aspartic acid) block copolymer. *Journal of Controlled Release, 11*(1-3), 269–278. doi:10.1016/0168-3659(90)90139-K

Yokoyama, M., Okano, T., Sakurai, Y., Ekimoto, H., Shibazaki, C., & Kataoka, K. (1991). Toxicity and antitumor activity against solid tumors of micelle-forming polymeric anticancer drug and its extremely long circulation in blood. *Cancer Research, 51*, 3229–3236. PMID:2039998

KEY TERMS AND DEFINITIONS

Nanomedicines: It is the branch of medicine concerned with the use of nanotechnology.

Nanopharmaceutical Aerosol: It can be defined as an aerosol product containing therapeutically active ingredients dissolved in a propellant solvent for oral administration into body.

Nanostructured Material: Nanoscale particles of organic and inorganic materialswhose diamensions are 1-100nm.

Quantum Dots: Quantum dots (QDs) are semiconductor nanoparticles whose optical and electronic properties differ from larger particles due to quantum mechanics.

Chapter 18
Implication of Nanoparticles in Drosophila Toxicology Research

Sumira Malik
https://orcid.org/0000-0001-5077-1493
Amity Institute of Biotechnology, Amity University, Ranchi, India

ABSTRACT

Homo sapiens and Drosophila malenogaster, a fruit fly, share genetic homology in development process regulated through fundamental biological pathways and conserved mechanisms conserved as a process of evolution among these species. Drosophila melanogaster is an eminent model organism to study diverse biological species. In this chapter, the use of wide variety of nano particles and their impact on Drosophila melanogastsr's development, longevity, characteristics of reproduction has been studied.

INTRODUCTION

Nanoparticles *and Drosophila melanogaster* as a model: A nanoparticle has vast potential applications in field of medicine where they are used in diagnostic techniques, tissue repair, drug delivery and antibacterial treatments (Krukemeyer et al., 2015). The small size of NPs aids them to facilitate the active ingredient in crossing cell membranes and penetrating the skin (Gupta et al., 2013). The nanotechnological practices include major application in field of cosmeceuticals for the delivery of formulated nanocosmeceuticals used for hair, nail, lips and skin (Kaul et al., 2018). However, NPs have some potential health risks as they possess increased solubility which allows them to more easily cross the membrane barrier leading to increasing toxicity (Brunner et al., 2006). Upon inhalation, these NPs can accumulate in the respiratory tract and move on to other organs through blood stream and cause them to accumulate in gastrointestinal tract, liver and brain. Nanoparticles are the remarkably small particles having a length of 1-100 nm in one or more dimensions imparting it a higher surface-area to volume ratio which accounts for their remarkable optical and electrical properties. The shape of NPs in form of tubes, chains and spheres contribute in their unique properties, which cannot be substituted by the bulky material. Nanoparticles (NPs) cover a developing aspect of our environmental, industrial and clinical economy. The model organism *Drosophila melanogaster* offers an effective example for investigating human dis-

DOI: 10.4018/978-1-7998-5563-7.ch018

eases and nano toxicity. Therefore it is accountable for specific human genetic diseases, which include immunological, auditory, visual, neurological, cardiovascular, developmental and metabolic disorders (Koh et al., 2006; Khurana et al., 2006; Wolf et al., 2006; Reiter et al., 2001). *Drosophila melanogaster* is also used as a fly model for the study of different genes involved in the molecular pathway of neurodegeneration relevant diseases and aging-associated diseases such as cancer, neurodegeneration and chronic inflammation (Sykiotis & Bohmann, 2008). It serves as an appropriate model organism for the cost effective and flexible experimental procedures to be performed in limited span of time with rapid results which eventually supports the rapid assessment of the large number of NP for the reproductive and chronic effects. It is a non-vertebrate organism shares the significant conservation of genetic and signaling pathways with humans and therefore it is preferred as model organism for nano particle studies.

BACKGROUND

***Drosophila melanogaster* as a model to study human disease and toxicity:** *Drosophila melanogaster* research has contributed in the study of human disease and the role of many genes such as α-synuclein function in development of Parkinson's has been elucidated in fly (Feany & Bender, 2000). The onset of Alzheimer's disease has been shown associated to Presenilin (McBride et al., 2010) from cancer (Rudrapatna et al., 2012) and drug addiction (Bainton et al., 2000) to sleep problems (Huber et al., 2004), therefore the knowledge about almost any human disease condition of significance has been benefited from *Drosophila melanogaster* research. This model has been used to study herbicide toxicity, to explore the mechanisms of genotoxicity of herbicides (Kaya et al., 2000) and also the toxicity of drugs such as cocaine (McClung & Hirsh, 1998). It is also considered as a high throughput assay due to its rapid reproduction in short span time, cheap maintenance, easily identifiable mutant phenotypes, and ability for high order screening. *Drosophila melanogaster* life cycle has four discrete parts: embryonic, larval, pupa, and adult and thus each phase provide accessibility for toxicity assays and their interpretations. It shows less redundancy in its genome as compared to mouse or zebra fish toxicity models. Therefore, this model acts as one of the in vivo model facilitating the rapid analysis of gene functions (Hsu & Schulz, 2000). *Drosophila melanogaster* fly can be manipulated experimentally much more readily than vertebrate models due to both ethical and technical issues.

***Drosophila melanogaster* as a model to study nanotoxicity:** The *Drosophila melanogaster* and mammalian systems shares a similarity and homology among the genome, gene response, and response to nanoparticle treatment. Currently, together in combination to genetics, *Drosophila melanogaster* fly has established an immense attractive system to study nano particle toxicity. Initially at the establishment phase, *Drosophila melanogaster* as one of the nanotoxicity model have been used to study the effect of nanoparticles on its life history and cycle traits.The most commonly used method of nano particle delivery to the fly is via ingestion. A previous studies showed that fly larvae fed upon carbon nano tubes (CNTs) show endophysical or reproductive effect but the adult flies exposed to dry powder forms of the two of the same CNTs experienced impaired locomotors function and mortality which demonstrated that flies were susceptible to nanoparticle exposure and thus they produced a significant different particle specific response. These studies signify the importance and specificity of nanoparticles size, dose, and material dependent toxicity. This also implies that feeding of different nanoparticles of various sizes may shows different reaction in flies. Another case has been reported in which silver nanoparticle fed fly larvae have decreased survivorship and fecundity, developmental delay, and a distinct adult phenotype (Gorth et al., 2011; Key et al., 2011; Panacek et al., 2011; Philbrook et al.,2011; Posgai et al.,2011). *Drosophila melanogaster* offers an advantage of genetic and physiological attribute making it accessible to variety of assays to study and explore the genotoxic, subacute, and chronic effects of nanomaterial exposure. The previous data reported the gene toxic affect of metallic nanoparticles through the wing somatic mutation test, recombination test, affecting life history traits in flies (Demir et al., 2011; Vales et al., 2013).The first nanomaterial based mutated organism named "nanomaterial-mutated" (NM-mut) was also isolated and maintained with distinctive feature of bisected eye with the abnormal presence of an extraneous structure in the middle with the use of gold nanoparticles (Vecchio et al., 2012). Currently, fly model is also used tool to evaluate the development of nanoparticle-based drug or gene delivery systems (Barandeh et al., 2012). Another approach of nanoparticle toxicity have been assessed through expression levels of genes and proteins, presence of DNA fragmentation, as well as a modification in the involved in stress responses, and apoptosis pathways in *Drosophila melanogaster* (Ahamed et al., 2010; Vecchio et al., 2012).

Methods and Mechanisms of Nanoparticles studies in *Drosophila melanogaster*

The general methods and mechanism involved in studying *Drosophila melanogaster* model are explained in figure 1 and 2.

TYPES OF NANOPARTICLES NPS AND THEIR APPLICATION IN FLY RESEARCH

1. **Gallium phosphide nanowires and their effect on *Drosophila melanogaster* immunity**: The effect of nanoparticles in form of Gallium phosphide nanowires has been used in *Drosophila melanogaster* for examination of immune system. These nanowires are used to determine which genetic networks and signaling pathways are active upon nanowire exposure and helps in investigating effect of Gallium phosphide nanowires on *Drosophila melanogaster* immune system. The toxic affect of nanowires on tissue was evaluated by genome-wide gene expression to study life span, fecundity, somatic mutation and activation of immune response. It was also reported that when the *Drosophila melanogaster* larvae or adults ingested gallium phosphide nanowires with food through the diet, these nanowires were are not taken up into tissues, and showed negligible response on any of the factors examined. This suggests that the *Drosophila melanogaster* intestinal tract is not only insensitive to nanowire exposure but it plays significant role in protection of adjoining tissues from environmental hazards. This study emphasizes upon the requirement of direct injection of nano materials into the hemolymph to facilitate the absorption of nanomaterials in *Drosophila melanogaster* immune system cells and tissues (Adolfsson et al., 2013).

Figure 1. General methods involved in studying Drosophila melanogaster model

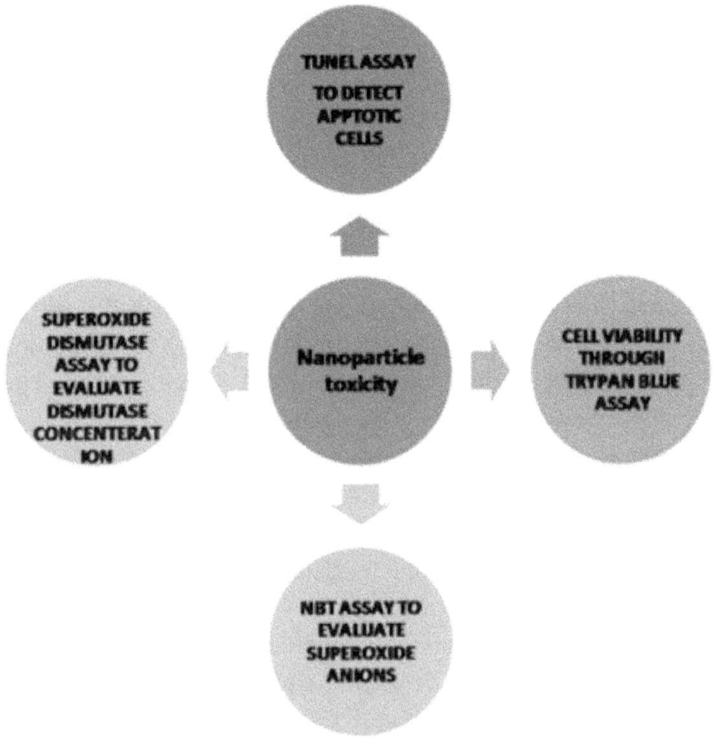

Figure 2. Mechanisms involved in studying Drosophila melanogaster model

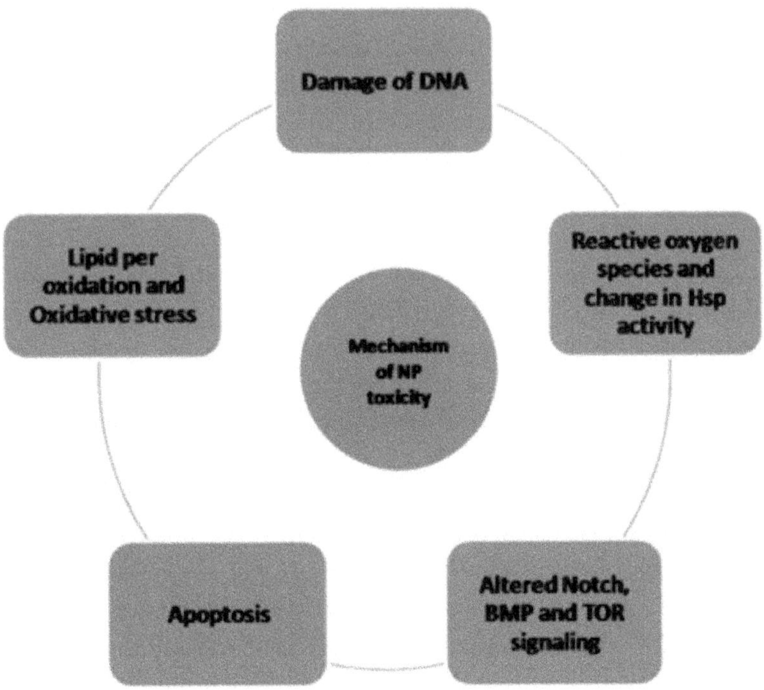

2. **Calcium Phosphate (CP) nanoparticles role in population studies of *Drosophila melanogaster*** - Calcium Phosphate nanoparticles with the variations in phase composition, crystalline behavior and the pathway of formation as calcium phosphate (CP) nano powder. These nanopowders were administered orally in population of *Drosophila melanogaster* from the egg to the adult organism for the evaluation of viability and fertility factors. CP nano particles possess identical sizes and shapes but they were differing in crystallinity (amorphous vs crystalline), chemical nature of the phosphate group (orthophosphate vs pyrophosphate), and pathway of formation. The result showed that each of these three variables affected the fertility and viability of the fruit flies (Wu & Uskoković, 2017).
   2. **Silver nanoparticles (AgNPs) dose-dependent effect on fertility and survival of *Drosophila melanogaster*-** Flies which were administered with AgNPs in the dose-dependent manner showed significantly lower egg laying capability along with impaired growth of ovary. At the larval stage dietary intake of AgNPs has more harmful effects that result in reduced ovary size, longevity and egg laying capability. The administration of higher doses of AgNPs at early development is detrimental to the reproductive health and survival of *Drosophila melanogaster* and its upcoming generation (Raj et al., 2017). Another study reported that Ag NPs may act may decrease dopamine levels directly by targeting dopamine pathway genes, enzymes, or localization of melanin. They may elicit the stress response, may generate ROS or a combination of both mechanisms (Chifiriuc et al., 2011). Further the exposure of AgNP may increase ROS levels in the *Drosophila melanogaster* testis that may lead to a reduction of GSC number by promoting premature GSC differentiation (Ong et al., 2016).It was also reported that Ag NPs induces apoptosis, DNA damage and oxidative stress in *Drosophila melanogaster* suggesting chronic exposure of silver nano particles can cause reproductive and developmental toxicity (Ahamed et al., 2010).
   3. **Nickel Oxide NPs** – Assessment of in vivo genotoxic potential of Cu-NPs and Ni-NPs in the *Drosophila melanogaster* model the characterization and evaluation of genotoxic potential of Nickel-based nanoparticles (NPs) and their industrial products is essential. The genotoxicity of NiO NPs in vivo and in vitro using the recombination test and somatic mutation induced a significant increase in DNA damage that indicates NiO NPs genotoxic and mutagenic effects (De Carli et al., 2018). However, Ni-NPs showed a significant increase of small single spots and total mutant spots at the highest dose assessed in the wing-spot assay in *Drosophila melanogaster* (Di Giacomo et al., 2017).
   4. **Copper Oxide NP in the *Drosophila melanogaster* model**-Upon oral administration of copper oxide nanoparticles, CuO NPs get accumulated and cause a dose-dependent decrease in egg-to-adult survivorship, delayed development, toxicity through inducing Reactive Oxygen species in *Drosophila melanogaster*. Gut homeostasis get disrupted and oxidative stress serves as one of the primary causes of CuO NP-induced toxicity in *Drosophila melanogaster* (Baeg et al., 2018).
   5. **Aluminum oxide (Al_2O_3) nanoparticles (NPs)**-Aluminum oxide (Al_2O_3) nanoparticles (NPs) have a wide applications which cause unintentional exposure to humans, making it important to study its nanobio interaction in *Drosophila melanogaster* tissue. In recent study, the chronic exposure of Al_2O_3 and evaluation of toxin with enrichment analysis of differentially expressed proteins showed significant alteration in striated muscle cell differentiation, digestive tract

morphogenesis, photo transduction, regulation of chromatin organization and DNA duplex unwinding (Carmona et al., 2018).

6. **Gold particles (Au NPs)-** Evaluation of the toxic effects of citrate-capped gold nanoparticles (Au NPs) upon ingestion on the model system *Drosophila melanogaster* showed a significant *in vivo* toxicity of Au NP, that elicited strong reduction of life span of flies, presence of DNA fragmentation and poor fertility, as well as a significant over expression of the stress proteins. Gold NPs induced toxicity in vivo caused the reduction of *Drosophila melanogaster* lifespan, low fertility performance, presence of DNA fragmentation and significant modification in the expression levels of genes involved in stress responses leading to DNA damage recognition and apoptosis pathway. The toxic effects in the exposed organisms were directly related to the concentration of the ingested AuNPs irrespective of their size (Vecchio et al., 2012).
7. **Zinc Oxide NPs**- Evaluation of genotoxicity in *Drosophila melanogaster* cells performed through evaluation of cytotoxicity, reactive oxygen species (ROS) formation, gene expression profiling and genotoxicity induced by ZnO NPs. They induced oxidative stress-related cytotoxicity and genotoxicity in *Drosophila melanogaster* in vivo. The safety issues related to increased usage of ZnO NPs by consumers needs to be verified (Ng et al., 2017). The genotoxic effects of these nanomaterials were evaluated through short term *vivo* bioassay, the somatic mutation and recombination test (SMART) in *Drosophila melanogaster* in which the *in vivo* exposure indicates that ZnO NPs are genotoxic to the somatic cells of *Drosophila melanogaster* (Cardozo et al., 2019).
8. **Carbon Nanotubes-** Carbon nanotubes were the tested for evaluation of the cytotoxicity on *D. melanogaster* model. *Drosophila melanogaster* diet supplemented with single-walled or multi-walled carbon nanotubes (CNT) at adult stage showed an intensive adherence of CNT to fly body surface with impairing in the grooming behavior, locomotion and increased mortality. These results suggests that superstructure and aggregation condition of nano material influence its adhesion and toxicity to the fly body surface and influence it's behavior leading to the nano particle transport inside the body (Liu et al., 2009; Lam et al., 2006).
9. **Titanium dioxide NPs-**Titanium dioxide nanoparticles are known to induce oxidative stress *in vitro* and *in vivo*. Feeding upon nano silver may result into oxidative stress, and consumption of antioxidants is the only remedy to nano silver toxicity. Ingestion of nanosilver particles imparts toxic effects on development, survivorship, and mating success in *Drosophila melanogaster* (Posgai et al., 2011). These nanoparticles also alter glucose transport across the intestinal epithelium, which may have physiological consequences (Richter et al., 2018).

The purpose and functions of different nanoparticles studied in *Drosophila melanogaster* are summarized in Table no.1.

Table 1. Summary of function of Nanoparticles involved in different research areas using Drosophila melanogaster model

S.No	Type of Nanoparticle (NPs)	Function of Nanoparticle in *D.melanogaster*
1	Gallium phosphide	Examination of immune system
2	Silver Oxide	Examination of fertility and survival
3	Nickel Oxide	Assessment of in vivo genotoxic potential
4	Copper Oxide	Assessment of toxicity through inducing Reactive Oxygen
5	Aluminum oxide	Evaluation of toxin with enrichment analysis
6	Gold	Evaluation of the toxic effects
7	Zinc Oxide	Evaluation of genotoxicity in cells performed through evaluation of cytotoxicity,
8	Carbon	Evaluation of the cytotoxicity
9	Titanium dioxide	Study of oxidative stress *in vitro* and *in vivo*

FUTURE RESEARCH DIRECTIONS

The current chapter focuses on summary of different research works performed to explore the effect of various nanoparticles toxicity which has major implementation in field of medical sciences and agricultural sciences. *Drosophila melanogaster* may be used as the model organism in toxicity based assays and studies as it's system is comprised of short life cycle and genetically tractable for various developmental stages in the study of different disease in human beings as well as in pest management in agricultural sciences.

CONCLUSION

In this chapter, application of metallic NPs in drug delivery, nano toxicology and cell tracking were discussed. Nanomaterials specifically interact with cell membranes via various mechanisms and after their internalized within the nucleus, the specific activation of crucial transcription factors and signaling pathway-associated molecules occurs. Here, we discussed the physical and chemical features of the NPs, as well as their functionalization in *Drosophila melanogaster* system. It was observed that metallic NPs showed differential activity towards various exposure dose and time. Accordingly, further research will be needed to determine the optimal NP exposure conditions required for their interaction with tissue and to perform appropriate function. In sum, different NPs are capable of modulating stem *Drosophila melanogaster* cellular and tissue system which highlights their potential to be used in toxicological research. However, intensive efforts are required to find the optimal exposure conditions of NPs in order to obtain good model for toxicological studies with minimal toxicity, which will allow the effective use of *Drosophila melanogaster* model as source of nanotoxiciology model to cure untreatable human diseases.

ACKNOWLEDGMENT

This research received no specific grant from any funding agency in the public, commercial, or not-for-profit sectors.

REFERENCES

Adolfsson, K., Schneider, M., Hammarin, G., Häcker, U., & Prinz, C. N. (2013). Ingestion of gallium phosphide nanowires has no adverse effect on Drosophila tissue function. *Nanotechnology*, *24*(28), 285101. doi:10.1088/0957-4484/24/28/285101 PMID:23787695

Ahamed, M., Posgai, R., Gorey, T. J., Nielsen, M., Hussain, S. M., & Rowe, J. J. (2010). Silver nanoparticles induced heat shock protein 70, oxidative stress and apoptosis in Drosophila melanogaster. *Toxicology and Applied Pharmacology*, *242*(3), 263–269. doi:10.1016/j.taap.2009.10.016 PMID:19874832

Baeg, E., Sooklert, K., & Sereemaspun, A. (2018). Copper Oxide Nanoparticles Cause a Dose-Dependent Toxicity via Inducing Reactive Oxygen Species in Drosophila. *Nanomaterials (Basel, Switzerland)*, *8*(10), 824. doi:10.3390/nano8100824 PMID:30322073

Bainton, R. J., Tsai, L. T., Singh, C. M., Moore, M. S., Neckameyer, W. S., & Heberlein, U. (2000). Dopamine modulates acute responses to cocaine, nicotine and ethanol in Drosophila. *Current Biology*, *10*(4), 187–194. doi:10.1016/S0960-9822(00)00336-5 PMID:10704411

Barandeh, F., Nguyen, P. L., Kumar, R., Iacobucci, G. J., Kuznicki, M. L., Kosterman, A., Bergey, E. J., Prasad, P. N., & Gunawardena, S. (2012). Organically modified silica nanoparticles are biocompatible and can be targeted to neurons in vivo. *PLoS One*, *7*(1), e29424. doi:10.1371/journal.pone.0029424 PMID:22238611

Brunner, T. J., Wick, P., Manser, P., Spohn, P., Grass, R. N., Limbach, L. K., Bruinink, A., & Stark, W. J. (2006). In vitro cytotoxicity of oxide nanoparticles: Comparison to asbestos, silica, and the effect of particle solubility. *Environmental Science & Technology*, *40*(14), 4374–4381. doi:10.1021/es052069i PMID:16903273

Cardozo, T. R., De Carli, R. F., Seeber, A., Flores, W. H., da Rosa, J., Kotzal, Q., Lehmann, M., da Silva, F. R., & Dihl, R. R. (2019). Genotoxicity of zinc oxide nanoparticles: An *in vivo* and *in silico* study. *Toxicology Research*, *8*(2), 277–286. doi:10.1039/C8TX00255J PMID:30997027

Carmona, E. R., García-Rodríguez, A., & Marcos, R. (2018). Genotoxicity of Copper and Nickel Nanoparticles in Somatic Cells of *Drosophila melanogaster. Journal of Toxicology*, *7278036*, 1–8. Advance online publication. doi:10.1155/2018/7278036 PMID:30111998

Chifiriuc, M. C., Ratiu, A. C., Popa, M., & Ecovoiu, A. A. (2016). Drosophotoxicology: An Emerging Research Area for Assessing Nanoparticles Interaction with Living Organisms. *International Journal of Molecular Sciences*, *17*(2), 36. doi:10.3390/ijms17020036 PMID:26907252

De Carli, R. F., Chaves, D., Cardozo, T. R., de Souza, A. P., Seeber, A., Flores, W. H., Honatel, K. F., Lehmann, M., & Dihl, R. R. (2018). Evaluation of the genotoxic properties of nickel oxide nanoparticles in vitro and in vivo. *Mutation research. Genetic toxicology and environmental mutagenesis, 836*(Pt B), 47–53. doi:10.1016/j.mrgentox.2018.06.003

Demir, E., Vales, G., Kaya, B., Creus, A., & Marcos, R. (2011). Genotoxic analysis of silver nanoparticles in Drosophila. *Nanotoxicology*, *5*(3), 417–424. doi:10.3109/17435390.2010.529176 PMID:21039182

Di Giacomo, S., Sollazzo, M., de Biase, D., Ragazzi, M., Bellosta, P., Pession, A., & Grifoni, D. (2017). Human Cancer Cells Signal Their Competitive Fitness Through MYC Activity. *Scientific Reports*, *7*(1), 12568. doi:10.103841598-017-13002-1 PMID:28974715

Feany, M. B., & Bender, W. W. (2000). A Drosophila model of Parkinson's disease. *Nature*, *404*(6776), 394–398. doi:10.1038/35006074 PMID:10746727

Gorth, D. J., Rand, D. M., & Webster, T. J. (2011). Silver nanoparticle toxicity in Drosophila: Size does matter. *International Journal of Nanomedicine*, *6*, 343–350. doi:10.2147/IJN.S16881 PMID:21383859

Gupta, S., Bansal, R., Gupta, S., Jindal, N., & Jindal, A. (2013). Nanocarriers and nanoparticles for skin care and dermatological treatments. *Indian Dermatology Online Journal*, *4*(4), 267–272. doi:10.4103/2229-5178.120635 PMID:24350003

Hsu, T., & Schulz, R. A. (2000). Sequence and functional properties of Ets genes in the model organism Drosophila. *Oncogene, 19*(55), 6409–6416. doi:10.1038j.onc.1204033

Huber, R., Hill, S. L., Holladay, C., Biesiadecki, M., Tononi, G., & Cirelli, C. (2004). Sleep homeostasis in Drosophila melanogaster. *Sleep*, *27*(4), 628–639. doi:10.1093leep/27.4.628 PMID:15282997

Kaul, S., Gulati, N., Verma, D., Mukherjee, S., & Nagaich, U. (2018). Role of Nanotechnology in Cosmeceuticals: A Review of Recent Advances. *Journal of Pharmaceutics*, *3420204*, 1–19. Advance online publication. doi:10.1155/2018/3420204 PMID:29785318

Kaya, B., Creus, A., Yanikoğlu, A., Cabré, O., & Marcos, R. (2000). Use of the Drosophila wing spot test in the genotoxicity testing of different herbicides. *Environmental and Molecular Mutagenesis*, *36*(1), 40–46. doi:10.1002/1098-2280(2000)36:1<40::AID-EM6>3.0.CO;2-K PMID:10918358

Khurana, V., Lu, Y., Steinhilb, M. L., Oldham, S., Shulman, J. M., & Feany, M. B. (2006). TOR-mediated cell-cycle activation causes neurodegeneration in a Drosophila tauopathy model. *Current Biology*, *16*(3), 230–241. doi:10.1016/j.cub.2005.12.042 PMID:16461276

Koh, K., Evans, J. M., Hendricks, J. C., & Sehgal, A. (2006). A Drosophila model for age-associated changes in sleep:wake cycles. *Proceedings of the National Academy of Sciences of the United States of America*, *103*(37), 13843–13847. doi:10.1073/pnas.0605903103 PMID:16938867

Krukemeyer, M. G., Krenn, V., Huebner, F., Wagner, W., & Resch, R. (2015). History and Possible Uses of Nanomedicine Based on Nanoparticles and Nanotechnological Progress. *Journal of Nanomedicine & Nanotechnology*, *6*, 1–7.

Lam, C. W., James, J. T., McCluskey, R., Arepalli, S., & Hunter, R. L. (2006). A review of carbon nanotube toxicity and assessment of potential occupational and environmental health risks. *Critical Reviews in Toxicology*, *36*(3), 189–217. doi:10.1080/10408440600570233 PMID:16686422

Liu, X., Vinson, D., Abt, D., Hurt, R. H., & Rand, D. M. (2009). Differential toxicity of carbon nanomaterials in Drosophila: Larval dietary uptake is benign, but adult exposure causes locomotor impairment and mortality. *Environmental Science & Technology*, *43*(16), 6357–6363. doi:10.1021/es901079z PMID:19746737

McBride, S. M., Choi, C. H., Schoenfeld, B. P., Bell, A. J., Liebelt, D. A., Ferreiro, D., Choi, R. J., Hinchey, P., Kollaros, M., Terlizzi, A. M., Ferrick, N. J., Koenigsberg, E., Rudominer, R. L., Sumida, A., Chiorean, S., Siwicki, K. K., Nguyen, H. T., Fortini, M. E., McDonald, T. V., & Jongens, T. A. (2010). Pharmacological and genetic reversal of age-dependent cognitive deficits attributable to decreased presenilin function. *The Journal of Neuroscience: The Official Journal of the Society for Neuroscience*, *30*(28), 9510–9522. doi:10.1523/JNEUROSCI.1017-10.2010 PMID:20631179

McClung, C., & Hirsh, J. (1998). Stereotypic behavioral responses to free-base cocaine and the development of behavioral sensitization in Drosophila. *Current Biology*, *8*(2), 109–112. doi:10.1016/S0960-9822(98)70041-7 PMID:9427649

Ng, C. T., Yong, L. Q., Hande, M. P., Ong, C. N., Yu, L. E., Bay, B. H., & Baeg, G. H. (2017). Zinc oxide nanoparticles exhibit cytotoxicity and genotoxicity through oxidative stress responses in human lung fibroblasts and *Drosophila melanogaster. International Journal of Nanomedicine*, *12*, 1621–1637. doi:10.2147/IJN.S124403 PMID:28280330

Ong, C., Lee, Q. Y., Cai, Y., Liu, X., Ding, J., Yung, L. Y., Bay, B. H., & Baeg, G. H. (2016). Silver nanoparticles disrupt germline stem cell maintenance in the Drosophila testis. *Scientific Reports*, *6*(1), 20632. doi:10.1038rep20632 PMID:26847594

Panacek, A., Prucek, R., Safarova, D., Dittrich, M., Richtrova, J., Benickova, K., Zboril, R., & Kvitek, L. (2011). Acute and chronic toxicity effects of silver nanoparticles (NPs) on Drosophila melanogaster. *Environmental Science & Technology*, *45*(11), 4974–4979. doi:10.1021/es104216b PMID:21553866

Philbrook, N. A., Winn, L. M., Afrooz, A. R., Saleh, N. B., & Walker, V. K. (2011). The effect of TiO(2) and Ag nanoparticles on reproduction and development of Drosophila melanogaster and CD-1 mice. *Toxicology and Applied Pharmacology*, *257*(3), 429–436. doi:10.1016/j.taap.2011.09.027 PMID:22005274

Posgai, R., Cipolla-McCulloch, C. B., Murphy, K. R., Hussain, S. M., Rowe, J. J., & Nielsen, M. G. (2011). Differential toxicity of silver and titanium dioxide nanoparticles on Drosophila melanogaster development, reproductive effort, and viability: Size, coatings and antioxidants matter. *Chemosphere*, *85*(1), 34–42. doi:10.1016/j.chemosphere.2011.06.040 PMID:21733543

Raj, A., Shah, P., & Agrawal, N. (2017). Dose-dependent effect of silver nanoparticles (AgNPs) on fertility and survival of Drosophila: An in-vivo study. *PLoS One*, *12*(5), e0178051. doi:10.1371/journal.pone.0178051 PMID:28542630

Reiter, L. T., Potocki, L., Chien, S., Gribskov, M., & Bier, E. (2001). A systematic analysis of human disease-associated gene sequences in Drosophila melanogaster. *Genome Research, 11*(6), 1114–1125. doi:10.1101/gr.169101 PMID:11381037

Richter, J. W., Shull, G. M., Fountain, J. H., Guo, Z., Musselman, L. P., Fiumera, A. C., & Mahler, G. J. (2018). Titanium dioxide nanoparticle exposure alters metabolic homeostasis in a cell culture model of the intestinal epithelium and Drosophila melanogaster. *Nanotoxicology, 12*(5), 390–406. doi:10.1080/17435390.2018.1457189 PMID:29600885

Rudrapatna, V. A., Cagan, R. L., & Das, T. K. (2012). Drosophila cancer models. *Developmental Dynamics, 241*(1), 107–118. doi:10.1002/dvdy.22771 PMID:22038952

Sykiotis, G. P., & Bohmann, D. (2008). Keap1/Nrf2 signaling regulates oxidative stress tolerance and lifespan in Drosophila. *Developmental Cell, 14*(1), 76–85. doi:10.1016/j.devcel.2007.12.002 PMID:18194654

Vales, G., Demir, E., Kaya, B., Creus, A., & Marcos, R. (2013). Genotoxicity of cobalt nanoparticles and ions in Drosophila. *Nanotoxicology, 7*(4), 462–468. doi:10.3109/17435390.2012.689882 PMID:22548285

Vecchio, G., Galeone, A., Brunetti, V., Maiorano, G., Rizzello, L., Sabella, S., Cingolani, R., & Pompa, P. P. (2012). Mutagenic effects of gold nanoparticles induce aberrant phenotypes in Drosophila melanogaster. *Nanomedicine; Nanotechnology, Biology, and Medicine, 8*(1), 1–7. doi:10.1016/j.nano.2011.11.001 PMID:22094122

Vecchio, G., Galeone, A., Brunetti, V., Maiorano, G., Sabella, S., Cingolani, R., & Pompa, P. P. (2012). Concentration-dependent, size-independent toxicity of citrate capped AuNPs in Drosophila melanogaster. *PLoS One, 7*(1), e29980. doi:10.1371/journal.pone.0029980 PMID:22238688

Wolf, M. J., Amrein, H., Izatt, J. A., Choma, M. A., Reedy, M. C., & Rockman, H. A. (2006). Drosophila as a model for the identification of genes causing adult human heart disease. *Proceedings of the National Academy of Sciences of the United States of America, 103*(5), 1394–1399. doi:10.1073/pnas.0507359103 PMID:16432241

Wu, V. M., & Uskoković, V. (2017). Population Effects of Calcium Phosphate Nanoparticles in *Drosophila melanogaster*: The Effects of Phase Composition, Crystallinity, and the Pathway of Formation. *ACS Biomaterials Science & Engineering, 3*(10), 2348–2357. doi:10.1021/acsbiomaterials.7b00540 PMID:29862315

Compilation of References

1 Wang, K., Peng, H., Thurecht, K. J., Puttick, S., & Whittaker, A. K. (2015). Segmented highly branched copolymers: Rationally designed macromolecules for improved and tunable 19f mri. *Biomacromolecules*, *16*(9), 2827–2839. doi:10.1021/acs.biomac.5b00800 PMID:26218187

Abbaspourrad, A., Datta, S. S., & Weitz, D. A. (2013). Controlling release from pH-responsive microcapsules. *Langmuir*, *29*(41), 12697–12702. doi:10.1021/la403064f PMID:24041287

Abdulhalim, I., Zourob, M., & Lakhtakia, A. (2008). Surface plasmon resonance for biosensing: A mini-review. *Electromagnetics*, *28*(3), 214–242. doi:10.1080/02726340801921650

Abu-Salah. (2010). DNA-based applications in nanobiotechnology. *Journal of Biomedicine & Biotechnology.*

Acharya, P., Jayaprakasha, G. K., Crosby, K. M., Jifon, J. L., & Patil, B. S. (2019). Green-Synthesized Nanoparticles Enhanced Seedling Growth, Yield, and Quality of Onion (*Allium cepa* L.). *ACS Sustainable Chemistry & Engineering*, *7*(17), 14580–14590. doi:10.1021/acssuschemeng.9b02180

Acharya, S., Dilnawaz, F., & Sahoo, S. K. (2009). Targeted epidermal growth factor receptor nanoparticle bioconjugates for breast cancer therapy. *Biomaterials*, *30*(29), 5737–5750. doi:10.1016/j.biomaterials.2009.07.008 PMID:19631377

Aderibigbe, B. A. (2017). Metal-Based Nanoparticles for the Treatment of Infectious Diseases. *Molecules (Basel, Switzerland)*, *22*(8), 1370. doi:10.3390/molecules22081370 PMID:28820471

Adisa, I. O., Pullagurala, V. L. R., Peralta-Videa, J. R., Dimkpa, C. O., Elmer, W. H., Gardea-Torresdey, J. L., & White, J. C. (2019). Recent advances in nano-enabled fertilizers and pesticides: A critical review of mechanisms of action. *Environmental Science. Nano*, *6*(7), 2002–2030. doi:10.1039/C9EN00265K

Adolfsson, K., Schneider, M., Hammarin, G., Häcker, U., & Prinz, C. N. (2013). Ingestion of gallium phosphide nanowires has no adverse effect on Drosophila tissue function. *Nanotechnology*, *24*(28), 285101. doi:10.1088/0957-4484/24/28/285101 PMID:23787695

Aenishanslins, N. A. O., Saona, L. A., Dura'n-Toro, V. M., Monra's, J. P., Bravo, D. M., & Donoso, J. M. P. (2014). Use of titanium dioxide nanoparticles biosynthesized by Bacillus mycoides in quantum dot sensitized solar cells. *Microbial Cell Factories*, *13*, 90. PMID:25027643

Agarwal, H., Kumar, S. V., & Rajeshkumar, S. (2017). A review on green synthesis of zinc oxide nanoparticles–An eco-friendly approach. *Resource-Efficient Technologies*, *3*(4), 406–413. doi:10.1016/j.reffit.2017.03.002

Agarwal, S., & Prajapati, Y. K. (2019). Multifunctional metamaterial surface for absorbing and sensing applications. *Optics Communications*, *439*, 304–307. doi:10.1016/j.optcom.2019.01.020

Agrawal, S., & Rathore, P. (2014). Article. *International Journal of Current Microbiology and Applied Sciences*, *3*, 43–55.

Ahamed, M., Posgai, R., Gorey, T. J., Nielsen, M., Hussain, S. M., & Rowe, J. J. (2010). Silver nanoparticles induced heat shock protein 70, oxidative stress and apoptosis in Drosophila melanogaster. *Toxicology and Applied Pharmacology*, *242*(3), 263–269. doi:10.1016/j.taap.2009.10.016 PMID:19874832

Ahmad, A., Senapati, S., Khan, M. I., Kumar, R., Ramani, R., Srinivas, V., & Sastry, M. (2003). Intracellular synthesis of gold nanoparticles by a novel alkalotolerant actinomycete, Rhodococcus species. *Nanotechnology*, *14*(7), 824–828. doi:10.1088/0957-4484/14/7/323

Ahmad, O. S., Bedwell, T. S., Esen, C., Garcia-Cruz, A., & Piletsky, S. A. (2019). Molecularly imprinted polymers in electrochemical and optical sensors. *Trends in Biotechnology*, *37*(3), 294–309. doi:10.1016/j.tibtech.2018.08.009 PMID:30241923

Ahmed, A., Baig, H., Sundaram, S., & Mallick, T. K. (2019). Use of Nanofluids in Solar PV/Thermal Systems. *International Journal of Photoenergy. Article ID*, *8039129*, 1–17.

Akbari, M. K., Derakhshan, R., & Mirzaee, O. (2015). Article. *Chemical Engineering Journal*, *259*, 918–926. doi:10.1016/j.cej.2014.08.053

Akerblom, L., Nara, P., Dunlop, N., Putney, S., & Morein, B. (1993). HIV experimental vaccines based on the iscom technology using envelope and GAG gene products. *Biotechnol. Ther.*, *4*, 145–161.

Akhoon, S. A., Rubab, S., & Shah, M. A. (2016). A Review of Various Nanostructures to Enhance the Efficiency of Solar-Photon-Conversions. *Renewable and Alternative Energy: Concepts, Methodologies, Tools, and Applications: Concepts, Methodologies, Tools, and Applications, 197.*

Akhoon, S. A., Rubab, S., & Shah, M. A. (2017). Enhanced cycling properties and better rate capabilities of Al-doped $LiMn_2O_4$ nanorods and nanospheres. *Materials Research Express*, *4*(10), 105016. doi:10.1088/2053-1591/aa8e58

Albert, D. (2016). *Nanomedicine*. Immune Rebalancing. The Future of Immunosuppression.

Alivisatos, A. P. (1996). Perspectives on the Physical Chemistry of Semiconductor Nanocrystals. *Journal of Physical Chemistry*, *100*(31), 13226–13239. doi:10.1021/jp9535506

Ali, Z. A., Yahya, R., Sekaran, S. D., & Puteh, R. (2016). Green synthesis of silver nanoparticles using apple extract and its antibacterial properties. *Adv. Mater. Sci. Eng.*, *4102196*, 6. doi:10.1155/2016/4102196

Allen, T. M., & Cullis, P. R. (2004). Drug delivery systems: Entering the mainstream. *Science*, *303*(5665), 1818–1822. doi:10.1126cience.1095833 PMID:15031496

Allouche, Y., Varga, S., Bouden, C., & Oliveira, A. C. (2017). Dynamic simulation of an integrated solar-driven ejector based air conditioning system with PCM cold storage. *Applied Energy*, *190*, 600–611. doi:10.1016/j.apenergy.2017.01.001

Altintas, Z., Guerreiro, A., Piletsky, S. A., & Tothill, I. E. (2015). NanoMIP based optical sensor for pharmaceuticals monitoring. *Sensors and Actuators. B, Chemical*, *213*, 305–313. doi:10.1016/j.snb.2015.02.043

Altintas, Z., Pocock, J., Thompson, K. A., & Tothill, I. E. (2015). Comparative investigations for adenovirus recognition and quantification: Plastic or natural antibodies? *Biosensors & Bioelectronics*, *74*, 996–1004. doi:10.1016/j.bios.2015.07.076 PMID:26264266

Alving, C. R., Richards, R. L., Moss, J., Alving, L. I., Clements, J. D., Shiba, T., Kotani, S., Wirtz, R. A., & Hockmeyer, W. T. (1986). Effectiveness of liposomes as potential carriers of vaccines: Applications to cholera toxin and human malaria sporozoite antigen. *Vaccine*, *4*(3), 166–172. doi:10.1016/0264-410X(86)90005-8 PMID:3532603

Alyautdin, R.N., Tezikov, E.B., Ramge, P., Kharkevich, D.A., Begley, D.J., & Kreuter, J. (1998). Significant entry of tubocurarine into the brain of rats by adsorption to polysorbate 80-coated poly butyl cyanoacrylate nanoparticles: an insitu brain perfusion study. *J Micro Encapsule, 15*, 67–74.

Amaral, F. A., Bocchi, N., Brocenschi, R. F., Biaggio, S. R., & Rocha-Filho, R. C. (2010). Structural and electrochemical properties of the doped spinels $Li_{1.05}M_{0.02}Mn_{1.98}O_{3.98}N_{0.02}$ (M= Ga^{3+}, Al^{3+}, or Co^{3+}; N= S^{2-} or F^{-}) for use as cathode material in lithium batteries. *Journal of Power Sources, 195*(10), 3293–3299. doi:10.1016/j.jpowsour.2009.12.002

Amatucci, G. G., Badway, F., Du Pasquier, A., & Zheng, T. (2001). An Asymmetric Hybrid Nonaqueous Energy Storage Cell. *Journal of the Electrochemical Society, 148*(8), A930–A939. doi:10.1149/1.1383553

Amendola, V., & Meneghetti, M. (2009). *Laser ablation synthesis in solution and size manipulation of noble metal nanoparticles*. Academic Press.

Ammons, M. C. (2010). Anti-biofilm strategies and the need for innovations in wound care. *Recent Patents on Anti-infective Drug Discovery, 5*(1), 10–17. doi:10.2174/157489110790112581 PMID:19807676

Ananthakumar, S., Kumar, J. R., Babu, S. M. (2019). Third-Generation Solar Cells: Concept, Materials and Performance - An Overview. *Emerging Nanostructured Materials for Energy and Environmental Science*, 305–339.

Anderson, M. E. (1998). Glutathione: An overview of biosynthesis and modulation. *Chemico-Biological Interactions, 111*, 1–14. doi:10.1016/S0009-2797(97)00146-4 PMID:9679538

Angelatos, A. S., Radt, B., & Caruso, F. (2005). Light-responsive polyelectrolyte/gold nanoparticle microcapsules. *The Journal of Physical Chemistry B, 109*(7), 3071–3076. doi:10.1021/jp045070x PMID:16851322

An, J., Zhang, M., Wang, S., & Tang, J. (2008). Physical, chemical and microbiological changes in stored green asparagus spears as affected by coating of silver nanoparticles-PVP. *Lebensmittel-Wissenschaft + Technologie, 41*(6), 1100–1107. doi:10.1016/j.lwt.2007.06.019

An, K. H., Jeon, K. K., Heo, J. K., Lim, S. C., Bae, D. J., & Lee, Y. H. (2002). High-Capacitance Supercapacitor Using a Nanocomposite Electrode of Single-Walled Carbon Nanotube and Polypyrrole. *Journal of the Electrochemical Society, 149*(8), A1058. doi:10.1149/1.1491235

An, K. H., Kim, W. S., Park, Y. S., Moon, J. M., Bae, D. J., Lim, S. C., Lee, Y. S., & Lee, Y. H. (2001). Electrochemical Properties of High-Power Supercapacitors Using Single-Walled Carbon Nanotube Electrodes. *Advanced Functional Materials, 11*(5), 387–392. doi:10.1002/1616-3028(200110)11:5<387::AID-ADFM387>3.0.CO;2-G

Ankamwar, B. (2010). Biosynthesis of gold nanoparticles (green-gold) using leaf extract of Terminalia catappa. *Journal of Chemistry, 7*, 1334–1339.

Aramesh, M., Pourfayaz, F., Haghir, M., Kasaeian, A., & Ahmadi, M. H. (2019). Investigating the effect of using nanofluids on the performance of a double-effect absorption refrigeration cycle combined with a solar collector. *Proceedings of the Institution of Mechanical Engineers, Part A: Journal of Power and Energy*. 10.1177/0957650919889811

Arangoa, M. A., Campanero, M. A., Renedo, M. J., Ponchel, G., & Irache, J. M. (2001). Gliadin nanoparticles as carriers for the oral administration of lipophilic drugs. Relationships between bioadhesion and pharmacokinetics. *Pharmaceutical Research, 18*(11), 1521–1527. doi:10.1023/A:1013018111829 PMID:11758758

Arayne, M. S., Sultana, N., & Qureshi, F. (2007). nanoparticles in delivery of cardiovascular drugs. *Pakistan Journal of Pharmaceutical Sciences, 20*, 340–348. PMID:17604260

Arbos, P., Campanero, M. A., Arangoa, M. A., & Irache, J. M. (2004). Nanoparticles with specific bioadhesive properties to circumvent the pre-systemic degradation of fluorinated pyrimidines. *Journal of Controlled Release*, *96*(1), 55–65. doi:10.1016/j.jconrel.2004.01.006 PMID:15063029

Aricò, A. S., Bruce, P., Scrosati, B., Tarascon, J. M., & van Schalkwijk, W. (2005). Nanostructured materials for advanced energy conversion and storage devices. *Nature Materials*, *4*(5), 366–377. doi:10.1038/nmat1368 PMID:15867920

Arun, D., Vimala, R., & Ramkumar, K. D. (2020). Investigating the microbial-influenced corrosion of UNS S32750 stainless-steel base alloy and weld seams by biofilm-forming marine bacterium Macrococcus equipercicus. *Bioelectrochemistry (Amsterdam, Netherlands)*, *135*, 107546. doi:10.1016/j.bioelechem.2020.107546 PMID:32413811

Arvizo, R. R., Bhattacharyya, S., Kudgus, R. A., Giri, K., Bhattacharya, R., & Mukherjee, P. (2012). Intrinsic therapeutic applications of noble metal nanoparticles: Past, present and future. *Chemical Society Reviews*, *41*(7), 2943–2970. doi:10.1039/c2cs15355f PMID:22388295

Ashby, M. F., Ferreira, P. J. S. G., & Schodek, D. L. (2009). *Nanomaterials, nanotechnologies and design: an introduction for engineers and architects*. Elsevier.

Ashkavand, P., Zarafshar, M., Tabari, M., Mirzaie, J., Nikpour, A., Bordbar, S. K., Struve, D., & Striker, G. G. (2018). Application of SiO2 nanoparticles as pretreatment alleviates the impact of drought on the physiological performance of Prunus mahaleb (Rosaceae). *Boletín de la Sociedad Argentina de Botánica*, *53*(2), 207–219. doi:10.31055/1851.2372.v53.n2.20578

Ashoori, R. C., Stormer, H. L., Weiner, J. S., Pfeiffer, N. L., Baldwin, K. W., & West, K. W. (1992). N-electron ground state energies of a quantum dot in magnetic field. *Physical Review Letters*, *71*(4), 613–616. doi:10.1103/PhysRevLett.71.613 PMID:10055320

Assadpour, E., & Mahdi Jafari, S. (2019). A systematic review on nanoencapsulation of food bioactive ingredients and nutraceuticals by various nanocarriers. *Critical Reviews in Food Science and Nutrition*, *59*(19), 3129–3151. doi:10.1080/10408398.2018.1484687 PMID:29883187

Atwater, H. A., & Polman, A. (2010). Erratum: Plasmonics for improved photovoltaic devices. *Nature Materials*, *9*(10), 865. doi:10.1038/nmat2866

Auría-Soro, C. (2011). Interactions of nanoparticles and biosystems: microenvironment of nanoparticles and biomolecules in nanomedicine. *Nanomaterials*, *9*(10), 1365.

Ayankojo, A. G., Reut, J., Öpik, A., Furchner, A., & Syritski, V. (2018). Hybrid molecularly imprinted polymer for amoxicillin detection. *Biosensors & Bioelectronics*, *118*, 102–107. doi:10.1016/j.bios.2018.07.042 PMID:30056300

Baca, E. M., Foldvari, M., Snider, M., Harding, K., Kournikakis, B., & Babiuk, L. A. (2000). Intra nasal immunization with liposome-formulated Yersinia pestis vaccine enhances mucosal immune responses. *Vaccine*, *18*(21), 2203–2211. doi:10.1016/S0264-410X(00)00019-0 PMID:10717339

Baeg, E., Sooklert, K., & Sereemaspun, A. (2018). Copper Oxide Nanoparticles Cause a Dose-Dependent Toxicity via Inducing Reactive Oxygen Species in Drosophila. *Nanomaterials (Basel, Switzerland)*, *8*(10), 824. doi:10.3390/nano8100824 PMID:30322073

Bagga, P., Ansari, T. M., Siddiqui, H. H., Syed, A., Bahkali, A. H., Rahman, M. A., & Khan, M. S. (2016). Bromelain capped gold nanoparticles as the novel drug delivery carriers to aggrandize effect of the antibiotic levofloxacin. *EXCLI Journal*, *15*, 772–780. PMID:28337108

Baghbani, F., Moztarzadeh, F., Mohandesi, J. A., Yazdian, F., & MokhtariDizaji, M. (2016), Novel alginate-stabilized doxorubicin-loaded nanodroplets for ultrasounic theranosis of breast cancer. *Int J Biol Macromol, 93*, 512–9.

Bai, B., Zhao, K., & Li, X. (2019). Application research of nano-storage materials in cold chain logistics of e-commerce fresh agricultural products. *Results in Physics, 13*, 102049. doi:10.1016/j.rinp.2019.01.083

Bai, H., Zhang, Z., Guo, Y., & Jia, W. (2009). Biological Synthesis of Size-Controlled Cadmium Sulfide Nanoparticles Using ImmobilizedRhodobacter sphaeroides. *Nanoscale Research Letters, 4*(7), 717–723. doi:10.100711671-009-9303-0 PMID:20596372

Bailey, R. E., Smith, A. M., & Nie, S. (2004). Quantum dots in biology and medicine. *Physica E, Low-Dimensional Systems and Nanostructures, 25*(1), 1–12.

Bainton, R. J., Tsai, L. T., Singh, C. M., Moore, M. S., Neckameyer, W. S., & Heberlein, U. (2000). Dopamine modulates acute responses to cocaine, nicotine and ethanol in Drosophila. *Current Biology, 10*(4), 187–194. doi:10.1016/S0960-9822(00)00336-5 PMID:10704411

Balagurunathan, R., Radhakrishnan, M., Rajendran, B. R., & Velmurugan, D. (2011). Biosyntheis of gold nanoparticles by actinomycetes *Streptomyces viridogens* strain HM10. *Indian Journal of Biochemistry & Biophysics, 48*, 331–335. PMID:22165291

Balaji, D. S., Basavaraja, S., Deshpande, R., Mahesh, D. B., Prabhakar, B. K., & Venkataraman, A. (2009). Extracellular biosynthesis of functionalized silver nanoparticles by strains of Cladosporium cladosporioides fungus. *Colloids and Surfaces. B, Biointerfaces, 68*(1), 88–92. doi:10.1016/j.colsurfb.2008.09.022 PMID:18995994

Balaji, S. R. K., Mutharasu, D., Shanmugan, S., Subramanian, N. S., & Ramanathan, K. (2010). Influence of Sm^{3+} ion in structural, morphological, and electrochemical properties of $LiMn_2O_4$ synthesized by microwave calcination. *Ionics, 16*(4), 351–360. doi:10.100711581-009-0400-y

Balaya, P., Bhattacharyya, A. J., Jamnik, J., Zhukovskii, Y. F., Kotomin, E. A., & Maier, J. (2006). Nano-ionics in the context of lithium batteries. *Journal of Power Sources, 159*(1), 171–178. doi:10.1016/j.jpowsour.2006.04.115

Banerjee, T., Sulthana, S., Shelby, T., Heckert, B., Jewell, J., Woody, K., Karimnia, V., McAfee, J., & Santra, S. (2016). Multiparametric Magneto-fluorescent Nanosensors for the Ultrasensitive Detection of *Escherichia coli* O157:H7. *ACS Infectious Diseases, 2*(10), 667–673. doi:10.1021/acsinfecdis.6b00108 PMID:27737552

Bangham, A. D., Standish, M. M., & Watkins, J. C. (1965). Diffusion of univalent ions across the lamellae of swollen phospholipids. *Journal of Molecular Biology, 13*(1), 238–252. doi:10.1016/S0022-2836(65)80093-6 PMID:5859039

Bao, N., Shen, L., Takata, T., Lu, D., & Domen, K. (2006). Highly ordered Pt loaded CdS nanowire assays for photocatalytic hydrogen production under visible light. *Chemistry Letters, 35*(3), 318–319. doi:10.1246/cl.2006.318

Bapat, A., Perrey, C. R., Campbell, S. A., Barry Carter, C., & Kortshagen, U. (2003). Synthesis of highly oriented, single-crystal silicon nanoparticles in a low-pressure, inductively coupled plasma. *Journal of Applied Physics, 94*(3), 1969–1974. doi:10.1063/1.1586957

Barandeh, F., Nguyen, P. L., Kumar, R., Iacobucci, G. J., Kuznicki, M. L., Kosterman, A., Bergey, E. J., Prasad, P. N., & Gunawardena, S. (2012). Organically modified silica nanoparticles are biocompatible and can be targeted to neurons in vivo. *PLoS One, 7*(1), e29424. doi:10.1371/journal.pone.0029424 PMID:22238611

Barlow, P. G., Donaldson, K., MacCallum, J., Clouter, A., & Stone, V. (2005). Serum exposed to nanoparticle carbon black displays increased potential to induce macrophage migration. *Toxicology Letters, 155*(3), 397–401. doi:10.1016/j.toxlet.2004.11.006 PMID:15649623

Barr, I. G., Sjolander, A., & Cox, J. C. (1998). ISCOMs and others aponin based adjuvants. *Advanced Drug Delivery Reviews*, *32*(3), 247–271. doi:10.1016/S0169-409X(98)00013-1 PMID:10837647

Bartolucci, C. (2017). Nanotechnology in Agriculture and Food Science. Academic Press.

Bartosova, L., & Bajgar, J. (2012). Transdermal drug delivery in vitro using diffusion cells. *Current Medicinal Chemistry*, *19*(27), 4671–4677. doi:10.2174/092986712803306358 PMID:22934776

Baruah, S., & Dutta, J. (2009). Nanotechnology applications in pollution sensing and degradation in agriculture: A review. *Environmental Chemistry Letters*, *7*(3), 191–204. doi:10.100710311-009-0228-8

Bastian, A. R., Nangarlia, A., Bailey, L. D., Holmes, A., Sundaram, R. V., Ang, C., Moreira, D. R., Freedman, K., Duffy, C., Contarino, M., & … . (2015). Mechanism of multivalent nanoparticle encounter with HIV-1 for potency enhancement of peptide triazole virus inactivation. *The Journal of Biological Chemistry*, *290*(1), 529–543. doi:10.1074/jbc.M114.608315 PMID:25371202

Basu, D. N., & Ganguly, A. (2016). Solar thermal–photovoltaic powered potato cold storage – Conceptual design and performance analyses. *Applied Energy*, *165*, 308–317. doi:10.1016/j.apenergy.2015.12.070

Baudrin, E., Cassaignon, S., Koesch, M., Jolivet, J. P., Dupont, L., & Tarascon, J. M. (2007). J. Structural Evolution During the Reaction of Li with NanoSized Rutile Type TiO2 at Room Temperature. *Electrochemistry Communications*, *9*(2), 337–342. doi:10.1016/j.elecom.2006.09.022

Bayal, N., & Jeevanandam, P. (2012). Synthesis of metal aluminate nanoparticles by sol–gel method and studies on their reactivity. *Journal of Alloys and Compounds*, *516*, 27–32. doi:10.1016/j.jallcom.2011.11.080

Beard, M. C., Midgett, A. G., Hanna, M. C., Luther, J. M., Hughes, B. K., & Nozik, A. J. (2010). Comparing multiple exciton generation in quantum dots to impact ionization in bulk semiconductors: Implications for enhancement of solar energy conversion. *Nano Letters*, *10*(8), 3019–3027. doi:10.1021/nl101490z PMID:20698615

Beatriz, P. (2017). Diverse applications of nanomedicine. *ACS Nano*. Doi:10.1021/acsnano.6b0604011

Beaulieu, L. Y., & Dahn, J. R. (2000). The reaction of lithium with Sn-Mn-C intermetallics prepared by mechanical alloying. *Journal of the Electrochemical Society*, *147*(9), 3237–3241. doi:10.1149/1.1393889

Benkovicova, M., Vegso, K., Siffalovic, P., Jergel, M., Luby, S., & Majkova, E. (2013). Preparation of gold nanoparticles for plasmonic applications. *Thin Solid Films*, *543*, 138–141. doi:10.1016/j.tsf.2013.01.048

Bernkop-Schnürch, A., Pinter, Y., Guggi, D., Kahlbacher, H., Schöffmann, G., Schuh, M., Schmerold, I., Del Curto, M. D., D'Antonio, M., Esposito, P., & Huck, C. (2005). The use of thiolated polymers as carrier matrix in oral peptide delivery—Proof of concept. *Journal of Controlled Release*, *106*(1-2), 26–33. doi:10.1016/j.jconrel.2005.04.004 PMID:15939501

Berr, M., Vaneski, A., Susha, A. S., Rodrıguez-Fernandez, J., Doblinger, M., Jackel, F., Rogach, A. L., & Feldmann, J. (2010). Colloidal CdS nanorods decorated with subnanometer sized Pt clusters for photocatalytic hydrogen generation. *Applied Physics Letters*, *97*(9), 093108. doi:10.1063/1.3480613

Beutler, J. A. (2009). Natural products as a foundation for drug discovery. *Current Protocols in Pharmacology*, *46*(1), 9–11. doi:10.1002/0471141755.ph0911s46 PMID:20161632

Beyth, N., Houri-Haddad, Y., Domb, A., Khan, W., & Hazan, R. (2015). *Alternative antimicrobial approach: nano-antimicrobial materials*. Evid Based Compl. Altern Med.

Bharadwaj, P., Deutsch, B., & Novotny, L. (2009). Optical Antennas. Adv. *Opt. Photonics*, *1*(3), 438–483. doi:10.1364/AOP.1.000438

Bharali, D. J., Khalil, M., Gurbuz, M., Simone, T. M., & Mousa, S. A. (2009). Nanoparticles and cancer therapy: A concise review with emphasis on dendrimers. *International Journal of Nanomedicine*, *4*, 1. PMID:19421366

Bhardwaj, P., Singh, S., Kharangarh, P. R., & Grace, A. N. (2020). Surfactant decorated polypyrrole-carbon materials composites electrodes for supercapacitor. *Diamond and Related Materials*, *108*, 107989. doi:10.1016/j.diamond.2020.107989

Bhattacharya, K., Mukherjee, S. P., Gallud, A., Burkert, S. C., Bistarelli, S., & Bellucci, S. (2016). Biological interactions of carbon-based nanomaterials: from coronation to degradation. *Nanomedicine, 12*, 333–351. doi: .nano.2015.11.011 doi:10.1016/j

Bhattacharya, R., & Mukherjee, P. (2008). Biological properties of "naked" metal nanoparticles. *Advanced Drug Delivery Reviews*, *60*(11), 1289–1306. doi:10.1016/j.addr.2008.03.013 PMID:18501989

Bhattacharyya, D., Singh, S., Satnalika, N., Khandelwal, A., & Jeon, S.-H. (2009). Nanotechnology, big things from a tiny world : A review. *Science and Technology*, *2*(3), 29–38.

Bhaviripudi, S., Mile, E., Iii, S A S., Zare, A. T., Dresselhaus, M. S., Belcher, A. M., & Kong, J. (2007). CVD Synthesis of Single-Walled Carbon Nanotubes from Gold Nanoparticle. *Catalysts*, *129*(6), 1516–1517. PMID:17283991

Bhumkar, D. R., Joshi, H. M., Sastry, M., & Pokharkar, V. B. (2007b). Chitosan reduced gold nanoparticles as novel carriers for transmucosal delivery of insulin. *Pharmaceutical Research*, *24*(8), 1415–1426. doi:10.100711095-007-9257-9 PMID:17380266

Bina, B., Pourzamani, H., Rashidi, A., & Amin, M. M. (2012). Ethylbenzene removal by carbon nanotubes from aqueous solution. *Journal of Environmental and Public Health*, *817187*, 1–8. doi:10.1155/2012/817187 PMID:22187576

Bindhu, M. R., Umadevi, M., Micheal, M. K., Arasu, M. V., & Al-Dhabi, N. A. (2016). Structural, morphological and optical properties of MgO nanoparticles for antibacterial applications. *Materials Letters*, *166*, 19–22. doi:10.1016/j.matlet.2015.12.020

Biricova, V., & Laznickova, A. (2009). Dendrimers: Analytical characterization and applications. *Bioorganic Chemistry*, *37*(6), 185–192. doi:10.1016/j.bioorg.2009.07.006 PMID:19703699

BlancoAndujar. C. (2014). *Sodium Carbonate Mediated Synthesis of Iron Oxide NPs to Improve Magnetic Hyperthermia Efficiency and Induce Apoptosis*. University College London.

Bleeker, E. A., de Jong, W. H., Geertsma, R. E., Groenewold, M., Heugens, E. H., Koers-Jacquemijns, M., van de Meent, D., Popma, J. R., Rietveld, A. G., Wijnhoven, S. W. P., Cassee, F. R., & Oomen, A. G. (2013). Considerations on the EU definition of a nanomaterial: Science to support policy making. *Regulatory Toxicology and Pharmacology*, *65*(1), 119–125. doi:10.1016/j.yrtph.2012.11.007 PMID:23200793

Bohunicky, B., & Mousa, S. A. (2011). Biosensors: The new wave in cancer diagnosis. *Nanotechnology, Science and Applications*, *4*, 1–10. doi:10.2147/NSA.S13465 PMID:24198482

Bollini, P., Didas, S. A., & Jones, C. W. (2011). Amine-oxide hybrid materials for acid gas separations. *Journal of Materials Chemistry*, *21*(39), 15100–15120. doi:10.1039/c1jm12522b

Bonino, F., Busani, L., Lazzari, M., Manstretta, M., Rivolta, B., & Scrosati, B. (1981). Anatase as a cathode material in lithium—Organic electrolyte rechargeable batteries. *Journal of Power Sources*, *6*(3), 261–270. doi:10.1016/0378-7753(81)80031-6

Boonyanitipong, P., Kositsup, B., Kumar, P., Baruah, S., & Dutta, J. (2011). Toxicity of ZnO and TiO2 Nanoparticles on Germinating Rice Seed Oryza sativa L. *International Journal of Bioscience, Biochemistry, Bioinformatics*, *1*, 282–285. doi:10.7763/IJBBB.2011.V1.53

Borgarello, E., Kiwi, J., Gratzel, M., Pelizzetti, E., & Visca, M. (1982). Visible light induced water cleavage in colloidal solutions of chromium-doped titanium dioxide particles. *Journal of the American Chemical Society*, *104*(11), 2996–3002. doi:10.1021/ja00375a010

Borghols, W. J. H., Wagemaker, M., Lafont, U., Kelder, E. M., & Mulder, F. M. (2009). Size Effects in the Li_4+xTi_5O_{12} Spinel. *Journal of the American Chemical Society*, *131*(49), 17786–17792. doi:10.1021/ja902423e PMID:19919072

Borgmann, S., Schulte, A., Neugebauer, S., & Schuhmann, W. (2012). Amperometric biosensors. In R. C. Alkire, D. M. Kolb, & J. Lipkowski (Eds.), *Bioelectrochemistry: Fundamentals, applications and recent developments* (Vol. 13, pp. 1–83)., doi:10.1002/9783527644117.ch1

Borse, V., Kaler, A., & Banerjee, U.C. (2015). Microbial synthesis of platinum nanoparticles and evaluation of their anticancer activity. *Int. J. Emerg. Trends Electr. Electron.*, *11*.

Boukamp, B. A., Lesh, G. C., & Huggins, R. A. (1981). All-Solid Lithium Electrodes with Mixed-Conductor Matrix. *Journal of the Electrochemical Society*, *128*(4), 725–729. doi:10.1149/1.2127495

Brakmane, G., Winslet, M., & Seifalian, A. M. (2012). Systematic review: The applications of nanotechnology in gastroenterology. *Alimentary Pharmacology & Therapeutics*, *36*(3), 213–221. doi:10.1111/j.1365-2036.2012.05179.x PMID:22686286

Bramhanwade, K., Shende, S., Bonde, S., Gade, A., & Rai, M. (2016). Article. *Environmental Chemistry Letters*, 14.

Brayner, R., Ferrari-Iliou, R., Brivois, N., Djediat, S., Benedetti, M. F., & Fievet, F. (2006). Toxicological impact studies based on *Escherichia coli* bacteria in ultrafine ZnO nanoparticles colloidal medium. *Nano Letters*, *6*(4), 866–870. doi:10.1021/nl052326h PMID:16608300

Bregoli, L., Movia, D., Gavigan-Imedio, J. D., Lysaght, J., Reynolds, J., & Prina-Mello, A. (2016). Nanomedicine applied to translational oncology: A future perspective on cancer treatment. *Nanomedicine; Nanotechnology, Biology, and Medicine*, *12*(1), 81–103. doi:10.1016/j.nano.2015.08.006 PMID:26370707

Brigger, I., Dubernet, C., & Couveur, P. (2002). Nanoparticles in cancer therapy and diagnosis. *Advanced Drug Delivery Reviews*, *54*(5), 631–651. doi:10.1016/S0169-409X(02)00044-3 PMID:12204596

Brinkmann, N., Giebel, D., Lohmer, G., Reetz, M. T., & Kragl, U. (1999). Allylic substitution with dendritic palladium catalysts in a continuously operating membrane reactor. *Journal of Catalysis*, *183*(2), 163–168. doi:10.1006/jcat.1999.2462

Broadley, M. R., White, P. J., Hammond, J. P., Zelko, I., & Lux, A. (2007). Zinc in plants. *The New Phytologist*, *173*(4), 677–702. doi:10.1111/j.1469-8137.2007.01996.x PMID:17286818

Brodd, R. J., Bullock, K. R., Leising, R. A., Middaugh, R. L., Miller, J. R., & Takeuchi, E. (2004). Batteries, 1977 to 2002. *Journal of the Electrochemical Society*, *151*(3), K1–K11. doi:10.1149/1.1641042

Brown, J. (1953). Artificial dielectrics having refractive indices less than unity. *Proceedings of the IEE - Part IV: Institution Monographs*, *100*(5), 51–62. doi:10.1049/pi-4.1953.0009

Bruce, P. G., Scrosati, B., & Tarascon, J.-M. (2008). Nanomaterials for rechargeable lithium batteries. *Angewandte Chemie International Edition*, *47*(16), 2930–2946. doi:10.1002/anie.200702505 PMID:18338357

Brunner, T. J., Wick, P., Manser, P., Spohn, P., Grass, R. N., Limbach, L. K., Bruinink, A., & Stark, W. J. (2006). In vitro cytotoxicity of oxide nanoparticles: Comparison to asbestos, silica, and the effect of particle solubility. *Environmental Science & Technology*, *40*(14), 4374–4381. doi:10.1021/es052069i PMID:16903273

Buchmann, I. (2001). *Will Lithium-Ion batteries power the new millennium.* Cadex Electronics Inc.

Budak, S., Smith, C., Chacha, J., Muntele, C., & Ila, D. (2012). Characterization of gold nanodots arrangements in SiO_2/ SiO_2 + Au nanostructured metamaterials. *Radiation Effects and Defects in Solids*, *167*(8), 607–611. doi:10.1080/1042 0150.2012.668697

Burda, C., Chen, X., Narayanan, R., & El-Sayed, M. A. (2005). Chemistry and properties of nanocrystals of different shapes. *Chemical Reviews*, *105*(4), 1025–1102. doi:10.1021/cr030063a PMID:15826010

Burke, A., & Arulepp, M. (2001). Recent Developments in Carbon-based Electrochemcial Capacitors: Status of the Technology and Future Prospects. *Electrochem. Soc. Proc.*, *21*, 576.

Burygin, G. L., Khlebtsov, B. N., Shantrokha, A. N., Dykman, L. A., Bogatyrev, V. A., & Khlebtsov, N. G. (2009). On the enhanced antibacterial activity of antibiotics mixed with gold nanoparticles. *Nanoscale Research Letters*, *4*(8), 794–801. doi:10.100711671-009-9316-8 PMID:20596384

Butterworth, K. T., Coulter, J. A., Jain, S., Forker, J., McMahon, S. J., Schettino, G., Prise, K. M., Currell, F. J., & Hirst, D. G. (2010). Evaluation of cytotoxicity and radiation enhancement using 1.9 nm gold particles: Potential application for cancer therapy. *Nanotechnology*, *21*(29), 295101. doi:10.1088/0957-4484/21/29/295101 PMID:20601762

Buxton, D. (2006). The Promise of nanotechnology for heart, lung and blood diseases. *Expert Opinion of Drug Deliver*, 173.

Cai, W., Gao, T., & Hong, H. (2008). Applications of gold nanoparticles in cancer nanotechnology, J. Nanotechnology. *Science and Applications*, *1*, 17–32. PMID:24198458

Cai, W., Gao, T., Hong, H., & Sun, J. (2008). Applications of gold nanoparticles in cancer nanotechnology. *Nanotechnology, Science and Applications*, *1*, 17–32. doi:10.2147/NSA.S3788 PMID:24198458

Cai, W., & Hong, H. (2012). In a "nutshell": Intrinsically radio-labeled quantum dots. *American Journal of Nuclear Medicine and Molecular Imaging*, *2*, 136–140. PMID:23133808

Cai, W., Hsu, A. R., Li, Z. B., & Chen, X. (2007). Are quantum dots ready for in vivo imaging in human subjects? *Nanoscale Research Letters*, *2*(6), 265–281. doi:10.100711671-007-9061-9 PMID:21394238

Calvo, P., Remuñan-López, C., Vila-Jato, J. L., & Alonso, M. J. (1997). Chitosan and chitosan/ethylene oxide-propylene oxide block copolymer nanoparticles as novel carriers for proteins and vaccines. *Pharmaceutical Research*, *14*(10), 1431–1436. doi:10.1023/A:1012128907225 PMID:9358557

Campbell, M. L., Guerra, F. D., Dhulekar, J., Alexis, F., & Whitehead, D. C. (2015). Target-Specific Capture of Environmentally Relevant Gaseous Aldehydes and Carboxylic Acids with Functional Nanoparticles. *Chemistry (Weinheim an der Bergstrasse, Germany)*, *21*(42), 14834–14842. doi:10.1002/chem.201502021 PMID:26331393

Cao, C., Zhang, J., Wen, X., Dodson, S. L., Dao, N. T., Wong, L. M., Wang, S., Li, S., Phan, A. T., & Xiong, Q. (2013). Metamaterials-based label-free nanosensor for conformation and affinity biosensing. *ACS Nano*, *7*(9), 7583–7591. doi:10.1021/nn401645t PMID:23952283

Caputoa, A. (2009). Induction of humoral and enhanced cellular immune responses by novel core-shell nanosphere-and microsphere-based vaccine formulations following systemic and mucosal administration. *Vaccine*, *27*(27), 3605–3615. doi:10.1016/j.vaccine.2009.03.047 PMID:19464541

Cardozo, T. R., De Carli, R. F., Seeber, A., Flores, W. H., da Rosa, J., Kotzal, Q., Lehmann, M., da Silva, F. R., & Dihl, R. R. (2019). Genotoxicity of zinc oxide nanoparticles: An *in vivo* and *in silico* study. *Toxicology Research*, *8*(2), 277–286. doi:10.1039/C8TX00255J PMID:30997027

Carlson, C., Hussain, S. M., Schrand, A. M., Braydich-Stolle, K., Hess, K. L., & … . (2008). Unique cellular interaction of silver nanoparticles: Size-dependent generation of reactive oxygen species. *The Journal of Physical Chemistry B*, *112*(43), 13608–13619. doi:10.1021/jp712087m PMID:18831567

Carmona, E. R., García-Rodríguez, A., & Marcos, R. (2018). Genotoxicity of Copper and Nickel Nanoparticles in Somatic Cells of *Drosophila melanogaster. Journal of Toxicology*, *7278036*, 1–8. Advance online publication. doi:10.1155/2018/7278036 PMID:30111998

Carrara, S., Baj-rossi, C., Boero, C., & De Micheli, G. (2014). Do carbon nanotubes contribute to electrochemical biosensing? *Electrochimica Acta*, *128*, 102–112. doi:10.1016/j.electacta.2013.12.123

Carrara, S., Shumyantseva, V. V., Archakov, A. I., & Samor, B. (2008). Screen-printed electrodes based on carbon nanotubes and cytochrome P450scc for highly sensitive cholesterol biosensors. *Biosensors & Bioelectronics*, *24*(1), 148–150. doi:10.1016/j.bios.2008.03.008 PMID:18455917

Cass, A. E. G., Davis, G., Francis, G. D., Allen, H., Hill, H. A. O., Aston, W. J., ... Turner, A. P. F. (1984). Ferrocene-mediated enzyme electrode for amperometric determination of glucose. *Analytical Chemistry*, *56*(4), 667–671. doi:10.1021/ac00268a018 PMID:6721151

Catchpole, K., & Polman, A. (2008). Design principles for particle plasmon enhanced solar cells. *Applied Physics Letters*, *93*(19), 191113. doi:10.1063/1.3021072

Cenci, L., Andreetto, E., Vestri, A., Bovi, M., Barozzi, M., Iacob, E., Busato, M., Castagna, A., Girelli, D., & Bossi, A. M. (2015). Surface plasmon resonance based on molecularly imprinted nanoparticles for the picomolar detection of the iron regulating hormone Hepcidin-25. *Journal of Nanobiotechnology*, *13*(1), 51. doi:10.118612951-015-0115-3 PMID:26311037

Chai, G. S., Yoon, S. B., Yu, J. S., Choi, J. H., & Sung, Y. E. (2004). Ordered porous carbons with tunable pore sizes as catalyst supports in direct methanol fuel cell. *The Journal of Physical Chemistry B*, *108*(22), 7074–7079. doi:10.1021/jp0370472

Chakravorty, A., & Abhishek, N. (2019). Processed Exudate of Pathogen Can Kill Wild Pathogens: Successful In Vitro Application of Newly Synthesized Novel Antimicrobial Therapeutic against Multiple Human Pathogens & Plant Pathogens. *Think India Journal, 22.*

Chakravorty, A., Biswas, B., Sana, S. S., Rayan, R. A., Lala, N. L., & Ramakrishna, S. (2020). A review on toxicity of turmeric derived Nano-Formulates against bacterial and fungal cells with special emphasis on electrospun nanofibers. *Materials Today: Proceedings*. Advance online publication. doi:10.1016/j.matpr.2020.05.820

Chakravorty, A., Rather, G. A., Ali, A., Bhat, B. A., Sana, S. S., Abhishek, N., & Nanda, A. (2020). *Nano Approach: Indian Spices as Antimicrobial Agents. In Ethnopharmacological Investigation of Indian Spices*. IGI Global.

Chaloupka, K. Y., Malam, A. M., & Seifalian, A. M. (2010). Seifalian, Nanosilver as a new generation of nanoproduct in biomedical applications. *Trends in Biotechnology*, *28*(11), 580–588. doi:10.1016/j.tibtech.2010.07.006 PMID:20724010

Chambers, J. P., Arulanandam, B. P., Matta, L. L., Weis, A., & Valdes, J. J. (2008). Biosensor recognition elements. *Current Issues in Molecular Biology*, *10*, 1–12. doi:10.21775/cimb.010.001 PMID:18525101

Chan, C. K., Patel, R. N., O'Connell, M. J., Korgel, B. A., & Cui, Y. (2010). Solution-grown silicon nanowires for lithium-ion battery anodes. *ACS Nano*, *4*(3), 1443–1450. doi:10.1021/nn901409q PMID:20201547

Chan, C. K., Peng, H., Liu, G., McIlwrath, K., Zhang, X. F., Huggins, R. A., & Cui, Y. (2007). High-performance lithium battery anodes using silicon nanowires. *Nature Nanotechnology*, *3*(1), 31–35. doi:10.1038/nnano.2007.411 PMID:18654447

Chan, H. W., Duh, J. G., & Sheen, S. R. (2004). Electrochemical performance of LBO-coated spinel lithium manganese oxide as cathode material for Li-ion battery. *Surface and Coatings Technology*, *188*, 116–119. doi:10.1016/j.surfcoat.2004.08.065

Chan, H. W., Duh, J. G., & Sheen, S. R. (2005). Surface treatment of the lithium boron oxide coated $LiMn_2O_4$ cathode material in Li-ion battery. *Key Engineering Materials*, *280*, 671–676.

Chan, W. C., & Nie, S. (1998). Quantum dot bioconjugates for ultrasensitive nonisotopic detection. *Science*, *281*(5385), 2016–2018. doi:10.1126cience.281.5385.2016 PMID:9748158

Chao, J., Cao, W., Su, S., Weng, L., Song, S., Fan, C., & Wang, L. (2016). Nanostructure-based surface-enhanced Raman scattering biosensors for nucleic acids and proteins. *Journal of Materials Chemistry. B, Materials for Biology and Medicine*, *4*(10), 1757–1769. doi:10.1039/C5TB02135A PMID:32263053

Chao, L. I., Yanliang, F. A. N., Shuzhong, L. I., Bing, X. I. E., Lei, B. I., & Shuting, Y. A. N. G. (2006). Synthesis and electrochemical properties of Th-doped $LiMn_2O_4$ powders for lithium-ion batteries. *Rare Metals*, *25*(6), 58–61. doi:10.1016/S1001-0521(07)60045-X

Chau, C. F., Wu, S. H., & Yen, G. C. (2007). The development of regulations for food nanotechnology. *Trends in Food Science & Technology*, *18*(5), 269–280. doi:10.1016/j.tifs.2007.01.007

Chaudhry, N., Dwivedi, S., Chaudhry, V., Singh, A., Saquib, Q., Azam, A., & Musarrat, J. (2018). Bio-inspired nanomaterials in agriculture and food: Current status, foreseen applications and challenges. *Microbial Pathogenesis*, *123*, 196–200. doi:10.1016/j.micpath.2018.07.013 PMID:30009970

Chaudhry, Q., Scotter, M., Blackburn, J., Ross, B., Boxall, A., Castle, L., Aitken, R., & Watkins, R. (2008). Applications and implications of nanotechnologies for the food sector. *Food Additives and Contaminants*, *25*(3), 241–258. doi:10.1080/02652030701744538 PMID:18311618

Chawengkijwanich, C., & Hayata, Y. (2008). Development of TiO_2 powder-coated food packaging film and its ability to inactivate *Escherichia coli in vitro* and in actual tests. *International Journal of Food Microbiology*, *123*(3), 288–292. doi:10.1016/j.ijfoodmicro.2007.12.017 PMID:18262298

Chen, B., Piletsky, S., & Turner, A. P. F. (2002). Molecular recognition: Design of "keys.". *Combinatorial Chemistry & High Throughput Screening*, *5*(6), 409–427. doi:10.2174/1386207023330129 PMID:12470272

Chen, F., Ehlerding, E. B., & Cai, W. (2014). Theranostic nanoparticles. *Journal of Nuclear Medicine*, *55*(12), 1919–1922. doi:10.2967/jnumed.114.146019 PMID:25413134

Cheng, B., Chen, X., Li, X., Xu, H., Yang, J., & Qian, Y. (2012). High Rate Performance of $LiM_{0.1}Mn_{1.9}O_4$ (M= Mn, Al, Fe) as Cathodes of Lithium Ion Battery at 25 C and 55 C. *International Journal of Electrochemical Science*, *7*, 6453–6464.

Cheng, F., Yang, X., & Gao, J. (2014). Enhancing intensity and refractive index sensing capability with infrared plasmonic perfect absorbers. *Optics Letters*, *39*(11), 3185–3188. doi:10.1364/OL.39.003185 PMID:24876008

Cheng, G., Dong, X., Wang, Y., Peng, D., Wang, X., Hao, H., Xie, S., Qu, W., Liu, Z., & Yuan, Z. (2014). Development of a novel genetically modified bioluminescent-bacteria-based assay for detection of fluoroquinolones in animal-derived foods. *Analytical and Bioanalytical Chemistry*, *406*(30), 7899–7910. doi:10.100700216-014-8228-3 PMID:25354889

Cheng, X., & Zhai, X. (2018). Thermal performance analysis of a cascaded cold storage unit using multiple PCMs. *Energy*, *143*, 448–457. doi:10.1016/j.energy.2017.11.009

Chen, J., Hong, M., Chen, J., Hu, T., & Xu, Q. (2018). Fabrication of hierarchical porous hollow carbon spheres with few-layer graphene framework and high electrochemical activity for supercapacitor. *Applied Surface Science*, *443*, 367–373. doi:10.1016/j.apsusc.2018.02.052

Chen, J., Yang, D., Jiang, J., Ma, A., & Song, D. (2014). Research Progress of Phase Change Materials (PCMs) Embedded with Metal Foam (a Review). *Procedia Materials Science*, *4*, 389–394. doi:10.1016/j.mspro.2014.07.579

Chen, K. S., Hung, T. S., Wu, H. M., Wu, J. Y., Lin, M. T., & Feng, C. K. (2010). Preparation of thermosensitive gold nanoparticles by plasma pretreatment and UV grafted polymerization. *Thin Solid Films*, *518*(24), 7557–7562. doi:10.1016/j.tsf.2010.05.043

Chen, S., Zhu, J., Wu, X., Han, Q., & Wang, X. (2010). Graphene oxide-MnO_2 nanocomposites for supercapacitors. *ACS Nano*, *4*(5), 2822–2830. doi:10.1021/nn901311t PMID:20384318

Chen, T., Li, S., & Sun, H. (2012). Metamaterials application in sensing. *Sensors (Basel)*, *12*(3), 2742–2765. doi:10.3390120302742 PMID:22736975

Chen, W., Fan, Z., Gu, L., Bao, X., & Wang, C. (2010). Enhanced capacitance of manganese oxide via confinement inside carbon nanotubes. *Chemical Communications (Cambridge)*, *46*(22), 3905–3907. doi:10.1039/c000517g PMID:20411189

Chen, X., Cen, C., Tang, Z., Zeng, W., Chen, D., Fang, P., & Chen, Z. (2013). The key role of pH value in the synthesis of titanate nanotubes-loaded manganese oxides as a superior catalyst for the selective catalytic reduction of NO with NH_3. *Journal of Nanomaterials*, *871528*, 1–7. doi:10.1155/2013/871528

Chen, X., Shen, S., Guo, L., & Mao, S. S. (2010). Semiconductor-based Photocatalytic Hydrogen Generation. *Chemical Reviews*, *110*(11), 6503–6570. doi:10.1021/cr1001645 PMID:21062099

Chen, X., Worall, M., Omer, S., Su, Y., & Riffat, S. (2014). Experimental investigation on PCM cold storage integrated with ejector cooling system. *Applied Thermal Engineering*, *63*(1), 419–427. doi:10.1016/j.applthermaleng.2013.11.029

Chen, Y. B., Hu, Y., Lian, F., & Liu, Q. G. (2010). Synthesis and characterization of spinel $Li_{1.05}Cr_{0.1}Mn_{1.9}O_{4-z}F_z$ as cathode materials for lithium-ion batteries. *International Journal of Minerals Metallurgy and Materials*, *17*(2), 220–224. doi:10.100712613-010-0217-8

Chen, Y. H., & Yeh, C. S. (2002). Laser ablation method: Use of surfactants to form the dispersed Ag nanoparticles. *Colloids and Surfaces. A, Physicochemical and Engineering Aspects*, *197*(1-3), 133–139. doi:10.1016/S0927-7757(01)00854-8

Chen, Y. S., Hung, Y. C., Lin, W. H., & Huang, G. S. (2010). Assessment of gold nanoparticles as a size-dependent vaccine carrier for enhancing the antibody response against synthetic foot and mouth disease virus peptide. *Nanotechnology*, *21*(19), 195101. doi:10.1088/0957-4484/21/19/195101 PMID:20400818

Chen, Y., & Ming, H. (2012). Review of surface plasmon resonance and localized surface plasmon resonance sensor. *Photonic Sensors*, *2*(1), 37–49. doi:10.100713320-011-0051-2

Chen, Y., Sheng, L., Gouda, M., & Ma, M. (2019). Impact of ultrasound treatment on the foaming and physicochemical properties of egg white during cold storage. *Lebensmittel-Wissenschaft + Technologie*, *13*, 108303. doi:10.1016/j.lwt.2019.108303

Cherchi, C., & Gu, A. Z. (2010). Impact of Titanium Dioxide Nanomaterials on Nitrogen Fixation Rate and Intracellular Nitrogen Storage in *Anabaena variabilis*. *Environmental Science & Technology*, *4*(21), 8302–8307. doi:10.1021/es101658p PMID:20853867

Chifiriuc, M. C., Ratiu, A. C., Popa, M., & Ecovoiu, A. A. (2016). Drosophotoxicology: An Emerging Research Area for Assessing Nanoparticles Interaction with Living Organisms. *International Journal of Molecular Sciences*, *17*(2), 36. doi:10.3390/ijms17020036 PMID:26907252

Chiodo, F., Marradi, M., Calvo, J., Yuste, E., & Penadés, S. (2014). Glycosystems in nanotechnology: Gold glyconanoparticles as carrier for anti-HIV prodrugs. *Beilstein Journal of Organic Chemistry*, *10*, 1339–1346. doi:10.3762/bjoc.10.136 PMID:24991287

Chithrani, D. B., Dunne, M., Stewart, J., Allen, C., & Jaffray, D. A. (2010). Cellular uptake and transport of gold nanoparticles incorporated in a liposomal carrier. *Nanomedicine; Nanotechnology, Biology, and Medicine*, *6*(1), 161–169. doi:10.1016/j.nano.2009.04.009 PMID:19447206

Cho, E. J., Holback, H., Liu, K. C., Abouelmagd, S. A., Park, J., & Yeo, Y. (2013). Nanoparticle characterization : State of the art, challenges and emerging technologies. *Molecular Pharmaceutics*, *10*(6), 2093–2110. doi:10.1021/mp300697h PMID:23461379

Choi, K.Y., Jeon, E.J., & Yoon, H.Y. (2012b). Theranostic nanoparticles based on PEGylated hyaluronic acid for the diagnosis, therapy and monitoring of colon cancer. *Biomaterials, 33*(26), 6186-6193.

Choi, K.Y., Liu, G., & Chen, X. (2012a). Theranostic nanoplatforms for simultaneous cancer imaging and therapy: current approaches and future perspectives. *Nanoscale, 4*(2), 330-342.

Choi, J.-H., Lee, C., Cho, S., Moon, G. D., kim, B., Chang, H., & Jang, H. D. (2018). High capacitance and energy density supercapacitor based on biomass-derived activated carbons with reduced graphene oxide binder. *Carbon*, *132*, 16–24. doi:10.1016/j.carbon.2018.01.105

Choi, O., Deng, K. K., Kim, N. J., Ross, L. Jr, Surampalli, R. Y., & Hu, Z. Q. (2008). The inhibitory effects of silver nanoparticles, silver ions, and silver chloride colloids on microbial growth. *Water Research*, *42*(12), 3066–3074. doi:10.1016/j.watres.2008.02.021 PMID:18359055

Choi, W. C., Woo, S. I., Jeon, M. K., Sohn, J. M., Kim, M. R., & Jeon, H. J. (2005). Platinum Nanoclusters Studded in the Microporous Nanowalls of Ordered Mesoporous Carbon. *Advanced Materials*, *17*(4), 446–451. doi:10.1002/adma.200400978

Cho, J. (2008). VO_x-coated $LiMn_2O_4$ nanorod clusters for lithium battery cathode materials. *Journal of Materials Chemistry*, *18*(19), 2257–2261. doi:10.1039/b719177d

Chopra, K. L., Paulson, P. D., & Dutta, V. (2004). Thin film solar cells: An overview. *Progress in Photovoltaics: Research and Applications*, *12*(2–3), 69–92. doi:10.1002/pip.541

Chumha, N., Kittiwachana, S., Thongtem, T., Thongtem, S., & Kaowphong, S. (2014). Synthesis and characterization of GdVO4 nanoparticles by a malic acid-assisted sol–gel method. *Materials Letters*, *136*, 18–21. doi:10.1016/j.matlet.2014.07.175

Chung, T., Lee, S. Y., Song, E. Y., Chun, H., & Lee, B. (2011). Plasmonic nanostructures for nano-scale bio-sensing. *Sensors (Basel)*, *11*(11), 10907–10929. doi:10.3390111110907 PMID:22346679

Clark, L. C. Jr, & Lyons, C. (1962). Electrode systems for continuous monitoring in cardiovascular surgery. *Annals of the New York Academy of Sciences*, *102*(1), 29–45. doi:10.1111/j.1749-6632.1962.tb13623.x PMID:14021529

Classen, I., & Osterhaus, A. (1992). The iscom structure as an immune enhancing moiety: Experiences in viral systems. *Australian Orthodontic Journal*, *15*, 260–268.

Clifford, J. N., Planells, M., & Palomares, E. (2012). Advances in high efficiency dye sensitized solar cells based on Ru(ii) free sensitizers and a liquid redox electrolyte. *Journal of Materials Chemistry*, *22*(46), 24195–24201. doi:10.1039/c2jm34289h

Cobb, M. D., & Macoubrie, J. (2004). Public perceptions about nanotechnology: Risks, benefits and trust. *Journal of Nanoparticle Research*, *6*(4), 395–405. doi:10.100711051-004-3394-4

Cobley, C. M., Chen, J., Cho, E. C., Wang, L. V., & Xia, Y. (2011). Gold nanostructures: A class of multifunctional materials for biomedical applications. *Chemical Society Reviews*, *40*(1), 44–56. doi:10.1039/B821763G PMID:20818451

Colangelo, G., Milanese, M., & Risi, A. D. (2019). Energy simulation of a nanofluid solar cooling system in Italy. *Proceedings of the Institution of Civil Engineers. Engineering Sustainability*, *172*(1), 32–39. doi:10.1680/jensu.16.00027

Cole, T. (1983). Thermoelectric energy conversion with solid electrolytes. *Science*, *221*(4614), 915–920. doi:10.1126cience.221.4614.915 PMID:17748444

Coma, V., Deschamps, A., & Martial-Gros, A. (2003). Bioactive packaging materials from edible chitosan polymer-antimicrobial activity assessment on dairy-related contaminants. *Journal of Food Science*, *68*(9), 2788–2792. doi:10.1111/j.1365-2621.2003.tb05806.x

Compton, O. C., & Nguyen, S. T. (2010). Graphene oxide, highly reduced graphene oxide, and graphene: Versatile building blocks for carbon-based materials. *Small*, *2010*(6), 711–723. doi:10.1002mll.200901934 PMID:20225186

Conroy, D. J. R., Millner, P. A., Stewart, D. I., & Pollmann, K. (2010). Biosensing for the environment and defence: Aqueous uranyl detection using bacterial surface layer proteins. *Sensors (Basel)*, *10*(5), 4739–4755. doi:10.3390100504739 PMID:22399904

Conway, B. E. (1999). *Electrochemical supercapacitors: scientific fundamentals and technological applications*. Plenum Press. doi:10.1007/978-1-4757-3058-6

Corley, E., Scheufele, D., & Hu, Q. (2009). Of risks and regulations: How leading U.S. nanoscientists form policy stances about nanotechnology. *Journal of Nanoparticle Research*, *11*(7), 1573–1585. doi:10.100711051-009-9671-5 PMID:21170136

Cormack, P. A. G., & Elorza, A. Z. (2004). Molecularly imprinted polymers: Synthesis and characterisation. *Journal of Chromatography. B, Analytical Technologies in the Biomedical and Life Sciences*, *804*(1), 173–182. doi:10.1016/j.jchromb.2004.02.013 PMID:15093171

Cormack, P. A. G., & Mosbach, K. (1999). Molecular imprinting: Recent developments and the road ahead. *Reactive & Functional Polymers*, *41*(1-3), 115–124. doi:10.1016/S1381-5148(99)00024-3

Cotterell, P. (2018). Parkinson's disease: Symptoms, treatment options and nursing care. *Nursing Standard*, *33*(7), 53–58. doi:10.7748/ns.2018.e11207 PMID:30198239

Couture, M., Zhao, S. S., & Masson, J. F. (2013). Modern surface plasmon resonance for bioanalytics and biophysics. *Physical Chemistry Chemical Physics*, *15*(27), 11190–11216. doi:10.1039/c3cp50281c PMID:23748491

Couvreur, P., Kante, B., Grislain, L., Roland, M., & Speiser, P. (1982). Toxicity of polyalkylcyanoacrylate nanoparticles II: Doxorubicin-loaded nanoparticles. *Journal of Pharmaceutical Sciences*, *71*(7), 790–792. doi:10.1002/jps.2600710717 PMID:7120064

Crabtree, G. W., & Lewis, N. S. (2007). Solar energy conversion. *Physics Today*, *60*(3), 37–42. doi:10.1063/1.2718755

Cromwell, W. A., Yang, J., Starr, J. L., & Jo, Y. K. (2014). Article. *Journal of Nematology*, *46*, 261–266. PMID:25275999

Cruz-Romero, M. C., Murphy, T., Morris, M., Cummins, E., & Kerry, J. P. (2013). Antimicrobial activity of chitosan, organic acids and nano-sized solubilisates for potential use in smart antimicrobially-active packaging for potential food applications. *Food Control*, *34*(2), 393–397. doi:10.1016/j.foodcont.2013.04.042

Cui, D., Tian, F., Ozkan, C. S., Wang, M., & Gao, H. (2005). Effect of single wall carbon nanotubes on human HEK293 cells. *Toxicology Letters*, *155*(1), 73–85. doi:10.1016/j.toxlet.2004.08.015 PMID:15585362

Cui, Y., Wei, Q., Park, H., & Lieber, C. M. (2001). Nanowire nanosensors for highly sensitive and selective detection of biological and chemical species. *Science*, *293*(5533), 1289–1292. doi:10.1126cience.1062711 PMID:11509722

Cushen, M., Kerry, J., Morris, M., Cruz-Romero, M., & Cummins, E. (2012). Nanotechnologies in the food industry – Recent developments, risks and regulation. *Trends in Food Science & Technology*, *24*(1), 30–46. doi:10.1016/j.tifs.2011.10.006

D'Amato, R., Falconieri, M., Gagliardi, S., Popovici, E., Serra, E., Terranova, G., & Borsella, E. (2013). Synthesis of ceramic nanoparticles by laser pyrolysis: From research to applications. *Journal of Analytical and Applied Pyrolysis*, *104*, 461–469. doi:10.1016/j.jaap.2013.05.026

da Silva, E. T. S. G., Souto, D. E. P., & Barragan, J. T. C., de F. Giarola, J., de Moraes, A. C. M., & Kubota, L. T. (. (2017). Electrochemical biosensors in point-of-care devices: Recent advances and future trends. *ChemElectroChem*, *4*(4), 778–794. doi:10.1002/celc.201600758

Dabrowski, M., Lach, P., Cieplak, M., & Kutner, W. (2018). Nanostructured molecularly imprinted polymers for protein chemosensing. *Biosensors & Bioelectronics*, *102*, 17–26. doi:10.1016/j.bios.2017.10.045 PMID:29101784

Dagar, G., & Bagchi, G. (2020). Nanoparticles as potential endocrine disruptive chemicals. In S. K. Saxena & S. M. P. Khurana (Eds.), *NanoBioMedicine* (pp. 411–429). Springer., doi:10.1007/978-981-32-9898-9_17

Dai, L., Chang, D. W., Baek, J-B., Lu, W. (2012). Carbon Nanomaterials for Advanced Energy Conversion and Storage. *Small*, *8*, 1130–1166.

Dai, L. (2006). *Carbon Nanotechnology: Recent Developments in Chemistry, Physics, Materials Science and Device Applications*. Elsevier Science.

Damm, C., Munstedt, H., & Rosch, A. (2008). The antimicrobial efficacy of polyamide6/silver-nano and microcomposites. *Materials Chemistry and Physics*, *108*(1), 61–66. doi:10.1016/j.matchemphys.2007.09.002

Dang, T. M. D., Le, T. T. T., Fribourg-Blanc, E., & Dang, M. C. (2011). The influence of solvents and surfactants on the preparation of copper nanoparticles by a chemical reduction method. *Advances in Natural Sciences: Nanoscience and Nanotechnology*, *2*(2), 025004. doi:10.1088/2043-6262/2/2/025004

Danilov, A., Tselikov, G., Wu, F., Kravets, V. G., Ozerov, I., Bedu, F., Grigorenko, A. N., & Kabashin, A. V. (2018). Ultra-narrow surface lattice resonances in plasmonic metamaterial arrays for biosensing applications. *Biosensors & Bioelectronics*, *104*, 102–112. doi:10.1016/j.bios.2017.12.001 PMID:29331424

Daraio, C., & Jin, S. (2012). Synthesis and patterning methods for nanostructures useful for biological applications. In *Nanotechnology for biology and medicine* (pp. 27–44). Springer. doi:10.1007/978-0-387-31296-5_2

Das, V. L., Thomas, R., Varghese, R. T., Soniya, E. V., Mathew, J., & Radhakrishnan, E. K. (2014). Extracellular synthesis of silver nanoparticles by the Bacillus strain CS 11 isolated from industrialized area. *3 Biotech*, *4*(2), 121-126.

Dasgupta, N., Ranjan, S., Mundekkad, D., Ramalingam, C., Shanker, R., & Kumar, A. (2015a). Nanotechnology in agro-food: From field to plate. *Food Research International*, *69*, 381–400. doi:10.1016/j.foodres.2015.01.005

Das, I., & Ansari, S. A. (2009). Nanomaterials in science and technology. *Journal of Scientific and Industrial Research, 68*(8), 657–667.

Das, S., Chakraborty, J., Chatterjee, S., & Kumar, H. (2018). Prospects of biosynthesized nanomaterials for remediation of organic and inorganic environmental contaminants. *Environmental Science. Nano, 5*(12), 2784–2808. doi:10.1039/C8EN00799C

Das, S., Li, J., & Hui, R. (2014, October). Impact of Electrode Surface/Volume Ratio on Li-ion Battery Performance. *Proceedings of the COMSOL Conference*, 8-10.

Davis, M. E., Chen, Z., & Shin, D. M. (2010). Nanoparticle therapeutics, an emerging treatment modality for cancer: in Nanoscience and technology. In A collection of reviews from nature journals, (pp. 239-250). Academic Press.

Davis, S. S. (1997). Biomedical applications of nanotechnology—Implications for drug targeting and gene therapy. *Trends in Biotechnology, 15*(6), 217–224. doi:10.1016/S0167-7799(97)01036-6 PMID:9183864

De Carli, R. F., Chaves, D., Cardozo, T. R., de Souza, A. P., Seeber, A., Flores, W. H., Honatel, K. F., Lehmann, M., & Dihl, R. R. (2018). Evaluation of the genotoxic properties of nickel oxide nanoparticles in vitro and in vivo. *Mutation research. Genetic toxicology and environmental mutagenesis, 836*(Pt B), 47–53. doi:10.1016/j.mrgentox.2018.06.003

De Carvalho, J. F., De Medeiros, S. N., Morales, M. A., Dantas, A. L., & Carriço, A. S. (2013). Synthesis of magnetite nanoparticles by high energy ball milling. *Applied Surface Science, 275*, 84–87. doi:10.1016/j.apsusc.2013.01.118

De Filpo, G., Palermo, A. M. F., Rachiele, F. P., & Nicoletta, F. P. (2013). Preventing fungal growth in wood by titanium dioxide nanoparticles. *Int. Biodeter. Biodegr., 85*, 217–222. doi:10.1016/j.ibiod.2013.07.007

De Jong, W. H., & Borm, P. J. (2008). Drug delivery and nanoparticles: Applications and hazards. *International Journal of Nanomedicine, 3*, 133. doi:10.2147/IJN.S596 PMID:18686775

de Kozak, Y., Andrieux, K., Villarroya, H., Klein, C., Thillaye Goldenberg, B., Naud, M. C., Garcia, E., & Couvreur, P. (2004). Intraocular injection of tamoxifen-loaded nanoparticles: A new treatment of experimental autoimmune uveoretinitis. *European Journal of Immunology, 34*(12), 3702–3712. doi:10.1002/eji.200425022 PMID:15517615

de la Escosura-Muñiz, A., Sánchez-Espinel, C., Díaz-Freitas, B., Gonzalez-Fernandez, A., Maltez-da Costa, M., & Merkoçi, A. (2009). Rapid identification and quantification of tumor cells using an electrocatalytic method based on gold nanoparticles. *Analytical Chemistry, 81*(24), 10268–10274. doi:10.1021/ac902087k PMID:19911778

De Windt, W., Aelterman, P., & Verstraete, W. (2005). Bioreductive deposition of palladium (0) nanoparticles on *Shewanella oneidensis* with catalytic activity towards reductive dechlorination of polychlorinated biphenyls. *Environmental Microbiology, 7*(3), 314–325. doi:10.1111/j.1462-2920.2005.00696.x PMID:15683392

De-Azeredo, H. M. C. (2013). Antimicrobial nanostructures in food packaging. *Trends in Food Science & Technology, 30*(1), 56–69. doi:10.1016/j.tifs.2012.11.006

Deb, A., & Vimala, R. (2017). Graphene Mediated Drug Delivery-A Boon to Cancer Therapy. *Research Journal of Pharmacy and Technology, 10*(5), 1571–1576. doi:10.5958/0974-360X.2017.00276.1

Deb, S., Patra, H. K., Lahiri, P., Dasgupta, A. K., Chakrabarti, K., & Chaudhuri, U. (2011). Multistability in platelets and their response to gold nanoparticles. *Nanomedicine; Nanotechnology, Biology, and Medicine, 7*(4), 376–384. doi:10.1016/j.nano.2011.01.007 PMID:21310267

Deerinck, T. J. (2008). The application of fluorescent quantum dots to confocal, multiphoton, and electron microscopic imaging. *Toxicologic Pathology, 36*(1), 112–116.

Delacourt, C., Poizot, P., Levasseur, S., & Masquelier, C. (2006). Size effects on carbon-free LiFePO. chem. *Solid-State Lett.*, *9*(7), A352. doi:10.1149/1.2201987

DeLong, R. K., Reynolds, C. M., Malcolm, Y., Schaeffer, A., Severs, T., & Wanekaya, A. (2010). Functionalized gold nanoparticles for the binding, stabilization, and delivery of therapeutic DNA, RNA, and other biological macromolecules. *Nanotechnology, Science and Applications*, *3*, 53. doi:10.2147/NSA.S8984 PMID:24198471

Demento, S. L., Cui, W., Criscione, J. M., Stern, E., Tulipan, J., Kaech, S. M., & Fahmy, T. M. (2012). Role of sustained antigen release from nanoparticle vaccines in shaping the T cell memory phenotype. *Biomaterials*, *33*(19), 4957–4964. doi:10.1016/j.biomaterials.2012.03.041 PMID:22484047

Demir, E., Vales, G., Kaya, B., Creus, A., & Marcos, R. (2011). Genotoxic analysis of silver nanoparticles in Drosophila. *Nanotoxicology*, *5*(3), 417–424. doi:10.3109/17435390.2010.529176 PMID:21039182

Deng, H., McShan, D., Zhang, Y., Sinha, S. S., Arslan, Z., Ray, P. C., & Yu, H. (2016). Mechanistic study of the synergistic antibacterial activity of combined silver nanoparticles and common antibiotics. *Environmental Science & Technology*, *50*(16), 8840–8848. doi:10.1021/acs.est.6b00998 PMID:27390928

des Rieux, A., Fievez, V., Garinot, M., Schneider, Y. J., & Préat, V. (2006). Nanoparticles as potential oral delivery systems of proteins and vaccines: A mechanistic approach. *Journal of Controlled Release*, *116*(1), 1–27. doi:10.1016/j.jconrel.2006.08.013 PMID:17050027

Deshpande, V. V., Chandra, B., Caldwell, R., Novikov, D. S., Hone, J., & Bockrath, M. (2009). Mott Insulating State in Ultraclean Carbon Nanotubes. *Science*, *323*(5910), 106–110. doi:10.1126cience.1165799 PMID:19119228

Dhand, C. (2015). Methods and strategies for the synthesis of diverse nanoparticles and their applications: A comprehensive overview. *RSC Advances*, *5*(127), 105003–105037.

Dhar, S., Daniel, W. L., Giljohann, D. A., Mirkin, C. A., & Lippard, S. J. (2009). Polyvalent oligonucleotide gold nanoparticle conjugates as delivery vehicles for platinum (IV) 0000 warheads. *Journal of the American Chemical Society*, *131*(41), 14652–14653. doi:10.1021/ja9071282 PMID:19778015

Di Giacomo, S., Sollazzo, M., de Biase, D., Ragazzi, M., Bellosta, P., Pession, A., & Grifoni, D. (2017). Human Cancer Cells Signal Their Competitive Fitness Through MYC Activity. *Scientific Reports*, *7*(1), 12568. doi:10.103841598-017-13002-1 PMID:28974715

Diallo, M. S., Christie, S., Swaminathan, P., Johnson, J. H., & Goddard, W. A. (2005). Dendrimer enhanced ultrafiltration.1. Recovery of Cu (II) from aqueous solutions using PAMAM dendrimers with ethylene diamine core and terminal NH_2 groups. *Environmental Science & Technology*, *39*(5), 1366–1377. doi:10.1021/es048961r PMID:15787379

Dincer, C., Bruch, R., Costa-Rama, E., Fernández-Abedul, M. T., Merkoçi, A., Manz, A., Urban, G. A., & Güder, F. (2019). Disposable sensors in diagnostics, food, and environmental monitoring. *Advanced Materials*, *31*(30), 1806739. doi:10.1002/adma.201806739 PMID:31094032

Ding, Y. L., Xie, J., Cao, G. S., Zhu, T. J., Yu, H. M., & Zhao, X. B. (2011). Enhanced elevated-temperature performance of Al-doped single-crystalline $LiMn_2O_4$ nanotubes as cathodes for lithium ion batteries. *The Journal of Physical Chemistry C*, *115*(19), 9821–9825. doi:10.1021/jp201669x

Diwan, M., Elamanchili, P., Lane, H., Gainer, A., & Samuel, J. (2003). Biodegradable nanoparticle mediated antigen delivery to human cord blood derived dendritic cells for induction of primary T cell responses. *Journal of Drug Targeting*, *11*(8-10), 495–507. doi:10.1080/10611860410001670026 PMID:15203918

Dobrucka, R., & Długaszewska, J. (2016). Biosynthesis and antibacterial activity of ZnO nanoparticles using Trifolium pratense flower extract. *Saudi Journal of Biological Sciences*, *23*(4), 517–523. doi:10.1016/j.sjbs.2015.05.016 PMID:27298586

Dong, X., Cao, Y., Wang, J., Chan-Park, M. B., Wang, L., Huang, W., & Chen, P. (2012). Hybrid structure of zinc oxide nanorods and three dimensional graphene foam for supercapacitor and electrochemical sensor applications. *RSC Advances*, *2*(10), 4364–4369. doi:10.1039/c2ra01295b

Dong, Z. G., Liu, H., Cao, J. X., Li, T., Wang, S. M., Zhu, S. N., & Zhang, X. (2010). Enhanced sensing performance by the plasmonic analog of electromagnetically induced transparency in active metamaterials. *Applied Physics Letters*, *97*(11), 10–13. doi:10.1063/1.3488020

Doung, T. G. (2003). *2002 Annual Progress Report for Energy Storage Research and Development*. Freedom Car & Vehicle Technologies Program.

Drabu, S., Khatri, S., Babu, S., & Verma, D. (2010). Nanotechnology: An introduction to future drug delivery system. *Journal of Chemical and Pharmaceutical Research*, *2*, 171–179.

Driscoll, K. E., Costa, D. L., Henderson, R., Oberdo¨ rster, G., Salem, H. Schlesinger, R. B. (2000). Intratracheal instillation as an exposure technique for the evaluation of respiratory tract toxicity: Uses and limitations, *Toxicological Sciences*, *55*, 24 – 35.

Du, G., Sharma, N., Peterson, V. K., Kimpton, J. A., Jia, D., & Guo, Z. (2011). Br-Doped $Li_4Ti_5O_{12}$ and Composite TiO_2 Anodes for Li-ion Batteries: Synchrotron X-Ray and in situ Neutron Diffraction Studies. *Advanced Functional Materials*, *21*(20), 3990–3997. doi:10.1002/adfm.201100846

Du, J., Liu, Z., Wu, W., Li, Z., Han, B., & Huang, Y. (2005). Preparation of single-crystal copper ferrite nanorods and nanodisks. *Materials Research Bulletin*, *40*(6), 928–935. doi:10.1016/j.materresbull.2005.03.002

Du, L., Zhang, X., Mei, T., & Yuan, X. (2010). Localized surface plasmons, surface plasmon polaritons, and their coupling in 2D metallic array for SERS. *Optics Express*, *18*(3), 1959–1965. doi:10.1364/OE.18.001959 PMID:20174025

Dulkeith, E., Morteani, A. C., Niedereichholz, T., Klar, T. A., Feldmann, J., Levi, S. A., van Veggel, F. C. J. M., Reinhoudt, D. N., Möller, M., & Gittins, D. I. (2002). Fluorescence quenching of dye molecules near gold nanoparticles: Radiative and nonradiative effects. *Physical Review Letters*, *89*(20), 203002. doi:10.1103/PhysRevLett.89.203002 PMID:12443474

Duverger, E., Frison, N., Roche, A. C., & Monsigny, M. (2003). Carbohydrate-lectin interactions assessed by surface plasmon resonance. *Biochimie*, *85*(1-2), 167–179. doi:10.1016/S0300-9084(03)00060-9 PMID:12765786

Dwivedi, A. D., & Gopal, K. (2010). Biosynthesis of silver and gold nanoparticles using Chenopodium album leafextract. *Colloids and Surfaces. A, Physicochemical and Engineering Aspects*, *369*(1-3), 27–33. doi:10.1016/j.colsurfa.2010.07.020

Dye, C. (2014). After 2015: Infectious diseases in a new era of health and development. *Philosophical Transactions of the Royal Society of London. Series B, Biological Sciences*, *369*(1645), 20130426. doi:10.1098/rstb.2013.0426 PMID:24821913

Ealias, A. M., & Saravanakumar, M. P. (2017, November). A review on the classification, characterization, synthesis of nanoparticles and their application. In IOP Conf. *Ser. Mater. Sci. Eng*, *263*, 032019.

Edelstein, R. L., Tamanaha, C. R., Sheehan, P. E., Miller, M. M., Baselt, D. R., Whitman, L. J., & Colton, R. J. (2000). The BARC biosensor applied to the detection of biological warfare agents. *Biosensors & Bioelectronics*, *14*(10-11), 805–813. doi:10.1016/S0956-5663(99)00054-8 PMID:10945455

Eftekhari, A., Moghaddam, A. B., & Solati-Hashjin, M. (2006). Electrochemical properties of $LiMn_2O_4$ cathode material doped with an actinide. *Journal of Alloys and Compounds*, *424*(1), 225–230. doi:10.1016/j.jallcom.2005.10.088

Ein-Eli, Y., Urian, R. C., Wen, W., & Mukerjee, S. (2005). Low temperature performance of copper/nickel modified $LiMn_2O_4$ spinels. *Electrochimica Acta*, *50*(9), 1931–1937. doi:10.1016/j.electacta.2004.09.002

El-Ansary, A., & Faddah, L. M. (2010). Nanoparticles as biochemical sensors. *Nanotechnology, Science and Applications*, *3*, 65–76. doi:10.2147/NSA.S8199 PMID:24198472

El-Badawy, H. (2012). Effect of Chitosan and Calcium Chloride Spraying on Fruits Quality of Florida Prince Peach Under Cold Storage. *Research Journal of Agriculture and Biological Sciences*, *8*, 272-281.

Elechiguerra, J. L., Burt, J. L., Morones, J. R., Camacho-Bragado, A., Gao, X., Lara, H. H., & Yacaman, M. J. (2005). Interaction of silver nanoparticles with HIV-1. *Journal of Nanobiotechnology*, *3*(1), 6. doi:10.1186/1477-3155-3-6 PMID:15987516

Ellingson, R. J., Beard, M. C., Johnson, J. C., Yu, P., Micic, O. I., Nozik, A. J., Shabaev, A., & Efros, A. L. (2005). Highly efficient multiple exciton generation in colloidal PbSe and PbS quantum dots. *Nano Letters*, *5*(5), 865–871. doi:10.1021/nl0502672 PMID:15884885

El, M., Akjouj, A., & Mir, A. (2020). Design of silver nanoparticles with graphene coatings layers used for LSPR biosensor applications. *Vacuum*, *180*, 109497-1, 109497–11. doi:10.1016/j.vacuum.2020.109497

El-Sayyad, G. S., Mosallam, F. M., & El-Batal, A. I. (2018). One-pot green synthesis of magnesium oxide nanoparticles using Penicillium chrysogenum melanin pigment and gamma rays with antimicrobial activity against multidrug-resistant microbes. *Advanced Powder Technology*, *29*(11), 2616–2625. doi:10.1016/j.apt.2018.07.009

El-Shabouri, M. H. (2002). Positively charged nanoparticles for improving the oral bioavailability of cyclosporin-A. *International Journal of Pharmaceutics*, *249*(1-2), 101–118. doi:10.1016/S0378-5173(02)00461-1 PMID:12433438

Eltarahony, M., Zaki, S., ElKady, M., & Abd-El-Haleem, D. (2018). Article. *Journal of Nanomaterials*, *2018*, 1–16.

Emadpour, M., Ghareyazie, B., & Kalaj, Y.REntesari, MBouzari, N. (2015). Effect of the potassium permanganate coated zeolite nanoparticles on the quality characteristic and shelf life of peach and nectarine. *Agricultural Technology (Thailand)*, *11*(5), 1263–1273.

Emamifar, A., Kadivar, M., Shahedi, M., & Soleimanian-Zad, S. (2011). Effect of nanocomposite packaging containing Ag and ZnO on inactivation of Lactobacillus plantarum in orange juice. *Food Control*, *22*(3–4), 408–413. doi:10.1016/j.foodcont.2010.09.011

Emerich, D. F., & Thanos, C. G. (2003). Nanotechnology and medicine. *Expert Opinion on Biological Therapy*, *3*(4), 655–663. doi:10.1517/14712598.3.4.655 PMID:12831370

Engin, K., Leeper, D. B., & Cater, J. R. (1995). a J. Thistlethwaite, L. Tupchong and JD McFarlane. *International Journal of Hyperthermia*, *11*, 211–216. doi:10.3109/02656739509022457 PMID:7790735

Erdem, Ö., Saylan, Y., Cihangir, N., & Denizli, A. (2019). Molecularly imprinted nanoparticles based plasmonic sensors for real-time Enterococcus faecalis detection. *Biosensors & Bioelectronics*, *126*, 608–614. doi:10.1016/j.bios.2018.11.030 PMID:30502683

Ersöz, A., Denizli, A., Özcan, A., & Say, R. (2005). Molecularly imprinted ligand-exchange recognition assay of glucose by quartz crystal microbalance. *Biosensors & Bioelectronics*, *20*(11), 2197–2202. doi:10.1016/j.bios.2004.07.030 PMID:15797316

Ertürk, G., Özen, H., Tümer, M. A., Mattiasson, B., & Denizli, A. (2016). Microcontact imprinting based surface plasmon resonance (SPR) biosensor for real-time and ultrasensitive detection of prostate specific antigen (PSA) from clinical samples. *Sensors and Actuators. B, Chemical*, *224*, 823–832. doi:10.1016/j.snb.2015.10.093

Ertürk, G., Uzun, L., Tümer, M. A., Say, R., & Denizli, A. (2011). Fab fragments imprinted SPR biosensor for real-time human immunoglobulin G detection. *Biosensors & Bioelectronics*, *28*(1), 97–104. doi:10.1016/j.bios.2011.07.004 PMID:21802938

Erzinger, G. S., Schmoeller, F., Pinto, L. H., Americo, L., Hemmersbach, R., Hauslage, J., & Hader, D.-P. (2018). Bioluminescence systems in environmental biosensors. In Bioassays (pp. 242–262). doi:10.1016/B978-0-12-811861-0.00012-7

Eshghi, S., Hashemi, M., Mohammadi, A., Badii, F., Mohammadhoseini, Z., & Ahmadi, K. (2014). Effect of nano-chitosan-based coating with and without copper loaded on physicochemical and bioactive components of fresh strawberry fruit (Fragaria x ananassa Duchesne) during storage. *Food and Bioprocess Technology*, *7*(8), 2397–2409. doi:10.100711947-014-1281-2

Etacheri, V., Marom, R., Elazari, R., Salitra, G., & Aurbach, D. (2011). Challenges in the development of advanced Li-ion batteries: A review. *Energy & Environmental Science*, *4*(9), 3243–3262. doi:10.1039/c1ee01598b

European Parliament and Council. (2015). Regulation (EC) 2015/2283 of the European parliament and of the Council of 25 November 2015 on novel foods. Author.

European Science Foundation. (2005). *Nanomedicine. Forward look on Nanomedicine*. Academic Press.

Ewert, K., Evans, H. M., Ahmad, A., Slack, N. L., Lin, A. J., Martin-Herranz, A., & Safinya, C. R. (2005). Lipoplex structures and their distinct cellular pathways. *Advances in Genetics*, *53*, 119–155. doi:10.1016/S0065-2660(05)53005-0 PMID:16240992

Fadi, E., Hartwig, S., & Muller, B. W. (2004). In vitro evaluation of Cyclosporin A (CsA) inhalation nanosuspension. *Respir Drug Deliv*, *9*(2), 433-6.

Fagan, R., McComack, D., Dionysiou, D., & Pillai, S. (2016). A review of solar visible light active TiO2 photocatalysis for treating bacteria, cyanotoxins and contaminants of emerging concern. *Materials Science in Semiconductor Processing*, *42*, 2–14. doi:10.1016/j.mssp.2015.07.052

Fang, Z., Qiu, X., Chen, J., & Qiu, X. (2011). Debromination of polybrominated diphenyl ethers by Ni/Fe bimetallic nanoparticles: Influencing factors, kinetics, and mechanism. *Journal of Hazardous Materials*, *185*(2-3), 958–969. doi:10.1016/j.jhazmat.2010.09.113 PMID:21035251

Fan, W., Sun, J., Chen, Y., Qiu, J., Zhang, Y., & Chi, Y. (2009). Effects of chitosan coating on quality and shelf life of silver carp during frozen storage. *Food Chemistry*, *115*(1), 66–70. doi:10.1016/j.foodchem.2008.11.060

Farias, I. A. P. (2018). Antimicrobial Activity of Cerium Oxide Nanoparticles on Opportunistic Microorganisms: A Systematic Review. *BioMedical Research International. Article ID*, *1923606*, 1–14.

Farokhzad, O. C., & Langer, R. (2006). Nanomedicine: Developing smarter therapeutic and diagnostic modalities. *Advanced Drug Delivery Reviews*, *58*(14), 1456–1459. doi:10.1016/j.addr.2006.09.011 PMID:17070960

Fartash, B., Tangerud, T., Silness, J., & Arvidson, K. (1996). Rehabilitation of mandibular edentulism by single crystal sapphire implants and over dentures: 3- year results in 86 patients. A dual center international study. *Clinical Oral Implants Research*, *7*(3), 220–229. doi:10.1034/j.1600-0501.1996.070304.x PMID:9151586

Farzin, L., & Shamsipur, M. (2018). Recent advances in design of electrochemical affinity biosensors for low level detection of cancer protein biomarkers using nanomaterial-assisted signal enhancement strategies. *Journal of Pharmaceutical and Biomedical Analysis*, *147*, 185–210. doi:10.1016/j.jpba.2017.07.042 PMID:28869052

Fathi, M., Mozafari, M. R., & Mohebbi, M. (2012). Nanoencapsulation of food ingredients using lipid based delivery systems. *Trends in Food Science & Technology*, *23*(1), 13–27. doi:10.1016/j.tifs.2011.08.003

Fawole, O. G., Cai, X., & Mackenzie, A. R. (2016). Gas flaring and resultant air pollution: A review focusing on black Environ. *Pollution*, *216*, 182–197. doi:10.1016/j.envpol.2016.05.075 PMID:27262132

Feany, M. B., & Bender, W. W. (2000). A Drosophila model of Parkinson's disease. *Nature*, *404*(6776), 394–398. doi:10.1038/35006074 PMID:10746727

Feizi, H., Moghaddam, P. R., Shahtahmassebi, N., & Fotovat, A. (2012). Impact of Bulk and Nanosized Titanium Dioxide (TiO2) on Wheat Seed Germination and Seedling Growth. *Biological Trace Element Research*, *146*(1), 101–106. doi:10.100712011-011-9222-7 PMID:21979242

Feng, C., Li, H., Zhang, P., Guo, Z., & Liu, H. (2010). Synthesis and modification of non-stoichiometric spinel ($Li_{1.02}Mn_{1.90}Y_{0.02}O_{4-y}F_{0.08}$) for lithium-ion batteries. *Materials Chemistry and Physics*, *119*(1), 82–85. doi:10.1016/j.matchemphys.2009.07.049

Feng, F., Sakoda, Y., Ohyanagi, T., Nagahori, N., Shibuya, H., Okamastu, M., Miura, N., Kida, H., & Nishimura, S. I. (2013). Novel thiosialosides tethered to metal nanoparticles as potent influenza A virus haemagglutinin blockers. *Antiviral Chemistry & Chemotherapy*, *23*(2), 59–65. doi:10.3851/IMP2553 PMID:23425865

Feng, L., Niu, M., Wen, Z., & Hao, X. (2018). Recent Advances of Plasmonic Organic Solar Cells: Photophysical Investigations. *Polymers*, *10*(2), 123. doi:10.3390/polym10020123 PMID:30966159

Feng, Q. L., Wu, J., Chen, G. Q., Cui, F. Z., Kim, T. N., & Kim, J. O. (2000). A mechanistic study of the antibacterial effect of silver ions on Escherichia coli and Staphylococcus aureus. *Journal of Biomedical Materials Research*, *52*(4), 662–668. doi:10.1002/1097-4636(20001215)52:4<662::AID-JBM10>3.0.CO;2-3 PMID:11033548

Feng, S. S., Mu, L., Win, K. Y., & Huang, G. (2004). Nanoparticles of biodegradable polymers for clinical administration of paclitaxel. *Current Medicinal Chemistry*, *11*(4), 413–424. doi:10.2174/0929867043455909 PMID:14965222

Feng, W., Li, Y., Du, J., Wang, W., & Zhong, X. (2016). Highly efficient and stable quasi-solid-state quantum dot-sensitized solar cells based on a superabsorbent polyelectrolyte. *Journal of Materials Chemistry. A, Materials for Energy and Sustainability*, *4*(4), 1461–1468. doi:10.1039/C5TA08209A

Feng, Y., Zhu, W., Guo, W., & Jiang, L. (2017). Bioinspired Energy Conversion in Nanofluidics: A Paradigm of Material Evolution. *Advanced Materials*, *29*(45), 1702773. doi:10.1002/adma.201702773

Ferdnandez, A., Soriano, E., Lopez-Carballo, G., Picouet, P., Lloret, E., Gavara, R., & ... . (2009). Preservation of aseptic conditions in absorbent pads by using silver nanotechnology. *Food Research International*, *42*(8), 1105–1112. doi:10.1016/j.foodres.2009.05.009

Feregrino-Pérez, A. A., Magaña-López, E., Guzmán, C., & Esquivel, K. (2018). A general overview of the benefits and possible negative effects of the nanotechnology in horticulture. *Scientia Horticulturae*, *238*, 126–137. doi:10.1016/j.scienta.2018.03.060

Fergus, J. W. (2010). Recent developments in cathode materials for lithium ion batteries. *Journal of Power Sources*, *195*(4), 939–954. doi:10.1016/j.jpowsour.2009.08.089

Fernandez, A., Manchanda, R., & McGoran, A. (2011). Theranostic applications of nanomaterials in cancer therapy: drug delivery, image-guided therapy and multifunctional platforms. *Appl Biochem Biotechnol.*, *165*(7-8), 1628-51.

Ferrari, M. (2005). Cancer Nanotechnology: Opportunities and Challenges. *Cancer*, *5*, 161–171. PMID:15738981

Ferrari, M. (2005). Cancer nanotechnology: Opportunities and challenges. *Nature Reviews. Cancer*, *5*(3), 161–171. doi:10.1038/nrc1566 PMID:15738981

Ferreira, L., Karp, J. M., Nobre, L., & Langer, R. (2008). New Opportunities: The Use of Nanotechnologies to Manipulate and Track Stem Cells. *Cell Stem Cell*, *3*(2), 136–146. doi:10.1016/j.stem.2008.07.020 PMID:18682237

Ferry, V. E., Munday, J. N., & Atwater, H. A. (2010). Design considerations for plasmonic photovoltaics. *Advanced Materials*, *22*(43), 4794–4808. doi:10.1002/adma.201000488 PMID:20814916

Fic, K., Frackowiak, E., & Beguin, F. (2012). Unusual energy enhancement in carbon-based electrochemical capacitors. *Journal of Materials Chemistry*, *22*(46), 24213–24223. doi:10.1039/c2jm35711a

Fine, P. E. (1995). Variation in protection by BCG: Implications of and for heterologous immunity. *Lancet*, *346*(8986), 1339–1345. doi:10.1016/S0140-6736(95)92348-9 PMID:7475776

Fishman, M. L., Chau, H. K., Hotchkiss, A. T. Jr, White, A., Garcia, R. A., & Cooke, P. H. (2019). Effect of long term cold storage and microwave extraction time on the physical and chemical properties of citrus pectin. *Food Hydrocolloids*, *92*, 104–116. doi:10.1016/j.foodhyd.2018.12.047

Forrest, S. R. (2004). The path to ubiquitous and low-cost organic electronic appliances on plastic. *Nature*, *428*(6986), 911–918. doi:10.1038/nature02498 PMID:15118718

Fowsiya, J., Asharani, I. V., Mohapatra, S., Eshapula, A., Mohi, P., Thakar, N., Monad, S., & Madhumitha, G. (2019). Aegle marmelos phytochemical stabilized synthesis and characterization of ZnO nanoparticles and their role against agriculture and food pathogen. *Green Process Synth.*, *8*(1), 488–495. doi:10.1515/gps-2019-0017

Fraceto, L. F., Grillo, R., de Medeiros, G. A., Scognamiglio, V., Rea, G., & Bartolucci, C. (2016). Nanotechnology in Agriculture: Which Innovation Potential Does It Have? *Frontiers in Environmental Science*, *4*. Advance online publication. doi:10.3389/fenvs.2016.00020

Frackowiak, E., & Beguin, F. (2001). Carbon materials for the electrochemical storage of energy in Capacitors. *Carbon*, *39*(6), 937–950. doi:10.1016/S0008-6223(00)00183-4

Freitas, M., Nouws, H. P. A., & Delerue-Matos, C. (2018). Electrochemical biosensing in cancer diagnostics and follow-up. *Electroanalysis*, *30*(8), 1584–1603. doi:10.1002/elan.201800193

Frenkel, V. (2008). Ultrasound mediated delivery of drugs and genes to solid tumors. *Advanced Drug Delivery Reviews*, *60*(10), 1193–1208. doi:10.1016/j.addr.2008.03.007 PMID:18474406

Fries, L. F., Gordon, D. M., Richards, R. L., Egan, J. E., Hollingdale, M. R., Gross, M., Silverman, C., & Alving, C. R. (1992). Liposomal malaria vaccine in humans: A safe and potent adjuvant strategy. *Proceedings of the National Academy of Sciences of the United States of America*, *89*(1), 358–362. doi:10.1073/pnas.89.1.358 PMID:1729706

Fu, G., Vary, P. S., & Lin, C. T. (2005). Anatase TiO_2 nanocomposites for antimicrobial coatings. *The Journal of Physical Chemistry B*, *109*(18), 8889–8898. doi:10.1021/jp0502196 PMID:16852057

Fujishima, A., & Honda, K. (1972). Electrochemical Photolysis of Water at a Semiconductor Electrode. *Nature*, *238*(5358), 37–38. doi:10.1038/238037a0 PMID:12635268

Fu, L., Liu, Z. H. I. M. I. N., Liu, Y., Han, B., Hu, P., Cao, L., & Zhu, D. A. O. B. E. N. (2005). Beaded cobalt oxide nanoparticles along carbon nanotubes: Towards more highly integrated electronic devices. *Advanced Materials*, *17*(2), 217–221. doi:10.1002/adma.200400833

Fymat, A. L. (2016). Recent developments in nanomedicine research. *Journal of Nanomedicine Research*, *4*(4), 12. doi:10.15406/jnmr.2016.04.00096

Fynan, E. F., Webster, R. G., Fuller, D. H., Haynes, J. R., Santoro, J. C., & Robinson, H. L. (1993). DNA vaccines: Protective immunizations by parenteral, mucosal, and gene-gun inoculations. *Proceedings of the National Academy of Sciences of the United States of America*, *90*(24), 11478–11482. doi:10.1073/pnas.90.24.11478 PMID:8265577

Gad, M. M., Zagzog, O. A., & Hemeda, O. M. (2016). Development of Nano-Chitosan Edible Coating for Peach Fruits Cv. Desert Red. *International Journal of Environment*, *05*(04), 43–55.

Ganachari, S. V., Yaradoddi, J. S., Somappa, S. B., Mogre, P., Tapaskar, R. P., Salimath, B., Venkataraman, A., & Viswanath, V. J. (2018). *Handbook of Ecomaterials*. Springer International Publishing AG., doi:10.1007/978-3-319-48281-1_184-1

Ganapathy, S., van Eck, E. R., Kentgens, A. P. M., Mulder, F. M., & Wagemaker, M. (2011). Equilibrium Lithium-Ion Transport Between Nanocrystalline Lithium- Inserted Anatase TiO2 and the Electrolyte. *Chemistry (Weinheim an der Bergstrasse, Germany)*, *17*(52), 14811–14816. doi:10.1002/chem.201101431 PMID:22120842

Gao, W., Hu, C. M. J., Fang, R. H., & Zhang, L. (2013). Liposome-like nanostructures for drug delivery. *Journal of Materials Chemistry. B, Materials for Biology and Medicine*, *1*(48), 6569–6585.

Gao, X., Cui, Y., Levenson, R. M., Chung, L. W. K., & Nie, S. (2004). In vivo cancer targeting and imaging with semiconductor quantum dots. *Nature Biotechnology*, *22*(8), 969–976. doi:10.1038/nbt994 PMID:15258594

Garca-Segura, S., Bellotindos, L. M., Huang, Y. H., Brillas, E., & Lu, M. C. (2016). Fluidized-bed Fenton process as alternative wastewater treatment technology—A review. *Journal of the Taiwan Institute of Chemical Engineers*, *67*, 211–225. doi:10.1016/j.jtice.2016.07.021

Garcia-Garcia, E., Gil, S., Andrieux, K., Desmaële, D., Nicolas, V., Taran, F., Georgin, D., Andreux, J. P., Roux, F., & Couvreur, P. (2005). A relevant in vitro rat model for the evaluation of blood–brain barrier translocation of nanoparticles. *Cellular and Molecular Life Sciences*, *62*(12), 1400–1408. doi:10.100700018-005-5094-3 PMID:15905957

Garnett, E., Mai, L., & Yang, P. (2019). *Introduction: 1D nanomaterials/nanowires*. Academic Press.

Garrido, C., Simpson, C. A., Dahl, N. P., Bresee, J., Whitehead, D. C., Lindsey, E. A., Harris, T. L., Smith, C. A., Carter, C. J., Feldheim, D. L., Melander, C., & Margolis, D. M. (2015). Gold nanoparticles to improve HIV drug delivery. *Future Medicinal Chemistry*, *7*(9), 1097–1107. doi:10.4155/fmc.15.57 PMID:26132521

Gaskell, G., Eyck, T. T., Jackson, J., & Veltri, G. (2005). Imagining nanotechnology: Cultural support for technological innovation in Europe and the United States. *Public Understanding of Science (Bristol, England)*, *14*(1), 81–90. doi:10.1177/0963662505048949

Ge, F., Li, M.-M., Ye, H., & Zhao, B.-X. (2012). Effective removal of heavy metal ions Cd^{2+}, Zn^{2+}, Pb^{2+}, Cu^{2+} from aqueous solution by polymermodified magnetic nanoparticles. *Journal of Hazardous Materials*, *211–212*, 366–372. doi:10.1016/j.jhazmat.2011.12.013 PMID:22209322

Geng, Z., Zhang, X., Fan, Z., Lv, X., & Chen, H. (2017). A route to terahertz metamaterial biosensor integrated with microfluidics for liver cancer biomarker testing in early stage. *Scientific Reports*, *7*(1), 16378-1-16378–11. doi:10.103841598-017-16762-y

Geng, Z., Guo, X., Cao, Y., Yang, Y., & Chen, H. (2015). Flexible, low-loss and large area metamaterials with high Q value. *Microelectronic Engineering*, *135*, 23–27. doi:10.1016/j.mee.2015.02.045

Geys, J., Nemery, B., & Hoet, P. H. M. (2010). Assay conditions can influence the outcome of cytotoxicity tests of nanomaterials: Better assay characterization is needed to compare studies. *Toxicology In Vitro*, *24*(2), 620–629. doi:10.1016/j.tiv.2009.10.007 PMID:19850119

Ge, Z. (2018). Graphene Family Nanomaterials: Properties and Potential Applications in Dentistry. *International Journal of Biomaterials. Article ID, 1539678*, 1–12.

Ghaemi, F., Abdullah, L. C., & Tahir, P. Md. (2017). Natural and synthetics nanomaterials: comparative study on their mechanical and thermal properties as nanofiller in polymer composite. *IOP Conf. Series: Journal of Physics: Conf. Series 914*. doi:10.1088/1742-6596/914/1/012014

Ghosh, P., Han, G., De, M., Kim, C. K., & Rotello, V. M. (2008). Gold nanoparticles in delivery applications. *Advanced Drug Delivery Reviews*, *60*(11), 1307–1315. doi:10.1016/j.addr.2008.03.016 PMID:18555555

Gibson, J. D., Khanal, B. P., & Zubarev, E. R. (2007). Paclitaxel-functionalized gold nanoparticles. *Journal of the American Chemical Society*, *129*(37), 11653–11661. doi:10.1021/ja075181k PMID:17718495

Göçenoğlu Sarıkaya, A., Osman, B., Çam, T., & Denizli, A. (2017). Molecularly imprinted surface plasmon resonance (SPR) sensor for uric acid determination. *Sensors and Actuators. B, Chemical*, *251*, 763–772. doi:10.1016/j.snb.2017.05.079

Goetzberger, A., Luther, J., & Willeke, G. (2002). Solar cells: Past, present, future. *Solar Energy Materials and Solar Cells*, *74*(1–4), 1–11. doi:10.1016/S0927-0248(02)00042-9

Gogoi, S. K., Gopinath, P., Paul, A., Ramesh, A., Ghosh, S. S., & Chattopadhyay, A. (2006). Green Fluorescent Protein-Expressing *Escherichia coli* as a Model System for Investigating the Antimicrobial Activities of Silver Nanoparticles. *Langmuir*, *22*(22), 9322–9328. doi:10.1021/la060661v PMID:17042548

Gokulakrishnan, R., Ravikumar, S., & Raj, J. A. (2012). In vitro antibacterial potential of metal oxide nanoparticles against antibiotic resistant bacterial pathogens. *Asian Pacific Journal of Tropical Disease*, *2*(5), 411–413. doi:10.1016/S2222-1808(12)60089-9

Gold, K., Slay, B., Knackstedt, M., & Gaharwar, A. K. (2018). Antimicrobial activity of metal and metal-oxide based nanoparticles. *Advanced Therapeutics*, *1*(3), 1700033. doi:10.1002/adtp.201700033

Goldstein, J. I., Newbury, D. E., Michael, J. R., Ritchie, N. W., Scott, J. H. J., & … . (2017). *Scanning Electron Microscopy and X-Ray Microanalysis*. Springer.

Gombotz, W. R., & Wee, S. (1998). Protein release from alginate matrices. *Advanced Drug Delivery Reviews*, *31*(3), 267–285. doi:10.1016/S0169-409X(97)00124-5 PMID:10837629

Goncalves, L. F., Kanodarwala, F. K., Stride, J. A., Silva, C. J., Pereira, M. R., & Gomes, M. J. (2014). One-pot synthesis of CdSe nanoparticles exhibiting quantum size effect within a sol–gel derived ureasilicate matrix. *Journal of Photochemistry and Photobiology A Chemistry*, *285*, 21–29. doi:10.1016/j.jphotochem.2014.04.005

Gonzalez, G., Freites, J. A., & Rojas, C. E. (2001). Synthesis and characterization of nanophase particles obtained by DC sputtering. *Scripta Materialia*, *44*(8-9), 1883–1887. doi:10.1016/S1359-6462(01)00805-3

Goodenough, J. B., & Kim, Y. (2010). Challenges for Rechargeable Li Batteries. *Chemistry of Materials*, *22*(3), 587–603. doi:10.1021/cm901452z

Gorrasi, G., & Bugatti, V. (2016). Edible bio-nano-hybrid coatings for food protection based on pectins and LDH-salicylate: Preparation and analysis of physical properties. *Lebensmittel-Wissenschaft + Technologie*, *69*, 139–145. doi:10.1016/j.lwt.2016.01.038

Gorth, D. J., Rand, D. M., & Webster, T. J. (2011). Silver nanoparticle toxicity in Drosophila: Size does matter. *International Journal of Nanomedicine*, *6*, 343–350. doi:10.2147/IJN.S16881 PMID:21383859

Govindaraju, K., Basha, S. K., Kumar, V. G., & Singaravelu, G. (2008). Silver, gold and bimetallic nanoparticles production using single-cell protein (*Spirulina platensis*) Geitler. *Journal of Materials Science*, *43*(15), 5115–5122. doi:10.100710853-008-2745-4

Govindaraju, K., Kiruthiga, V., Kumar, V. G., & Singaravelu, G. (2009). Extracellular synthesis of silver nanoparticles by a marine alga, Sargassum wightii Grevilli and their antibacterial effects. *Journal of Nanoscience and Nanotechnology*, *9*(9), 5497–5501. doi:10.1166/jnn.2009.1199 PMID:19928252

Graham, J. H., Johnson, E. G., Myers, M. E., Young, M., Rajasekaran, P., Das, S., & Santra, S. (2016). Potential of Nano-Formulated Zinc Oxide for Control of Citrus Canker on Grapefruit Trees. *Plant Disease*, *100*(12), 2442–2447. doi:10.1094/PDIS-05-16-0598-RE PMID:30686171

Grahn, H. T. (1999). *Introduction to semiconductor physics*. World Scientific Pub Co Inc. doi:10.1142/3631

Grande, C. J., Torres, F. G., Gomez, C. M., & Carmen Bañó, M. (2009). Bañó, Nanocomposites ofbacterial cellulose/hydroxyapatite for biomedical applications. *Acta Biomaterialia*, *5*(5), 1605–1615. doi:10.1016/j.actbio.2009.01.022 PMID:19246264

Gratzel, M. (2003), Dye-Sensitized Solar Cells. *J. Photochem. Photobiol., C, 4*, 145–153.

Gratzel, M. (2004). Conversion of sunlight to electric power by nanocrystalline dye-sensitized solar cells. *Journal of Photochemistry and Photobiology A Chemistry*, *164*(1-3), 3–14. doi:10.1016/j.jphotochem.2004.02.023

Gref, R., Minamitake, Y., Peracchia, M. T., Trubetskoy, V., Torchilin, V., & Langer, R. (1994). Biodegradable long-circulating polymeric nanospheres. *Science*, *263*(5153), 1600–1603. doi:10.1126cience.8128245 PMID:8128245

Grgacic, E. V. L., & Anderson, D. A. (2006). Virus-likeparticles: Passporttoimmunerecognition. *Methods (San Diego, Calif.)*, *40*(1), 60–65. doi:10.1016/j.ymeth.2006.07.018 PMID:16997714

Guccione, S., Li, K. C., & Bednarski, M. D. (2004). Vascular-targeted nanoparticles for molecular imaging and therapy. *Methods in Enzymology*, *386*, 219–236. doi:10.1016/S0076-6879(04)86010-5 PMID:15120254

Guerra, F., Attia, M., Whitehead, D., & Alexis, F. (2018). Nanotechnology for environmental remediation: Materials and applications. *Molecules (Basel, Switzerland)*, *23*(7), 1760. doi:10.3390/molecules23071760 PMID:30021974

Gunnarsdottir, S., Rucki, M., & Elfarra, A. A. (2002). Novel glutathione-dependent thiopurine prodrugs: Evidence for enhanced cytotoxicity in tumor cells and for decreased bone marrow toxicity in mice. *The Journal of Pharmacology and Experimental Therapeutics*, *301*(1), 77–86. doi:10.1124/jpet.301.1.77 PMID:11907160

Gunther, N. W. IV, Abdul-Wakeel, A., Scullen, O. J., & Sommers, C. (2019). The evaluation of gamma irradiation and cold storage for the reduction of Campylobacter jejuni in chicken livers. *Food Microbiology*, *82*, 249–253. doi:10.1016/j.fm.2019.02.014 PMID:31027780

Guo, D., Chang, Z., Li, B., Tang, H., Yuan, X. Z., & Wang, H. (2013). Synthesis of high-purity $LiMn_2O_4$ with enhanced electrical properties from electrolytic manganese dioxide treated by sulfuric acid-assisted hydrothermal method. *Journal of Solid State Electrochemistry*, *17*(11), 2849–2856. doi:10.100710008-013-2199-8

Guo, L., Yuan, W., Lu, Z., & Li, C. M. (2013). Polymer/nanosilver composite coatings for antibacterial applications. *Colloids and Surfaces. A, Physicochemical and Engineering Aspects*, *439*(0), 69–83. doi:10.1016/j.colsurfa.2012.12.029

Guo, X. (2012). Surface plasmon resonance based biosensor technique: A review. *Journal of Biophotonics*, *5*(7), 483–501. doi:10.1002/jbio.201200015 PMID:22467335

Guo, X., Lu, X., Fang, X., Mao, Y., Wang, Z., Chen, L., Xu, X., Yang, H., & Liu, Y. (2010). Lithium storage in hollow spherical $ZnFe_2O_4$ as anode materials for lithium ion batteries. *Electrochemistry Communications*, *12*(6), 847–850. doi:10.1016/j.elecom.2010.04.003

Guo, Y. G., Hu, Y. S., Sigle, W., & Maier, J. (2007). Superior Electrode Performance of Nanostructured Mesoporous TiO_2 (Anatase) through Efficient Hierarchical Mixed Conducting Networks. *Advanced Materials*, *19*(16), 2087–2091. doi:10.1002/adma.200602828

Guo, Y.-G., Hu, J.-S., & Wan, L.-J. (2008). Nanostructured Materials for Electrochemical Energy Conversion and Storage Devices. *Advanced Materials*, *20*(15), 2878–2887. doi:10.1002/adma.200800627

Gupta, A., Joia, J., Sood, A., Sood, R., & Sidhu, C. (2016). Microbes as Potential Tool for Remediation of Heavy Metals: A Review. *Journal of Microbial & Biochemical Technology*, *8*(4), 364–372. doi:10.4172/1948-5948.1000310

Gupta, S., Bansal, R., Gupta, S., Jindal, N., & Jindal, A. (2013). Nanocarriers and nanoparticles for skin care and dermatological treatments. *Indian Dermatology Online Journal*, *4*(4), 267–272. doi:10.4103/2229-5178.120635 PMID:24350003

Gür, S. D., Bakhshpour, M., & Denizli, A. (2019). Selective detection of Escherichia coli caused UTIs with surface imprinted plasmonic nanoscale sensor. *Materials Science and Engineering C*, *104*, 109869. doi:10.1016/j.msec.2019.109869 PMID:31500013

Gu, W., Tang, G., & Tao, W. (2015). High efficiency thermophotovoltaic emitter by metamaterial-based nano-pyramid array. *Optics Express*, *23*(24), 30681–30694. doi:10.1364/OE.23.030681 PMID:26698700

Guy, B. (2007). The perfect mix: Recent progress in adjuvant research. *Nature Reviews. Microbiology*, *5*(7), 505–517. doi:10.1038/nrmicro1681 PMID:17558426

Ha, H. W., Yun, N. J., & Kim, K. (2007). Improvement of electrochemical stability of $LiMn_2O_4$ by CeO_2 coating for lithium-ion batteries. *Electrochimica Acta*, *52*(9), 3236–3241. doi:10.1016/j.electacta.2006.09.066

Haider, A., & Kang, I.-K. (2015). Preparation of Silver Nanoparticles and Their Industrial and Biomedical Applications: A Comprehensive Review. *Advances in Materials Science and Engineering*, 1–16.

Hainfeld, J. F., Slatkin, D. N., & Smilowitz, H. M. (2005). *The use of gold nanoparticles to enhance radiotherapy in mice*. Academic Press.

Hajipour, M. J., Fromm, K. M., Akbar Ashkarran, A., Jimenez de Aberasturi, D., Larramendi, I. R., Rojo, T., Serpooshan, V., Parak, W. J., & Mahmoudi, M. (2012). Antibacterial properties of nanoparticles. *Trends in Biotechnology*, *30*(10), 499–511. doi:10.1016/j.tibtech.2012.06.004 PMID:22884769

Hall, P. J., Mirzaeian, M., Fletcher, S. I., Sillars, F. B., Rennie, A. J. R., Shitta-Bey, G. O., Wilson, G., Cruden, A., & Carter, R. (2010). Energy storage in electrochemical capacitors: Designing functional materials to improve performance. *Energy & Environmental Science*, *3*(9), 1238–1251. doi:10.1039/c0ee00004c

Hammond, J. L., Formisano, N., Estrela, P., Carrara, S., & Tkac, J. (2016). Electrochemical biosensors and nanobiosensors. *Essays in Biochemistry*, *60*(June), 69–80. doi:10.1042/EBC20150008 PMID:27365037

Handy, R. D., & Shaw, B. J. (2007). Toxic effects of nanoparticles and nanomaterials: Implications for public health, risk assessment and the public perception of nanotechnology. *Health Risk & Society*, *9*(2), 125–144. doi:10.1080/13698570701306807

Han, J. H. (2005). *Innovations in food packaging* (2nd ed.). Academic Press.

Han, L., Islam, A., Chen, H., Malapaka, C., Chiranjeevi, B., Zhang, S., Yang, A., & Yanagida, M. (2012). High-efficiency dye-sensitized solar cell with a novel co-adsorbent. *Energy & Environmental Science*, *5*(3), 6057–6060. doi:10.1039/c2ee03418b

Hanna, M., & Nozik, A. J. (2006). Solar conversion efficiency of photovoltaic and photoelectrolysis cells with carrier multiplication absorbers. *Journal of Applied Physics*, *100*(7), 074510. doi:10.1063/1.2356795

Han, S., Lin, J., Zhou, F., & Vellanoweth, R. L. (2000). Oligonucleotide-capped gold nanoparticles for improved atomic force microscopic imaging and enhanced selectivity in polynucleotide detection. *Biochemical and Biophysical Research Communications*, *279*(1), 265–269. doi:10.1006/bbrc.2000.3943 PMID:11112450

Hansen, K. M., & Thundat, T. (2005). Microcantilever biosensors. *Methods (San Diego, Calif.)*, *37*(1), 57–64. doi:10.1016/j.ymeth.2005.05.011 PMID:16199177

Hao, Y.-M., Man, C., & Hu, Z.-B. (2010). Effective removal of Cu (II) ions from aqueous solution by amino-functionalized magnetic nanoparticles. *Journal of Hazardous Materials*, *184*(1-3), 392–399. doi:10.1016/j.jhazmat.2010.08.048 PMID:20837378

Harandi, A. M., Medaglini, D., & Shattock, R. J. (2010). Vaccine adjuvants: Apriority for vaccine research. *Vaccine*, *28*(12), 2363–2366. doi:10.1016/j.vaccine.2009.12.084 PMID:20064476

Haran, G., Cohen, R., Bar, L. K., & Barenholz, Y. (1993). Transmembrane ammonium sulfate gradients in liposomes produce efficient and stable entrapment of amphipathic weak bases. *Biochimica et Biophysica Acta*, *1151*(2), 201–215. doi:10.1016/0005-2736(93)90105-9 PMID:8373796

Harris, P. J. F. (2001). *Carbon Nanotubes and Related Structures – New Materials for the Twenty-First Century*. Cambridge University Express.

Hart, S. L. (2005). Lipid carriers for gene therapy. *Current Drug Delivery*, *2*(4), 423–428. doi:10.2174/156720105774370230 PMID:16305445

Hart, S. L. (2010). Multifunctional nanocomplexes for gene transfer and gene therapy. *Cell Biology and Toxicology*, *26*(1), 69–81. doi:10.100710565-009-9141-y PMID:20127400

Hasan, S. (2015). A review on nanoparticles: Their synthesis and types. *Research Journal of Recent Sciences ISSN*, *2277*, 2502.

Hassanzadeh, P., Fullwood, I., Sothi, S., & Aldulaimi, D. (2011). Cancer nanotechnology. *Gastroenterology and Hepatology from Bed To Bench*, *4*(2), 63.

Haupt, K., & Mosbach, K. (2000). Molecularly imprinted polymers and their use in biomimetic sensors. *Chemical Reviews*, *100*(7), 2495–2504. doi:10.1021/cr990099w PMID:11749293

Hébert, E. M., Debouttière, P. J., Lepage, M., Sanche, L., & Hunting, D. J. (2010). Preferential tumour accumulation of gold nanoparticles, visualised by Magnetic Resonance Imaging: Radiosensitisation studies in vivo and in vitro. *International Journal of Radiation Biology*, *86*(8), 692–700. doi:10.3109/09553001003746067 PMID:20586540

Hedayati, M. K., Faupel, F., & Elbahri, M. (2014). Review of plasmonic nanocomposite metamaterial absorber. *Materials (Basel)*, *7*(2), 1221–1248. doi:10.3390/ma7021221 PMID:28788511

He, J., Yang, X., Men, B., & Wang, D. (2016). Interfacial mechanisms of Heterogenous Fenton reactions catalyzed by iron based materials: A review. *Journal of Environmental Sciences (China)*, *39*, 97–109. doi:10.1016/j.jes.2015.12.003 PMID:26899649

Helan, M., Berchmans, L. J., Syamala Kumari, V. S., RaviSankar, R., & Shanmugam, V. M. (2011). Molten salt synthesis of $LiGd_{0.01}Mn_{1.99}O_4$ using chloride–carbonate melt. *Materials Research Innovations*, *15*(2), 130–134. doi:10.1179/143307511X12998222918958

Helgert, C., Pshenay-Severin, E., Falkner, M., Menzel, C., Rockstuhl, C., Kley, E. B., Tünnermann, A., Lederer, F., & Pertsch, T. (2011). Chiral metamaterial composed of three-dimensional plasmonic nanostructures. *Nano Letters*, *11*(10), 4400–4404. doi:10.1021/nl202565e PMID:21853984

Henriksen-Lacey, M., Korsholm, K. S., Andersen, P., Perrie, Y., & Christensen, D. (2011). Liposomal vaccine delivery systems. *Expert Opinion on Drug Delivery*, *8*(4), 505–519. doi:10.1517/17425247.2011.558081 PMID:21413904

He, S., Cui, Y., Ye, Y., Zhang, P., & Jin, Y. (2009). Optical nano-antennas and metamaterials. *Materials Today*, *12*(12), 16–24. doi:10.1016/S1369-7021(09)70313-X

Heurtault, B., Frisch, B., & Pons, F. (2010). Liposomes as delivery systems for nasal vaccination: Strategies and outcomes. *Expert Opinion on Drug Delivery*, *7*(7), 829–844. doi:10.1517/17425247.2010.488687 PMID:20459361

He, X. (2015). Tunable terahertz graphene metamaterials. *Carbon*, *82*, 229–237. doi:10.1016/j.carbon.2014.10.066

He, Y., Deng, H., Jiao, X., He, S., Gao, J., & Yang, X. (2013). Infrared perfect absorber based on nanowire metamaterial cavities. *Optics Letters*, *38*(7), 1179–1181. doi:10.1364/OL.38.001179 PMID:23546283

He, Y., Ingudam, S., Reed, S., Gehring, A., Strobaugh, T. P. Jr, & Irwin, P. (2016). Study on the mechanism of antibacterial action of magnesium oxide nanoparticles against foodborne pathogens. *Journal of Nanobiotechnology*, *14*(1), 54. doi:10.118612951-016-0202-0 PMID:27349516

Hibino, M., Abe, K., Mochizuki, M., & Miyayama, M. (2004). Amorphous titanium oxide electrode for high-rate discharge and charge. *Journal of Power Sources*, *126*(1-2), 139–143. doi:10.1016/j.jpowsour.2003.08.025

Hirsch, L. R., Gobin, A. M., Lowery, A. R., Tam, F., Drezek, R. A., Halas, N. J., & West, J. L. (2006). Metal nanoshells. *Annals of Biomedical Engineering*, *34*(1), 15–22.

Hirvikorpi, T., Vaha-Nissi, M., Harlin, A., & Karppinen, M. (2010). Comparison of some coating techniques to fabricate barrier layers on packaging materials. *Thin Solid Films*, *518*(19), 5463–5466. doi:10.1016/j.tsf.2010.04.018

Ho, C. J., & Gao, J. Y. (2009). Preparation and Thermophysical Properties of Nanoparticle-in-Paraffin Emulsion as Phase Change Material. *International Communications in Heat and Mass Transfer*, *36*(5), 467–470. doi:10.1016/j.icheatmasstransfer.2009.01.015

Hochella, M. F. Jr, Spencer, M. G., & Jones, K. L. (2015). Nanotechnology: Nature's gift or scientists' brainchild? *Environmental Science. Nano*, *2*(2), 114–119. doi:10.1039/C4EN00145A

Hoel, S., Vadstein, O., & Jakobsen, A. N. (2018). Growth of mesophilic Aeromonas salmonicida in an experimental model of nigiri sushi during cold storage. *International Journal of Food Microbiology*, *285*, 1–6. doi:10.1016/j.ijfoodmicro.2018.07.008 PMID:30005315

Hokari, R., Kurihara, K., Higurashi, E., & Hiroshima, H. (2019). Optical evaluation of nanocomposite metamaterials fabricated by nano-printing technique utilizing silver nanoink. *Microelectronic Engineering*, *211*, 44–49. doi:10.1016/j.mee.2019.03.024

Holzapfel, M., Buqa, H., Scheifele, W., Novák, P., & Petrat, F. M. (2005). A new type of nano-sized silicon/carbon composite electrode for reversible lithium insertion. *Chemical Communications (Cambridge)*, *28*(12), 1566–1568. doi:10.1039/B417492E PMID:15770261

Holzhauser, T., & Röder, M. (2015). Polymerase chain reaction (PCR) methods for detecting allergens in foods. In *Handbook of Food Allergen Detection and Control*. Woodhead Publishing Limited., doi:10.1533/9781782420217.2.245

Holzinger, M., Le Gof, A., & Cosnier, S. (2014). Nanomaterials for biosensing applications: A review. *Frontiers in Chemistry*, *2*, 63. doi:10.3389/fchem.2014.00063 PMID:25221775

Homola, J. (2008). Surface plasmon resonance sensors for detection of chemical and biological species. *Chemical Reviews*, *108*(2), 462–493. doi:10.1021/cr068107d PMID:18229953

Homola, J., Dostálek, J., Chen, S., Rasooly, A., Jiang, S., & Yee, S. S. (2002). Spectral surface plasmon resonance biosensor for detection of staphylococcal enterotoxin B in milk. *International Journal of Food Microbiology*, *75*(1-2), 61–69. doi:10.1016/S0168-1605(02)00010-7 PMID:11999118

Homola, J., Yee, S. S., & Gauglitz, G. (1999). Surface plasmon resonance sensors [Review]. *Sensors and Actuators. B, Chemical*, *54*(1-2), 3–15. doi:10.1016/S0925-4005(98)00321-9

Hone, D. C., Walker, P. I., Evans-Gowing, R., FitzGerald, S., Beeby, A., Chambrier, I., Cook, M. J., & Russell, D. A. (2002). Generation of cytotoxic singlet oxygen via phthalocyanine-stabilized gold nanoparticles: A potential delivery vehicle for photodynamic therapy. *Langmuir*, *18*(8), 2985–2987. doi:10.1021/la0256230

Hong, H., Gao, T., & Cai, W. (2009). Molecular imaging with single-walled carbon nanotubes. *Nano Today*, *4*(3), 252–261. doi:10.1016/j.nantod.2009.04.002 PMID:21754949

Hong, R., Han, G., Fernández, J. M., Kim, B. J., Forbes, N. S., & Rotello, V. M. (2006). Glutathione-mediated delivery and release using monolayer protected nanoparticle carriers. *Journal of the American Chemical Society*, *128*(4), 1078–1079. doi:10.1021/ja056726i PMID:16433515

Hossain, M. I., Faruque, M. R. I., Islam, M. T., & Ullah, M. H. (2015). A new wide-band double-negative metamaterial for C- and S-Band applications. *Materials (Basel)*, *8*(1), 57–71. doi:10.3390/ma8010057 PMID:28787924

Hostetler, M. J., Wingate, J. E., Zhong, C. J., Harris, J. E., Vachet, R. W., Clark, M. R., ... Glish, G. L. (1998). Alkanethiolate gold cluster molecules with core diameters from 1.5 to 5.2 nm: Core and monolayer properties as a function of core size. *Langmuir*, *14*(1), 17–30. doi:10.1021/la970588w

Hou, J., Shao, Y., Ellis, M. W., Moore, R. B., & Yi, B. (2011). Graphene-based electrochemical energy conversion and storage, fuel cells, supercapacitors and lithium ion batteries. *Physical Chemistry Chemical Physics*, *13*(34), 15384–15402. doi:10.1039/c1cp21915d PMID:21799983

Hsu, T., & Schulz, R. A. (2000). Sequence and functional properties of Ets genes in the model organism Drosophila. *Oncogene*, *19*(55), 6409–6416. doi:10.1038j.onc.1204033

Hsueh, Y. H., Ke, W. J., Hsieh, C. T., Lin, K. S., Tzou, D. Y., & Chiang, C. L. (2015). ZnO nanoparticles affect Bacillus subtilis cell growth and biofilm formation. *PLoS One*, *10*(6), e0128457. doi:10.1371/journal.pone.0128457 PMID:26039692

Hu, A. W., & Fu, Z. H. (2003). Nanotechnology and its applications in packaging and packaging machinery. *Packaging Engineering*, *24*, 22–24.

Huang, H. Y., Yang, R. T., Chinn, D., & Munson, C. L. (2003). Amine-Grafted MCM-48 and Silica Xerogel as Superior Sorbents for Acidic Gas Removal from Natural Gas. *Industrial & Engineering Chemistry Research*, *42*(12), 2427–2433. doi:10.1021/ie020440u

Huang, J., Cao, Y., Liu, Z., Deng, Z., Tang, F., & Wang, W. (2012). Efficient removal of heavy metal ions from water system by titanate nanoflowers. *Chemical Engineering Journal*, *180*, 75–80. doi:10.1016/j.cej.2011.11.005

Huang, J., Wang, X., Phuah, X. L., Lu, P., Qi, Z., & Wang, H. (2019). Plasmonic Cu nanostructures in ZnO as hyperbolic metamaterial thin films. *Materials Today Nano*, *8*, 100052-1, 100052–100056. doi:10.1016/j.mtnano.2019.100052

Huang, S. Y., Pooyan, S., Wang, J., Choudhury, I., Leibowitz, M. J., & Stein, S. (1998). A polyethylene glycol copolymer for carrying and releasing multiple copies of cysteine-containing peptides. *Bioconjugate Chemistry*, *9*(5), 612–617. doi:10.1021/bc980038p PMID:9736495

Huang, X., Boey, F., & Zhang, H. U. A. (2010). Graphene-nanoparticle. *Composites*, *6*, 159–166.

Huang, X., Jain, P. K., & Ivan, H. (2008). El-Sayed and Mostafa A. El-Sayed, Plasmonic photothermal therapy (PPTT). *Lasers in Medical Science*, *23*, 217–228. doi:10.100710103-007-0470-x PMID:17674122

Huang, X., Yin, Z., Wu, S., Qi, X., He, Q., Zhang, Q., Yan, Q., Boey, F., & Zhang, H. (2011). Graphene-based materials: Synthesis, characterization, properties, and applications. *Small*, *7*(14), 1876–1902. doi:10.1002mll.201002009 PMID:21630440

Huber, R., Hill, S. L., Holladay, C., Biesiadecki, M., Tononi, G., & Cirelli, C. (2004). Sleep homeostasis in Drosophila melanogaster. *Sleep*, *27*(4), 628–639. doi:10.1093leep/27.4.628 PMID:15282997

Huff, T.B., Tong, L., Zhao, Y., Hansen, M.N., Cheng, J.X., & Wei, A. (2007). Hyperthermic effects of gold nanorods on tumor cells. *Nanomedicine, 2*(1), 125-132.

Huh, A. J., & Kwon, Y.J. (2011) Nanoantibiotics: A new paradigm for treating infectious diseases using nanomaterials in the antibiotics resistant era. *J. Control Release., 156*(2), 128–45.

Hu, L., Tang, X., & Cui, F. (2004). Solid lipid nanoparticles (SLNs) to improve oral bioavailability of poorly soluble drugs. *The Journal of Pharmacy and Pharmacology*, *56*(12), 1527–1535. doi:10.1211/0022357044959 PMID:15563759

Hu, R. L., Li, S. R., Kong, F. J., Hou, R. J., Guan, X. L., & Guo, F. (2014). Inhibition effect of silver nanoparticles on herpes simplex virus 2. *Genetics and Molecular Research*, *13*(3), 7022–7028. doi:10.4238/2014.March.19.2 PMID:24682984

Hussain, M., Bensaid, S., Geobaldo, F., Saracco, G., & Russo, N. (2011). Photocatalytic Degradation of Ethylene Emitted by Fruits with TiO_2 Nanoparticles. *Industrial & Engineering Chemistry Research*, *50*(5), 2536–2543. doi:10.1021/ie1005756

Husseiny, M. I., El-Aziz, M. A., Badr, Y., & Mahmoud, M. A. (2007). Biosynthesis of gold nanoparticles using Pseudomonas aeruginosa. *Spectrochimica Acta. Part A: Molecular Spectroscopy*, *67*(3-4), 1003–1006. doi:10.1016/j.saa.2006.09.028 PMID:17084659

Hu, X., Xu, G., Wen, L., Wang, H., Zhao, Y., Zhang, Y., Cumming, D. R. S., & Chen, Q. (2016). Metamaterial absorber integrated microfluidic terahertz sensors. *Laser & Photonics Reviews*, *10*(6), 962–969. doi:10.1002/lpor.201600064

Hu, Y. (2011). Nanodevices in diagnostics. *Wiley Interdisciplinary Reviews. Nanomedicine and Nanobiotechnology*, *3*(1), 11–32.

Hu, Y. C. (2005). Baculo virus as a highly efficient expression vector in insect and mammalian cells. Act a Pharmacol. Sin. 26, 405–416. folding in vivo by anonlytic baculovirus. *The Biochemical Journal*, *382*, 695–702.

Hu, Y. S., Lorenz, K., Guo, Y. G., & Maier, J. (2006). High lithium electroactivity of nanometer-sized rutile TiO2. *Advanced Materials*, *18*(11), 1421–1426. doi:10.1002/adma.200502723

Hu, Z., & Gänzle, M. G. (2019). Challenges and opportunities related to the use of chitosan as a food preservative. *Journal of Applied Microbiology*, *1269*(5), 1318–1331. doi:10.1111/jam.14131 PMID:30325559

Ibrahim, R., Hayyan, M., AlSaadi, M., Hayyan, A., & Ibrahim, S. (2016). Environmental application of nanotechnology: Air, soil and water. *Environmental Science and Pollution Research International*, *23*(14), 13754–13788. doi:10.100711356-016-6457-z PMID:27074929

Idil, N., Hedström, M., Denizli, A., & Mattiasson, B. (2017). Whole cell based microcontact imprinted capacitive biosensor for the detection of Escherichia coli. *Biosensors & Bioelectronics*, *87*, 807–815. doi:10.1016/j.bios.2016.08.096 PMID:27657842

Idota, Y., Kabuto, T., Matsufuji, A., Maekawa, Y., & Miyasaki, T. (1997). Tin-Based Amorphous Oxide: A High-Capacity Lithium-Ion-Storage. *Materials Science*, *276*, 1395–1397.

Idrees, M. (2015). Role of nanotechnology in medical sciences: A review. *Int. J. Drug Discovery*, *5*, 14–24.

Idumah, C. I., Zurina, M., Ogbu, J., Ndem, J. U., & Igba, E. C. (2019). A review on innovations in polymeric nanocomposite packaging materials and electrical sensors for food and agriculture. *Composite Interfaces*, *27*(1), 1–72. doi:10.1080/09276440.2019.1600972

Ijaz, M., Zafar, M., Afsheen, S., & Iqbal, T. (2020). A Review on Ag-Nanostructures for Enhancement in Shelf Time of Fruits. *Journal of Inorganic and Organometallic Polymers*, *30*(5), 1475–1482. doi:10.100710904-020-01504-x

Iqbal, M. J., & Ahmad, Z. (2008). Electrical and dielectric properties of lithium manganate nanomaterials doped with rare-earth elements. *Journal of Power Sources*, *179*(2), 763–769. doi:10.1016/j.jpowsour.2007.12.115

Iravani, S. (2014). Bacteria in nanoparticle synthesis: Current status and future prospects. *Int. Sch. Res. Not., 359316.*

Iravani, S. (2011). Green synthesis of metal nanoparticles using plants. *Green Chemistry*, *13*(10), 2638–2650. doi:10.1039/c1gc15386b

Irvine, D. J., Swartz, M. A., & Szeto, G. L. (2013). Engineering synthetic vaccines using cues from natural immunity. *Nature Materials*, *12*(11), 978–990. doi:10.1038/nmat3775 PMID:24150416

Ishida, T., Wang, X., Shimizu, T., Nawata, K., & Kiwada, H. (2007). PEGylated liposomes elicit an anti-PEG IgM response in a T cell-independent manner. *Journal of Controlled Release*, *122*(3), 349–355. doi:10.1016/j.jconrel.2007.05.015 PMID:17610982

Ishikawa, A., & Tanaka, T. (2006). Negative magnetic permeability of split ring resonators in the visible light region. *Optics Communications*, *258*(2), 300–305. doi:10.1016/j.optcom.2005.07.076

Jabir, N. R., Tabrez, S., Ashraf, G. M., Shakil, S., Damanhouri, G. A., & Kamal, M. A. (2012). Nanotechnology-based approaches in anticancer research. *International Journal of Nanomedicine*, *7*, 4391–4408. PMID:22927757

Jadhav, S., Gaikwad, S., Nimse, M., & Rajbhoj, A. (2011). Copper oxide nanoparticles: Synthesis, characterization and their antibacterial activity. *Journal of Cluster Science*, *22*(2), 121–129. doi:10.100710876-011-0349-7

Jaejung, S., Jeesu, K., Sekyu, H., Mansik, J., Sanghwa, J., Chulhong, K., & Sungjee, K. (2016). "Smart" Gold Nanoparticles for Photoacoustic Imaging: Imaging Contrast Agent Responsive to Cancer Microenvironment and Signal Amplification by pH-induced Aggregation. *Chemical Communications*, *52*(53), 8287–8290. Advance online publication. doi:10.1039/C6CC03100E PMID:27292365

Jafari, A. R., Mosavi, T., Mosavari, N., Majid, A., Movahedzade, F., Tebyaniyan, M., & Arastoo, S. (2016). Mixed metal oxide nanoparticles inhibit growth of Mycobacterium tuberculosis into THP-1 cells. *International Journal of Mycobacteriology*, *5*, S181–S183. doi:10.1016/j.ijmyco.2016.09.011 PMID:28043541

Jahangirian, H., Lemraski, E. G., Webster, T. J., Rafee-Moghaddam, R., & Abdollahi, Y. (2017). A review of drug delivery systems based on nanotechnology and green chemistry: Green nanomedicine. *International Journal of Nanomedicine, 12*, 2957–2978. doi:10.2147/IJN.S127683 PMID:28442906

Jain, K. K., (2012). Role of nano diagnostics in personalized cancer therapy. *Clin Lab Med., 32*, 15-31.

Jain, P. K., El-Sayed, I. H., & El-Sayed, M. A. (2007). Au nanoparticles target cancer. *Nano Today, 2*(1), 18-29.

Jain, A., Ranjan, S., Dasgupta, N., & Ramalingam, C. (2018). Nanomaterials in food and agriculture: An overview on their safety concerns and regulatory issues. *Critical Reviews in Food Science and Nutrition, 58*(2), 297–317. doi:10.1080/10408398.2016.1160363 PMID:27052385

Jain, K. K. (2005). Nanotechnology in clinical laboratory diagnostics. *Clinica Chimica Acta, 358*(1-2), 37–54. doi:10.1016/j.cccn.2005.03.014 PMID:15890325

Jain, K. K. (2005). The role of nanobiotechnology in drug discovery. *Drug Discovery Today, 10*(21), 1435–1442. doi:10.1016/S1359-6446(05)03573-7 PMID:16243263

Jain, S., Hirst, D. G., & O'sullivan, J. M. (2012). Gold nanoparticles as novel agents for cancer therapy. *The British Journal of Radiology, 85*(1010), 101–113. doi:10.1259/bjr/59448833 PMID:22010024

James, S. J., & James, C. (2010). The Food Cold-Chain and Climate Change. *Food Research International, 43*(7), 1944–1956. doi:10.1016/j.foodres.2010.02.001

Jamnik, J., & Maiera, J. (2003). Nanocrystallinity effects in lithium battery materials Aspects of nano-ionics. Part IV. *Physical Chemistry Chemical Physics, 5*(23), 5215. doi:10.1039/b309130a

Jang, H., Lee, C., Nam, G. E., Quan, B., Choi, H. J., Yoo, J. S., & Piao, Y. (2016). In vivo magnetic resonance and fluorescence: Dual imaging of tumor sites by using dye-doped silica-coated iron oxide nanoparticles. *Journal of Nanoparticle Research, 18*(2), 41. doi:10.100711051-016-3353-x

Janib, S.M., Moses, A.S., & MacKay, J.A. (2010). Imaging and drug delivery using theranostic nanoparticles. *Adv. Drug Deliv. Rev., 62*(11), 1052-1063.

Jayanta, K., Patra, Gitishree, D., & Fernandes, F. (2018). Nano based drugdelivery systems: recent developments and future prospects. *J. Nanobiotechnol, 16.*

Jayaprakash, J., Srinivasan, N., & Chandrasekaran, P. (2014). Surface modifications of CuO nanoparticles using Ethylenediamine tetra acetic acid as a capping agent by sol–gel routine. *Spectrochimica Acta. Part A: Molecular and Biomolecular Spectroscopy, 123*, 363–368. doi:10.1016/j.saa.2013.12.080 PMID:24412789

Jayaprakash, N., Kalaiselvi, N., Doh, C. H., & Bhuvaneswari, D. (2010). A new class of Sol–gel derived $LiM_{1x}M_{2y}Mn_{2-x-y}O_{3.8}F_{0.2}$ (M_1= Cr, M_2= V; x= y= 0.2) cathodes for lithium batteries. *Journal of Applied Electrochemistry, 40*(12), 2193–2202. doi:10.100710800-010-0187-6

Jayaseelana, C., Rahumana, A. A., Kirthi, A. V., Marimuthua, S., Santhoshkumara, T., & Bagavana, A. (2012). Novel microbial route to synthesize ZnO nanoparticles using Aeromonas hydrophila and their activity against pathogenic bacteria and fungi. *Spectrochimica Acta Part A, 90*, 78–84. doi:10.1016/j.saa.2012.01.006 PMID:22321514

Jayaseelan, C., Rahuman, A. A., Roopan, S. M., Kirthi, A. V., Venkatesan, J., Kim, S. K., Iyappan, M., & Siva, C. (2013). Biological approach to synthesize TiO_2 nanoparticles using *Aeromonas hydrophila* and its antibacterial activity. *Spectrochimica Acta. Part A: Molecular and Biomolecular Spectroscopy, 107*, 82–89. doi:10.1016/j.saa.2012.12.083 PMID:23416912

Jeevanandam, J. (2018). Review on nanoparticles and nanostructured materials: history, sources, toxicity and regulations. *Beilstein Journal of Nanotechnology*, *9*(1), 1050-1074.

Jeevanandam, J., Barhoum, A., Yen, S. C., Dufresne, A., & Danquah, M. K. (2018). Review on nanoparticles and nanostructured materials: History, sources, toxicity and regulations. *Beilstein Journal of Nanotechnology*, *9*, 1050–1074. doi:10.3762/bjnano.9.98 PMID:29719757

Jeevanandam, J., Chan, Y. S., & Danquah, M. K. (2016). *Biosynthesis of Metal and Metal Oxide Nanoparticles. Chem. Bio. Eng. Rev.*, *3*(2), 55–67.

Jena, M., Mishra, S., Jena, S., & Mishra, S. S. (2013). Nanotechnology-future prospect in recent medicine: A review. *International Journal of Basic and Clinical Pharmacology*, *2*(4), 353.

Jeong, W. T., Joo, J. H., & Lee, K. S. (2003). Improvement of electrode performances of spinel $LiMn_2O_4$ prepared by mechanical alloying and subsequent firing. *Journal of Power Sources*, *119*, 690–694. doi:10.1016/S0378-7753(03)00229-5

Jerónimo, P. C. A., Araújo, A. N., & Conceição, M. (2007). Optical sensors and biosensors based on sol-gel films. *Talanta*, *72*(1), 13–27. doi:10.1016/j.talanta.2006.09.029 PMID:19071577

Jia, M., Zhang, Z., Li, J., Ma, X., Chen, L., & Yang, X. (2018). Molecular imprinting technology for microorganism analysis. *Trends in Analytical Chemistry*, *106*, 190–201. doi:10.1016/j.trac.2018.07.011

Jiang, J. (2018). The Advancing of Zinc Oxide Nanoparticles for Biomedical Applications. Bioinorganic Chemistry and Applications. *Article ID*, *1062562*, 1–18.

Jiang, J.-F., Li, S.-F., & Liu, Z.-H. (2018). Study on heat transfer and cold storage characteristics of a falling film type of cold energy regenerator with PCM. *Applied Thermal Engineering*, *143*, 676–687. doi:10.1016/j.applthermaleng.2018.07.127

Jiang, W., Kim, B. Y., Rutka, J. T., & Chan, W. C. (2008). Nanoparticle-mediated cellular response is size-dependent. *Nature Nanotechnology*, *3*(3), 145–150. doi:10.1038/nnano.2008.30 PMID:18654486

Jiao, A., Dong, X., Zhang, H., Xu, L., Tian, Y., Liu, X., & Chen, M. (2019). Construction of pure worm-like AuAg nanochains for ultrasensitive SERS detection of pesticide residues on apple surfaces. *Spectrochimica Acta. Part A: Molecular and Biomolecular Spectroscopy*, *209*, 241–247. doi:10.1016/j.saa.2018.10.051

Jin, Y. (2012). Engineering plasmonic gold nanostructures and metamaterials for biosensing and nanomedicine. *Advanced Materials*, *24*(38), 5153–5165. doi:10.1002/adma.201200622 PMID:22760939

Jiu, J., Isoda, S., Wang, F., & Adachi, M. (2006). Dye-sensitized solar cells based on a single-crystalline TiO2 nanorod film. *The Journal of Physical Chemistry B*, *110*(5), 2087–2092. doi:10.1021/jp055824n PMID:16471788

Johnson, C. J., Zhukovsky, N., Cass, A. E. G., & Nagy, J. M. (2008). Proteomics, nanotechnology and molecular diagnostics. *Proteomics*, *8*(4), 715–730. doi:10.1002/pmic.200700665 PMID:18297650

Johnston, J. H., Borrmann, T., Rankin, D., Cairns, M., Grindrod, J. E., & McFarlane, A. (2008). Nano-structured composite calcium silicate and some novel applications. *Current Applied Physics*, *8*(3-4), 504–507. doi:10.1016/j.cap.2007.10.060

Jones, D. P., Carlson, J. L., Mody, V. C. Jr, Cai, J., Lynn, M. J., & Sternberg, P. Jr. (2000). Redox state of glutathione in human plasma. *Free Radical Biology & Medicine*, *28*(4), 625–635. doi:10.1016/S0891-5849(99)00275-0 PMID:10719244

Jones, D. P., Carlson, J. L., Samiec, P. S., Sternberg, P. Jr, Mody, V. C. Jr, Reed, R. L., & Brown, L. A. S. (1998). Glutathione measurement in human plasma: Evaluation of sample collection, storage and derivatization conditions for analysis of dansyl derivatives by HPLC. *Clinica Chimica Acta*, *275*(2), 175–184. doi:10.1016/S0009-8981(98)00089-8 PMID:9721075

Jonoobi, M., Harun, J., Mishra, M., & Oksman, K. (2009). Chemical composition, crystallinity and thermal degradation of bleached and unbleached kenaf bast (*Hibiscus cannabinus*) pulp and nanofibers. *BioResources*, *4*(2), 626–639.

Joo, H. S., & Otto, M. (2012). Molecular basis of in vivo biofilm formation by bacterial pathogens. *Chemistry & Biology*, *19*(12), 1503–1513. doi:10.1016/j.chembiol.2012.10.022 PMID:23261595

Joseph, R. R., & Venkatraman, S. S. (2017). Drug delivery to the eye: What benefits do nanocarriers offer? *Nanomedicine (London)*, *12*(6), 683–702. doi:10.2217/nnm-2016-0379 PMID:28186436

Joshi, M., & Adak, B. (2018). *Advances in Nanotechnology Based Functional, Smart and Intelligent Textiles: A Review* (2nd ed.). Comprehensive Nanoscience and Nanotechnology., doi:10.1016/B978-0-12-803581-8.10471-0

Jozefowicz, M., & Jozefonvicz, J. (1997). Randomness and biospecificity: Random copolymers are capable of biospecific molecular recognition in living systems. *Biomaterials*, *18*(24), 1633–1644. doi:10.1016/S0142-9612(97)00145-2 PMID:9613811

Jung, J. H., Kim, S. W., Min, J. S., Kim, Y. J., Lamsal, K., Kim, K. S., & Lee, Y. S. (2010). The Effect of Nano-Silver Liquid against the White Rot of the Green Onion Caused by *Sclerotium cepivorum*. *Mycobiology*, *38*(1), 39–45. doi:10.4489/MYCO.2010.38.1.039 PMID:23956623

Jurmanovic, S., Kordi, S., & Steinberg, M. D. (2010). Organically modified silicate thin films doped with colourimetric pH indicators methyl red and bromocresol green as pH responsive sol–gel hybrid materials. *Thin Solid Films*, *518*(8), 2234–2240. doi:10.1016/j.tsf.2009.07.158

Ju, S. H., Kang, Y. C., Sun, Y. K., & Kim, D. W. (2012). Synthesis and electrochemical properties of nanorod-shaped $LiMn_{1.5}Ni_{0.5}O_4$ cathode materials for lithium-ion batteries. *Materials Chemistry and Physics*, *132*(1), 223–227. doi:10.1016/j.matchemphys.2011.11.042

Kaatz, F. H., Chow, G. M., & Edelstein, A. S. (1993). Narrowing sputtered nanoparticle size distributions. *Journal of Materials Research*, *8*(5), 995–1000. doi:10.1557/JMR.1993.0995

Kabashin, A. V., Evans, P., Pastkovsky, S., Hendren, W., Wurtz, G. A., Atkinson, R., Pollard, R., Podolskiy, V. A., & Zayats, A. V. (2009). Plasmonic nanorod metamaterials for biosensing. *Nature Materials*, *8*(11), 867–871. doi:10.1038/nmat2546 PMID:19820701

Kairyte, K., Kadys, A., & Luksiene, Z. (2013). Antibacterial and antifungal activity of photoactivated ZnO nanoparticles in suspension. *Journal of Photochemistry and Photobiology. B, Biology*, *128*, 78–84. doi:10.1016/j.jphotobiol.2013.07.017 PMID:24035847

Kakiage, K., Aoyama, Y., Yano, T., Oya, K., Fujisawa, J. I., & Hanaya, M. (2015). Highly-efficient dye-sensitized solar cells with collaborative sensitization by silyl-anchor and carboxy-anchor dyes. *Chemical Communications (Cambridge)*, *51*(88), 15894–15897. doi:10.1039/C5CC06759F PMID:26393334

Kale, A., Bao, Y., Zhou, Z., Prevelige, P. E., & Gupta, A. (2013). Directed self-assembly of CdS quantum dots on bacteriophage P22 coat protein templates. *Nanotechnology*, *24*(4), 045603. doi:10.1088/0957-4484/24/4/045603 PMID:23296127

Kalyanasundaram, K. (2010). *EPFL Press*. CRC Press.

Kalyani, P., Kalaiselvi, N., & Muniyandi, N. (2002). A new solution combustion route to synthesize $LiCoO_2$ and $LiMn_2O_4$. *Journal of Power Sources*, *111*(2), 232–238. doi:10.1016/S0378-7753(02)00307-5

Kamaly, N., Xiao, Z., Valencia, P. M., Radovic-Moreno, A. F., & Farokhzad, O. C. (2012). Targeted polymeric therapeutic nanoparticles: Design, development and clinical translation. *Chemical Society Reviews*, *41*(7), 2971–3010. doi:10.1039/c2cs15344k PMID:22388185

Kamarulzaman, N., Osman, Z., Muhamad, M. R., Ibrahim, Z. A., Arof, A. K., & Mohamed, N. S. (2001). Performance characteristics of $LiMn_2O_4$/polymer/carbon electrochemical cells. *Journal of Power Sources*, *97*, 722–725. doi:10.1016/S0378-7753(01)00647-4

Kamat, P. V. (2012). Boosting the Efficiency of Quantum Dot Sensitized Solar Cells Through Modulation of Interfacial Charge Transfer. *Accounts of Chemical Research*, *45*(11), 1906–1915. doi:10.1021/ar200315d PMID:22493938

Kamat, P. V. (2013). Quantum dot solar cells. The next big thing in photovoltaics. *The Journal of Physical Chemistry Letters*, *4*(6), 908–918. doi:10.1021/jz400052e PMID:26291355

Kaminskas, L. M., Kelly, B. D., McLeod, V. M., Boyd, B. J., Krippner, G. A., Williams, E. D., & Porter, C. J. H. (2009). Pharmacokinetics and tumor disposition of PEGylated, Methotrexate conjugated Poly-l-lysine Dendrimers. *Molecular Pharmaceutics*, *6*(4), 1190–1204. doi:10.1021/mp900049a PMID:19453158

Kandah, M. I., & Meunier, J. L. (2007). Removal of nickel ions from water bymulti-walled carbon nanotubes. *Journal of Hazardous Materials*, *146*(1-2), 283–288. doi:10.1016/j.jhazmat.2006.12.019 PMID:17196328

Kang, C. Y., Luo, L., Wainberg, M. A., & Li, Y. (1999). Development of HIV/AIDS vaccine using chimeric gag env virus-like particles. *Biological Chemistry*, *380*(3), 353–364. doi:10.1515/BC.1999.047 PMID:10223338

Kang, S., Pinault, M., Pfefferle, L. D., & Elimelech, M. (2007). Single-walled carbon nanotubes exhibit strong antimicrobial activity. *Langmuir*, *23*(17), 8670–8673. doi:10.1021/la701067r PMID:17658863

Kanmani, P., & Rhim, J. W. (2014). Physicochemical properties of gelatin/silver nanoparticle antimicrobial composite films. *Food Chemistry*, *148*, 162–169. doi:10.1016/j.foodchem.2013.10.047 PMID:24262541

Kaphle, A., Navya, P. N., Umapathi, A., & Daima, H. K. (2018). Nanomaterials for agriculture, food and environment: Applications, toxicity and regulation. *Environmental Chemistry Letters*, *16*(1), 43–58. doi:10.100710311-017-0662-y

Karami, P., Bagheri, H., Johari-Ahar, M., Khoshsafar, H., Arduini, F., & Afkhami, A. (2019). Dual-modality impedimetric immunosensor for early detection of prostate-specific antigen and myoglobin markers based on antibody-molecularly imprinted polymer. *Talanta*, *202*, 111–122. doi:10.1016/j.talanta.2019.04.061 PMID:31171159

Karimi, M. (2016). Smart micro/nanoparticles in stimulus-responsive drug/gene delivery systems. *Chemical Society Reviews*, *45*(5), 1457–1501.

Karkada, M., Weir, G. M., Quinton, T., Fuentes-Ortega, A., & Mansour, M. (2011). Aliposome-based platform, Vacci Max, and its modified water-free platform DepoVax enhance efficacy of in vivo nucleic acid delivery. *Vaccine*, *28*(38), 6176–6182. doi:10.1016/j.vaccine.2010.07.025 PMID:20656034

Karlssonz, R., & Fält, A. (1997). Experimental design for kinetic analysis of protein-protein interactions with surface plasmon resonance biosensors. *Journal of Immunological Methods*, *200*(1-2), 121–133. doi:10.1016/S0022-1759(96)00195-0 PMID:9005951

Karmakar, P. (2007). In Vitro structural and functional evaluation of gold nanoparticles conjugated antibiotics. *Nanoscale Research Letters*, *2*(12), 614–622. doi:10.100711671-007-9104-2

Karn, B., Kuiken, T., & Otto, M. (2009). Nanotechnology and in situ remediation: A review of the benefits and potential risks. *Environmental Health Perspectives*, *117*(12), 1813–1831. doi:10.1289/ehp.0900793 PMID:20049198

Karthik, K., Dhanuskodi, S., Kumar, S. P., Gobinath, C., & Sivaramakrishnan, S. (2017). Microwave assisted green synthesis of MgO nanorods and their antibacterial and anti-breast cancer activities. *Materials Letters*, *206*, 217–220. doi:10.1016/j.matlet.2017.07.004

Karthik, K., Jaya, N. V., & Kanagaraj, M. (2011). Arumugam, S. Temperature-dependent magnetic anomalies of CuO nanoparticles. *Solid State Communications*, *151*(7), 564–568. doi:10.1016/j.ssc.2011.01.008

Kathiresan, K., Manivannan, S., Nabeel, M. A., & Dhivya, B. (2009). Studies on silver nanoparticles synthesized by a marine fungus, Penicillium fellutanum isolated from coastal mangrove sediment. *Colloids and Surfaces. B, Biointerfaces*, *71*(1), 133–137. doi:10.1016/j.colsurfb.2009.01.016 PMID:19269142

Katsamba, P. S., Park, S., & Laird-Offringa, I. A. (2002). Kinetic studies of RNA-protein interactions using surface plasmon resonance. *Methods (San Diego, Calif.)*, *26*(2), 95–104. doi:10.1016/S1046-2023(02)00012-9 PMID:12054886

Kaul, S., Gulati, N., Verma, D., Mukherjee, S., & Nagaich, U. (2018). Role of Nanotechnology in Cosmeceuticals: A Review of Recent Advances. *Journal of Pharmaceutics*, *3420204*, 1–19. Advance online publication. doi:10.1155/2018/3420204 PMID:29785318

Kavitha, S., & Raghavan, V. (2018). Isolation and characterization of marine biofilm forming bacteria from a ship's hull. *Frontiers in Biology*, *13*(3), 208–214. doi:10.100711515-018-1496-0

Kawaoka, H., Hibino, M., Zhou, H., & Honma, I. (2004). Sonochemical synthesis of amorphous manganese oxide coated on carbon and application to high power battery. *Journal of Power Sources*, *125*(1), 85–89. doi:10.1016/S0378-7753(03)00823-1

Kaya, B., Creus, A., Yanikoğlu, A., Cabré, O., & Marcos, R. (2000). Use of the Drosophila wing spot test in the genotoxicity testing of different herbicides. *Environmental and Molecular Mutagenesis*, *36*(1), 40–46. doi:10.1002/1098-2280(2000)36:1<40::AID-EM6>3.0.CO;2-K PMID:10918358

Kazanji, M., Laurent, F., & Pery, P. (1994). Immune responses and protective effect in mice vaccinated orally with surface sporozoite protein of Eimeria falciformis in ISCOMs. *Vaccine*, *12*(9), 798–804. doi:10.1016/0264-410X(94)90288-7 PMID:7975858

Kearns, H., Goodacre, R., Jamieson, L. E., Graham, D., & Faulds, K. (2017). SERS Detection of Multiple Antimicrobial-Resistant Pathogens Using Nanosensors. *Analytical Chemistry*, *89*(23), 12666–12673. doi:10.1021/acs.analchem.7b02653 PMID:28985467

Kebede, M. A., Phasha, M. J., Kunjuzwa, N., Le Roux, L. J., Mkhonto, D., Ozoemena, K. I., & Mathe, M. K. (2014). Structural and electrochemical properties of aluminium doped $LiMn_2O_4$ cathode materials for Li battery: Experimental and ab initio calculations. *Sustainable Energy Technologies and Assessments*, *5*, 44–49. doi:10.1016/j.seta.2013.11.005

Kebede, M. A., Phasha, M. J., Kunjuzwa, N., Mathe, M. K., & Ozoemena, K. I. (2015). Solution-combustion synthesized aluminium-doped spinel ($LiAl_xMn_{2-x}O_4$) as a high-performance lithium-ion battery cathode material. *Applied Physics. A, Materials Science & Processing*, *121*(1), 51–57. doi:10.100700339-015-9311-0

Kelly, J. A., Shukaliak, A. M., Cheung, C. C., Shopsowitz, K. E., Hamad, W. Y., & MacLachlan, M. J. (2013). Responsive Photonic Hydrogels Based on Nanocrystalline Cellulose. *Angewandte Chemie International Edition*, *52*(34), 8912–8916. doi:10.1002/anie.201302687 PMID:23881841

Kelson, A. B., Carnevali, M., & Truong-Le, V. (2013). Gallium-based anti-infectives: Targeting microbial iron-uptake mechanisms. *Current Opinion in Pharmacology*, *13*(5), 707–716. doi:10.1016/j.coph.2013.07.001 PMID:23876838

Kersten, G. F., & Crommelin, D. J. (1995). Liposomes and ISCOMS as vaccine formulations. *Biochimica et Biophysica Acta*, *1241*(2), 117–138. doi:10.1016/0304-4157(95)00002-9 PMID:7640293

Kersten, G. F., Teerlink, T., Derks, H. J., Verkleij, A. J., van Wezel, T. L., Crommelin, D. J., & Beuvery, E. C. (1988). Incorporation of the major outer membrane protein of Neisseria gonorrhoeae in saponin-lipid complexes (iscoms): Chemical analysis, some structural features, and comparison of their immunogenicity with three other antigen delivery systems. *Infection and Immunity*, *56*(2), 432–438. doi:10.1128/IAI.56.2.432-438.1988 PMID:3123391

Kesarkar, R., Shroff, S., Yeole, M., Chowdhary, A. (2015). L-Cysteine Functionalized Gold Nanocargos Potentiates Anti-HIV Activity of Azidothymydine against HIV-1Ba-L Virus. *J. Immunol. Virol.*, *1*.

Kesarkar, R., Oza, G., Pandey, S., Dahake, R., Mukherjee, S., Chowdhary, A., & Sharon, M. (2017). Gold nanoparticles: Effective as both entry inhibitors and virus neutralizing agents against HIV. *Journal of Microbiology and Biotechnology Research*, *2*, 276–283.

Keshavarz, A., & Vafapour, Z. (2019). Water-based terahertz metamaterial for skin cancer detection application. *IEEE Sensors Journal*, *19*(4), 1519–1524. doi:10.1109/JSEN.2018.2882363

Khan, A.A., Fox, E.K., Gorzny, M.L., Nikulina, E., Brougham, D.F., Wege, C., & Bittner, A.M. (2013). pH control of the electrostatic binding of gold and iron oxide nanoparticles to tobacco mosaic virus. *Langmuir, 29*, 2094–2098.

Khan, M. M., Adil, S. F., & Al-Mayouf, A. (2015). Metal oxides as photocatalysts. *Journal of Saudi Chemical Society*, *19*(5), 462–464. doi:10.1016/j.jscs.2015.04.003

Khanra, P., Kuila, T., Bae, S. H., Kim, N. H., & Lee, J. H. (2012). b, Electrochemically exfoliated graphene using 9-anthracene carboxylic acid for supercapacitor application. *Journal of Materials Chemistry*, *22*(46), 24403. Advance online publication. doi:10.1039/c2jm34838a

Khan, S. A., & Ahmad, A. (2013). Fungus mediated synthesis of biomedically important cerium oxide nanoparticles. *Materials Research Bulletin*, *48*(10), 4134–4138. doi:10.1016/j.materresbull.2013.06.038

Khansili, N., Rattu, G., & Krishna, P. M. (2018). Label-free optical biosensors for food and biological sensor applications. *Sensors and Actuators. B, Chemical*, *265*, 35–49. doi:10.1016/j.snb.2018.03.004

Khare, P., Yadav, A., Ramkumar, J., & Verma, N. (2016). Microchannel-embedded metal–carbon–polymer nanocomposite as a novel support for chitosan for efficient removal of hexavalent chromium from water under dynamic conditions. *Chemical Engineering Journal*, *293*, 44–54. doi:10.1016/j.cej.2016.02.049

Kharisov, B. I., Rasika Dias, H. V., Kharissova, O. V., Manuel Jiménez-Pérez, V., Olvera Pérez, B., & Muñoz Flores, B. (2012). Iron-containing nanomaterials: Synthesis, properties, and environmental applications. *Royal Society of Chemistry Advances*, *2*(25), 9325–9358. doi:10.1039/c2ra20812a

Khasanova, N. R., Drozhzhin, O. A., Fedotov, S. S., Storozhilova, D. A., Panin, R. V., & Antipov, E. V. (2013). Synthesis and electrochemical performance of $Li_2Co_{1-x}M_xPO_4F$ (M= Fe, Mn) cathode materials. *Beilstein Journal of Nanotechnology*, *4*, 860–867. doi:10.3762/bjnano.4.97 PMID:24367755

Khin, M. M., Nair, A. S., Babu, V. J., Murugan, R., & Ramakrishna, S. A. (2012). Review on nanomaterials for environmental remediation. *Energy & Environmental Science*, *5*(8), 8075–8109. doi:10.1039/c2ee21818f

Khlebtsov, B., Zharov, V., Melnikov, A., Tuchin, V., & Khlebtsov, N. (2006). Optical amplification of photothermal therapy with gold nanoparticles and nanoclusters. *Nanotechnology, 17*(20), 5167-5179.

Khodadadi, J. M., & Hosseinizadeh, S. F. (2007). Nanoparticle-enhanced phase change materials (NEPCM) with great potential for improved thermal energy storage. *International Communications in Heat and Mass Transfer*, *34*(5), 534–543. doi:10.1016/j.icheatmasstransfer.2007.02.005

Khurana, C., & Chudasama, B. (2018). Nanoantibiotics: strategic assets in the fight against drug-resistant superbugs. *International Journal of nanomedicine, 13*, 3.

Khurana, V., Lu, Y., Steinhilb, M. L., Oldham, S., Shulman, J. M., & Feany, M. B. (2006). TOR-mediated cell-cycle activation causes neurodegeneration in a Drosophila tauopathy model. *Current Biology, 16*(3), 230–241. doi:10.1016/j.cub.2005.12.042 PMID:16461276

Kim, M., & Rho, J. (2015). Metamaterials and imaging. *Nano Convergence, 2*(1), 22-1-22–16. doi:10.118640580-015-0053-7

Kim, T. S., Lee, J. H., & Yoon, D. S. (2006). Nanomechanical cantilever devices for biological sensors. In Micromanufacturing and Nanotechnology (pp. 299–321). Academic Press.

Kim, C. K., Ghosh, P., & Rotello, V. M. (2009). Multimodal drug delivery using gold nanoparticles. *Nanoscale, 1*(1), 61–67. doi:10.1039/b9nr00112c PMID:20644861

Kim, C. S., Duncan, B., Creran, B., & Rotello, V. M. (2013). Triggered nanoparticles as therapeutics. *Nano Today, 8*(4), 439–447. doi:10.1016/j.nantod.2013.07.004 PMID:24159362

Kim, D. K., Muralidharan, P., Lee, H. W., Ruffo, R., Yang, Y., Chan, C. K., Peng, H., Huggins, R. A., & Cui, Y. (2008). Spinel $LiMn_2O_4$ nanorods as lithium ion battery cathodes. *Nano Letters, 8*(11), 3948–3952. doi:10.1021/nl8024328 PMID:18826287

Kim, H. S., Kang, H. S., Chu, G. J., & Byun, H. S. (2008). Antifungal Effectiveness of Nanosilver Colloid against Rose Powdery Mildew in Greenhouses. *Diffusion and Defect Data, Solid State Data. Part B, Solid State Phenomena, 135*, 15–18. doi:10.4028/www.scientific.net/SSP.135.15

Kim, J. S., Kuk, E., Yu, K., Kim, J. H., Park, S. J., Lee, H. J., Kim, S. H., Park, Y. K., Park, Y. H., Hwang, C. Y., Kim, Y.-K., Lee, Y.-S., Jeong, D. H., & Cho, M.-H. (2007). Antimicrobial effects of silver nanoparticles. *Nanomedicine (London), 3*(1), 95–101. doi:10.1016/j.nano.2006.12.001 PMID:17379174

Kim, K. W., Lee, S. W., Han, K. S., Chung, H. J., & Woo, S. I. (2003). Characterization of Al-doped spinel $LiMn_2O_4$ thin film cathode electrodes prepared by liquid source misted chemical deposition (LSMCD) technique. *Electrochimica Acta, 48*(28), 4223–4231. doi:10.1016/S0013-4686(03)00608-X

Kim, S., & Chung, B. H. (2016). Antioxidant activity of levan coated cerium oxide nanoparticles. *Carbohydrate Polymers, 150*, 400–407. doi:10.1016/j.carbpol.2016.05.021 PMID:27312651

Kim, T. H., Cho, K. S., Lee, E. K., Lee, S. J., Chae, J., Kim, J. W., Kwon, J. Y., Amaratunga, G., Lee, S. Y., & Choi, B. L. (2011). Full-colour quantum dot displays fabricated by transfer printing. *Nature Photonics, 5*(3), 176–182. doi:10.1038/nphoton.2011.12

Kingsman, S. M., & Kingsman, A. J. (1988). Polyvalent recombinant antigens; a new vaccine strategy. *Vaccine, 6*(4), 304–306. doi:10.1016/0264-410X(88)90174-0 PMID:2847436

Klimov, V. V., & Guzatov, D. V. (2012). Using chiral nano-meta-particles to control chiral molecule radiation. *Physics Uspekhi, 55*(10), 1054–1058. doi:10.3367/UFNe.0182.201210k.1130

Kneipp, J., Kneipp, H., Wittig, B., & Kneipp, K. (2010). Novel optical nanosensors for probing and imaging live cells. *Nanomedicine; Nanotechnology, Biology, and Medicine, 6*(2), 214–226. doi:10.1016/j.nano.2009.07.009 PMID:19699322

Kneipp, K., Kneipp, H., & Kneipp, J. (2006). Surface-enhanced Raman scattering in local optical fields of silver and gold nanoaggregates from single-molecule Raman spectroscopy to ultrasensitive probing in live cells. *Accounts of Chemical Research, 39*(7), 443–450. doi:10.1021/ar050107x PMID:16846208

Kobljanskyj, Y., Melkov, G., Guslienko, K., Novosad, V., Bader, S. D., Kostylev, M., & Slavin, A. (2012). Nano-structured magnetic metamaterial with enhanced nonlinear properties. *Scientific Reports, 2*, 478-1-478–6. doi:10.1038rep00478

Koh, K., Evans, J. M., Hendricks, J. C., & Sehgal, A. (2006). A Drosophila model for age-associated changes in sleep:wake cycles. *Proceedings of the National Academy of Sciences of the United States of America, 103*(37), 13843–13847. doi:10.1073/pnas.0605903103 PMID:16938867

Konate, A., Wang, Y., He, X., Adeel, M., Zhang, P., Ma, Y., Ding, Y., Zhang, J., Yang, J., Kizito, S., Rui, Y., & Zhang, Z. (2018). Comparative effects of nano and bulk-Fe3O4 on the growth of cucumber (Cucumis sativus). *Ecotoxicology and Environmental Safety, 165*, 547–554. doi:10.1016/j.ecoenv.2018.09.053 PMID:30223168

Kong, B., Tang, J., Wu, Z., Selomulya, C., Wang, H., Wei, J., Wang, Y., Zheng, G., & Zhao, D. (2014). Bio-inspired porous antenna-like nanocube/nanowire heterostructure as ultra-sensitive cellular interfaces. *NPG Asia Materials, 6*(8), e117. doi:10.1038/am.2014.56

Koping-Hoggard, M., Sanchez, A., & Alonso, M. J. (2005). Nanoparticles as carriers for nasal vaccine delivery. *Expert Review of Vaccines, 4*(2), 185–196. doi:10.1586/14760584.4.2.185 PMID:15889992

Kosaraju, S. L. (2005). Colon targeted delivery systems: Review of polysaccharides for encapsulation and delivery. *Critical Reviews in Food Science and Nutrition, 45*(4), 251–258. doi:10.1080/10408690490478091 PMID:16047493

Kou, R., Shao, Y., Mei, D., Nie, Z., Wang, D., Wang, C., Viswanathan, V. V., Park, S., Aksay, I. A., Lin, Y., Wang, Y., & Liu, J. (2011). Stabilization of Electrocatalytic Metal Nanoparticles at Metal–Metal Oxide–Graphene Triple Junction Points. *Journal of the American Chemical Society, 133*(8), 2541–2547. doi:10.1021/ja107719u PMID:21302925

Kozak, Y., Farid, M., & Ziskind, G. (2017). Experimental and comprehensive theoretical study of cold storage packages containing PCM. *Applied Thermal Engineering, 115*, 899–912. doi:10.1016/j.applthermaleng.2016.12.127

Kreibig, U., & Vollmer, M. (1995). *Optical Properties of Metal Clusters* (Vol. 25). Springer. doi:10.1007/978-3-662-09109-8

Kruis, F. E., Fissan, H., & Peled, A. (1998). Synthesis of nanoparticles in the gas phase for electronic, optical and magnetic applications—A review. *Journal of Aerosol Science, 29*(5-6), 511–535. doi:10.1016/S0021-8502(97)10032-5

Krukemeyer, M. G., Krenn, V., Huebner, F., Wagner, W., & Resch, R. (2015). History and Possible Uses of Nanomedicine Based on Nanoparticles and Nanotechnological Progress. *Journal of Nanomedicine & Nanotechnology, 6*, 1–7.

Krupa, A. N. D., & Vimala, R. (2017). AgNPs doped TEOS sol–gel coatings to prevent the adhesion of marine fouling organisms. *IET Nanobiotechnology / IET, 12*(2), 99–105. doi:10.1049/iet-nbt.2017.0047

Krupa, N. D., Grace, A. N., & Raghavan, V. (2019). Process optimisation for green synthesis of ZnO nanoparticles and evaluation of its antimacrofouling activity. *IET Nanobiotechnology / IET, 13*(5), 510–514. doi:10.1049/iet-nbt.2018.5396

Kryscio, D. R., & Peppas, N. A. (2012). Critical review and perspective of macromolecularly imprinted polymers. *Acta Biomaterialia, 8*(2), 461–473. doi:10.1016/j.actbio.2011.11.005 PMID:22100344

Kudo, T., Ikedaa, Y., Watanabea, T., Hibinoav, M., Miyayamaa, M., Abeb, H., & Kajitab, K. (2002). Amorphous V_2O_5/carbon composites as electrochemical supercapacitor electrodes. *Solid State Ionics, 833*, 152–153. doi:10.1016/S0167-2738(02)00383-1

Kukoswka-Latallo, J. F., Candido, K. A., Cao, Z., Nigavekar, S. S., Majoros, I. J., Thomas, T. P., & … . (2005). Nanoparticle targeting of anticancer drug improves therapeutic response in animal model of human epithelial cancer. *Cancer Research, 65*(12), 5317–5324. doi:10.1158/0008-5472.CAN-04-3921 PMID:15958579

Kulkarni, N., & Muddapur, U. (2014). Biosynthesis of metal nanoparticles: A review. *Journal of Nanotechnology*, *2014*, 510246. doi:10.1155/2014/510246

Kullmann, F., Hollerbach, S., Dollinger, M. M., Harder, J., Fuchs, M., Messmann, H., Trojan, J., Gäbele, E., Hinke, A., Hollerbach, C., & Endlicher, E. (2009). Cetuximab plus gemcitabine/oxaliplatin (GEMOXCET) in first-line metastatic pancreatic cancer: A multicentre phase II study. *British Journal of Cancer*, *100*(7), 1032–1036. doi:10.1038j.bjc.6604983 PMID:19293797

Kumar, A., Gupta, K., Dixit, S., Mishra, K., & Srivastava, S. (2019). A review on positive and negative impacts of nanotechnology in agriculture. *International Journal of Environmental Science and Technology*, *16*(4), 2175–2184. doi:10.100713762-018-2119-7

Kumari, A., Kumar, V., & Yadav, S. (2012). Nanotechnology: A tool to enhance therapeutic values of natural plant products. *Trends Med Res*, *7*(2), 34–42. doi:10.3923/tmr.2012.34.42

Kumaria, A., Yadava, S. K., & Yadav, S. C. (2010). Biodegradable polymeric nanoparticles based drug delivery systems. *Colloids and Surfaces. B, Biointerfaces*, *75*(1), 1–18. doi:10.1016/j.colsurfb.2009.09.001 PMID:19782542

Kumari, M., Mukherjee, A., & Chandrasekaran, N. (2009). Genotoxicity of silver nanoparticles in Allium cepa. *The Science of the Total Environment*, *407*(19), 5243–5246. doi:10.1016/j.scitotenv.2009.06.024 PMID:19616276

Kumarn, N. A., Choi, H.-J., & Shin, Y. R. (2012). Polyaniline-grafted reduced graphene oxide for efficient electrochemical supercapacitors. *ACS Nano*, *6*(2), 1715–1723. doi:10.1021/nn204688c PMID:22276770

Kumar, R., & Munstedt, H. (2005). Silver ion release from antimicrobial polyamide/silver composites. *Biomaterials*, *26*(14), 2081–2088. doi:10.1016/j.biomaterials.2004.05.030 PMID:15576182

Kumar, S., Harrison, N., Richards-Kortum, R., & Sokolov, K. (2007). Plasmonic nanosensors for imaging intracellular biomarkers in live cells. *Nano Letters*, *7*(5), 1338–1343. doi:10.1021/nl070365i PMID:17439187

Kumar, S., & Varela, M. F. (2003). Molecular mechanisms of bacterial resistance to antimicrobial agents. In A. Méndez-Vilas (Ed.), *Microbial Pathogens and Strategies for Combating Them: Science, Technology and Education* (Vol. 1, pp. 522–534). Formatex Research Centre.

Kuppusamy, P., Yusoff, M. M., Maniam, G. P., & Govindan, N. (2016). Biosynthesis of metallic nanoparticles using plant derivatives and their new avenues in pharmacological applications – an updated report. *Saudi Pharmaceutical Journal*, *24*(4), 473–484. doi:10.1016/j.jsps.2014.11.013 PMID:27330378

Ladd, J., Boozer, C., Yu, Q., Chen, S., Homola, J., & Jiang, S. (2004). DNA-directed protein immobilization on mixed self-assembled monolayers via a streptavidin bridge. *Langmuir*, *20*(19), 8090–8095. doi:10.1021/la049867r PMID:15350077

Lai, C., Wang, G., Ling, T., Wang, T., & Chiu, P. (2017). Near infrared surface-enhanced Raman scattering based on star-shaped gold/ silver nanoparticles and hyperbolic metamaterial. *Scientific Reports*, *7*, 5446-1-5446–5448. doi:10.103841598-017-05939-0

Lam, C. W., James, J. T., McCluskey, R., Arepalli, S., & Hunter, R. L. (2006). A review of carbon nanotube toxicity and assessment of potential occupational and environmental health risks. *Critical Reviews in Toxicology*, *36*(3), 189–217. doi:10.1080/10408440600570233 PMID:16686422

Lam, C. W., James, J. T., McCluskey, R., & Hunter, R. L. (2004). Pulmonary toxicity of single-wall carbon nanotubes in mice 7 and 90 days after intratracheal instillation. *Toxicological Sciences*, *77*(1), 126–134. doi:10.1093/toxsci/kfg243 PMID:14514958

Lam, P. L., Wong, W. Y., Bian, Z., Chui, C. H., & Gambari, R. (2017). Recent advances in green nanoparticulate systems for drug delivery: Efficient delivery and safety concern. *Nanomedicine (London), 12*(4), 357–385. doi:10.2217/nnm-2016-0305 PMID:28078952

Landy, N. I., Sajuyigbe, S., Mock, J. J., Smith, D. R., & Padilla, W. J. (2008). Perfect metamaterial absorber. *Physical Review Letters, 100*(20), 1–4. doi:10.1103/PhysRevLett.100.207402 PMID:18518577

Lange, P., Kewes, G., Severin, N., Benson, O., & Rabe, J. P. (2014), Evidence for Graphene Plasmons in the Visible Spectral Range Probed by Molecules. arXiv, arXiv:1404.

Langer, R., & Folkman, J. (1976). Polymers for the sustained release of proteins and other macromolecules. *Nature, 263*(5580), 797–800. doi:10.1038/263797a0 PMID:995197

Lara, H. H., Nilda, V. A., Liliana, I. T., & Cristina, R. P. (2010). Mode of antiviral action of silver nanoparticles against HIV-1. *Journal of Nanobiotechnology, 8*(1), 1. doi:10.1186/1477-3155-8-1 PMID:20145735

LaVan, D. A., Lynn, D. M., & Langer, R. (2002). Timeline: Moving Smaller in drug discovery and delivery. *Nature Reviews. Drug Discovery, 1*(1), 77–84. doi:10.1038/nrd707 PMID:12119612

Law, M., Greene, L. E., Johnson, J. C., Saykally, R., & Yang, P. (2005). Nanowire dye-sensitized solar cells. *Nature Materials, 4*(6), 455–459. doi:10.1038/nmat1387 PMID:15895100

Lee, D. K., Kang, J. H., Lee, J. S., Kim, H. S., Kim, C., Hun Kim, J., Lee, T., Son, J. H., Park, Q. H., & Seo, M. (2015). Highly sensitive and selective sugar detection by terahertz nano-antennas. *Scientific Reports, 5*, 15459-1-15459–7. doi:10.1038rep15459

Lee, C. M., Jang, D., Kim, J., Cheong, S. J., Kim, E. M., Jeong, M. H., Kim, S. H., Kim, D. W., Lim, S. T., Sohn, M. H., Jeong, Y. Y., & Jeong, H.-J. (2011). Oleyl-Chitosan nanoparticles based on a dual probe for Optical/MR imaging in vivo. *Bioconjugate Chemistry, 22*(2), 186–192. doi:10.1021/bc100241a PMID:21243999

Lee, D., Kang, J., Kwon, J., Lee, J., Lee, S., Woo, D. H., Kim, J. H., Song, C., Park, Q., & Seo, M. (2017). Nano metamaterials for ultrasensitive terahertz biosensing. *Scientific Reports, 7*(1), 1–6. doi:10.103841598-017-08508-7 PMID:28811551

Lee, D., Kim, G., Kim, C., Jhon, Y. M., Kim, J. H., Lee, T., Son, J., & Seo, M. (2016). Ultrasensitive detection of residual pesticides using THz near-field enhancement. *IEEE Transactions on Terahertz Science and Technology, 6*(3), 389–395. doi:10.1109/TTHZ.2016.2538731

Lee, H.-M., Kwac, L.-K., An, K.-H., Park, S.-J., & Kim, B.-J. (2016). Electrochemical behavior of pitch-based activated carbon fibers for electrochemical capacitors. *Energy Conversion and Management, 125*, 347–352. doi:10.1016/j.enconman.2016.06.006

Lee, J. H., Wu, Q., & Park, W. (2009). Metal nanocluster metamaterial fabricated by the colloidal self-assembly. *Optics Letters, 34*(4), 443–445. doi:10.1364/OL.34.000443 PMID:19373335

Lee, K. Y., & Mooney, D. J. (2012). Alginate: Properties and biomedical applications. *Progress in Polymer Science, 37*(1), 106–126. doi:10.1016/j.progpolymsci.2011.06.003 PMID:22125349

Lee, K., Lee, H., Bae, K. H., & Park, T. G. (2010). Heparin immobilized gold nanoparticles for targeted detection and apoptotic death of metastatic cancer cells. *Biomaterials, 31*(25), 6530–6536. doi:10.1016/j.biomaterials.2010.04.046 PMID:20537379

Lee, M. M., Teuscher, J., Miyasaka, T., Murakami, T. N., & Snaith, H. (in press). J. Science, (2012). *Efficient Hybrid Solar Cells Based on Meso-Superstructured Organometal Halide Perovskites.* Advance online publication. doi:10.1126cience.1228604 PMID:23042296

Lee, P.-W., Hsu, S.-H., Tsai, J.-S., Chen, F.-R., Huang, P.-J., Ke, C.-J., Liao, Z.-X., Hsiao, C.-W., Lin, H.-J., & Sung, H.-W. (2010). Multifunctional core-shell polymeric nanoparticles for transdermal DNA delivery and epidermal Langerhans cell stracking. *Biomaterials, 31*(8), 2425–2434. doi:10.1016/j.biomaterials.2009.11.100 PMID:20034662

Lee, S. B., Kim, H. L., Jeong, H. J., Lim, S. T., Sohn, M. H., & Kim, D. W. (2013). Mesoporous silica nanoparticle pretargeting for PET imaging based on a rapid bio-orthogonal reaction in a living body. *Angewandte Chemie, 125*(40), 10743–10746. doi:10.1002/ange.201304026

Lee, S. H., Park, C. M., Seo, Y. M., & Kim, C. K. (2010). Reversed Doppler effect in double negative metamaterials. *Physical Review B: Condensed Matter and Materials Physics, 81*(24), 241102-1, 241102–241104. doi:10.1103/PhysRevB.81.241102

Lee, S. W., Mao, C., Flynn, C. E., & Belcher, A. M. (2002). Ordering of quantum dots using genetically engineered viruses. *Science, 296*(5569), 892–895. doi:10.1126cience.1068054 PMID:11988570

Lee, S., Chon, H., Lee, M., Choo, J., Shin, S. Y., Lee, Y. H., Rhyu, I. J., Son, S. W., & Oh, C. H. (2009). Surface-enhanced Raman scattering imaging of HER2 cancer markers overexpressed in single MCF7 cells using antibody conjugated hollow gold nanospheres. *Biosensors & Bioelectronics, 24*(7), 2260–2263. doi:10.1016/j.bios.2008.10.018 PMID:19056254

Lee, W. M., An, Y. J., Yoon, H., & Kwbon, H. S. (2008). Toxicity and bioavailability of copper nanoparticles to the terrestrial plants mung bean (phaseolus radiatus) and wheat (triticum aestivum): plant agar test for water-insoluble nanoparticles. *Environmental Toxicology and Chemistry, 27*(9), 1915–1921. doi:10.1897/07-481.1 PMID:19086317

Lee, Y. S., Kumada, N., & Yoshio, M. (2001). Synthesis and characterization of lithium aluminum-doped spinel ($LiAl_xMn_{2-x}O_4$) for lithium secondary battery. *Journal of Power Sources, 96*(2), 376–384. doi:10.1016/S0378-7753(00)00652-2

Lei, J. P., Dong, X. L., Zhu, X., Lei, G. M., Huang, K. H., Zhang, X. F., Lu, B., Park, W. J., & Chung, H. S. (2007). Formation and characterization of intermetallic Fe–Sn nanoparticles synthesized by an arc discharge method. *Intermetallics, 15*(12), 1589–1594. doi:10.1016/j.intermet.2007.06.010

Levsen, K. (1995). Chronic inhalation exposure of wistar rats and 2 different strains of mice to diesel-engine exhaust, carbon-black, titanium dioxide. *Inhalation Toxicology, 7*(4), 533–556. doi:10.3109/08958379509015211

Lewandowski, A., & Agnieszka, S. M. (2009). Ionic liquids as electrolytes for Li-ion batteries-An overview of electrochemical studies. *Journal of Power Sources, 194*(2), 601–609. doi:10.1016/j.jpowsour.2009.06.089

Lewinski, N., Colvin, V., & Drezek, R. (2008). Cytotoxicity of nanoparticles. *Small, 4*(1), 26-49.

Lewis, N. S. (2007). Toward Cost-Effective Solar Energy Use. *Science, 315*, 798–801.

Lewis, N. S., & Crabtree, G. (2005). *Basic research needs for solar energy utilization. Office of Science*. U. S. Department of Energy.

Li Jia'en. (2011). *Cytotoxicity of Gold Nanoparticles in vitro* (Doctoral dissertation).

Liang, C., Dai, X., Zhou, B., & Zhang, Y. (2014). Application of zero-valent iron nanoparticles for the removal of aqueous zinc ions under various experimental conditions. *PLoS One, 9*(1), e85686. doi:10.1371/journal.pone.0085686 PMID:24416439

Liang, J., Yu, M., Guo, L., Cui, B., Zhao, X., Sun, C., Wang, Y., Liu, G., Cui, H., & Zeng, Z. (2018). Bioinspired Development of P(St–MAA)–Avermectin Nanoparticles with High Affinity for Foliage To Enhance Folia Retention. *Journal of Agricultural and Food Chemistry, 66*(26), 6578–6584. doi:10.1021/acs.jafc.7b01998 PMID:28727420

Li, C., Zhang, H. P., Fu, L. J., Liu, H., Wu, Y. P., Rahm, E., Holze, R., & Wu, H. Q. (2006). Cathode materials modified by surface coating for lithium ion batteries. *Electrochimica Acta*, *51*(19), 3872–3883. doi:10.1016/j.electacta.2005.11.015

Lichter, J. A., Van Vliet, K. J., & Rubner, M. F. (2009). Design of antibacterial surfaces and interfaces: Polyelectrolyte multilayers as a multifunctional platform. *Macromolecules*, *42*(22), 8573–8586. doi:10.1021/ma901356s

Liedberg, B., Nylander, C., & Lunström, I. (1983). Surface plasmon resonance for gas detection and biosensing. *Sensors and Actuators*, *4*, 299–304. doi:10.1016/0250-6874(83)85036-7

Li, G., Hwang, Y., Radermacher, R., & Chun, H.-H. (2013). Review of cold storage materials for subzero applications. *Energy*, *51*, 1–17. doi:10.1016/j.energy.2012.12.002

Li, H., Li, F., Wang, L., Sheng, J., Xin, Z., Zhao, L., Xiao, H., Zheng, Y., & Hu, Q. (2009). Effect of nano-packing on preservation quality of Chinese jujube. *Food Chemistry*, *114*(2), 547–562. doi:10.1016/j.foodchem.2008.09.085

Li, J., Zeng, H. S., Sun, S., Liu, J. P., & Wang, Z. L. (2004). Analyzing the Structure of CoFe−Fe_3O_4 Core−Shell Nanoparticles by Electron Imaging and Diffraction. *The Journal of Physical Chemistry B*, *108*(37), 14005–14008. doi:10.1021/jp047602f

Li, L., Fan, M., Brown, R., Van, L. J., Wang, J., Wang, W., Song, Y., & Zhang, P. (2006). Synthesis, properties, and environmental applications of nanoscale iron-based materials: A review. *Critical Reviews in Environmental Science and Technology*, *36*(5), 405–431. doi:10.1080/10643380600620387

Lim, Y. T., Kim, S., Nakayama, A., Stott, N. E., Bawendi, M. G., & Frangioni, J. V. (2003). Selection of quantum dot wavelengths for biomedical assays and imaging. *Molecular Imaging*, *2*(1), 50–64. doi:10.1162/15353500200303100 PMID:12926237

Lin, D., & Xing, B. (2007). Phytotoxicity of nanoparticles: Inhibition of seed germination and root growth. *Environmental Pollution*, *150*(2), 243–250. doi:10.1016/j.envpol.2007.01.016 PMID:17374428

Link, S., & El-Sayed, M. A. (2000). Shape and size dependence of radiative, non-radiative and photothermal properties of gold nanocrystals. *International Reviews in Physical Chemistry*, *19*(3), 409–453. doi:10.1080/01442350050034180

Lin, L. P., Huang, L. S., Lin, C. W., Lee, C. K., Chen, J. L., Hsu, S. M., & Lin, S. (2005). Determination of binding constant of DNA-binding drug to target DNA by surface plasmon resonance biosensor technology. *Current Drug Targets. Immune, Endocrine and Metabolic Disorders*, *5*(1), 61–72. doi:10.2174/1568008053174697 PMID:15777205

Linman, M. J., Taylor, J. D., Yu, H., Chen, X., & Cheng, Q. (2008). Surface plasmon resonance study of protein-carbohydrate interactions using biotinylated sialosides. *Analytical Chemistry*, *80*(11), 4007–4013. doi:10.1021/ac702566e PMID:18461973

Linsebigler, A. L., Lu, G., & Yates, J. T. (1995). Photocatalysis on TiO2 Surfaces: Principles, Mechanisms, and Selected Results. *Chemical Reviews*, *95*(3), 735–758. doi:10.1021/cr00035a013

Li, P., Li, J., Wu, C., Wu, Q., & Li, J. (2005). Synergistic antibacterial effects of _-lactam antibiotic combined with silver nanoparticles. *Nanotechnology*, *16*(9), 1912–1917. doi:10.1088/0957-4484/16/9/082

Li, Q., Lv, S., Lu, M., Lin, Z., & Tang, D. (2016). Potentiometric competitive immunoassay for determination of aflatoxin B1 in food by using antibody-labeled gold nanoparticles. *Mikrochimica Acta*, *183*(10), 2815–2822. doi:10.100700604-016-1929-x

Li, Q., Mahendra, S., Lyon, D. Y., Brunet, L., Liga, M. V., Li, D., & Alvarez, P. (2008). Antimicrobial nanomaterials for water disinfection and microbial control: Potential applications and implications. *Water Research*, *42*(18), 4591–4602. doi:10.1016/j.watres.2008.08.015 PMID:18804836

Lithoxoos, G. P., Labropoulos, A., Peristeras, L. D., Kanellopoulos, N., Samios, J., & Economou, I. G. (2010). Adsorption of N_2, CH_4, CO and CO_2 gases in single walled carbon nanotubes: A combined experimental and Monte Carlo molecular simulation study. *The Journal of Supercritical Fluids*, *55*(2), 510–523. doi:10.1016/j.supflu.2010.09.017

Liu, C., Li, B. Q., & Mi, C. C. (2009). Fast transient thermal analysis of gold nanoparticles in tissue-like medium. *IEEE Transactions on Nanobioscience*, *8*(3), 271–280. doi:10.1109/TNB.2009.2028885 PMID:20051339

Liu, C., Li, F., Ma, L. P., & Cheng, H. M. (2010). Advanced Materials for Energy Storage. *Advanced Materials*, *22*(8), E28–E62. doi:10.1002/adma.200903328 PMID:20217798

Liu, D. Q., He, Z. Z., & Liu, X. Q. (2007). Synthesis and characterization of $LiGa_xMn_{2-x}O_4$ ($0 \leq x \leq 0.05$) by triethanolamine-assisted sol–gel method. *Journal of Alloys and Compounds*, *440*(1), 69–73. doi:10.1016/j.jallcom.2006.09.013

Liu, D. Q., Liu, X. Q., & He, Z. Z. (2007). The elevated temperature performance of $LiMn_2O_4$ coated with $Li_4Ti_5O_{12}$ for lithium ion battery. *Materials Chemistry and Physics*, *105*(2), 362–366. doi:10.1016/S0254-0584(03)00268-2

Liu, D., & Cao, G. (2010). Engineering nanostructured electrodes and fabrication of film electrodes for efficient lithium ion intercalation. *Energy & Environmental Science*, *3*(9), 1218–1237. doi:10.1039/b922656g

Liu, D., Wang, H., Du, P., & Liu, P. (2017). Independently double-crosslinked carbon nanotubes/polyaniline composite films as flexible and robust free-standing electrodes for high-performance supercapacitors. *Carbon*, *122*, 761–774. doi:10.1016/j.carbon.2017.06.097

Liu, D., Zhang, Y., Xiao, P., Garcia, B. B., Zhang, Q., Zhou, X., Jeong, Y.-H., & Cao, G. (2009). TiO_2 nanotube arrays annealed in CO exhibiting high performance for lithium ion intercalation. *Electrochimica Acta*, *54*(27), 6816–6820. doi:10.1016/j.electacta.2009.06.090

Liu, H., Cheng, C., & Zhang, K. (2007). The effect of ZnO coating on $LiMn_2O_4$ cycle life in high temperature for lithium secondary batteries. *Materials Chemistry and Physics*, *101*(2), 276–279. doi:10.1016/j.matchemphys.2006.05.006

Liu, H., Dong, H., Chen, Z., Lin, L., Chen, H., Li, S., & Deng, Y. (2017). Magnetic nanoparticles enhanced microarray detection of multiple foodborne pathogens. *Journal of Biomedical Nanotechnology*, *13*(10), 1333–1343. doi:10.1166/jbn.2017.2418

Liu, J., Cao, G., Yang, Z., Wang, D., Dubois, D., Zhou, X., Graff, G. L., Pederson, L. R., & Zhang, J. G. (2008). Oriented nanostructures for energy conversion and storage. *ChemSusChem*, *1*(8-9), 676–697. doi:10.1002/cssc.200800087 PMID:18693284

Liu, N., Weiss, T., Mesch, M., Langguth, L., Eigenthaler, U., Hirscher, M., Sönnichsen, C., & Giessen, H. (2010). Planar metamaterial analogue of electromagnetically induced transparency for plasmonic sensing. *Nano Letters*, *10*(4), 1103–1107. doi:10.1021/nl902621d PMID:20017551

Liu, Q., Wang, S., Tan, H., Yang, Z., & Zeng, J. (2013). Preparation and doping mode of doped $LiMn_2O_4$ for Li-ion batteries. *Energies*, *6*(3), 1718–1730. doi:10.3390/en6031718

Liu, R., & Lal, R. (2015). Potentials of engineered nanoparticles as fertilizers for increasing agronomic productions. *The Science of the Total Environment*, *514*, 131–139. doi:10.1016/j.scitotenv.2015.01.104 PMID:25659311

Liu, T., Sreekumar, T. V., Kumar, S., Hauge, R. H., & Smalley, R. E. (2003). SWNT/PAN composite film-based supercapacitors. *Carbon*, *41*(12), 2440–2442. doi:10.1016/S0008-6223(03)00245-8

Liu, X., Vinson, D., Abt, D., Hurt, R. H., & Rand, D. M. (2009). Differential toxicity of carbon nanomaterials in Drosophila: Larval dietary uptake is benign, but adult exposure causes locomotor impairment and mortality. *Environmental Science & Technology*, *43*(16), 6357–6363. doi:10.1021/es901079z PMID:19746737

Liu, Y., Clark, M., Zhang, Q., Yu, D., Liu, D., Liu, J., & Cao, G. (2011). V_2O_5 Nano-Electrodes with High Power and Energy Densities for Thin Film Li-Ion Batteries. *Advanced Energy Materials*, *1*(2), 194–202. doi:10.1002/aenm.201000037

Liu, Y., He, L., Mustapha, A., Li, H., Hu, Z. Q., & Lin, M. (2009). Antibacterial activities of zinc oxide nanoparticles against Escherichia coli O157: H7. *Journal of Applied Microbiology*, *107*(4), 1193–1201. doi:10.1111/j.1365-2672.2009.04303.x PMID:19486396

Liu, Y., Liu, D., Zhang, Q., Yu, D., Liu, J., & Cao, G. (2011). Lithium iron phosphate/carbon nanocomposite film cathodes for high energy lithium ion batteries. *Electrochimica Acta*, *56*(5), 2559–2565. doi:10.1016/j.electacta.2010.11.050

Liu, Y., Yan, D., Li, Y., Wu, Z., Zhuo, R., Li, S., Feng, J., Wang, J., Yan, P., & Geng, Z. (2014). Manganese dioxide nanosheet arrays grown on graphene oxide as an advanced electrode material for supercapacitors. *Electrochimica Acta*, *117*, 528–533. doi:10.1016/j.electacta.2013.11.121

Liu, Y., Zhang, P., Du, Q., Peng, X., Liu, T., Wang, Z., Xia, Y., Zhang, W., Wang, K., & Zhu, H. (2011). Adsorption of fluoride from aqueous solution by graphene. *Journal of Colloid and Interface Science*, *363*(1), 348–354. doi:10.1016/j.jcis.2011.07.032 PMID:21821258

Li, X. H., Xing, Y. G., Li, W. L., Jiang, Y. H., & Ding, Y. L. (2010). Antibacterial and physical properties of poly (vinyl chloride)-based film coated with ZnO nanoparticles. *Food Science & Technology International*, *16*(3), 225–232. doi:10.1177/1082013209353986 PMID:21339138

Li, X., Cheng, F., Guo, B., & Chen, J. (2005). Template-synthesized $LiCoO_2$, $LiMn_2O_4$, and $LiNi_{0.8}Co_{0.2}O_2$ nanotubes as the cathode materials of lithium ion batteries. *The Journal of Physical Chemistry B*, *109*(29), 14017–14024. doi:10.1021/jp051900a PMID:16852760

Li, X., Deng, X., Yuan, M., Xiong, C., Huang, Z., Zhang, Y., & Jia, W. (2000). In vitro degradation and release profiles of poly-DL-lactide- poly(ethyleneglycol) microspheres with entrapped proteins. *Journal of Applied Polymer Science*, *78*(1), 140–148. doi:10.1002/1097-4628(20001003)78:1<140::AID-APP180>3.0.CO;2-P

Li, X., Robinson, S. M., Gupta, A., Saha, K., Jiang, Z., Moyano, D. F., Sahar, A., Riley, M. A., & Rotello, V. M. (2014). Functional gold nanoparticles as potent antimicrobial agents against multi-drug-resistant bacteria. *ACS Nano*, *8*(10), 10682–10686. doi:10.1021/nn5042625 PMID:25232643

Li, X., Xu, H., Chen, Z. S., & Chen, G. (2011). Biosynthesis of nanoparticles by microorganisms and their applications. *Journal of Nanomaterials*, *2011*, 270974. doi:10.1155/2011/270974

Li, X., & Xu, Y. (2008). Enhanced cycling performance of spinel $LiMn_2O_4$ coated with $ZnMn_2O_4$ shell. *Journal of Solid State Electrochemistry*, *12*(7-8), 851–855. doi:10.100710008-007-0426-x

Li, Y., Hu, Y., Zhao, Y., Shi, G., Deng, L., Hou, Y., & Qu, L. (2011). An electrochemical avenue to green-luminescent graphene quantum dots as potential electron-acceptors for photovoltaics. *Advanced Materials*, *6*(6), 776–780. doi:10.1002/adma.201003819 PMID:21287641

Li, Y., Lin, Z., Zhao, M., Guo, M., Xu, T., Wang, C., Xia, H., & Zhu, B. (2016). Reversal of H1N1 influenza virus-induced apoptosis by silver nanoparticles functionalized with amantadine. *RSC Advances*, *6*(92), 89679–89686. doi:10.1039/C6RA18493F

Li, Y., Liu, F., Xia, B., Du, Q., Zhang, P., Wang, D., Wang, Z., & Xia, Y. (2010). Removal of copper from aqueous solution by carbon nanotube/calcium alginate composites. *Journal of Hazardous Materials*, *177*(1–3), 876–880. doi:10.1016/j.jhazmat.2009.12.114 PMID:20083351

Li, Z., Yang, J., Wang, J., Tang, J., Lei, G., & Xiao, Q. (2012). A phase-inversion process to prepare porous $LiAl_{0.1}Mn_{1.9}O_4$ spinel for aqueous rechargeable lithium batteries. *Microporous and Mesoporous Materials*, *162*, 44–50. doi:10.1016/j.micromeso.2012.06.001

Llorens, A., Lloret, E., Picouet, P. A., Trbojevich, R., & Fernandez, A. (2012). Metallic-based micro and nanocomposites in food contact materials and active food packaging. *Trends in Food Science & Technology*, *24*(1), 19–29. doi:10.1016/j.tifs.2011.10.001

Loo, C., Lowery, A., Halas, N., West, J., & Drezek, R. (2005). Immunotargeted nanoshells for integrated cancer imaging and therapy. *Nano Letters*, *5*(4), 709–711.

Lotierzo, M., Henry, O. Y. F., Piletsky, S., Tothill, I., Cullen, D., Kania, M., Hock, B., & Turner, A. P. F. (2004). Surface plasmon resonance sensor for domoic acid based on grafted imprinted polymer. *Biosensors & Bioelectronics*, *20*(2), 145–152. doi:10.1016/j.bios.2004.01.032 PMID:15308215

Lou, X. W., Wang, Y., Yuan, C., Lee, J. Y., & Archer, L. A. (2006). Template-free synthesis of SnO_2 hollow nanostructures with high lithium storage capacity. *Advanced Materials*, *18*(17), 2325–2329. doi:10.1002/adma.200600733

Lovgren, K., & Morein, B. (1988). The requirement of lipids for the formation of immuno- stimulating complexes (iscoms). *Biotechnology and Applied Biochemistry*, *10*, 161–172. PMID:2838046

Lugscheider, E., Bärwulf, S., Barimani, C., Riester, M., & Hilgers, H. (1998). Magnetron-sputtered hard material coatings on thermoplastic polymers for clean room applications Surf. *CoatingsTechnol.*, *108-109*, 398–402.

Lu, H., Wang, J., Stoller, M., Wang, T., Bao, Y., & Hao, H. (2016). An overview of nanomaterials for water and wastewater treatment. *Advances in Materials Science and Engineering*, *4964828*, 1–10. doi:10.1155/2016/4964828

Lu, H., Wang, J., Wang, T., Zhong, J., Bao, Y., & Hao, H. (2016). Recent progress on nanostructures for drug delivery applications. *Journal of Nanomaterials*, *2016*, 2016–2020. doi:10.1155/2016/5762431

Lu, J. M., Wang, X., Marin-Muller, C., Wang, H., Lin, P. H., Yao, Q., & Chen, C. (2009). Current advances in research and clinical applications of PLGA-based nanotechnology. *Expert Review of Molecular Diagnostics*, *9*(4), 325–341. doi:10.1586/erm.09.15 PMID:19435455

Lu, J., & Bowles, M. (2013). Article. *Int. Food Agribus. Manag. Assoc.*, *16*, 21–42.

Lunge, S., Singh, S., & Sinha, A. (2014). Magnetic iron oxide (Fe_3O_4) nanoparticles from tea waste for arsenic removal. *Journal of Magnetism and Magnetic Materials*, *356*, 21–31. doi:10.1016/j.jmmm.2013.12.008

Luo, F., Chen, Z., Megharaj, M., & Naidu, R. (2016). Simultaneous removal of trichloroethylene and hexavalent chromium by green synthesized agarose-Fe nanoparticles hydrogel. *Chemical Engineering Journal*, *294*, 290–297. doi:10.1016/j.cej.2016.03.005

Luo, J., Cheng, L., & Xia, Y. (2007). $LiMn_2O_4$ hollow nanosphere electrode material with excellent cycling reversibility and rate capability. *Electrochemistry Communications*, *9*(6), 1404–1409. doi:10.1016/j.elecom.2007.01.058

Luoma, S. N. (2008). Silver Nanotechnologies and the Environment: Old Problems or New Challenges? Project on emerging Nanotechnologies, Woodrow Wilson International Center for Scholars.

Luo, Q., & Manthiram, A. (2009). Effect of Low-Temperature Fluorine Doping on the Properties of Spinel $LiMn_{2-2y}Li_yM_yO_{4-\eta}F_\eta$ (M= Fe, Co, and Zn) Cathodes. *Journal of the Electrochemical Society*, *156*(2), A84–A88. doi:10.1149/1.3028317

Luo, Q., Yu, N., Shi, C., Wang, X., & Wu, J. (2016). Surface plasmon resonance sensor for antibiotics detection based on photo-initiated polymerization molecularly imprinted array. *Talanta*, *161*, 797–803. doi:10.1016/j.talanta.2016.09.049 PMID:27769483

Lutsiak, M. E., Robinson, D. R., Coester, C., Kwon, G. S., & Samuel, J. (2002). Analysis of poly (d, l-lactic-co-glycolic acid) nanosphere uptake by human dendritic cells and macrophages in vitro. *Pharmaceutical Research*, *19*(10), 1480–1487. doi:10.1023/A:1020452531828 PMID:12425465

Lu, W., Belharouak, I., Liu, J., & Amine, K. (2007). Thermal properties of $Li_{4/3}Ti_{5/3}O_{4/}$ $LiMn_2O_4$ cell. *Journal of Power Sources*, *174*(2), 673–677. doi:10.1016/j.jpowsour.2007.06.199

Lu, Z., Rong, K., Li, J., Yang, H., & Chen, R. (2013). Size-dependent antibacterial activities of silver nanoparticles against oral anaerobic pathogenic bacteria. *Journal of Materials Science. Materials in Medicine*, *24*(6), 1465–1471. doi:10.100710856-013-4894-5 PMID:23440430

Lv, Y., Tahir, I. I., & Olsson, M. E. (2019). Effect of ozone application on bioactive compounds of apple fruit during short-term cold storage. *Scientia Horticulturae*, *253*, 49–60. doi:10.1016/j.scienta.2019.04.021

Lyons, K., & Whelan, J. (2010). Community engagement to facilitate, legitimize and accelerate the advancement of nanotechnologies in Australia. *NanoEthics*, *4*(1), 53–66. doi:10.100711569-009-0070-2

Machado, S., Pacheco, J. G., Nouws, H. P. A., Albergaria, J. T., & Delerue-Matos, C. (2015). Characterization of green zero-valent iron nanoparticles produced with tree leaf extracts. *The Science of the Total Environment*, *53*, 76–81. doi:10.1016/j.scitotenv.2015.06.091 PMID:26151651

Madamsetty, V. S., Mukherjee, A., & Mukherjee, S. (2019). Recent trends of the bio-inspired nanoparticles in cancer theranostics. *Frontiers in Pharmacology*, 10.

Madima, N., Mishra, S., Inamuddin, I., & Mishra, A. (2020). Carbon-based nanomaterials for remediation of organic and inorganic pollutants from wastewater: A review. *Environmental Chemistry Letters*, *18*(4), 1169–1191. doi:10.100710311-020-01001-0

Maeda, H., Wu, J., Sawa, T., Matsumura, Y., & Hori, K. (2000). Tumor vascular permeability and the EPR effect in macromolecular therapeutics: A review. *Journal of Controlled Release*, *65*(1-2), 271–284. doi:10.1016/S0168-3659(99)00248-5 PMID:10699287

Ma, F., Li, Y., Tang, B., & Zhang, C. (2016). Fluorescent biosensors based on single-molecule counting. *Accounts of Chemical Research*, *49*(9), 1722–1730. doi:10.1021/acs.accounts.6b00237 PMID:27583695

Mahtab, R., Rogers, J. P., & Murphy, C. J. (1995). Protein-sized quantum dot luminescence can distinguish between “straight”, “bent”, and “kinked” oligonucleotides. *Journal of the American Chemical Society*, *117*(35), 9099–9100. doi:10.1021/ja00140a040

Maicu, M., Schmittgens, R., Hecker, D., Glöß, D., Frach, P., & Gerlach, G. (2014). Synthesis and deposition of metal nanoparticles by gas condensation process. *Journal of Vacuum Science & Technology A: Vacuum, Surfaces, and Films*, *32*(2), 02B113.

Ma, J., Wong, H., Kong, L. B., & Peng, K. W. (2003). Biomimetic processing of nanocrystallite bioactive apatite coating on titanium. *Nanotechnology*, *14*(6), 619–623. doi:10.1088/0957-4484/14/6/310

Majeed, K., Jawaid, M., Hassan, A., Abu Bakar, A., Abdul Khalil, H. P. S., Salema, A. A., & Inuwa, I. (2013). Potential materials for food packaging from nanoclay/natural fibres filled hybrid composites. *Materials & Design*, *46*(0), 391–410. doi:10.1016/j.matdes.2012.10.044

Majka, J., & Speck, C. (2006). Analysis of protein-DNA interactions using surface plasmon resonance. In H. Seitz (Ed.), *Analytics of protein–DNA interactions. Advances in biochemical engineering/biotechnology* (Vol. 104, pp. 13–36). Springer., doi:10.1007/10_026

Makarenko, N. A., & Makarenko, V. V. (2019). Nanotechnologies in crop cultivation: Ecotoxicological aspects. *Biosystems Diversity*, *27*(2), 148–155. doi:10.15421/011920

Makarov, V. V., Love, A. J., Sinitsyna, O. V., Makarova, S. S., Yaminsky, I. V., Taliansky, M. E., & Kalinina, N. O. (2014). "Green" nanotechnologies: Synthesis of metal nanoparticles using plants. *Acta Naturae*, *6*(1 (20)), 35–44. doi:10.32607/20758251-2014-6-1-35-44 PMID:24772325

Makhluf, S., Dror, R., Nitzan, Y., Abramovich, Y., Jelinek, R., & Gedanken, A. (2005). Microwave-assisted synthesis of nanocrystalline MgO and its use as a bacteriocide. *Advanced Functional Materials*, *15*(10), 1708–1715. doi:10.1002/adfm.200500029

Malhotra, B. D., Kumar, S., & Pandey, C. M. (2016). Nanomaterials based biosensors for cancer biomarker detection. *Journal of Physics: Conference Series*, *704*(1), 012011. doi:10.1088/1742-6596/704/1/012011

Malusá, E., Sas-Paszt, L., & Ciesielska, J. (2012). *Transfus*. Apher. Sci.

Malyovanyi, S. M., Andriiko, A. A., & Monko, A. P. (2003). Synthesis and electrochemical behavior of Fe-doped overstoichiometric $LiMn_2O_4$-based spinels. *Journal of Solid State Electrochemistry*, *8*(1), 7–10. doi:10.100710008-003-0414-8

Manasreh, M. O. (2012). *Introduction to Nanomaterials and Devices*. Wiley Online Library.

Manavalan, R., Lal Pal, S., Jana, U., Manna, P. K., & Mohanta, G. P. (2011). Nanoparticle: An overview of preparation and characterization. *Journal of Applied Pharmaceutical Science*, *01*(06), 228–234.

Manjunatha, S. B., Biradar, D. P., & Aladakatti, Y. R. (2016). Article. *J. Farm Sci.*, *29*, 1–13.

Mansouri, S., & Schultz, J. S. (1984). A miniature optical glucose sensor based on affinity binding. *Nature Biotechnology*, *2*(10), 885–890. doi:10.1038/nbt1084-885

Manzoor, A. Mir., Umar, M., Bashir, A. S., & Syed, S. H. (2019). Nanobodies: The "magic bullets" in therapeutics, drug delivery and diagnostics. *Human Antibodies*, 1–23. doi:10.3233/HAB-190390

Mao, O., & Dahn, J. R. (1999). Mechanically alloyed Sn-Fe(-C) powders as anode materials for Li-ion batteries: I. The Sn2Fe-C system. *Journal of the Electrochemical Society*, *146*, 423–427.

Maqbool, M., Ali, A., Alderson, P. G., Zahid, N., & Siddiqui, Y. (2011). Effect of a Novel Edible Composite Coating Based on Gum Arabic and Chitosan on Biochemical and Physiological Responses of Banana Fruits during Cold Storage. *Journal of Agricultural and Food Chemistry*, *59*(10), 5474–5482. doi:10.1021/jf200623m PMID:21476593

Marchiol, L. (2018). *New Visions in Plant Science*. doi:10.5772/intechopen.74425

Mariani, S., & Minunni, M. (2014). Surface plasmon resonance applications in clinical analysis. *Analytical and Bioanalytical Chemistry*, *406*(9-10), 2303–2323. doi:10.100700216-014-7647-5 PMID:24566759

Mark, T. (2003). Vapor-phase synthesis of nanoparticles. *Current Opinion in Colloid & Interface Science*, *8*(1), 127–133. doi:10.1016/S1359-0294(03)00007-4

Martin, C. R. (2006). Welcome to nanomedicine. *Nanomedicine (London)*, *1*(1), 5. doi:10.2217/17435889.1.1.5

Martinez-Abad, A., Lagaron, J. M., & Ocio, M. J. (2012). Development and characterization of silver-based antimicrobial ethylene-vinyl alcohol copolymer (EVOH) films for food-packaging applications. *Agricultural and Food Chemistry, 60*(21), 5350–5359. doi:10.1021/jf300334z PMID:22577863

Martinho, N., Damgé, C., & Reis, C. P. (2011). Recent advances in drug delivery systems. *Journal of Biomaterials and Nanobiotechnology, 2*(05), 510–526. doi:10.4236/jbnb.2011.225062

Martins, T. D., Ribeiro, A. C. C., de Camargo, H. S., da Costa Filho, P. A., Cavalcante, H. P. M., & Dias, D. L. (2013). New insights on optical biosensors: Techniques, construction and application. In T. Rinken (Ed.), *State of the art in biosensors - General aspects* (pp. 111–139). IntechOpen. doi:10.5772/52330

Martis Elvis, A., Badve Rewa, R., Degwekar Mukta, D. (2012). Nanotechnology based devices and applications in medicine: An overview. *Nanotechnology Devices and Applications, 3*(1), 68-73. . doi:10.4103/2229-5186.94320

Marty, J. D., & Mauzac, M. (2005). Molecular imprinting: State of the art and perspectives. *Advances in Polymer Science, 172*, 1–35. doi:10.1007/b97573

Masiá, A., Suarez-Varela, M. M., Llopis-Gonzalez, A., & Picó, Y. (2016). Determination of pesticides and veterinary drug residues in food by liquid chromatography-mass spectrometry: A review. *Analytica Chimica Acta, 936*, 40–61. doi:10.1016/j.aca.2016.07.023 PMID:27566339

Matea, C. T., Mocan, T., Tabaran, F., Pop, T., Mosteanu, O., Puia, C., ... Mocan, L. (2017). Quantum dots in imaging, drug delivery and sensor applications. *International Journal of Nanomedicine, 12*, 5421.

Matsumura, Y., & Maeda, H. (1986). A new concept for macromolecular therapeutics in cancer chemotherapy: Mechanism of tumoritropic accumulation of proteins and the antitumor agent smancs. *Cancer Research, 46*, 6387–6392. PMID:2946403

Mauter, M., & Elimelech, M. (2008). Environmental applications of carbon-based nanomaterials. *Environmental Science & Technology, 42*(16), 5843–5859. doi:10.1021/es8006904 PMID:18767635

Ma, X., & Mao, R. (2018). Fuzzy Control of Cold Storage Refrigeration System with Dynamic Coupling Compensation. *Journal of Control Science and Engineering, 18*, 1–7. doi:10.1155/2018/6836129

Maynard, A., & Michelson, E. (2014). *The nanotechnology consumer products Inventory*. Retrieved 26/06/2014, from http://www. nanotechproject.org/cpi/

McBride, S. M., Choi, C. H., Schoenfeld, B. P., Bell, A. J., Liebelt, D. A., Ferreiro, D., Choi, R. J., Hinchey, P., Kollaros, M., Terlizzi, A. M., Ferrick, N. J., Koenigsberg, E., Rudominer, R. L., Sumida, A., Chiorean, S., Siwicki, K. K., Nguyen, H. T., Fortini, M. E., McDonald, T. V., & Jongens, T. A. (2010). Pharmacological and genetic reversal of age-dependent cognitive deficits attributable to decreased presenilin function. *The Journal of Neuroscience: The Official Journal of the Society for Neuroscience, 30*(28), 9510–9522. doi:10.1523/JNEUROSCI.1017-10.2010 PMID:20631179

McClung, C., & Hirsh, J. (1998). Stereotypic behavioral responses to free-base cocaine and the development of behavioral sensitization in Drosophila. *Current Biology, 8*(2), 109–112. doi:10.1016/S0960-9822(98)70041-7 PMID:9427649

Mcgrath, T. F., Andersson, K., Campbell, K., Fodey, T. L., & Elliott, C. T. (2013). Development of a rapid low cost fluorescent biosensor for the detection of food contaminants. *Biosensors & Bioelectronics, 41*, 96–102. doi:10.1016/j.bios.2012.07.081 PMID:22939510

McManus, M. C. (1995). Mechanisms of bacterial resistance to antimicrobial agents. *American Journal of Health-System Pharmacy, 54*(12), 1420–1433. doi:10.1093/ajhp/54.12.1420 PMID:9194989

McNamara, K., & Tofail, S. A. (2015). Nanosystems: The use of nanoalloys, metallic, bimetallic, and magnetic nanoparticles in biomedical applications. *Physical Chemistry Chemical Physics*, *17*(42), 27981–27995. doi:10.1039/C5CP00831J PMID:26024211

Md, F., Zakir, H., & Hafsa, A. (2012). Prospects and applications of nanobiotechnology: A medical perspective. *Journal of Nanobiotechnology*.

Medda, S., Hajra, A., Dey, U., Bose, P., & Mondal, N. K. (2014). Biosynthesis of silver nanoparticles from Aloe vera leaf extract and antifungal activity against Rhizopus sp. and Aspergillus sp. *Appl. Nanosci.*, *5*, 875–880. doi:10.100713204-014-0387-139

Medley, C. D., Smith, J. E., Tang, Z., Wu, Y., Bamrungsap, S., & Tan, W. (2008). Gold nanoparticle-based colorimetric assay for the direct detection of cancerous cells. *Analytical Chemistry*, *80*(4), 1067–1072. doi:10.1021/ac702037y PMID:18198894

Mehndiratta, P., Jain, A., Srivastava, S., & Gupta, N. (2013). Environmental pollution and nanotechnology. *Environment and Pollution*, *2*(2), 49–58. doi:10.5539/ep.v2n2p49

Mehrotra, P. (2016). Biosensors and their applications - a review. *Journal of Oral Biology and Craniofacial Research*, *6*(2), 153–159. doi:10.1016/j.jobcr.2015.12.002 PMID:27195214

Mellman, I., Fuchs, R., & Helenius, A. (1986). Acidification of the endocytic and exocytic pathways. *Annual Review of Biochemistry*, *55*(1), 663–700. doi:10.1146/annurev.bi.55.070186.003311 PMID:2874766

Melville, S., & Craig, L. (2013). Type IV pili in Gram-positive bacteria. *Microbiology and Molecular Biology Reviews*, *77*(3), 323–341. doi:10.1128/MMBR.00063-12 PMID:24006467

Metkar, S. K., & Girigoswami, K. (2019). Diagnostic biosensors in medicine - a review. *Biocatalysis and Agricultural Biotechnology*, *17*, 271–283. doi:10.1016/j.bcab.2018.11.029

Michalet, X., Pinaud, F. F., Bentolila, L. A., Tsay, J. M., Doose, S., Li, J. J., Sundaresan, G., Wu, A. M., Gambhir, S. S., & Weiss, S. (2005). Quantum dots for live cells, in vivo imaging, and diagnostics.Science. *Science*, *307*(5709), 538–544. doi:10.1126cience.1104274 PMID:15681376

Mills, A., & Hazafy, D. (2008). A solvent-based intelligence ink for oxygen. *Analyst (London)*, *133*(2), 213–218. doi:10.1039/B713450A PMID:18227944

Mills, A., & Hazafy, D. (2009). Nanocrystalline SnO_2-based, UVB-activated, colourimetric oxygen indicator. *Sensors and Actuators. B, Chemical*, *136*(2), 344–349. doi:10.1016/j.snb.2008.12.048

Mirela, I., & Apetrei, C. (2013). Amperometric biosensor based on polypyrrole and tyrosinase for the detection of tyramine in food samples. *Sensors and Actuators. B, Chemical*, *178*, 40–46. doi:10.1016/j.snb.2012.12.064

Mirkin, C. A., Letsinger, R. L., Mucic, R. C., & Storhoff, J. J. (1996). A DNA-based method for rationally assembling nanoparticles into macroscopic materials. *Nature*, *382*(6592), 607–609. doi:10.1038/382607a0 PMID:8757129

Mirza, A. Z., & Siddiqui, F. A. (2014). Nanomedicine and drug delivery: A mini review. *International Nano Letters*, *4*(1), 94. doi:10.100740089-014-0094-7

Mishra, M., Dashora, K., Srivastava, A., Fasake, V. D., & Nag, R. H. (2019). Prospects, challenges and need for regulation of nanotechnology with special reference to India. *Ecotoxicology and Environmental Safety*, *171*, 677–682. doi:10.1016/j.ecoenv.2018.12.085 PMID:30658303

Mishra, P. K., Mishra, H., Ekielski, A., Talegaonkar, S., & Vaidya, B. (2017). Zinc oxide nanoparticles: A promising nanomaterial for biomedical applications. *Drug Discovery Today*, *22*(12), 1825–1834. doi:10.1016/j.drudis.2017.08.006 PMID:28847758

Mitchell, S. J., & Wu, Y. (2010). Surface plasmon resonance biosensors for highly sensitive detection of small biomolecules. In P. A. Serra (Ed.), *Biosensors* (pp. 151–168). IntechOpen., doi:10.5772/7208

Mittal, A. K., Chisti, Y., & Banerjee, U. C. (2013). Synthesis of metallic nanoparticles using plant extracts. *Biotechnology Advances*, *31*(2), 346–356. doi:10.1016/j.biotechadv.2013.01.003 PMID:23318667

Mittal, S., Kaur, H., Gautam, N., & Mantha, A. K. (2017). Biosensors for breast cancer diagnosis: A review of bioreceptors, biotransducers and signal amplification strategies. *Biosensors & Bioelectronics*, *88*, 217–231. doi:10.1016/j.bios.2016.08.028 PMID:27567264

Mocellin, S., Bronte, V., & Nitti, D. (2007). Nitric oxide, a double edged sword in cancer biology: Searching for therapeutic opportunities. *Medicinal Research Reviews*, *27*(3), 317–352. doi:10.1002/med.20092 PMID:16991100

Moczko, E., Guerreiro, A., Cáceres, C., Piletska, E., Sellergren, B., & Piletsky, S. A. (2019). Epitope approach in molecular imprinting of antibodies. *Journal of Chromatography. B, Analytical Technologies in the Biomedical and Life Sciences*, *1124*, 1–6. doi:10.1016/j.jchromb.2019.05.024 PMID:31176265

Moffatt, S. (2016). Nanotechnology to nanomedicine: Reconciling ethical implications and public health. *MOJ Proteomics Bioinform.*, *3*(4), 77–79. doi:10.15406/mojpb.2016.03.00090

Moghimi, S. M., Hunter, A.C., & Murray, J. C. (2005). Nanomedicine: current status and future prospects. *FASEB J.*, *19*, 311-30.

Moghimi, S. M., Hunter, A. C., & Murray, J. C. (2001). Long-circulating and target-specific nanoparticles: Theory to practice. *Pharmacological Reviews*, *53*, 283. PMID:11356986

Mohamed, M. M., Fouad, S. A., Elshoky, H. A., Mohammed, G. M., & Salaheldin, T. A. (2017). Antibacterial effect of gold nanoparticles against Corynebacterium pseudotuberculosis. *International Journal of Veterinary Science and Medicine*, *5*(1), 23–29. doi:10.1016/j.ijvsm.2017.02.003 PMID:30255044

Molenda, J., & Molenda, M. (2011). *Composite Cathode Material for Li-Ion Batteries Based on $LiFePO_4$ System*. INTECH Open Access Publisher. doi:10.5772/21635

Molenda, M., Dziembaj, R., Podstawka, E., Proniewicz, L. M., & Piwowarska, Z. (2007). An attempt to improve electrical conductivity of the pyrolysed carbon- $LiMn_2O_{4-y}S_y$ ($0 \leq y \leq 0.5$) composites. *Journal of Power Sources*, *174*(2), 613–618. doi:10.1016/j.jpowsour.2007.06.117

Monica, J. C. (2010). *G. V. CalsterMatthew Hull and Diana Bowman publisher*. Elsevier.

Monošík, R., Streďanský, M., & Šturdík, E. (2012). Biosensors - classification, characterization and new trends. *Acta Chimica Slovenica*, *5*(1), 109–120. doi:10.2478/v10188-012-0017-z PMID:24061179

Montes, A., Bisson, M. A., Gardella, J. A. Jr, & Aga, D. S. (2017). Uptake and transformations of engineered nanomaterials: Critical responses observed in terrestrial plants and the model plant Arabidopsis thaliana. *The Science of the Total Environment*, *607-608*, 1497–1516. doi:10.1016/j.scitotenv.2017.06.190 PMID:28793406

Monticone, F., & Alu, A. (2017). Metamaterial, plasmonic and nanophotonic devices. *Reports on Progress in Physics*, *80*(3), 036401-1-036401–036437. doi:10.1088/1361-6633/aa518f

Morales, M. A., & Halpern, J. M. (2018). Guide to selecting a biorecognition element for biosensors. *Bioconjugate Chemistry*, *29*(10), 3231–3239. doi:10.1021/acs.bioconjchem.8b00592 PMID:30216055

Morein, B., Lövgren, K., Rönnberg, B., Sjölander, A., & Villacrés-Eriksson, M. (1995). Immunostimulating complexes. Clinical potential in vaccine development. *Clinical Immunotherapeutics*, *3*(6), 461–475. doi:10.1007/BF03259065

Morein, B., & Simons, K. (1985). Subunit vaccines against enveloped viruses: Virosomes, micelles and other protein complexes. *Vaccine*, *3*(2), 83–93. doi:10.1016/0264-410X(85)90055-6 PMID:3898625

Morfa, A. J., Rowlen, K. L., Reilly, T. H. III, Romero, M. J., & Lagemaatb, J. (2008). Plasmon-enhanced solar energy conversion in organic bulk heterojunction photovoltaics. *Applied Physics Letters*, *92*(1), 013504. doi:10.1063/1.2823578

Mor, G. K., Shankar, K., Paulose, M., Varghese, O. K., & Grimes, C. A. (2006). Use of highly-ordered TiO(2) nanotube arrays in dye-sensitized solar cells. *Nano Letters*, *6*(2), 215–218. doi:10.1021/nl052099j PMID:16464037

Moriguchi, I., Hidaka, R., Yamada, H., Kudo, T., Murakami, H., & Nakashima, N. (2006). A Mesoporous Nanocomposite of TiO_2 and Carbon Nanotubes as a High-Rate Li-Intercalation Electrode Material. *Advanced Materials*, *18*(1), 69–73. doi:10.1002/adma.200501366

Morones, J. R., Elechiguerra, J. L., Camacho, A., Holt, K., Kouri, J. B., Ramirez, J. T., & Yacaman, M. J. (2005). The bactericidal effect of silver nanoparticles. *Nanotechnology*, *16*(10), 2346–2353. doi:10.1088/0957-4484/16/10/059 PMID:20818017

Mostofizadeh, A., Li, Y., Song, B., & Huang, Y. (2011). Synthesis, properties, and applications of low-dimensional carbon-related nanomaterials. *Journal of Nanomaterials*, *685081*, 1–21. Advance online publication. doi:10.1155/2011/685081

Mottram, P. L., Leong, D., Crimeen-Irwin, B., Gloster, S., Xiang, S. D., Meanger, J., Ghildyal, R., Vardaxis, N., & Plebanski, M. (2007). Type 1 and 2 immunity following vaccination is influenced by nanoparticle size: Formulation of a model vaccine for respiratory syncytial virus. *Molecular Pharmaceutics*, *4*(1), 73–84. doi:10.1021/mp060096p PMID:17274665

Muhammad, T., Nur, Z., Piletska, E. V., Yimit, O., & Piletsky, S. A. (2012). Rational design of molecularly imprinted polymer: The choice of cross-linker. *Analyst (London)*, *137*(11), 2623. doi:10.1039/c2an35228a PMID:22534800

Mukherjee, P., Ahmad, A., Mandal, D., Senapati, S., Sainkar, S. R., Khan, M. I., Parishcha, R., Ajaykumar, P. V., Alam, M., Kumar, R., & Sastry, M. (2001). Fungus-mediated synthesis of silver nanoparticles and their immobilization in the mycelial matrix: A novel biological approach to nanoparticle synthesis. *Nano Letters*, *1*(10), 515–519. doi:10.1021/nl0155274

Mukherjee, P., Bhattacharya, R., Wang, P., Wang, L., Basu, S., Nagy, J. A., ... Soker, S. (2005). Antiangiogenic properties of gold nanoparticles. *Clinical Cancer Research*, *11*(9), 3530–3534. doi:10.1158/1078-0432.CCR-04-2482 PMID:15867256

Mukhopadhyay, S. S. (2014). Nanotechnology in agriculture: Prospects and constraints. *Nanotechnology, Science and Applications*, *7*, 63–71. doi:10.2147/NSA.S39409 PMID:25187699

Munita, J. M., & Arias, C. A. (2016). Mechanisms of antibiotic resistance. *Microbiology Spectrum*, *4*(2). Advance online publication. doi:10.1128/microbiolspec.VMBF-0016-2015 PMID:27227291

Munro, I. C., Haighton, L. A., Lynch, B. S., & Tafazoli, S. (2009). Technological challenges of addressing new and more complex migrating products from novel food packaging materials. *Food Additives and Contaminants*, *26*(12), 1534–1546. doi:10.1080/02652030902995277 PMID:19938328

Munuswamy, D. B., Madhavan, V. R., & Mohan, M. (2015). Synthesis and Surface Area Determination of Alumina Nanoparticles by Chemical Combustion Method. *International Journal of Chemtech Research*, *8*(11), 413–419.

Muraliganth, T., Murugan, A. V., & Manthiram, A. (2008). Nanoscale networking of $LiFePO_4$nanorods synthesized by a microwave-solvothermal route with carbon nanotubes for lithium ion batteries. *Journal of Materials Chemistry*, *18*(46), 5661–5668. doi:10.1039/b812165f

Murugan, A., & Kumara, K., & Shanmugasundaram. (2014). Biosynthesis and characterization of silver nanoparticles using the aqueous extract of vitexnegundo.linn. *World Journal of Pharmacy and Pharmaceutical Sciences*, *3*(8), 1385–1393.

Mustafa, G., Tahir, H., Sultan, M., & Akhtar, N. (2013). Synthesis and characterization of cupric oxide (CuO) nanoparticles and their application for the removal of dyes. *African Journal of Biotechnology*, *12*(47), 6650–6660. doi:10.5897/AJB2013.13058

Musumeci, T., Ventura, C. A., Giannone, I., Ruozi, B., Montenegro, L., Pignatello, R., & Puglisi, G. (2006). PLA/PLGA nanoparticles for sustained release of docetaxel. *International Journal of Pharmaceutics*, *325*(1-2), 172–179. doi:10.1016/j.ijpharm.2006.06.023 PMID:16887303

Muthu, M.S., Leong, D.T., Mei, L., & Feng, S.S. (2014). Nanotheranostics—application and further development of nanomedicine strategies for advanced theranostics. *Theranostics, 4*(6), 660-677.

Nadaroglu, H., Gungor, A.A., Ince, S., Babagil, A., (2017). Green synthesis and characterisation of platinum nanoparticles using quail egg yolk. *Spectrochimica Acta Part a-Molecular and Biomolecular Spectros-copy, 172*, 43–7. . doi:10.1016/j.saa.2016.05.023

Nagaura, T., & Tozawa, K. (1990). Lithium-ion rechargeable battery. *Prog. Batter. Sol. Cells*, *9*, 209–212.

Nagesha, D., Laevsky, G. S., Lampton, P., Banyal, R., Warner, C., DiMarzio, C., & Sridhar, S. (2007). In vitro imaging of embryonic stem cells using multiphoton luminescence of gold nanoparticles. *International Journal of Nanomedicine*, *2*(4), 813. PMID:18203448

Nahrendorf, M., Keliher, E., Marinelli, B., Waterman, P., Feruglio, P. F., Fexon, L., Pivovarov, M., Swirski, F. K., Pittet, M. J., Vinegoni, C., & Weissleder, R. (2010). Hybrid PET-optical imaging using targeted probes. *Proceedings of the National Academy of Sciences of the United States of America*, *107*(17), 7910–7915. doi:10.1073/pnas.0915163107 PMID:20385821

Naikaa, H. R., Lingarajua, K., Manjunathb, K., Kumar, D., Nagarajuc, G., Sureshd, D., & Nagabhushanae, H. (2015). Green synthesis of CuO nanoparticles using Gloriosa superba L. extract andtheir antibacterial activity. *Journal of Taibah University for Science: JTUSCI*, *9*(1), 7–12. doi:10.1016/j.jtusci.2014.04.006

Naik, G. V., Shalaev, V. M., & Boltasseva, A. (2013). Alternative plasmonic materials: Beyond gold and silver. *Advanced Materials*, *25*(24), 3264–3294. doi:10.1002/adma.201205076 PMID:23674224

Nakamura, C., Hasegawa, M., Nakamura, N., & Miyake, J. (2003). Rapid and specific detection of herbicides using a self-assembled photosynthetic reaction center from purple bacterium on an SPR chip. *Biosensors & Bioelectronics*, *18*(5-6), 599–603. doi:10.1016/S0956-5663(03)00030-7 PMID:12706568

Nak-Hyung, L., Jung-Ah, L., & Seung-Yong, P. (2012). A review of vaccine development and research for industry animals in Korea. *Clinical and Experimental Vaccine Research*, *1*(1), 18–34. doi:10.7774/cevr.2012.1.1.18 PMID:23596575

Naknaen, P. (2014). Utilization possibilities of antimicrobial biodegradable packaging produced by poly (butylene succinate) modified with zinc oxide nanoparticles in fresh-cut apple slices. *International Food Research Journal*, *21*(6), 2413–2420.

Nalawade, P., Mukherjee, T., & Kapoor, S. (2012). High-yield synthesis of multispiked gold nanoparticles: Characterization and catalytic reactions. *Colloids and Surfaces. A, Physicochemical and Engineering Aspects*, *396*, 336–340. doi:10.1016/j.colsurfa.2012.01.018

Nam, J. M., Thaxton, C. C., & Mirkin, C. A. (2003). Nanoparticles-based bio-bar codes for the ultrasensitive detection of proteins. *Science*, *301*(5641), 1884–1886. doi:10.1126cience.1088755 PMID:14512622

Nanotechnology and Human Health. (2013). Scientific evidence and risk governance. Report of the WHO expert meeting. *WHO Regional Office for Europe*.

Nanotubes and Asbestos. (n.d.). *Nutrition and the Nintendo Wii*. Available from: https://trickledown.wordpress.com/2008/05/27/nanotubes-and-asbestos-nutrition-and-the nintendo-wii/

Narasimha, G., Sridevi, A., Devi Prasad, B., & Praveen Kumar, B. (2014). Chemical synthesis of Zinc Oxide (ZnO) nanoparticles and their antibacterial activity against a clinical isolate Staphylococcus aureus. *International Journal of Nanodimension*, *5*, 337–340.

Narayanan, K. B., & Sakthivel, N. (2010). Biological synthesis of metal nanoparticles by microbes. *Advances in Colloid and Interface Science*, *156*(1-2), 1–13. doi:10.1016/j.cis.2010.02.001 PMID:20181326

Naser-moghadasi, M., Nia, A. Z., Toolabi, M., & Heydari, S. (2017). Microwave metamaterial absorber based on Jerusalem Cross with meandered load for bandwidth enhancement. *Optik (Stuttgart)*, *140*, 515–522. doi:10.1016/j.ijleo.2017.04.007

Nasir, M. E., Dickson, W., Wurtz, G. A., Wardley, W. P., & Zayats, A. V. (2014). Hydrogen detected by the naked eye: Optical hydrogen gas sensors based on core/shell plasmonic nanorod metamaterials. *Advanced Materials*, *26*(21), 3532–3537. doi:10.1002/adma.201305958 PMID:24643991

Nautiyal, P., Seikh, M. M., Lebedev, O. I., & Kundu, A. K. (2015). Sol–gel synthesis of Fe–Co nanoparticles and magnetization study. *Journal of Magnetism and Magnetic Materials*, *377*, 402–405. doi:10.1016/j.jmmm.2014.10.157

Nazarov, M. M., Khaydukov, E. V., Sokolov, V. I., Panchenko, V. Y., & Shkurinov, A. P. (2013, september). *Polymer matrix with nanoparticles as a high refraction material for the waveguides*. Paper presented at the Infrared, Millimeter, and Terahertz Waves (IRMMW-THz), 2013 38th International Conference. 10.1109/IRMMW-THz.2013.6665809

Nazarov, G. V., Galan, S. E., Nazarova, E. V., Karkishchenko, N. N., Muradov, M. M., & Stepanov, V. A. (2009). Nano-sized forms of drugs (a review). *Pharmaceutical Chemistry Journal*, *43*(3), 163–170. doi:10.100711094-009-0259-2

Nehru, K., & Sivakumar, M. (2012). Biosynthesis of Ag nanoparticles using Amaranthus tristis extract for the fabrication of nanoparticle embedded PVA membrane. *Current Nanoscience*, *8*, 703–708. doi:10.2174/157341312802884436

Nelson, P. A., & Owen, J. R. (2003). A high-performance supercapacitor/battery hybrid incorporating templated mesoporous electrodes. *Journal of the Electrochemical Society*, *150*(10), A1313–A1317. doi:10.1149/1.1603247

Ng, C. T., Yong, L. Q., Hande, M. P., Ong, C. N., Yu, L. E., Bay, B. H., & Baeg, G. H. (2017). Zinc oxide nanoparticles exhibit cytotoxicity and genotoxicity through oxidative stress responses in human lung fibroblasts and *Drosophila melanogaster. International Journal of Nanomedicine*, *12*, 1621–1637. doi:10.2147/IJN.S124403 PMID:28280330

Ng, S. M. (2019). Carbon dots as optical nanoprobes for biosensors. In S. C. B. Gopinath & T. Lakshmipriya (Eds.), *Nanobiosensors for biomolecular targeting* (pp. 269–300). Elsevier., doi:10.1016/B978-0-12-813900-4.00012-9

NICNAS. (2010). National industrial chemicals notification and assessment scheme. Australian Government. *Gazette*.

Nie, S., Xing, Y., Kim, G. J., & Simons, J. W. (2007). Nanotechnology applications in cancer. *Annual Review of Biomedical Engineering*, *9*(1), 257–288. doi:10.1146/annurev.bioeng.9.060906.152025 PMID:17439359

Nikolovska-Coleska, Z. (2015). Studying protein-protein interactions using surface plasmon resonance. In C. L. Meyerkord & H. Fu (Eds.), *Methods in molecular biology* (Vol. 1278, pp. 109–138). Humana Press., doi:10.1007/978-1-4939-2425-7_7

Nisar, M. S., Kang, S., & Zhao, X. (2020). Photothermal effect in plasmonic nanotip for LSPR sensing. *Sensors, 20*(3), 671-1-671–13. doi:10.339020030671

Nithya, K., Yuvasree, P., Neelakandeswari, N., Rajasekaran, N., Uthayarani, K., Chitra, M., & Kumar, S. S. (2014). Preparation and characterization of copper oxide nanoparticles. *International Journal of Chemtech Research*, *6*, 2220–2222.

Nitta, N., Wu, F., Lee, J. T., & Yushin, G. (2015). Li-ion battery materials: Present and future. *Materials Today*, *18*(5), 252–264. doi:10.1016/j.mattod.2014.10.040

Niu, C., Sichjel, E. K., Hoch, R., Hoi, D., & Tennent, H. (1997). High power electrochemical capacitors based on carbon nanotube electrodes. *Applied Physics Letters*, *70*(11), 1480–1482. doi:10.1063/1.118568

Nivetha, R., Gothandapani, K., Raghavan, V., Jacob, G., Sellappan, R., Bhardwaj, P., ... Grace, A. N. (2020). Highly Porous MIL-100 (Fe) for the Hydrogen Evolution Reaction (HER) in Acidic and Basic Media. *ACS Omega*.

Nkosi, F. P., Jafta, C. J., Kebede, M., le Roux, L., Mathe, M. K., & Ozoemena, K. I. (2015). Microwave-assisted optimization of the manganese redox states for enhanced capacity and capacity retention of $LiAl_xMn_{2-x}O_4$ (x= 0 and 0.3) spinel materials. *RSC Advances*, *5*(41), 32256–32262. doi:10.1039/C5RA02643A

Nobile, M. A., Cannarsi, M., Altieri, C., Sinigaglia, M., Favia, P., Iacoviello, G., & D'Agostino, R. (2004). Effect of Ag-containing nanocomposite active packaging system on Survival of Alicyclobacillus acidoterrestris. *Journal of Food Science*, *69*(8), E379–E383. doi:10.1111/j.1365-2621.2004.tb09899.x

Nomura, A., & Jones, C. W. (2013). Amine-functionalized porous silicas as adsorbents for aldehyde abatement. *ACS Applied Materials & Interfaces*, *5*(12), 5569–5577. doi:10.1021/am400810s PMID:23716505

Nourafkan, E., Asachi, M., Jin, H., Wen, D., & Ahmed, W. (2019). Stability and photo-thermal conversion performance of binary nanofluids for solar absorption refrigeration systems. *Renewable Energy*, *140*, 264–273. doi:10.1016/j.renene.2019.01.081

Nozik, A. J. (1975). Photoelectrolysis of water using semiconducting TiO_2 crystals. *Nature*, *257*(5525), 383–386. doi:10.1038/257383a0

Nozik, A. J. (2008). Multiple exciton generation in semiconductor quantum dots. *Chemical Physics Letters*, *457*(1-3), 3–11. doi:10.1016/j.cplett.2008.03.094

Nurmi, J. T., Tratnyek, P. G., Sarathy, V., Baer, D. R., Amonette, J. E., Pecher, K., Wang, C., Linehan, J. C., Matson, D. W., Penn, R. L., & Driessen, M. D. (2005). Characterization and properties of metallic iron nanoparticles: Spectroscopy, electrochemistry, and kinetics. *Environmental Science & Technology*, *39*(5), 1221–1230. doi:10.1021/es049190u PMID:15787360

Nyika, J. M. (2020a). The use of microorganism derived enzymes for bioremediation of soils pollutants. In S. Dey & B. Acharya (Eds.), *Recent advances in bioremediation of metal contaminants*. IGI Global.

Nyika, J. M. (2020b). Tolerance of microorganisms to heavy metals. In S. Dey & B. Acharya (Eds.), *Recent advances in bioremediation of metal contaminants*. IGI Global.

Nylander, C., Liedberg, B., & Lind, T. (1982). Gas detection by means of surface plasmon resonance. *Sensors and Actuators*, *3*, 79–88. doi:10.1016/0250-6874(82)80008-5

O'Donnell, P. B., & McGinity, J. W. (1997). Preparation of microspheres by the solvent evaporation technique. *Advanced Drug Delivery Reviews*, *28*(1), 25–42. doi:10.1016/S0169-409X(97)00049-5 PMID:10837563

O'Regan, B., & Gratzel, M. (1991). A low-cost, high-efficiency solar cell based on dye-sensitized colloidal TiO_2 films. *Nature*, *353*(6346), 737–740. doi:10.1038/353737a0

Ocsoy, I., Paret, M. L., Ocsoy, M. A., Kunwar, S., Chen, T., You, M., & Tan, W. (2013). Nanotechnology in Plant Disease Management: DNA-Directed Silver Nanoparticles on Graphene Oxide as an Antibacterial against *Xanthomonas perforans*. *ACS Nano*, *7*(10), 8972–8980. doi:10.1021/nn4034794 PMID:24016217

Ohara, S., Suzuki, J., Sekine, K., & Takamura, T. (2004). A thin film silicon anode for Li-ion batteries having a very large specific capacity and long cycle life. *Journal of Power Sources*, *136*(2), 303–306. doi:10.1016/j.jpowsour.2004.03.014

Ohzuku, T., Wakamatsu, H., Takehara, Z., & Yoshizawa, S. (1979). Nonaqueous lithium/pyromellitic dianhydride cell. *Electrochimica Acta*, *24*, 219–312. doi:10.1016/0013-4686(79)80028-6

Okuyama, K., & Lenggoro, I. W. (2003). Preparation of nanoparticles via spray route. *Chemical Engineering Science*, *58*(3-6), 537–547. doi:10.1016/S0009-2509(02)00578-X

Oliveira, O. N. Jr, Iost, R. M., Siqueira, J. R. Jr, Crespilho, F. N., & Caseli, L. (2014). Nanomaterials for diagnosis: Challenges and applications in smart devices based on molecular recognition. *ACS Applied Materials & Interfaces*, *6*(17), 14745–14766. doi:10.1021/am5015056 PMID:24968359

Olsson, S. E., Villa, L. L., Costa, R. L. R., Petta, C. A., Andrade, R. P., Malm, C., Iversen, O.-E., Høye, J., Steinwall, M., Riis-Johannessen, G., Andersson-Ellstrom, A., Elfgren, K., von Krogh, G., Lehtinen, M., Paavonen, J., Tamms, G. M., Giacoletti, K., Lupinacci, L., Esser, M. T., ... Barr, E. (2007). Induction of immune memory following administration of a prophylactic quadrivalent human papilloma virus (HPV) types 6/11/16/18 L1 virus-like particle (VLP)vaccine. *Vaccine*, *25*(26), 4931–4939. doi:10.1016/j.vaccine.2007.03.049 PMID:17499406

Oluwole, D. O., & Nyokong, T. (2015). Physicochemical behavior of nanohybrids of mono and tetra substituted carboxyphenoxy phthalocyanine covalently linked to GSH-CdTe/CdS/ZnS quantum dots. *Polyhedron*, *87*, 8–16. doi:10.1016/j.poly.2014.10.024

Omedi, Y., (2011). Smart multifunctional theranostics: simultaneous diagnosis and therapy of cancer. *Bioimpacts, 1*(3), 145-7.

Omlor, A. J., Nguyen, J., Bals, R., & Dinh, Q. T. (2015). Nanotechnology in respiratory medicine. *Respiratory Research*, *16*(1), 64. doi:10.118612931-015-0223-5 PMID:26021823

Ong, C., Lee, Q. Y., Cai, Y., Liu, X., Ding, J., Yung, L. Y., Bay, B. H., & Baeg, G. H. (2016). Silver nanoparticles disrupt germline stem cell maintenance in the Drosophila testis. *Scientific Reports*, *6*(1), 20632. doi:10.1038rep20632 PMID:26847594

Osman, B., Uzun, L., Beşirli, N., & Denizli, A. (2013). Microcontact imprinted surface plasmon resonance sensor for myoglobin detection. *Materials Science and Engineering C*, *33*(7), 3609–3614. doi:10.1016/j.msec.2013.04.041 PMID:23910256

Ossa, D. (2014). *Quality Aspects of Nano-Based Medicines.* SME Workshop: Focus on Quality for Medicines Containing Chemical Entities, London.

Ouattara, B., Simard, R. E., Piette, G., Begin, A., & Holley, R. A. (2000). Diffusion of Acetic and Propionic Acids from Chitosanbased Antimicrobial Packaging Films. *Journal of Food Science*, *65*(5), 768–773. doi:10.1111/j.1365-2621.2000.tb13584.x

Ouda, S. M. (2014). Antifungal Activity of Silver and Copper Nanoparticles on Two Plant Pathogens, Alternaria alternata and Botrytis cinerea. *Res. J. Microbiol.*, *9*(1), 34–42. doi:10.3923/jm.2014.34.42

Ou, J. Y., Plum, E., Jiang, L., & Zheludev, N. I. (2011). Reconfigurable photonic metamaterials. *Nano Letters*, *11*(5), 2142–2144. doi:10.1021/nl200791r PMID:21480583

Ouyang, C. Y., Zeng, X. M., Sljivancanin, Z., & Baldereschi, A. (2010). Oxidation states of Mn atoms at clean and Al2O3-covered LiMn2O4 (001) surfaces. *The Journal of Physical Chemistry C*, *114*(10), 4756–4759. doi:10.1021/jp911746g

Oyelere, A. K., Chen, P. C., Huang, X., El-Sayed, I. H., & El-Sayed, M. A. (2007). Peptide-conjugated gold nanorods for nuclear targeting. *Bioconjugate Chemistry*, *18*(5), 1490–1497. doi:10.1021/bc070132i PMID:17630680

Ozden, K., Mert, O., & Kocer, H. (2016). Metamaterial based broadband RF absorber at X-band. *International Journal of Electronics and Communications*, *70*(8), 1062–1070. doi:10.1016/j.aeue.2016.05.002

Özgür, E., Topçu, A. A., Yılmaz, E., & Denizli, A. (2020). Surface plasmon resonance based biomimetic sensor for urinary tract infections. *Talanta*, *212*, 120778. doi:10.1016/j.talanta.2020.120778 PMID:32113541

Ozturk, B., Uzun, S., & Karakaya, O. (2019). Combined effects of aminoethoxyvinylglycine and MAP on the fruit quality of kiwifruit during cold storage and shelf life. *Scientia Horticulturae*, *251*, 209–214. doi:10.1016/j.scienta.2019.03.034

Paiva, L. B., Morales, A. R., & Diaz, F. R. V. (2008). Organoclays: Properties preparation and applications. *Applied Clay Science*, *42*(1-2), 8–24. doi:10.1016/j.clay.2008.02.006

Pal, R., Panigrahi, S., Bhattacharyya, D., & Chakraborti, A. S. (2013). Characterization of citrate capped gold nanoparticle-quercetin complex: Experimental and quantum chemical approach. *Journal of Molecular Structure*, *1046*, 153–163. doi:10.1016/j.molstruc.2013.04.043

Pal, S. L. (2011). Nanoparticle: An overview of preparation and characterization. *Journal of Applied Pharmaceutical Science*, *1*(6), 228–234.

Pal, S., Tak, Y. K., & Song, J. M. (2007). Does the antibacterial activity of silver nanoparticles depend on the shape of the nanoparticle? A study of the gram-negative bacterium *Escherichia coli. Applied and Environmental Microbiology*, *73*(6), 1712–1720. doi:10.1128/AEM.02218-06 PMID:17261510

Panacek, A., Prucek, R., Safarova, D., Dittrich, M., Richtrova, J., Benickova, K., Zboril, R., & Kvitek, L. (2011). Acute and chronic toxicity effects of silver nanoparticles (NPs) on Drosophila melanogaster. *Environmental Science & Technology*, *45*(11), 4974–4979. doi:10.1021/es104216b PMID:21553866

Panatarotto, D., Prtidos, C. D., Hoebeke, J., Brown, F., Kramer, E., Briand, J. P., Muller, S., Prato, M., & Bianco, A. (2003). Immunization with peptide-functionalized carbon nanotubes enhances virus-specific neutralizing antibody responses. *Chemistry & Biology*, *10*(10), 961–966. doi:10.1016/j.chembiol.2003.09.011 PMID:14583262

Pan, B., & Xing, B. (2008). Adsorption mechanisms of organic chemicals on carbon nanotubes. *Environmental Science & Technology*, *42*(24), 9005–9013. doi:10.1021/es801777n PMID:19174865

Pander, A., Hatta, A., & Furuta, H. (2017). FIB secondary etching method for fabrication of fine CNT forest metamaterials. *Nano-Micro Letters*, *9*(4), 44-1-44-48. doi:10.100740820-017-0145-5

Pandey, G. (2018). Prospects of nanobioremediation in environmental clean-up. *Oriental Journal of Chemistry*, *34*(6), 2828–2840. doi:10.13005/ojc/340622

Pandey, H., Khare, P., Singh, S., & Singh, S. P. (2020). Carbon nanomaterials integrated molecularly imprinted polymers for biological sample analysis: A critical review. *Materials Chemistry and Physics*, *239*, 121966. doi:10.1016/j.matchemphys.2019.121966

Pandey, R., & Khuller, G. K. (2006). Nanotechnology Based Drug Delivery System(s) for the Management of Tuberculosis. *Indian Journal of Experimental Biology*, *44*, 357–366. PMID:16708887

Pandey, S., Kumari, M., Singh, S. P., Bhattacharya, A., Mishra, S. K., Chauhan, P. S., & Mishra, A. (2015). Bioremediation via Nanoparticles: An Innovative Microbial Approach. In S. Singh & K. Srivastava (Eds.), *Handbook of research on uncovering new methods for ecosystem management through bioremediation*. IGI Global. doi:10.4018/978-1-4666-8682-3.ch019

Pan, X.-L., Xu, C.-Y., & Zhen, L. (2012). Synthesis of $LiMnPO_4$ microspheres assembled by plates, wedges and prisms with different crystallographic orientations and their electrochemical performance. *CrystEngComm*, *14*(20), 6412. doi:10.1039/c2ce25593f

Panyam, J., & Labhasetwar, V. (2003). Biodegradable nanoparticles for drug and gene delivery to cells and tissue. *Advanced Drug Delivery Reviews*, *55*(3), 329–347. doi:10.1016/S0169-409X(02)00228-4 PMID:12628320

Pan, Z., Xie, S., Chang, B., Wang, C., Lu, L., Liu, W., Zhou, W., Li, W., & Qian, L. (1998). Very long carbon nanotubes. *Nature*, *394*(6694), 631–632. doi:10.1038/29206

Parak, W. J., Boudreau, R., Gros, M. L., Gerion, D., Zanchet, D., Micheel, C. M., Willams, S. C., Alivisatos, A. P., & Larabell, C. A. (2002). Cell motility and metastatic potential studies based on quantum dot imaging of phagokinetic tracks. *Advanced Materials*, *14*(12), 882–885. doi:10.1002/1521-4095(20020618)14:12<882::AID-ADMA882>3.0.CO;2-Y

Paret, M. L., Vallad, E. G., Averett, R. D., Jones, B. J., & Olson, M. S. (2013). Photocatalysis: Effect of Light-Activated Nanoscale Formulations of TiO_2 on *Xanthomonas perforans* and Control of Bacterial Spot of Tomato. *Phytopathology*, *103*(3), 228–236. doi:10.1094/PHYTO-08-12-0183-R PMID:23190116

Park, S. J., Hong, J. T., Choi, S. J., Kim, H. S., Park, W. K., Han, S. T., Park, J. Y., Lee, S., Kim, D. S., & Ahn, Y. H. (2014). Detection of microorganisms using terahertz metamaterials. *Scientific Reports*, *4*, 4988-1-4988–7. doi:10.1038rep04988

Park, B. K., Jeong, S., Kim, D., Moon, J., Lim, S., & Kim, J. S. (2007). Synthesis and size control of monodisperse copper nanoparticles by polyol method. *Journal of Colloid and Interface Science*, *311*(2), 417–424. doi:10.1016/j.jcis.2007.03.039 PMID:17448490

Park, J., & Lee, I. H. (2014). Photocatalytic degradation of 2-chlorophenol using Ag-doped TiO2 nanofibers and a near-UV light-emitting diode system. *Journal of Nanomaterials*, *250803*, 1–8.

Park, J., Seo, J. H., Plett, G., Lu, W., & Sastry, A. M. (2011). Numerical simulation of the effect of the dissolution of LiMn2O4 particles on Li-ion battery performance. *Electrochemical and Solid-State Letters*, *14*(2), A14–A18. doi:10.1149/1.3516619

Park, S. H., Lee, Y. S., & Sun, Y. K. (2003). Synthesis and electrochemical properties of sulfur doped-$Li_xMnO_{2-y}S_y$ materials for lithium secondary batteries. *Electrochemistry Communications*, *5*(2), 124–128. doi:10.1016/S1388-2481(03)00005-5

Park, S. J., Cha, S. H., Shin, G. A., & Ahn, Y. H. (2017). Sensing viruses using terahertz nano-gap metamaterials. *Biomedical Optics Express*, *8*(8), 3551–3558. doi:10.1364/BOE.8.003551 PMID:28856034

Park, S., Marsh, K. S., & Dawson, P. (2010). Application of chitosanincorporated LDPE film to sliced fresh red meats for shelf life extension. *Meat Science*, *85*(3), 493–499. doi:10.1016/j.meatsci.2010.02.022 PMID:20416821

Park, S., Sung, H. K., & Kim, Y. (2016). Green Synthesis of Metal Nanoparticles Using Sprout Plants: Pros and Cons. *Journal of Nanoscience and Nanotechnology*, *16*(5), 4444–4449. doi:10.1166/jnn.2016.10970 PMID:27483771

Parveen, S., Rana, S., & Fangueiro, R. (2013). A Review on Nanomaterial Dispersion, Microstructure, and Mechanical Properties of Carbon Nanotube and Nanofiber Reinforced Cementitious Composites. *Journal of Nanomaterials*. *Article ID*, *710175*, 1–19. doi:10.1155/2013/710175

Parveen, S., & Sahoo, S. K. (2008). Polymeric nanoparticles for cancer therapy. *Journal of Drug Targeting*, *16*(2), 108–123. doi:10.1080/10611860701794353 PMID:18274932

Patel, A. R., & Vavia, P. R. (2007). Nanotechnology and pharmaceutical inhalation aerosols. *Indian Journal of Experimental Biology*, *45*, 166–174. PMID:17375556

Patel, P., & Patel, J. (2017). Biosensors and biomarkers: Promising tools for cancer diagnosis. *International Journal of Biosensors & Bioelectronics*, *3*(4), 313–316. doi:10.15406/ijbsbe.2017.03.00072

Patel, S., Bhirde, A. A., Rusling, J. F., Chen, X., Gutkind, J. S., & Patel, V. (2011). Nano Delivers Big: Designing Molecular Missiles for Cancer Therapeutics. *Pharmaceutics*, *3*(1), 34–52. doi:10.3390/pharmaceutics3010034 PMID:21949900

Patel, V., Berthold, D., Puranik, P., & Gantar, M. (2015). Screening of cyanobacteria and micro algae for their ability to synthesize silver nanoparticles with antibacterial activity. *Biotechnology Reports (Amsterdam, Netherlands)*, *5*, 112–119. doi:10.1016/j.btre.2014.12.001 PMID:28626689

Patey, T. J., Ng, S. H., Büchel, R., Tran, N., Krumeich, F., Wang, J., Liu, H. K., & Novák, P. (2008). Electrochemistry of LiV3O8 nanoparticles made by flame spray pyrolysis. *Electrochemical and Solid-State Letters*, *11*(4), A46–A50. doi:10.1149/1.2836741

Patil, M., Mehta, D. S., & Guvva, S. S. (2008). Future impact of nanotechnology on medicine and dentistry. *Journal of Indian Society of Periodontology*, *12*(2), 34. doi:10.4103/0972-124X.44088 PMID:20142942

Pati, R., Shevtsov, M., & Sonawane, A. (2018). Nanoparticle Vaccines Against Infectious Diseases. *Frontiers in Immunology*, *9*, 2224. Advance online publication. doi:10.3389/fimmu.2018.02224 PMID:30337923

Patra, C. R., Bhattacharya, R., Wang, E., Katarya, A., Lau, J. S., Dutta, S., ... Yaszemski, M. J. (2008). Targeted delivery of gemcitabine to pancreatic adenocarcinoma using cetuximab as a targeting agent. *Cancer Research*, *68*(6), 1970–1978. doi:10.1158/0008-5472.CAN-07-6102 PMID:18339879

Patra, J. K., & Baek, K. H. (2014). Green nanobiotechnology: Factors affecting synthesis and characterization techniques. *Journal of Nanomaterials*, *2014*, 219. doi:10.1155/2014/417305

Patskovsky, S., Kabashin, A. V., Meunier, M., & Luong, J. H. T. (2004). Near-infrared surface plasmon resonance sensing on a silicon platform. *Sensors and Actuators. B, Chemical*, *97*(2-3), 409–414. doi:10.1016/j.snb.2003.09.023

Paul, A. M., Sajeev, A., Nivetha, R., Gothandapani, K., Bhardwaj, P., Govardhan, K., ... Grace, A. N. (2020). Cuprous oxide (Cu2O)/graphitic carbon nitride (g-C3N4) nanocomposites for electrocatalytic hydrogen evolution reaction. *Diamond and Related Materials*, *107*, 107899. doi:10.1016/j.diamond.2020.107899

Paulose, M., Shankar, K., Varghese, O. K., Mor, G. K., & Grimes, C. A. (2006 a). Application of highly-ordered TiO2 nanotube-arrays in heterojunction dye-sensitized solar cells. *Journal of Physics. D, Applied Physics*, *39*(12), 2498–2503. doi:10.1088/0022-3727/39/12/005

Paulose, M., Shankar, K., Varghese, O. K., Mor, G. K., Hardin, B., & Grimes, C. A. (2006b). Backside illuminated dye-sensitized solar cells based on titania nanotube array electrodes. *Nanotechnology*, *17*(5), 1446–1448. doi:10.1088/0957-4484/17/5/046

Pautler, M., & Sara, B. (2010). Nanomedicine: Promises and challenges for the future of public health. *International Journal of Nanomedicine*, *5*, 803–809. PMID:21042425

Peer, D., Karp, J. M., & Hong, S. (2007). Nanocarriers as an emerging platform for cancer therapy. *Nat Nanotechnol.*, *2*, 751-60.

Peer, D., Karp, J. M., Hong, S., Farokhzad, Q. C., Margalit, R., & Langer, R. (2007). Nanocarriers as an emerging platform for cancer therapy. *Nature Nanotechnology*, *2*(12), 751–760. doi:10.1038/nnano.2007.387 PMID:18654426

Pelemiš, S., & Hut, I. (2013). Nanotechnology materials for solar energy conversion. *Contemporary Materials Renewable Energy Sources, IV*, *2*, 145–151.

Peng, Z. D., Jiang, Q. L., Du, K., Wang, W. G., Hu, G. R., & Liu, Y. X. (2010). Effect of Cr-sources on performance of $Li_{1.05}Cr_{0.04}Mn_{1.96}O_4$ cathode materials prepared by slurry spray drying method. *Journal of Alloys and Compounds*, *493*(1), 640–644. doi:10.1016/j.jallcom.2009.12.172

Perçin, I., Idil, N., Bakhshpour, M., Yılmaz, E., Mattiasson, B., & Denizli, A. (2017).. . *Sensors and Actuators. B, Chemical*, *17*, 1375.

Perrault, S. D., & Chan, W. C. (2010). In vivo assembly of nanoparticle components to improve targeted cancer imaging. *Proceedings of the National Academy of Sciences of the United States of America*, *107*(25), 11194–11199. doi:10.1073/pnas.1001367107 PMID:20534561

Peters, R. J. B., Bouwmeester, H., Gottardo, S., Amenta, V., Arena, M., Brandhoff, P., Marvin, H. J. P., Mech, A., Moniz, F. B., Pesudo, L. Q., Rauscher, H., Schoonjans, R., Undas, A. K., Vettori, M. V., Weigel, S., & Aschberger, K. (2016). Nanomaterials for products and application in agriculture, feed and food. *Trends in Food Science & Technology*, *54*, 155–164. doi:10.1016/j.tifs.2016.06.008

Philbrook, N. A., Winn, L. M., Afrooz, A. R., Saleh, N. B., & Walker, V. K. (2011). The effect of TiO(2) and Ag nanoparticles on reproduction and development of Drosophila melanogaster and CD-1 mice. *Toxicology and Applied Pharmacology*, *257*(3), 429–436. doi:10.1016/j.taap.2011.09.027 PMID:22005274

Pillai, G., & Coronel, M. L. C. (2013). Science and technology of the emerging nanomedicines in cancer therapy: A primer for physicians and pharmacists. *SAGE Open Medicine*, *1*. Advance online publication. doi:10.1177/2050312113513759 PMID:26770691

Piriyawong, V. (2012). Preparation and Characterization of Alumina Nanoparticles in Deionized Water Using Laser Ablation Technique. *Journal of Nanomaterials. Article ID*, *819403*, 1–6.

Pita, R., Ehmann, F., & Papaluca, M. (2016). Nanomedicines in the EU—Regulatory overview. *The AAPS Journal*, *18*(6), 1576–1582. doi:10.120812248-016-9967-1 PMID:27527889

Piwek, L., Ellis, D. A., Andrews, S., & Joinson, A. (2016). The rise of consumer health wearables: Promises and barriers. *PLoS Medicine*, *13*(2), 1001953. doi:10.1371/journal.pmed.1001953 PMID:26836780

Pizarro-Cerda, J., & Cossart, P. (2006). Bacterial adhesion and entry into host cells. *Cell*, *124*(4), 715–727. doi:10.1016/j.cell.2006.02.012 PMID:16497583

Pleskova, S., Mikheeva, E., & Gornostaeva, E. (2018). Using of Quantum Dots in Biology and Medicine. *Advances in Experimental Medicine and Biology*, *1048*, 323–334. Advance online publication. doi:10.1007/978-3-319-72041-8_19 PMID:29453547

Polizzi, M. A., Stasko, N. A., & Schoenfisch, M. H. (2007). Water-soluble nitric oxide-releasing gold nanoparticles. *Langmuir*, *23*(9), 4938–4943. doi:10.1021/la0633841 PMID:17375944

Portet, C., Taberna, P., Simon, P., & Flahaut, E. (2005). Influence of carbon nanotubes addition on carbon-carbon supercapacitor performances in organic electrolyte. *Journal of Power Sources*, *139*(1-2), 371–378. doi:10.1016/j.jpowsour.2004.07.015

Posgai, R., Cipolla-McCulloch, C. B., Murphy, K. R., Hussain, S. M., Rowe, J. J., & Nielsen, M. G. (2011). Differential toxicity of silver and titanium dioxide nanoparticles on Drosophila melanogaster development, reproductive effort, and viability: Size, coatings and antioxidants matter. *Chemosphere*, *85*(1), 34–42. doi:10.1016/j.chemosphere.2011.06.040 PMID:21733543

Poursaberi, T., Hassanisadi, M., Torkestani, K., & Zare, M. (2012). Development of zirconium (IV)-metalloporphyrin grafted Fe3O4 nanoparticles for efficient fluoride removal. *Chemical Engineering Journal*, *189–190*, 117–125. doi:10.1016/j.cej.2012.02.039

Prabhu, S., & Poulose, E. K. (2012). Silver nanoparticles: Mechanism of antimicrobial action, synthesis, medical applications, and toxicity effects. *International Nano Letters*, *2*(1), 32. doi:10.1186/2228-5326-2-32

Prasad, K., & Jha, A. K. (2009). ZnO nanoparticles: Synthesis and adsorption study. *Nature and Science*, *1*(02), 129.

Prathna, T. C., & Lazar Mathew, N. (2010). Biomimetic synthesis of nanoparticles: science, technology & applicability. In Biomimetics, learning from nature. InTechOpen.

Prego, C., Paolicelli, P., Díaz, B., Vicente, S., Sánchez, A., González-Fernández, Á., & Alonso, M. J. (2010). Chitosan-based nanoparticles for improving immunization against hepatitis B infection. *Vaccine*, *28*(14), 2607–2614. doi:10.1016/j.vaccine.2010.01.011 PMID:20096389

Presnova, G., Presnov, D., Krupenin, V., Grigorenko, V., Trifonov, A., Andreeva, I., Ignatenko, O., Egorov, A., & Rubtsova, M. (2017). Biosensor based on a silicon nanowire field-effect transistor functionalized by gold nanoparticles for the highly sensitive determination of prostate specific antigen. *Biosensors & Bioelectronics*, *88*, 283–289. doi:10.1016/j.bios.2016.08.054 PMID:27567265

Priya, S., & Bernice, S. (2016). Defining Nano, Nanotechnology and Nanomedicine: Why Should It Matter? *Science and Engineering Ethics*, *22*(5), 1255–1276. doi:10.100711948-015-9705-6 PMID:26373718

Pröll, J., Kohler, R., Torge, M., Ulrich, S., Ziebert, C., Bruns, M., Seifert, H. J., & Pfleging, W. (2011). Laser microstructuring and annealing processes for lithium manganese oxide cathodes. *Applied Surface Science*, *257*(23), 9968–9976. doi:10.1016/j.apsusc.2011.06.117

Prosini, P. P., Carewska, M., Scaccia, S., Wisniewski, P., & Pasquali, M. (2003). Long-term cyclability of nanostructured $LiFePO_4$. *Electrochimica Acta*, *48*(28), 4205–4211. doi:10.1016/S0013-4686(03)00606-6

Pugazhendhi, A., Prabhu, R., Muruganantham, K., Shanmuganathan, R., & Natarajan, S. (2019). Anticancer, antimicrobial and photocatalytic activities of green synthesized magnesium oxide nanoparticles (MgONPs) using aqueous extract of Sargassum wightii. *Journal of Photochemistry and Photobiology. B, Biology*, *190*, 86–97. doi:10.1016/j.jphotobiol.2018.11.014 PMID:30504053

Puri, A., Loomis, K., Smith, B., Lee, J. H., Yavlovich, A., Heldman, E., & Blumenthal, R. (2009). Lipid-based nanoparticles as pharmaceutical drug carriers: From concepts to clinic. *Critical Reviews in Therapeutic Drug Carrier Systems*, *26*(6), 523–580. doi:10.1615/CritRevTherDrugCarrierSyst.v26.i6.10 PMID:20402623

Pusic, K., Aguilar, Z., McLoughlin, J., Kobuch, S., Xu, H., Tsang, M., Wang, A., & Hui, G. (2013). Iron oxide nanoparticles as a clinically acceptable delivery platform for a recombinant blood-stage human malaria vaccine. *The FASEB Journal*, *27*(3), 1153–1166. doi:10.1096/fj.12-218362 PMID:23195035

Putheti, R. R., & Okigbo, R. N., Sai Advanapu, M., & Chavanpatil, S. (2008). Nanotechnology importance in the pharmaceutical industry. *Afr J Pure Applied Chem*, *2*, 27–31.

Qamar, S. A., Asgher, M., Khalid, N., & Sadaf, M. (2019). Nanobiotechnology in health sciences: Current applications and future perspectives. *Biocatalysis and Agricultural Biotechnology*, *22*, 101388. doi:10.1016/j.bcab.2019.101388

Qian, X., Peng, X. H., Ansari, D. O., Yin-Goen, Q., Chen, G. Z., Shin, D. M., Yang, L., Young, A. N., Wang, M. D., & Nie, S. (2008). In vivo tumor targeting and spectroscopic detection with surface-enhanced Raman nanoparticle tags. *Nature Biotechnology*, *26*(1), 83–90. doi:10.1038/nbt1377 PMID:18157119

Qin, B., Li, Z., Hu, F., Hu, C., Chen, T., Zhang, H., & Zhao, Y. (2018). Highly sensitive detection of carbendazim by using terahertz time-domain spectroscopy combined with metamaterial. *IEEE Transactions on Terahertz Science and Technology*, *8*(2), 149–154. doi:10.1109/TTHZ.2017.2787458

Qing, C., Bai, Y., Yang, J., & Zhang, W. (2011). Enhanced cycling stability of $LiMn_2O_4$ cathode by amorphous $FePO_4$ coating. *Electrochimica Acta*, *56*(19), 6612–6618. doi:10.1016/j.electacta.2011.04.131

Quan, F. S., Huang, C., Compans, R. W., & Kang, S. M. (2007). Virus-like particle vaccine induces protective immunity against homologous and heterologous strains of influenza virus. *Journal of Virology*, *81*(7), 3514–3524. doi:10.1128/JVI.02052-06 PMID:17251294

Quan, X., Yang, S., Ruan, X., & Zhao, H. (2005). Preparation of Titania Nanotubes and Their Environmental Applications as Electrode. *Environmental Science & Technology*, *39*(10), 3770–3775. doi:10.1021/es048684o PMID:15952384

Quintana, M., Haro-Poniatowski, E., Morales, J., & Batina, N. (2002). Synthesis of selenium nanoparticles by pulsed laser ablation. *Applied Surface Science*, *195*(1-4), 175–186. doi:10.1016/S0169-4332(02)00549-4

Rachid, S., Lee, B., David, Q., Brajesh, K., & Luis, C. (2019). Nanoparticles for Environment, Engineering, and Nanomedicine. Hindawi *Journal of Nanotechnology*.

Rafque, M., Jahangir, J., Amin, B. A. Z., Tahir, M. B., Nabi, G., Khan, M. I., Khalid, N. R., Gillani, S. S. A., & Sadaf, I. (2019). Article. *Journal of Inorganic and Organometallic Polymers and Materials*, *29*, 2133–2144. doi:10.100710904-019-01173-5

Raghavan, V., Deb, A., & Grace, A. N. (2020). *Honokiol-Camptothecin loaded graphene oxide nanoparticle towards combinatorial anti-cancer drug delivery*. IET Nanobiotechnology.

Rahman, M. S., & Rashid, M. A. (2008). Antimicrobial activity and cytotoxicity of Eclipta prostrata. *Oriental Pharmacy and Experimental Medicine*, *8*(1), 47–52. doi:10.3742/OPEM.2008.8.1.047

Rai, A., Prabhune, A., & Perry, C. C. (2010). Antibiotic mediated synthesis of gold nanoparticles with potent antimicrobial activity and their application in antimicrobial coatings. *Journal of Materials Chemistry*, *20*(32), 6789–6798. doi:10.1039/c0jm00817f

Raj, A., Shah, P., & Agrawal, N. (2017). Dose-dependent effect of silver nanoparticles (AgNPs) on fertility and survival of Drosophila: An in-vivo study. *PLoS One*, *12*(5), e0178051. doi:10.1371/journal.pone.0178051 PMID:28542630

Rajakumar, G., Rahumana, A. A., Roopan, S. M., Khannac, V. G., Elangoa, G., Kamaraja, C., & … . (2012). Fungus-mediated biosynthesis and characterization of TiO2 nanoparticles and their activity against pathogenic bacteria. *Spectrochimica Acta Part A*, *9*, 123–129. doi:10.1016/j.saa.2012.01.011

Rajeev, P. V., Gnanasekar, S., Sellappan, R., & Grace, A. N. (2019). Synthesis and analysis of Mo2N as efficient counter electrodes for dye sensitized solar cells. *Materials Today: Proceedings*. Advance online publication. doi:10.1016/j.matpr.2019.05.438

Rajendra, R., Balakumar, C., Ahammed, H. A. M., Jayakumar, S., Vaideki, K., & Rajesh, E. (2010). Use of zinc oxide nano particles for production of antimicrobial textiles. *International Journal of Engineering Science and Technology*, *2*(1), 202–208. doi:10.4314/ijest.v2i1.59113

Rajesh, Y. B. R. D., & Dubey, R. S. (2013). Sol-Gel Synthesis and Characterization of Nanocrystalline Spinel $LiMn_2O_4$ For Battery Applications. *Nanoscience and Nanoengineering*, *1*(3), 139–141.

Rajput, N. (2015). Methods of preparation of nanoparticles-a review. *International Journal of Advances in Engineering and Technology*, *7*(6), 1806.

Ramachandran, R., & Shanmughavel, P. (2010). Preparation and characterization of biopolymeric nanoparticles used in drug delivery. *Indian Journal of Biochemistry & Biophysics*, *47*, 56–59. PMID:21086757

Ramesh, P., Rajendran, A., & Shisundaram, M. M. (2014). Green synthesisof zinc oxide nanoparticles using flower extract cassia. *Journal of Nanoscience and Nanotechnology*, *2*, 41–45.

Ranjan, S., Dasgupta, N., Ganesh, S. A., Ramalingam, C., & Kumar, A. (2016). Microwave-irradiation-assisted hybrid chemical approach for titanium dioxide nanoparticle synthesis: Microbial and cytotoxicological evaluation. *Environmental Science and Pollution Research International*, *23*(12), 12287–12302. doi:10.100711356-016-6440-8 PMID:26976013

Rasalingam, S., Peng, R., & Koodali, R. T. (2014). Removal of hazardous pollutants from wastewaters: Applications of TiO2-SiO2 mixed oxide materials. *Journal of Nanomaterials*, *617405*, 1–10. doi:10.1155/2014/617405

Rashmirekha, P., Maxim, S., & Avinash, S. (2018). Nanoparticle Vaccines against Infectious Diseases. *Frontiers in Immunology*. PMID:30337923

Rathod, K. B., Patel, M. B., Parmar, P. K., Kharadi, S. R., Patel, P. V., & Patel, K. S. (2011). Glimpses of Current Advances of Nanotechnology in Therapeutics. *International Journal of Pharmacy and Pharmaceutical Sciences*, *3*, 8–12.

Ratlamwala, T. A., & Abid, M. (2018). Performance analysis of solar assisted multi-effect absorption cooling systems using nanofluids: A comparative analysis. *International Journal of Energy Research*, *42*(9), 2901–2915. doi:10.1002/er.3980

Ravichandran, R. (2010). Nanotechnology Applications in Food and Food Processing: Innovative Green Approaches, Opportunities and Uncertainties for Global Market. *Int. J. Green Nanotechnol. Phys. Chem.*, *1*(2), 72–P96. doi:10.1080/19430871003684440

Ravindran, R. (2011). Nanotechnology in cancer diagnosis and treatment: An overview. *Oral Maxillofac Pathol J.*, *2*, 101–106.

Ra, W., Nakayama, M., Uchimoto, Y., & Wakihara, M. (2005). Experimental and computational study of the electronic structural changes in $LiTi_2O_4$ spinel compounds upon electrochemical Li insertion reactions. *The Journal of Physical Chemistry B*, *109*(3), 1130–1134. doi:10.1021/jp040499+ PMID:16851071

Raza, M.A., Kanwal, Z., Rauf, A., Sabri, A.N., Riaz, S., Naseem, S. (2016). Size-and shape-dependent antibacterial studies of silver nanoparticles synthesized by wet chemical routes. *Nanomater., 6*.

Reda, S. M. (2010). Synthesis of ZnO and Fe2O3 nanoparticles by sol–gel method and their application in dye-sensitized solar cells. *Materials Science in Semiconductor Processing*, *13*(5-6), 417–425. doi:10.1016/j.mssp.2011.09.007

Reddy, L. S., Nisha, M. M., Joice, M., & Shilpa, P. N. (2014). Antimicrobial activity of zinc oxide (ZnO) nanoparticle against Klebsiella pneumonia. *Pharmaceutical Biology*, *52*(11), 1388–1397. doi:10.3109/13880209.2014.893001 PMID:25026353

Reibold, M., Paufler, P., Levin, A. A., Kochmann, W., Pätzke, N., & Meyer, D. C. (2006). Materials: Carbon nanotubes in an ancient Damascus sabre. *Nature*, *444*(7117), 286. doi:10.1038/444286a PMID:17108950

Reiter, L. T., Potocki, L., Chien, S., Gribskov, M., & Bier, E. (2001). A systematic analysis of human disease-associated gene sequences in Drosophila melanogaster. *Genome Research*, *11*(6), 1114–1125. doi:10.1101/gr.169101 PMID:11381037

Ren, M., Pan, C., Li, Q., Cai, W., Zhang, X., Wu, Q., Fan, S., & Xu, J. (2013). Isotropic spiral plasmonic metamaterial for sensing large refractive index change. *Optics Letters*, *38*(16), 3133–3136. doi:10.1364/OL.38.003133 PMID:24104668

Ren, X., Chen, C., Nagatsu, M., & Wang, X. (2011). Carbon nanotubes as adsorbents in environmental pollution management: A review. *Chemical Engineering Journal*, *170*(2-3), 395–410. doi:10.1016/j.cej.2010.08.045

Rezaii Kalaj, Y., Ghareyazie, B., Emadpour, M., & Omrani, A. (2009). Effect of the Removal of Ethylen Hormone by Potassium Permangenate Coated Zeolite Nanoparticles on the Increased Quality and Quantity of Storage of Iceberg Lettuce (Lactuca sativa L.) and Chinese Cabbage (Brassica pekinensis). *Journal of Agricultural Sciences and Natural Resources*, *15*, 1–11.

Rezende, T. S., Andrade, G. R., Barreto, L. S., Costa, N. B. Jr, Gimenez, I. F., & Almeida, L. E. (2010). Facile preparation of catalytically active gold nanoparticles on a thiolated chitosan. *Materials Letters*, *64*(7), 882–884. doi:10.1016/j.matlet.2010.01.051

Rhim, J. W., Hong, S. I., Park, H. M., & Ng, P. K. W. (2006). Preparation and characterization of chitosan-based nanocomposite films with antimicrobial activity. *Journal of Agricultural and Food Chemistry*, *54*(16), 5814–5822. doi:10.1021/jf060658h PMID:16881682

Rhim, J. W., Park, H. M., & Ha, C.-S. (2013). Bio-nanocomposites for food packaging applications. *Progress in Polymer Science*, *38*(10-11), 1629–1652. doi:10.1016/j.progpolymsci.2013.05.008

Riaz, M. (1996). Liposomes preparation methods. *Pakistan Journal of Pharmaceutical Sciences*, *19*, 65–77. PMID:16414777

Ribet, D., & Cossart, P. (2015). How bacterial pathogens colonize their hosts and invade deeper tissues. *Microbes and Infection*, *17*(3), 173–183. doi:10.1016/j.micinf.2015.01.004 PMID:25637951

Rich, R. L., & Myszka, D. G. (2002). Survey of the year 2001 commercial optical biosensor literature. *Journal of Molecular Recognition*, *15*(6), 352–376. doi:10.1002/jmr.598 PMID:12501157

Richter, J. W., Shull, G. M., Fountain, J. H., Guo, Z., Musselman, L. P., Fiumera, A. C., & Mahler, G. J. (2018). Titanium dioxide nanoparticle exposure alters metabolic homeostasis in a cell culture model of the intestinal epithelium and Drosophila melanogaster. *Nanotoxicology*, *12*(5), 390–406. doi:10.1080/17435390.2018.1457189 PMID:29600885

Rimmelzwaan, G. F., Siebelink, K. H., Huisman, R. C., Moss, B., Francis, M. J., & Osterhaus, A. D. (1994). Removal of the cleavage site of recombinant feline immunodeficiency virus envelope protein facilitates incorporation of the surface glycoprotein in immune- stimulating complexes. *The Journal of General Virology*, *75*(Pt 8), 2097–2102. doi:10.1099/0022-1317-75-8-2097 PMID:8046415

Ritzefeld, M., & Sewald, N. (2012). Real-time analysis of specific protein-DNA interactions with surface plasmon resonance. *Journal of Amino Acids*, *2012*, 1–19. doi:10.1155/2012/816032 PMID:22500214

Rizeq, B. R., Younes, N. N., Rasool, K., & Nasrallah, G. K. (2019). Article. *International Journal of Molecular Sciences*, *20*(5776), 1–24.

Rizvi, S. A. A., & Saleh, A. M. (2018). Applications of nanoparticle systems in drug delivery technology. *Saudi Pharmaceutical Journal*, *26*(1), 64–70. doi:10.1016/j.jsps.2017.10.012 PMID:29379334

Rizwan, M., Singh, M., Mitra, C. & Morve, R. (2014). Eco-friendly application of nanomaterials: nanobioremediation. *Journal of Nanoparticles*, 1-7.

Roberts, M. C. (2005). Update on acquired tetracycline resistance genes. *FEMS Microbiology Letters*, *245*(2), 195–203. doi:10.1016/j.femsle.2005.02.034 PMID:15837373

Robledo, N., López, L., Bunger, A., Tapia, C., & Abugoch, L. (2018). Effects of Antimicrobial Edible Coating of Thymol Nanoemulsion/Quinoa Protein/Chitosan on the Safety, Sensorial Properties, and Quality of Refrigerated Strawberries (Fragaria × ananassa) Under Commercial Storage Environment. *Food and Bioprocess Technology*, *11*(8), 1566–1574. doi:10.100711947-018-2124-3

Robles-García, M. A., Rodríguez-Félix, F., Márquez-Ríos, E., Aguilar, J. A., Barrera Rodríguez, A., Aguilar, J., Ruiz-Cruz, S., & Lizette Del-Toro-Sánchez, C. (2016). Applications of Nanotechnology in the Agriculture, Food, and Pharmaceuticals. *Journal of Nanoscience and Nanotechnology*, *16*(8), 8188–8207. doi:10.1166/jnn.2016.12925

Roduner, E. (2006). *Nanoscopic materials size-dependent phenomena*. The Royal Society of Chemistry.

Rohmawati, L., Sholicha, S. P., Holisa, S. S., & Setyarsih, W. (2019, December). Identification of Phase CaCO3/MgO in Bangkalan Dolomite Sand as An Antibacterial Substance. *Journal of Physics: Conference Series*, *1417*(1), 012001. doi:10.1088/1742-6596/1417/1/012001

Roldao, A., Mellado, M. C., Castilho, L. R., Carrondo, M. J., & Alves, P. M. (2010). Virus-like particles in vaccine development. *Expert Review of Vaccines*, *9*(10), 1149–1176. doi:10.1586/erv.10.115 PMID:20923267

Roszek, B., De Jong, W.H., & Geertsma, R.E. (2005). *Nanotechnology in medical applications: state-of-the-art in materials and devices*. Academic Press.

Roy, R., Pal, A., & Chaudhuri, A. N. (2015). Antimicrobial Effect of Silver Nanoparticle on Pathogenic Organisms Isolated from East Kolkata Wetland. *International Journal of Applied Research*, *1*, 745–752.

Ruales-lonfat, C., Barona, J. F., Sienkiewicz, A., Bensimon, M., & Vélez-colmenares, J. (2015). Applied Catalysis B : Environmental Iron oxides semiconductors are efficients for solar water disinfection : A comparison with photo-Fenton processes at neutral pH, *Applied Catalyst. B. Environment*, *166-167*, 497–508.

Rudge, A., Davey, J., Raistrick, I., Gottesfeld, S., & Ferraris, J. P. (1994). Conducting polymers as active materials in electrochemical capacitors. *Journal of Power Sources*, *47*(1-2), 89–107. doi:10.1016/0378-7753(94)80053-7

Rudramurthy, G. R., Swamy, M. K., Sinniah, U. R., & Ghasemzadeh, A. (2016). Nanoparticles: Alternatives against drug-resistant pathogenic microbes. *Molecules (Basel, Switzerland)*, *21*(7), 836. doi:10.3390/molecules21070836 PMID:27355939

Rudrapatna, V. A., Cagan, R. L., & Das, T. K. (2012). Drosophila cancer models. *Developmental Dynamics*, *241*(1), 107–118. doi:10.1002/dvdy.22771 PMID:22038952

Rukh, S., Sofi, A. H., Shah, M. A., & Yousuf, S. (2019). Antibacterial activity of magnesium oxide nanostructures prepared by hydrothermal method. *Asian Journal of Nanosciences and Materials*, *2*(4), 425–430.

Ruzzin, J. (2012). Public health concern behind the exposure to persistent organic pollutants and the risk of metabolic diseases. *BMC Public Health*, *12*(1), 298. doi:10.1186/1471-2458-12-298 PMID:22520265

Rychoudhury, T., & Scheytt, T. (2013). Potential of zerovalent iron nanoparticles for remediation of environmental organic contaminants in water: A review. *Water Science and Technology*, *68*(7), 1425–1439. doi:10.2166/wst.2013.358 PMID:24135090

Ryu, W. H., Eom, J. Y., Yin, R. Z., Han, D. W., Kim, W. K., & Kwon, H. S. (2011). Synergistic effects of various morphologies and Al doping of spinel $LiMn_2O_4$ nanostructures on the electrochemical performance of lithium-rechargeable batteries. *Journal of Materials Chemistry*, *21*(39), 15337–15342. doi:10.1039/c1jm10146c

Saadeh, Y., & Vyas, D. (2014). Nanorobotic applications in medicine: Current proposals and designs. *American Journal of Robotic Surgery*, *1*(1), 4–11. doi:10.1166/ajrs.2014.1010 PMID:26361635

Sabir, S., Muhammad, A., & Chaudhari, S. K. (2014). Zinc Oxide Nanoparticles for Revolutionizing Agriculture: Synthesis and Applications, *Scientific World Journal. Article ID*, *925494*, 8. doi:10.1155/2014/925494 PMID:25436235

Sadeghi, B., Sarraf-Mamoory, R., & Shahverdi, H. R. (2012). The Effect of $LiFePO_4$ Coating on Electrochemical Performance of $LiMn_2O_4$ Cathode Material. *Iranian Journal of Chemistry and Chemical Engineering*, *31*(4), 29–33.

Sahoo, D., Mandal, A., Mitra, T., Chakraborty, K., Bardhan, M., & Dasgupta, A. K. (2018). Nanosensing of Pesticides by Zinc Oxide Quantum Dot: An Optical and Electrochemical Approach for the Detection of Pesticides in Water. *Journal of Agricultural and Food Chemistry*, *66*(2), 414–423. doi:10.1021/acs.jafc.7b04188 PMID:29239610

Sahoo, S. K., & Labhasetwar, V. (2003). Nanotech approaches to drug delivery and imaging. *Drug Discovery Today*, *8*(24), 1112–1120. doi:10.1016/S1359-6446(03)02903-9 PMID:14678737

Sahoo, S. K., Panyam, J., Prabha, S., & Labhasetwar, V. (2002). Residual polyvinyl alcohol associated with poly (d,l-lactide-co-glycolide) nanoparticles affects their physical properties and cellular uptake. *Journal of Controlled Release*, *82*(1), 105–114. doi:10.1016/S0168-3659(02)00127-X PMID:12106981

Sahoo, S. K., Parveen, S., & Panda, J. J. (2007). The present and future of nanotechnology in human health care. *Nanomedicine; Nanotechnology, Biology, and Medicine*, *3*(1), 20–31. doi:10.1016/j.nano.2006.11.008 PMID:17379166

Sahraei Khosh Gardesh, A., Badii, F., Hashemi, M., & Ardakani, A. YMaftoonazad, NGorji, A. M. (2016). Effect of nano-chitosan based coating on climacteric behavior and postharvest shelf-life extension of apple cv. *Golab Kohanz. Lebensmittel-Wissenschaft + Technologie*, *70*, 33–40.

Saifuddin, N. (2013). Carbon Nanotubes: A Review on Structure and Their Interaction with Proteins. *Journal of Chemistry. Article ID*, *676815*, 1–18.

Sailaja, G., Skountzou, I., Quan, F. S., Compans, R. W., & Kang, S. M. (2007). Human immunodeficiency virus like particles activate multiple types of immune cells. *Virology*, *362*(2), 331–341. doi:10.1016/j.virol.2006.12.014 PMID:17276476

Sait, H. H. (2018). Design and analysis of a flooded tube for cold energy storage. *International Journal of Refrigeration*, *94*, 151–160. doi:10.1016/j.ijrefrig.2018.07.018

Saito, G., Swanson, J. A., & Lee, K. D. (2003). Drug delivery strategy utilizing conjugation via reversible disulfide linkages: Role and site of cellular reducing activities. *Advanced Drug Delivery Reviews*, *55*(2), 199–215. doi:10.1016/S0169-409X(02)00179-5 PMID:12564977

Saji, V. S., Choe, H. C., & Young, K. W. K. (2010). Nanotechnology in biomedical applications—A review. *Int J Nano Biomater*, *3*(2), 119–139. doi:10.1504/IJNBM.2010.037801

Salant, A., Shalom, M., Hod, I., Faust, A., Zaban, A., & Banin, U. (2010). Quantum dot sensitized solar cells with improved efficiency prepared using electrophoretic deposition. *ACS Nano*, *4*(10), 5962–5968. doi:10.1021/nn1018208 PMID:20866044

Salata, O. V. (2004). Applications of nanoparticles in biology and medicine. *Journal of Nanobiotechnology*, *2*(1), 3.

Salavati-niasari, M., Davar, F., & Mir, N. (2008). Synthesis and characterization of metallic copper nanoparticles via thermal decomposition. *Polyhedron*, *27*(17), 3514–3518. doi:10.1016/j.poly.2008.08.020

Salem, E. H., Nawito, M A S., & El-Raouf Ahmed, A. E. A. (2019). Effect of Silver Nano-Particles on Gray Mold of Tomato Fruits. *Journal of Nanotechnology Research*, *1*, 108–118.

Salman, J. A. S., Ibrahem, K. H., & Ali, F. A. (2014). Effect of culture media on biosynthesis of titanium dioxide nanoparticles using Lactobacillus crispatus. *International Journal of Advanced Research*, *2*, 1014–1021.

Salouti, Mojtaba, Ahangari, & Azam. (2014). *Nanoparticle based Drug Delivery Systems for Treatment of Infectious Diseases, Application of Nanotechnology in Drug Delivery*. Academic Press.

Salvia-Trujillo, L., Rojas-Graü, M. A., Soliva-Fortuny, R., & Martín-Belloso, O. (2015). Use of antimicrobial nanoemulsions as edible coatings: Impact on safety and quality attributes of fresh-cut Fuji apples. *Postharvest Biology and Technology*, *105*, 8–16. doi:10.1016/j.postharvbio.2015.03.009

Salzemann, C., Lisiecki, I., Brioude, A., Urban, J., & Pileni, M. P. (2004). Collections of copper nanocrystals characterized by different sizes and shapes: Optical response of these nanoobjects. *The Journal of Physical Chemistry B*, *108*(35), 13242–13248. doi:10.1021/jp048491n

Samad, A., Sultana, Y., & Aqil, M. (2007). Liposomal drug delivery systems: Anul date review. *Current Drug Delivery*, *4*(4), 297–305. doi:10.2174/156720107782151269 PMID:17979650

Samanta, A., & Medintz, I. L. (2016). Nanoparticles and DNA – a powerful and growing functional combination in bionanotechnology. *Nanoscale*, *8*(17), 9037–9095.

Santhosh, C., Velmurugan, V., Jacob, G., Jeong, S. K., Grace, A. N., & Bhatnagar, A. (2016). Role of nanomaterials in water treatment applications: A review. *Chemical Engineering Journal*, *306*, 1116–1137. doi:10.1016/j.cej.2016.08.053

Santhoshkumar, T., Rahuman, A. A., Rajakumar, G., Marimuthu, S., Bagavan, A., Jayaseelan, C., Zahir, A. A., Elango, G., & Kamaraj, C. (2011). Synthesis of silver nanoparticles using Nelumbo nucifera leaf extract and its larvicidal activity against malaria and filariasis vectors. *Parasitology Research*, *108*(3), 693–702. doi:10.100700436-010-2115-4 PMID:20978795

Sapozhnikova, Y., & Lehotay, S. J. (2015). Review of recent developments and applications in low-pressure (vacuum outlet) gas chromatography. *Analytica Chimica Acta*, *899*, 13–22. doi:10.1016/j.aca.2015.10.003 PMID:26547491

Sapsford, K. E., Berti, L., & Medintz, I. L. (2006). Materials for fluorescence resonance energy transfer analysis: Beyond traditional donor–acceptor combinations. *Angewandte Chemie International Edition*, *45*(28), 4562–4589. doi:10.1002/anie.200503873 PMID:16819760

Sapsford, K. E., Bradburne, C., Delehanty, J. B., & Medintz, I. L. (2008). Sensors for detecting biological agents. *Materials Today*, *11*(3), 38–49. doi:10.1016/S1369-7021(08)70018-X

Saratale, R. G., Saratale, G. D., Shin, H. S., Jacob, J. M., Pugazhendhi, A., Bhaisare, M., & Kumar, G. (2018). New insights on the green synthesis of metallic nanoparticles using plant and waste biomaterials: Current knowledge, their agricultural and environmental applications. *Environmental Science and Pollution Research International*, *25*(11), 10164–10183. doi:10.100711356-017-9912-6 PMID:28815433

Sari, E., Üzek, R., Duman, M., & Denizli, A. (2016). Fabrication of surface plasmon resonance nanosensor for the selective determination of erythromycin via molecular imprinted nanoparticles. *Talanta*, *150*, 607–614. doi:10.1016/j.talanta.2015.12.043 PMID:26838449

Sari, E., Üzek, R., Duman, M., & Denizli, A. (2018). Detection of ciprofloxacin through surface plasmon resonance nanosensor with specific recognition sites. *Journal of Biomaterials Science. Polymer Edition, 29*(11), 1302–1318. doi:10.1080/09205063.2018.1457417 PMID:29607779

Sarwar, H., Khalid, H., Basher, M. K., Mia, M. N. H., Rahman, M. T., & Jalal Uddin, M. (2019). Smart nanocarrier-based drug delivery systems for cancer therapy and toxicity studies: A review. *Journal of Advanced Research, 15*, 1–18. doi:10.1016/j.jare.2018.06.005 PMID:30581608

Satija, J., Bharadwaj, R., Sai, V., & Mukherji, S. (2010). Emerging use of nanostructure films containing capped gold nanoparticles in biosensors. *Nanotechnology, Science and Applications, 3*, 171-88.

Sato, A. C. K., Quintas, M. A., Vincente, A. A., & Cunha, R. L. (2011). *Food Grade nanoparticles obtained from natural source ingredients.* Paper presented at the ICEF 11th International Congress on Engineering and Food.

Satyanarayana, T., & Sudhakar Reddy, S. (2018). A Review on Chemical and Physical Synthesis Methods of Nanomaterials. *International Journal for Research in Applied Science & Engineering Technology, 6*(1).

Saupe, A., McBurney, W., Rades, T., & Hook, S. (2006). Immunostimulatory colloidal delivery systems for cancer vaccines. *Expert Opinion on Drug Delivery, 3*(3), 345–354. doi:10.1517/17425247.3.3.345 PMID:16640495

Savolainen, K., Alenius, H., Norppa, H., Pylkkänen, L., Tuomi, T., & Kasper, G. (2010). Risk assessment of engineered nanomaterials and nanotechnologies—A review. *Toxicology, 269*(2-3), 92–104. doi:10.1016/j.tox.2010.01.013 PMID:20105448

Saxena, S. K., Nyodu, R., Kumar, S., & Maurya, V. K. (2020). Current advances in nanotechnology and medicine. In S. K. Saxena & S. M. P. Khurana (Eds.), *NanoBioMedicine* (pp. 3–16). Springer., doi:10.1007/978-981-32-9898-9_1

Saylan, Y., Akgönüllü, S., Çimen, D., Derazshamshir, A., Bereli, N., Yılmaz, F., & Denizli, A. (2017). Development of surface plasmon resonance sensors based on molecularly imprinted nanofilms for sensitive and selective detection of pesticides. *Sensors and Actuators. B, Chemical, 241*, 446–454. doi:10.1016/j.snb.2016.10.017

Saylan, Y., Yılmaz, F., Derazshamshir, A., Yılmaz, E., & Denizli, A. (2017). Synthesis of hydrophobic nanoparticles for real-time lysozyme detection using surface plasmon resonance sensor. *Journal of Molecular Recognition, 30*(9), e2631. doi:10.1002/jmr.2631 PMID:28322473

Say, R., Ersöz, A., Türk, H., & Denizli, A. (2004). Selective separation and preconcentration of cyanide by a column packed with cyanide-imprinted polymeric microbeads. *Separation and Purification Technology, 40*(1), 9–14. doi:10.1016/j.seppur.2003.12.021

Scarisoreanu, M., Morjan, I., Alexandrescu, R., Fleaca, C. T., Badoi, A., Dutu, E., ... Bouhadoun, S. (2014). Enhancing the visible light absorption of titania nanoparticles by S and C doping in a single-step process. *Applied Surface Science, 302*, 11–18. doi:10.1016/j.apsusc.2014.01.135

Schurig, D., Mock, J. J., & Smith, D. R. (2006). Electric-field-coupled resonators for negative permittivity metamaterials. *Applied Physics Letters, 88*(4), 1–3. doi:10.1063/1.2166681

Sclar, H., Haik, O., Menachem, T., Grinblat, J., Leifer, N., Meitav, A., Luski, S., & Aurbach, D. (2012). The effect of ZnO and MgO coatings by a sono-chemical method, on the stability of $LiMn_{1.5}Ni_{0.5}O_4$ as a cathode material for 5 V Li-ion batteries. *Journal of the Electrochemical Society, 159*(3), A228–A237. doi:10.1149/2.032203jes

Scrosati, B. (1995). Challenge of portable power. *Nature, 373*, 557–558.

Scrosati, B. (2007). Nanomaterials: Paper powers battery breakthrough. *Nature Nanotechnology, 2*(10), 598–599. doi:10.1038/nnano.2007.318 PMID:18654380

Scrosati, B., & Garche, J. (2010). Lithium batteries: Status, prospects and future. *Journal of Power Sources, 195*(9), 2419–2430. doi:10.1016/j.jpowsour.2009.11.048

Sekhon, B. S. (2010). *Nanotechnology, Science and Applications*. Academic Press. PMID:24198465

Sekhon, B. S. (2014). Nanotechnology in agri-food production: An overview. *Nanotechnology, Science and Applications, 7*, 31–53. doi:10.2147/NSA.S39406 PMID:24966671

Selin, C. (2007). Expectations and the Emergence of Nanotechnology. *Human Values, 32*(2), 196–220. doi:10.1177/0162243906296918

Selvolini, G., & Marrazza, G. (2017). MIP-based sensors: Promising new tools for cancer biomarker determination. *Sensors (Basel), 17*(4), 718. doi:10.339017040718 PMID:28353669

Senapati, T., Senapati, D., Singh, A. K., Fan, Z., Kanchanapally, R., & Ray, P. C. (2011). Highly selective SERS probe for Hg(ii) detection using tryptophan-protected popcorn shaped gold nanoparticles. *Chemical Communications (Cambridge), 47*(37), 10326–10328. doi:10.1039/c1cc13157e

Sener, G., Uzun, L., Say, R., & Denizli, A. (2011). Use of molecular imprinted nanoparticles as biorecognition element on surface plasmon resonance sensor. *Sensors and Actuators. B, Chemical, 160*(1), 791–799. doi:10.1016/j.snb.2011.08.064

Sengupta, S., Eavarone, D., Capila, I., Zhao, G., Watson, N., Kiziltepe, T., & Sasisekharan, R. (2005). Temporal targeting of tumour cells and neovasculature with a nanoscale delivery system. *Nature, 436*(7050), 568–572. doi:10.1038/nature03794 PMID:16049491

Senthilkumar, S. R., & Sivakumar, T. (2014). Green tea (Camelli sinensis) mediated synthesis of zinc oxide (ZnO) nanoparticles and studies on their antimicrobial activities. *International Journal of Pharmacy and Pharmaceutical Sciences, 6*, 461–465.

Service, R. F. (2005). Solar energy. Is it time to shoot for the sun? *Science, 309*(5734), 548–551. doi:10.1126cience.309.5734.548 PMID:16040683

Servin, A. D., & White, J. C. (2016). Nanotechnology in agriculture: Next steps for understanding engineered nanoparticle exposure and risk. *NanoImpact, 1*, 9–12. doi:10.1016/j.impact.2015.12.002

Shafiq, S. A., Al-Shammari, R. H., & Majeed, H. Z. (2016). Study of Biosynthesis silver nanoparticles by Fusarium graminaerum and test their antimicrobial activity. *International Journal of Innovation and Applied Studies, 15*, 4.

Shah, P., & Gavrin, A. (2006). Synthesis of nanoparticles using high-pressure sputtering for magnetic domain imaging. *Journal of Magnetism and Magnetic Materials, 301*(1), 118–123. doi:10.1016/j.jmmm.2005.06.023

Shah, S. W. A., Jahangir, M., Qaisar, M., Khan, S. A., Mahmood, T., Saeed, M., Farid, A., & Liaquat, M. (2015). Storage Stability of Kinnow Fruit (Citrus reticulata) as Affected by CMC and Guar Gum-Based Silver Nanoparticle Coatings. *Molecules (Basel, Switzerland), 2015*(20), 22645–22661. doi:10.3390/molecules201219870 PMID:26694344

Shaibani, A. R., Keshtkar, M. M., & Sardari, P. T. (2019). Thermo-economic analysis of a cold storage system in full and partial modes with two different scenarios: A case study. *Journal of Energy Storage, 24*, 100783. doi:10.1016/j.est.2019.100783

Shailesh, S., Neelam, S., Sandeep, K., & Gupta, G. D. (2009). Liposomes: A review. *Journal of Pharmacy Research, 2*, 1163–1167.

Shamaila, S., Zafar, N., Riaz, S., Sharif, R., Nazir, J., & Naseem, S. (2016). Gold nanoparticles: An efficient antimicrobial agent against enteric bacterial human pathogen. *Nanomater, 6*.

Shan, G., Xing, J., Zhang, H., & Liu, H. (2005). Biodesulfurization of Dibenzothiophene by Microbial Cells Coated with Magnetite Nanoparticles. *Applied and Environmental Microbiology*, *71*(8), 4497–4502. doi:10.1128/AEM.71.8.4497-4502.2005 PMID:16085841

Shao, Y. Y., Liu, J., Wang, Y., & Lin, Y. H. (2009). Novel catalyst support materials for PEMfuelcells: Current status and future prospects. *Journal of Materials Chemistry*, *19*(1), 46–49. doi:10.1039/B808370C

Shao, Y. Y., Yin, G. P., Wang, J. J., Gao, Y. Z., & Shi, P. F. (2006). Multi-walled carbon nanotubes based Pt electrodes prepared with in situ ion exchange method for oxygen reduction. *Journal of Power Sources*, *161*(1), 47–53. doi:10.1016/j.jpowsour.2006.03.064

Sharma, V. K., Filip, J., Zboril, R., & Varma, R. S. (2015). Natural inorganic nanoparticles—Formation, fate, and toxicity in the environment. *Chemical Society Reviews*, *44*(23), 8410–8423. doi:10.1039/C5CS00236B PMID:26435358

Sharp, G. J., Khan, S. I., Khokhar, A. Z., De La Rue, R. M., & Johnson, N. P. (2014). Negative index fishnet with nanopillars formed by direct nano-imprint lithography. *Materials Research Express*, *1*(4), 045802-1-045802–045811. doi:10.1088/2053-1591/1/4/045802

Shelby, R. A., Smith, D. R., & Schultz, S. (2001). Experimental verification of a negative index of refraction. *Science*, *292*(April), 77–79. doi:10.1126cience.1058847 PMID:11292865

Shellhart, W. C., & Oesterle, L. J. (1999). Uprighting molars without extrusion. *The Journal of the American Dental Association*, *130*(3), 381–385. doi:10.14219/jada.archive.1999.0208 PMID:10085661

Shi, F., Zhou, X., Yao, M.-M., Tan, Z., Zhou, Q., Zhang, L., & Ji, S.-J. (2018). miRNAs play important roles in aroma weakening during the shelf life of 'Nanguo' pear after cold storage. *Energy Research*, *116*, 942–952. PMID:30717027

Shi, J. Y., Yi, C. W., & Kim, K. (2010). Improved electrochemical performance of $AlPO_4$-coated $LiMn_{1.5}Ni_{0.5}O_4$ electrode for lithium-ion batteries. *Journal of Power Sources*, *195*(19), 6860–6866. doi:10.1016/j.jpowsour.2010.02.063

Shi, M., Lan, F., Mazumder, P., Aghadjani, M., Yang, Z., Meng, L., & Zhou, J. (2018). Enhanced quadruple-resonant terahertz metamaterial with asymmetric hybrid resonators. *Optical Materials*, *75*, 533–537. doi:10.1016/j.optmat.2017.11.011

Shi, S., Wang, W., Liu, L., Wu, S., Wei, Y., & Li, W. (2013). Effect of chitosan/nano-silica coating on the physicochemical characteristics of longan fruit under ambient temperature. *Journal of Food Engineering*, *118*(1), 125–131. doi:10.1016/j.jfoodeng.2013.03.029

Shobha, G., Moses, V., & Ananda, S. (2014). Biological synthesis of copper nanoparticles and its impact. *International Journal of Pharmaceutical Science Invention*, *3*(8), 6–28.

Shukla, S. K., Kumar, R., Mishra, R. K., Pandey, A., Pathak, A., Zaidi, M. G. H., Srivastava, S. K., & Dikshit, A. (2015). Prediction and validation of gold nanoparticles (GNPs) on plant growth promoting rhizobacteria (PGPR): A step toward development of nano-biofertilizers. *Nanotechnology Reviews*, *4*(5), 439–448. doi:10.1515/ntrev-2015-0036

Shvedova, A. A., Kisin, E. R., Mercer, R., Murray, A. R., Johnson, V. J., & Potapovich, A. I. (2005). Unusual inflammatory and fibrogenic pulmonary responses to singlewalled carbon nanotubes in mice. *Am J Physiol Cell Mol Physiol.*, *289*, L698–708. . doi:10.1152/ajplung.00084.2005

Shvedova, A. A., Castranova, V., Kisin, E. R., Schwegler-Berry, D., Murray, A. R., Gandelsman, V. Z., Maynard, A., & Baron, P. (2003). Exposure to carbon nanotube material: Assessment of nanotube cytotoxicity using human keratinocyte cells. *Journal of Toxicology and Environmental Health. Part A.*, *66*(20), 1909–1926. doi:10.1080/713853956 PMID:14514433

Siddiqi, K. S., & Husen, A. (2016). Fabrication of metal and metal oxide nanoparticles by algae and their toxic effects. *Nanoscale Research Letters*, *11*(1), 363. doi:10.118611671-016-1580-9 PMID:27530743

Siddiqi, K. S., Husen, A., & Rao, R. A. K. (2018). A Review on Biosynthesis of Silver Nanoparticles and Their Biocidal Properties. *Journal of Nanobiotechnology*, *16*(1), 14. doi:10.118612951-018-0334-5 PMID:29452593

Siddiqui, I. A., & Sanna, V. (2016). Impact of nanotechnology on the delivery of natural products for cancer prevention and therapy. *Molecular Nutrition & Food Research*, *60*(6), 1330–1341. doi:10.1002/mnfr.201600035 PMID:26935239

Siegrist, M., Cousin, M.-E., Kastenholz, H., & Wiek, A. (2007). Public acceptance of nanotechnology foods and food packaging: The influence of affect and trust. *Appetite*, *49*(2), 459–466.

Sies, H. (1999). Glutathione and its role in cellular functions. *Free Radical Biology & Medicine*, *27*(9-10), 916–921. doi:10.1016/S0891-5849(99)00177-X PMID:10569624

Sikder, M. A. A., Kaisar, M. A., & Parvez, M. M., Hossian, A. N., Akhter, F., & Rashid, M. A. (2011). Preliminary antimicrobial activity and cytotoxicity of leaf extracts of Mesua nagassarium (Burm. f.). *Boletín Latinoamericano y del Caribe de Plantas Medicinales y Aromáticas*, *10*(1), 83–87.

silver-polyvinyl pyrrolidone (Ag-PVP) nanoparticles in mouse macrophages infected with live Chlamydia trachomatis. *Int. J. Nanomed.*, *8*, 2421–2432.

Silvestre, C., Duraccio, D., & Cimmino, S. (2011). Food packaging based on polymer nanomaterials. *Progress in Polymer Science*, *36*(12), 1766–1782.

Sim, M. S., You, K. Y., & Esa, F. (2017). Broadband metamaterial microwave absorber for X-Ku band usingplanar split ring-slot structures. *Progress in Electromagnetics Research Symposium-Fall (PIERS-FALL)*, 215–221. 10.1109/PIERS-FALL.2017.8293138

Sim, M. S., You, K. Y., & Esa, F. (2020). Electromagnetic metamaterials in microwave regime. In Handbook of Research on Recent Developments in Electrical and Mechanical Engineering (pp. 64–86). doi:10.4018/978-1-7998-0117-7.ch002

Sim, M. S., You, K. Y., Esa, F., Dimon, M. N., & Khamis, N. H. (2018). Multiband metamaterial microwave absorbers using split ring and multiwidth slot structure. *International Journal of RF and Microwave Computer-Aided Engineering*, *28*(7), 1–13. doi:10.1002/mmce.21473

Simon, P., Chaudhry, Q., & Bakos, D. (2008). Migration of engineered nanoparticles from polymer packaging to food - a physicochemical view. *Journal of Food and Nutrition Research*, *47*(3), 105–113.

Singhal, G., Bhavesh, R., Kasariya, K., Sharma, A. R., & Singh, R. P. (2011). Biosynthesis of silver nanoparticles using Ocimum sanctum (Tulsi) leaf extract and screening its antimicrobial activity. *Journal of Nanoparticle Research*, *13*(7), 2981–2988. doi:10.100711051-010-0193-y

Singhal, R., Das, S. R., Tomar, M. S., Ovideo, O., Nieto, S., Melgarejo, R. E., & Katiyar, R. S. (2007). Synthesis and characterization of Nd doped $LiMn_2O_4$ cathode for Li-ion rechargeable batteries. *Journal of Power Sources*, *164*(2), 857–861. doi:10.1016/j.jpowsour.2006.09.098

Singh, D., Gautam, R. K., Kumar, R., Shukla, B. K., Shankar, V., & Krishna, V. (2014). Citric acid coated magnetic nanoparticles: Synthesis, characterization and application in removal of Cd (II) ions from aqueous solution. *Journal of Water Process Engineering*, *4*, 233–241. doi:10.1016/j.jwpe.2014.10.005

Singh, M., Manikandan, S., & Kumaraguru, A. K. (2011). Nanoparticles: A new technology with wide applications. *Res. J. Nanosci. Nanotechnol.*, *1*(1), 1–11. doi:10.3923/rjnn.2011.1.11

Singh, P., Sil, A., Nath, M. A. L. A., & Ray, S. (2010). Synthesis and characterisation of Li $(Mn_{2-X}mg_x)o_4$(x= 0. 0-0. 3) prepared by sol-gel synthesis. *Ceramics-Silikáty*, *54*(1), 38–46.

Singh, P., Sil, A., Nath, M., & Ray, S. (2009). Preparation and Characterization of Li $(Mn_{2-x}Fe_x)O_4$ (x= 0.0-0.6) Spinel Nanoparticles as Cathode Materials for Lithium Ion Battery. (). Trans Tech Publications.). *Advanced Materials Research*, *67*, 233–238. doi:10.4028/www.scientific.net/AMR.67.233

Singh, R., Misra, V., & Singh, R. P. (2012). Removal of hexavalent chromium from contaminated ground water using zerovalent iron nanoparticles. *Environmental Monitoring and Assessment*, *184*(6), 3643–3651. doi:10.100710661-011-2213-5 PMID:21769560

Singh, R., Nawale, L. U., Arkile, M., Shedbalkar, U. U., Wadhwani, S. A., Sarkar, D., & Chopade, B. A. (2015). Chemical and biological metal nanoparticles as antimycobacterial agents: A comparative study. *International Journal of Antimicrobial Agents*, *46*(2), 183–188. doi:10.1016/j.ijantimicag.2015.03.014 PMID:26009020

Singh, S. C., & Gopal, R. (2007). Zinc nanoparticles in solution by laser ablation technique. *Bulletin of Materials Science*, *30*(3), 291–293. doi:10.100712034-007-0048-z

Singh, S., Dhanjal, D. S., Thotapalli, S., Kumar, V., Datta, S., Kumar, V., Kumar, M., & Singh, J. (2020). An insight in bacteriophage based biosensors with focus on their detection methods and recent advancements. *Environmental Technology & Innovation*, *20*, 101081. doi:10.1016/j.eti.2020.101081

Sitaaraman, S. R., Santhosh, R., Kollu, P., Jeong, S. K., Sellappan, R., Raghavan, V., ... Grace, A. N. (2020). Role of graphene in NiSe2/graphene composites-Synthesis and testing for electrochemical supercapacitors. *Diamond and Related Materials*.

Situ, C., Mooney, M. H., Elliott, C. T., & Buijs, J. (2010). Advances in surface plasmon resonance biosensor technology towards high-throughput, food-safety analysis. *Trends in Analytical Chemistry*, *29*(11), 1305–1315. doi:10.1016/j.trac.2010.09.003

Skirtach, A. G., Munoz Javier, A., Kreft, O., Köhler, K., Piera Alberola, A., Möhwald, H., Parak, W. J., & Sukhorukov, G. B. (2006). Laser-induced release of encapsulated materials inside living cells. *Angewandte Chemie International Edition*, *45*(28), 4612–4617. doi:10.1002/anie.200504599 PMID:16791887

Slavkin, H. C. (1999). Entering the era of molecular dentistry. *The Journal of the American Dental Association*, *130*(3), 413–417. doi:10.14219/jada.archive.1999.0212 PMID:10085665

Slupetzky, K., Gambhira, R., Culp, T. D., Shafti Keramat, S., Schellenbacher, C., Christensen, N. D., Roden, R. B. S., & Kirnbauer, R. (2007). A papilloma virus like particle (VLP) vaccine displaying HPV 16 L2 epitopes induces cross neutralizing antibodies to HPV 11. *Vaccine*, *25*(11), 2001–2010. doi:10.1016/j.vaccine.2006.11.049 PMID:17239496

Smekalova, M., Aragon, V., Panacek, A., Prucek, R., Zboril, R., & Kvitek, L. (2016). Enhanced antibacterial effect of antibiotics in combination with silver nanoparticles against animal pathogens. *Veterinary Journal (London, England)*, *209*, 174–179. doi:10.1016/j.tvjl.2015.10.032 PMID:26832810

Smith, D. M., Simon, J. K., & Baker, J. R. Jr. (2013). Applications of nanotechnology for immunology. *Nature Reviews. Immunology*, *13*(8), 592–605. doi:10.1038/nri3488 PMID:23883969

Smith, D. R., Padilla, W. J., Vier, D. C., & Schultz, S. (2000). Composite Medium with Simultaneously Negative Permeability and Permittivity. *Physical Review Letters*, *84*(18), 1–4. doi:10.1103/PhysRevLett.84.4184 PMID:10990641

Smolander, M., Hurme, E., Koivisto, M., & Kivinen, S. (2004). *Indicator*. International Patent WO2004/102185 A1.

Sohail, M. I., Waris, A. A., Ayub, M. A., Usman, M., Rehman, M. Z., Sabir, M., & Faiz, T. (2019). Article. *Comprehensive Analytical Chemistry*, 1–54.

Soheilifar, M. R., & Sadeghzadeh, R. A. (2015). Design, fabrication and characterisation of scaled and stacked layers planar metamaterial absorber. *IET Microwaves, Antennas & Propagation*, *9*(1), 86–93. doi:10.1049/iet-map.2014.0350

Sonaje, K., Chuang, E.-Y., Lin, K.-J., Yen, T.-C., Su, F.-Y., Tseng, M. T., & Sung, H.-W. (2012). Opening of epithelial tight junctions and enhancement of paracellular permeation by chitosan: Microscopic, ultrastructural, and computed-tomographic observations. *Molecular Pharmaceutics*, *9*(5), 1271–1279. doi:10.1021/mp200572t PMID:22462641

Song, A.-X., Mao, Y.-H., Siu, K.-C., Tai, W. C. S., & Wu, J.-Y. (2019). Protective effects of exopolysaccharide of a medicinal fungus on probiotic bacteria during cold storage and simulated gastrointestinal conditions. *International Journal of Biological Macromolecules*, *133*, 957–963. doi:10.1016/j.ijbiomac.2019.04.108 PMID:31028812

Song, H., Yuan, W., Jin, P., Wang, W., Wang, X., Yang, L., & Zhang, Y. (2016). Effects of chitosan/nano-silica on postharvest quality and antioxidant capacity of loquat fruit during cold storage. *Postharvest Biology and Technology*, *119*, 41–48. doi:10.1016/j.postharvbio.2016.04.015

Song, M. Y., Ahn, Y. R., Jo, S. M., Kim, D. Y., & Ahn, J.-P. (2005). TiO_2 single-crystalline nanorod electrode for quasi-solid-state dye-sensitized solar cells. *Applied Physics Letters*, *87*(11), 113113. doi:10.1063/1.2048816

Song, T., Xia, J., Lee, J.-H., Lee, D. H., Kwon, M.-S., Choi, J.-M., Wu, J., Doo, S. K., Chang, H., Park, W. I., Zang, D. S., Kim, H., Huang, Y., Hwang, K.-C., Rogers, J. A., & Paik, U. (2010). Arrays of sealed silicon nanotubes as anodes for lithium ion batteries. *Nano Letters*, *10*(5), 1710–1716. doi:10.1021/nl100086e PMID:20369889

Song, X., Sun, S., Zhang, W., & Yin, Z. (2004). A method for the synthesis of spherical copper nanoparticles in the organic phase. *Journal of Colloid and Interface Science*, *273*(2), 463–469. doi:10.1016/j.jcis.2004.01.019 PMID:15082381

Son, J. T., Park, K. S., Kim, H. G., & Chung, H. T. (2004). Surface-modification of $LiMn_2O_4$ with a silver-metal coating. *Journal of Power Sources*, *126*(1), 182–185. doi:10.1016/j.jpowsour.2003.07.010

Sonkaew, P., Sane, A., & Suppakul, P. (2012). Antioxidant activities of curcumin and ascorbyl dipalmitate nanoparticles and their activities after incorporation into cellulose-based packaging films. *Journal of Agricultural and Food Chemistry*, *60*(21), 5388–5399.

Sonkaria, S., Ahn, S.-H., & Khare, V. (2012). *Recent Patents on Food, Nutrition & Agriculture*. Academic Press. PMID:22316269

Soper, S. A., Brown, K., Ellington, A., Frazier, B., Garcia-Manero, G., Gau, V., Gutman, S. I., Hayes, D. F., Korte, B., Landers, J. L., Larson, D., Ligler, F., Majumdar, A., Mascini, M., Nolte, D., Rosenzweig, Z., Wang, J., & Wilson, D. (2006). Point-of-care biosensor systems for cancer diagnostics/prognostics. *Biosensors & Bioelectronics*, *21*(10), 1932–1942. doi:10.1016/j.bios.2006.01.006 PMID:16473506

Sosnik, A., Carcaboso, A. M., Glisoni, R. J., Moretton, M. A., & Chiappetta, D. A. (2010). New old challenges in tuberculosis: Potentially effective nanotechnologies in drug delivery. *Advanced Drug Delivery Reviews*, *62*(4-5), 547–559. doi:10.1016/j.addr.2009.11.023 PMID:19914315

Souery, W. N., & Bishop, C. J. (2018). Clinically advancing and promising polymer-based therapeutics. *Acta Biomaterialia*, *67*, 1–20. doi:10.1016/j.actbio.2017.11.044 PMID:29246651

Sparreboom, A., Scripture, C. D., Trieu, V., Williams, P. J., De, T., Yang, A., ... Desai, N. (2005). Comparative preclinical and clinical pharmacokinetics of a cremophor-free, nanoparticle albumin-bound paclitaxel (ABI-007) and paclitaxel formulated in Cremophor (Taxol). *Clinical Cancer Research*, *11*(11), 4136–4143. doi:10.1158/1078-0432.CCR-04-2291 PMID:15930349

Sperling, R. A., Gil, P. R., Zhang, F., Zanella, M., & Parak, W. J. (2008). Biological applications of gold nanoparticles. *Chemical Society Reviews*, *37*(9), 1896–1908. doi:10.1039/b712170a PMID:18762838

Sreekanth, K. V., Alapan, Y., Elkabbash, M., Ilker, E., Hinczewski, M., Gurkan, U. A., De Luca, A., & Strangi, G. (2016a). Extreme sensitivity biosensing platform based on hyperbolic metamaterials. *Nature Materials*, *15*(6), 621–627. doi:10.1038/nmat4609 PMID:27019384

Sreekanth, K. V., Alapan, Y., ElKabbash, M., Wen, A. M., Ilker, E., Hinczewski, M., Gurkan, U. A., Steinmetz, N. F., & Strangi, G. (2016b). Enhancing the angular sensitivity of plasmonic sensors using hyperbolic metamaterials. *Advanced Optical Materials*, *4*(11), 1767–1772. doi:10.1002/adom.201600448 PMID:28649484

Sreethawong, T., Ngamsinlapasathian, S., & Yoshikawa, S. (2013). Facile surfactant-aided sol–gel synthesis of mesoporous-assembled Ta2O5 nanoparticles with enhanced photocatalytic H2 production. *Journal of Molecular Catalysis A Chemical*, *374*, 94–101. doi:10.1016/j.molcata.2013.04.003

Srinivasan, K., Samuel, E. J. J., Poopathi, V., & Grace, A. N. (2019). Investigation on energy dependency of dose enhancement factor produced by gold nanoparticle. *Materials Today: Proceedings*, *9*, 446–449. doi:10.1016/j.matpr.2019.02.174

Stampoulis, D., Sinha, S. K., & White, J. C. (2009). Assay-Dependent Phytotoxicity of Nanoparticles to Plants. *Environmental Science & Technology*, *43*(24), 9473–9479. doi:10.1021/es901695c PMID:19924897

Stasyuk, N., Gayda, G., Zakalskiy, A., Zakalska, O., Serkiz, R., & Gonchar, M. (2019). Amperometric biosensors based on oxidases and PtRu nanoparticles as artificial peroxidase. *Food Chemistry*, *285*(January), 213–220. doi:10.1016/j.foodchem.2019.01.117 PMID:30797337

Steiner, G. (2004). Surface plasmon resonance imaging. *Analytical and Bioanalytical Chemistry*, *379*(3), 328–331. doi:10.100700216-004-2636-8 PMID:15127177

Stigter, E. C. A., De Jong, G. J., & Van Bennekom, W. P. (2005). An improved coating for the isolation and quantitation of interferon-γ in spiked plasma using surface plasmon resonance (SPR). *Biosensors & Bioelectronics*, *21*(3), 474–482. doi:10.1016/j.bios.2004.11.008 PMID:16076437

Stoller, M. D., Park, S., Zhu, Y., An, J., & Ruoff, R. S. (2008). (. Graphene-based ultracapacitors. *Nano Letters*, *8*(10), 3498–3502. doi:10.1021/nl802558y PMID:18788793

Strangi, G., Sreekanth, K. V., & Elkabbash, M. (2017). Hyperbolic metamaterial-based ultrasensitive plasmonic biosensors for early-stage cancer detection. In Next Generation Point-of-care Biomedical Sensors Technologies for Cancer Diagnosis (pp. 155–172). doi:10.1007/978-981-10-4726-8_7

Strasfeld, L., & Chou, S. (2010). Antiviral drug resistance: Mechanisms and clinical implications. *Infectious Disease Clinics of North America*, *24*(3), 809–833. doi:10.1016/j.idc.2010.07.001 PMID:20674805

Stritih, U., & Butala, V. (2007). Energy saving in building with PCM cold storage. *International Journal of Energy Research*, *31*(15), 1532–1544. doi:10.1002/er.1318

Stroh, M., Zimmer, J. P., Duda, D. G., Levchenko, T. S., Cohen, K. S., Brown, E. B., Scadden, D. T., Torchilin, V. P., Bawendi, M. G., Fukumura, D., & Jain, R. K. (2005). Quantum dots spectrally distinguish multiple species within the tumor milieu in vivo. *Nature Medicine*, *11*(6), 678–682. doi:10.1038/nm1247 PMID:15880117

Stuart, H. R., & Hall, D. G. (1998). Island size effects in nanoparticle-enhanced photodetectors. *Applied Physics Letters, 73*(26), 3815–3817. doi:10.1063/1.122903

Stylianakis, M.M., Konios, D., Petridis, C., Kakavelakis, G., Stratakis, E., Kymakis, E. (2017). Ternary solution-processed organic solar cells incorporating 2D materials. *2D Mater., 4*, 042005.

Subhankari, I., & Nayak, P. L. (2013). Antimicrobial activity of copper nanoparticles synthesised by ginger (Zingiber officinale) extract. *World J. Nano Sci. Technol., 2*, 10–13.

Sudakaran, S. V., Venugopal, J. R., Vijayakumar, G. P., Abisegapriyan, S., Grace, A. N., & Ramakrishna, S. (2017). Sequel of MgO nanoparticles in PLACL nanofibers for anti-cancer therapy in synergy with curcumin/β-cyclodextrin. *Materials Science and Engineering C, 71*, 620–628. doi:10.1016/j.msec.2016.10.050 PMID:27987753

Su, F. B., Zeng, J., Bao, X., Yu, Y., Lee, J. Y., & Zhao, X. S. (2005). Preparation and characterization of highly ordered graphitic mesoporous as a Pt catalyst support for direct methanol fuel cells. *Chemistry of Materials, 17*(15), 3960–3967. doi:10.1021/cm0502222

Sugan, A., & Dutta, J. (2004). Nanoparticles for nanotechnology. *PSI Jilid, 50.*

Sugumaran, S., Jamlos, M. F., Ahmad, M. N., Bellan, C. S., & Schreurs, D. (2018). Nanostructured materials with plasmonic nanobiosensors for early cancer detection: A past and future prospect. *Biosensors & Bioelectronics, 100*, 361–373. doi:10.1016/j.bios.2017.08.044 PMID:28946108

Sun, A., Chai, J., Xiao, T., Shi, X., Li, X., Zhao, Q., Li, D., & Chen, J. (2018). Development of a selective fluorescence nanosensor based on molecularly imprinted-quantum dot optosensing materials for saxitoxin detection in shellfish samples. *Sensors and Actuators. B, Chemical, 258*, 408–414. doi:10.1016/j.snb.2017.11.143

Sundar, S., Prajapati, V. K. (2012). Drug targeting to infectious diseases by nanoparticles surface functionalized with special biomolecules. *Curr Med Chem., 1*(19), 3196–3202.

Sun, H., Chen, Y., Xu, C., Zhu, D., & Huang, L. (2012). Electrochemical performance of rare-earth doped $LiMn_2O_4$ spinel cathode materials for Li-ion rechargeable battery. *Journal of Solid State Electrochemistry, 16*(3), 1247–1254. doi:10.100710008-011-1514-5

Sunkar, S., & Nachiyar, C. V. (2012). Biogenesis of antibacterial silver nanoparticles using the endophytic bacterium Bacillus cereus isolated from Garcinia xanthochymu. *Asian Pacific Journal of Tropical Biomedicine, 12*(12), 953–959. doi:10.1016/S2221-1691(13)60006-4 PMID:23593575

Sun, Q. H., Radosz, M., & Shen, Y. Q. (2012). Challenges in Design of Translational Nanocarriers. *Journal of Controlled Release, 164*(2), 156–169. doi:10.1016/j.jconrel.2012.05.042 PMID:22664472

Sun, Q. H., Sun, X. R., Ma, X. P., Zhou, Z. X., Jin, E. L., Zhang, B., Shen, Y. Q., Van Kirk, E. A., Murdoch, W. J., Lott, J. R., Lodge, T. P., Radosz, M., & Zhao, Y. L. (2014). Integration of Nanoassembly Functions for an Effective Delivery Cascade for Cancer Drugs. *Advanced Materials, 26*(45), 7615–7621. doi:10.1002/adma.201401554 PMID:25328159

Sun, T., Zhang, Y. S., Pang, B., Hyun, D. C., Yang, M., & Xia, Y. (2014). Engineered nanoparticles for drug delivery in cancer therapy. *Angewandte Chemie International Edition, 53*(46), 12320–12364. doi:10.1002/anie.201403036 PMID:25294565

Sun, Y., Fang, L., Wan, Y., & Gu, Z. (2018). Pathogenic detection and phenotype using magnetic nanoparticle-urease nanosensor. *Sensors and Actuators. B, Chemical, 259*, 428–432. doi:10.1016/j.snb.2017.12.095

Sun, Y., Singh, Z., Tokala, V. Y., & Heather, B. (2019). Harvest maturity stage and cold storage period influence lemon fruit quality. *Scientia Horticulturae, 249*, 322–328. doi:10.1016/j.scienta.2019.01.056

Suryakala, K., Marikkannu, K. R., Kalaignan, G. P., & Vasudevan, T. (2008). Synthesis and electrochemical characterization of LiMn2O4 and LiNd0. 3Mn1. 7O4 as cathode for lithium ion battery. *International Journal of Electrochemical Science, 3*, 136–144.

Sutradhar, K. B., & Amin, M. L. (2014). Nanotechnology in cancer drug delivery and selective targeting. *ISRN Nanotechnology*. doi. doi:Org /10.1155 / 2014 / 939378

Suvith, V. S., & Philip, D. (2014). Catalytic degradation of methylene blue using biosynthesized gold and silver nanoparticles. *Spectrochimica Acta. Part A: Molecular and Biomolecular Spectroscopy, 118*, 526–532. doi:10.1016/j.saa.2013.09.016 PMID:24091344

Su, X. D., Zhao, J. Z., Bala, H., Zhu, Y. C., Gao, Y., Ma, S. S., & Wang, Z. C. J. (2007). Article. *PhysChemComm, 111*(40), 14689–1469.

Swamy, M. K., & Sinniah, U. R. (2016). Patchouli (Pogostemon Cablin Benth.): Botany, agrotechnology, and biotechnological aspects. *Industrial Crops and Products, 87*, 161–176. doi:10.1016/j.indcrop.2016.04.032

Swierczewska, M., Han, H., Kim, K., Park, J., & Lee, S. (2016). Polysaccharide-based nanoparticles for theranostic nanomedicine. *Advanced Drug Delivery Reviews, 99*, 70–84. doi:10.1016/j.addr.2015.11.015 PMID:26639578

Syedmoradi, L., Daneshpour, M., Alvandipour, M., Gomez, F. A., Hajghassem, H., & Omidfar, K. (2017). Point of care testing: The impact of nanotechnology. *Biosensors & Bioelectronics, 87*, 373–387. doi:10.1016/j.bios.2016.08.084 PMID:27589400

Sykiotis, G. P., & Bohmann, D. (2008). Keap1/Nrf2 signaling regulates oxidative stress tolerance and lifespan in Drosophila. *Developmental Cell, 14*(1), 76–85. doi:10.1016/j.devcel.2007.12.002 PMID:18194654

Szentirmay, Z. (1992). Surface plasmon spectroscopy of metal/dielectric structures. *Spectrochimica Acta. Part A: Molecular Spectroscopy, 48*(1), 9–17. doi:10.1016/0584-8539(92)80192-Y

Taatjes, D. J., Schrader, M., Koji, T., & Roth, J. (2019). *Histochemistry and Cell Biology: 61 years and not tired at all.* Academic Press.

Tai, C. Y., Tai, C., Chang, M., & Liu, H. (2007). *Synthesis of Magnesium Hydroxide and Oxide Nanoparticles Using a Spinning Disk Reactor.* Academic Press.

Takamura, S., Niikura, M., Li, T. C., Takeda, N., Kusagawa, S., Takebe, Y., Miyamura, T., & Yasutomi, Y. (2004). DNA vaccine encapsulated virus like particles derived from an orally transmissible virus stimulate mucosal and systemic immune responses by oral administration. *Gene Therapy, 11*(7), 628–635. doi:10.1038j.gt.3302193 PMID:14973544

Takeuchi, H., Yamamoto, H., & Kawashima, Y. (2001). Mucoadhesive nanoparticulate systems for peptide drug delivery. *Advanced Drug Delivery Reviews, 47*(1), 39–54. doi:10.1016/S0169-409X(00)00120-4 PMID:11251244

Tallury, P., Malhotra, A., Byrne, L., & Santra, S. (2010). Nanobioimaging and sensing of infectious diseases. *Advanced Drug Delivery Reviews, 62*(4-5), 424–437. doi:10.1016/j.addr.2009.11.014 PMID:19931579

Talukdar, S., Afroz, H. M. M., Hossain, M. A., Aziz, M., & Hossain, M. M. (2019). Heat transfer enhancement of charging and discharging of phase change materials and size optimization of a latent thermal energy storage system for solar cold storage application. *Journal of Energy Storage, 24*, 100797. doi:10.1016/j.est.2019.100797

Tanaka, T., & Ishikawa, A. (2017). Towards three-dimensional optical metamaterials. *Nano Convergence, 4*(1), 34-1-34–39. doi:10.118640580-017-0129-7

Tanaka, S., Nishi, M., Yamaguchi, M., Bataev, I., & Hokamoto, K. (2020). Simultaneous Initiation of Nitromethane in Two Holes by Pulsed Wire Discharge for Crack Control of a Concrete Block. *Journal of Dynamic Behavior of Materials*, *6*(1), 53–63. doi:10.100740870-019-00227-6

Tang, S. B., Lai, M. O., & Lu, L. (2006). Properties of nano-crystalline $LiMn_2O_4$ thin films deposited by pulsed laser deposition. *Electrochimica Acta*, *52*(3), 1161–1168. doi:10.1016/j.electacta.2006.07.014

Tang, W., Wang, X. J., Hou, Y. Y., Li, L. L., Sun, H., Zhu, Y. S., Bai, Y., Wu, Y. P., Zhu, K., & Van Ree, T. (2012). Nano $LiMn_2O_4$ as cathode material of high rate capability for lithium ion batteries. *Journal of Power Sources*, *198*, 308–311. doi:10.1016/j.jpowsour.2011.09.106

Tang, X., Tan, L., Shi, K., Peng, J., Xiao, Y., Li, W., Chen, L., Yang, Q., & Qian, Z. (2018). Gold nanorods together with HSP inhibitor-VER-155008 micelles for colon cancer mild-temperature photothermal therapy. *Acta Pharmaceutica Sinica. B*, *8*(4), 587–601. doi:10.1016/j.apsb.2018.05.011 PMID:30109183

Taniguchi, N. (1974). On the basic concept of nano-technology. *Proc. Intl. Conf. Prod. Eng. Tokyo, Part II, 10*, 5-10.

Tao, H., Brenckle, M. A., Yang, M., Zhang, J., Liu, M., Siebert, S. M., Averitt, R. D., Mannoor, M. S., McAlpine, M. C., Rogers, J. A., Kaplan, D. L., & Omenetto, F. G. (2012). Silk-based conformal, adhesive, edible food sensors. *Advanced Materials*, *24*(8), 1067–1072. doi:10.1002/adma.201103814 PMID:22266768

Tarascon, J.-M., & Armand, M. (2001). Issues and challenges facing rechargeable lithium batteries. *Nature*, *414*(6861), 359–367. doi:10.1038/35104644 PMID:11713543

Tarnawski, R., & Ulbricht, M. (2011). Amphiphilic gold nanoparticles: Synthesis, characterization and adsorption to PEGylated polymer surfaces. *Colloids and Surfaces. A, Physicochemical and Engineering Aspects*, *374*(1-3), 13–21. doi:10.1016/j.colsurfa.2010.10.027

Taylor, A. D., Ladd, J., Yu, Q., Chen, S., Homola, J., & Jiang, S. (2006). Quantitative and simultaneous detection of four foodborne bacterial pathogens with a multi-channel SPR sensor. *Biosensors & Bioelectronics*, *22*(5), 752–758. doi:10.1016/j.bios.2006.03.012 PMID:16635568

Temmerman, R., Huys, G., & Swings, J. (2004). Identification of lactic acid bacteria: Culture-dependent and culture-independent methods. *Trends in Food Science & Technology*, *15*(7–8), 348–359. doi:10.1016/j.tifs.2003.12.007

Thackeray, M. M. (1997). Manganese oxides for lithium batteries. *Progress in Solid State Chemistry*, *25*(1), 1–71. doi:10.1016/S0079-6786(97)81003-5

Thakur, H., Nirmala Grace, A., & Vimala, R. (2015). Biosorption of di-butyl phthalate from aqueous solutions using Pleurotus ostreatus: Isotherm and Kinetic study. *Journal of Chemical and Pharmaceutical Research*, *7*(4), 697–706.

The European Commission, Commission Regulation (EU) No 10/2011 of 14 January. (2011). 2011 on plastic materials and articles intended to come into contact with food Text with EEA relevance Official J. *European Union*, *12*, 1–89.

Theron, J., Walker, J.A., & Cloete, T.E. (2008). Nanotechnology and water treatment: applications and emerging opportunities. *Critical Reviews in Microbiology, 34*(1), 43-69.

Thirumurugan, G., Rao, J. S., & Dhanaraju, M. D. (2016). Elucidating pharmacodynamic interaction of silver nanoparticle-topical deliverable antibiotics. *Scientific Reports*, *6*(1), 29982. doi:10.1038rep29982 PMID:27427207

Thirunakaran, R., Kim, K. T., Kang, Y. M., & Lee, J. Y. (2004). Solution synthesis of boron substituted $LiMn_2O_4$ spinel oxide for use in lithium rechargeable battery. *Ionics*, *10*(3), 188–192. doi:10.1007/BF02382815

Thirunakaran, R., Ravikumar, R., Gopukumar, S., & Sivashanmugam, A. (2013). Electrochemical evaluation of dual-doped $LiMn_2O_4$ spinels synthesized via co-precipitation method as cathode material for lithium rechargeable batteries. *Journal of Alloys and Compounds*, *556*, 266–273. doi:10.1016/j.jallcom.2012.12.053

Thirunakaran, R., Sivashanmugam, A., Gopukumar, S., & Rajalakshmi, R. (2009). Cerium and zinc: Dual-doped $LiMn_2O_4$ spinels as cathode material for use in lithium rechargeable batteries. *Journal of Power Sources*, *187*(2), 565–574. doi:10.1016/j.jpowsour.2008.10.134

Thrall, J.H. (2004). Nanotechnology and medicine. *Radiology, 230*, 315–318.

Tian, S., Shao, S., & Liu, B. (2019). Investigation on transient energy consumption of cold storages: Modeling and a case study. *Energy*, *180*, 1–9. doi:10.1016/j.energy.2019.04.217

Tian, X., Ning, L., & Andre, E. (2009). Potential health impact of nanoparticles. *Annual Review of Public Health*, *30*(1), 137–150. doi:10.1146/annurev.publhealth.031308.100155 PMID:19705557

Tiede, K., Boxall, A. B. A., Tear, S. P., Lewis, J., David, H., & Hassellov, M. (2008). Detection and characterization of engineered nanoparticles in food and the environment. *Food Additives and Contaminants*, *25*, 795–821.

Tinkle, S., McNeil, S. E., Mühlebach, S., Bawa, R., Borchard, G., Barenholz, Y. C., Tamarkin, L., & Desai, N. (2014). Nanomedicines: Addressing the scientific and regulatory gap. *Annals of the New York Academy of Sciences*, *1313*(1), 35–56. doi:10.1111/nyas.12403 PMID:24673240

Tippayawat, P., Phromviyo, N., Boueroy, P., & Chompoosor, A. (2016). Green synthesis of silver nanoparticles in aloe vera plant extract prepared by a hydrothermal method and their synergistic antibacterial activity. *PeerJ*, *4*, 4. doi:10.7717/peerj.2589 PMID:27781173

Tisa, A., Raman, A., & Daud, W. (2014). Applicability of fluidized bed reactor in recalcitrant compound degradation through advanced oxidation processes: A review. *Journal of Environmental Management*, *146*, 260–275. doi:10.1016/j.jenvman.2014.07.032 PMID:25190594

Tiwari, A., & Turner, A. P. F. (2014). *Biosensors Nanotechnology*. doi:10.1002/9781118773826

Tiwari, M., Sharma, N. C., Fleischmann, P., Burbage, J., Venkatachalam, P., & Sahi, S. V. (2017). Nanotitania exposure causes alterations in physiological, nutritional and stress responses in tomato (Solanum lycopersicum). *Front. Plant Sci.*, *8*, 8. doi:10.3389/fpls.2017.00633 PMID:28484486

Tollamadugu, K. V., Prasad, T., Kambala, V. S., & Naidu, R. (2011). A critical review on biogenic silver nanoparticles and their antimicrobial activity. *Current Nanoscience*, *7*, 531–544. doi:10.2174/157341311796196736

Topçu, A. A., Özgür, E., Yılmaz, F., Bereli, N., & Denizli, A. (2019). Real time monitoring and label free creatinine detection with artificial receptors. *Materials Science and Engineering B*, *244*, 6–11. doi:10.1016/j.mseb.2019.04.018

Torchilin, V. P. (2006). Multifunctional nanocarriers. *Adv Drug Deliv Rev., 58*, 1532-55.

Tosi, G., Constantino, L., Ruozi, B., Forni, F., & Vandelli, M.A. (2008). Polymeric nanoparticles for drug delivery to central nervous system. *Exp Opin Drug Deliv., 5*(2), 155-74.

Tothill, I. E. (2009). Biosensors for cancer markers diagnosis. *Seminars in Cell & Developmental Biology*, *20*(1), 55–62. doi:10.1016/j.semcdb.2009.01.015 PMID:19429492

Toumey, C. (2009). Plenty of room, plenty of history. *Nature Nanotechnology*, *4*(12), 783–784. doi:10.1038/nnano.2009.357 PMID:19966818

Tretyakov, S., Barois, P., Scharf, T., Kruglay, V., & Bergmair, I. (2010). Nanostructured metamaterials: exchange between experts in electromagnetics and material science. Publications Office of the European Union. doi:10.2777/54953

Tripathi, S., Singh, D. K., Singh, S., Dubey, S., & Chauhan, N. K. (2016). Impact of nanoparticles on photosynthesis: Challenges and opportunities. *Mater. Focus*, *5*(5), 405–411. doi:10.1166/mat.2016.1327

Tsai, C. H., Chang, W. C., Saikia, D., Wu, C. E., & Kao, H. M. (2016). Functionalization of cubic mesoporous silica SBA-16 with carboxylic acid via one-pot synthesis route for effective removal of cationic dyes. *Journal of Hazardous Materials*, *309*, 236–248. doi:10.1016/j.jhazmat.2015.08.051 PMID:26906434

Tsai, W. C., & Hsu, Y. H. (2012). Development of a surface plasmon resonance-based DNA sensor and its application for screening DNA-targeted anticancer drugs. *Analytical Letters*, *45*(11), 1495–1505. doi:10.1080/00032719.2012.675496

Tsé, C., Gauchez, A. S., Jacot, W., & Lamy, P. J. (2012). HER2 shedding and serum HER2 extracellular domain: Biology and clinical utility in breast cancer. *Cancer Treatment Reviews*, *38*(2), 133–142. doi:10.1016/j.ctrv.2011.03.008 PMID:21549508

Tu, J., Zhao, X. B., Cao, G. S., Tu, J. P., & Zhu, T. J. (2006). Improved performance of $LiMn_2O_4$ cathode materials for lithium ion batteries by gold coating. *Materials Letters*, *60*(27), 3251–3254. doi:10.1016/j.matlet.2006.02.089

Tu, J., Zhao, X. B., Xie, J., Cao, G. S., Zhuang, D. G., Zhu, T. J., & Tu, J. P. (2007). Enhanced low voltage cycling stability of $LiMn_2O_4$ cathode by ZnO coating for lithium ion batteries. *Journal of Alloys and Compounds*, *432*(1), 313–317. doi:10.1016/j.jallcom.2006.06.016

Tungittiplakorn, W., Lion, L. W., Cohen, C., & Kim, J. Y. (2004). Engineered Polymeric Nanoparticles for Soil Remediation. *Environmental Science & Technology*, *38*(5), 1605–1610. doi:10.1021/es0348997 PMID:15046367

Türkoğlu, E. A., Yavuz, H., Uzun, L., Akgöl, S., & Denizli, A. (2013). The fabrication of nanosensor-based surface plasmon resonance for IgG detection. *Artificial Cells, Nanomedicine, and Biotechnology*, *41*(3), 213–221. doi:10.3109/10731199.2012.716066 PMID:23110360

U.S. FDA Inventory of effective food contact substance (FCS) notifications Administration USFaD (2018).

Uekawa, N. (2012). Characterization of Titanium Oxide Nanoparticles Obtained by Hydrolysis Reaction of Ethylene Glycol Solution of Alkoxide. *Journal of Nanotechnology. Article ID*, *102361*, 1–8.

ul Ain, N., Anis, I., Ahmed, F., Shah, M. R., Parveen, S., Faizi, S., & Ahmed, S. (2018). Colorimetric detection of amoxicillin based on querecetagetin coated silver nanoparticles. *Sensors and Actuators B, 265,* 617-624. doi:10.1016/j.snb.2018.03.079

Ullah, H., Wahid, F., Santos, H. A., & Khan, T. (2016). Advances in biomedical and pharmaceutical applications of functional bacterial cellulose-based nanocomposites. *Carbohydrate Polymers*, *150*, 330–352. doi:10.1016/j.carbpol.2016.05.029 PMID:27312644

Umer, Naveed, & Naveedramzan. (2012). Selection of a suitable method for the synthesis of copper nanoparticles. *World Sci. Publ.Company*, *7*(5), 18.

UNAIDS. (2019). *Global HIV & AIDS statistics — 2019 fact sheet*. https://www.unaids.org/en/resources/fact-sheet

Ure, D., & Harris, J. (2003). Nanotechnology in dentistry: Reduction to practice. *Dental Update*, *30*(1), 10–15. doi:10.12968/denu.2003.30.1.10 PMID:12619307

Uzun, L., Say, R., Ünal, S., & Denizli, A. (2009). Production of surface plasmon resonance based assay kit for hepatitis diagnosis. *Biosensors & Bioelectronics*, *24*(9), 2878–2884. https://doi.org/10.1016/j.bios.2009.02.021

Vafapour, Z. (2019). Polarization-independent perfect optical metamaterial absorber as a glucose sensor in food industry applications. *IEEE Transactions on Nanobioscience*, *18*(4), 622–627. doi:10.1109/TNB.2019.2929802 PMID:31329124

Vales, G., Demir, E., Kaya, B., Creus, A., & Marcos, R. (2013). Genotoxicity of cobalt nanoparticles and ions in Drosophila. *Nanotoxicology*, *7*(4), 462–468. doi:10.3109/17435390.2012.689882 PMID:22548285

Vallhov, H., Qin, J., Johansson, S. M., Ahlborg, N., Muhammed, M. A., Scheynius, A., & Gabrielsson, S. (2006). The importance of an endotoxin-free environment during the production of nanoparticles used in medical applications. *Nano Letters*, *6*(8), 1682–1686. doi:10.1021/nl060860z PMID:16895356

Van Gosen, B. S., Blitz, T. A., Plumlee, G. S., Meeker, G. P., & Pierson, M. P. (2013). Geologic occurrences of erionite in the United States: An emerging national public health concern for respiratory disease. *Environmental Geochemistry and Health*, *35*(4), 419–430. https://doi.org/10.1007/s10653-012-9504-9

Van Viet, P., Nguyen, H. N., Cao, T. M., & Van Hieu, L. (2016). Article. *Nanomaterials (Basel, Switzerland)*, *2016*, 1957–612.

Vandergheynst, J., Scher, H., Guo, H. Y., & Schultz, D. (2007). Water-in-oil emulsions that improve the storage and delivery of the biolarvacide Lagenidium giganteum. *BioControl*, *52*(2), 207–229. doi:10.100710526-006-9021-9

Vargas, M., Albors, A., Chiralt, A., & González-Martínez, C. (2006). Quality of cold-stored strawberries as affected by chitosan–oleic acid edible coatings. Post. *Bio/Technology*, *41*, 164–171.

Vasilescu, A., Gáspár, S., Gheorghiu, M., David, S., Dinca, V., & Peteu, S. … Szunerits, S. (2017). Surface plasmon resonance based sensing of lysozyme in serum on Micrococcus lysodeikticus-modified graphene oxide surfaces. *Biosensors and Bioelectronics, 89,* 525-531. doi:10.1016/j.bios.2016.03.040

Vasir, J. K., & Labhasetwar, V. (2005). Targeted drug delivery in cancer therapy. *Technology in Cancer Research & Treatment*, *4*(4), 363–374. doi:10.1177/153303460500400405 PMID:16029056

Vasir, J. K., & Labhasetwar, V. (2007). Biodegradable nanoparticles for cytosolic delivery of therapeutics. *Advanced Drug Delivery Reviews*, *59*(8), 718–728. doi:10.1016/j.addr.2007.06.003 PMID:17683826

Vasir, J. K., Reddy, M. K., & Labhasetwar, V. (2005). Nanosystems in drug targeting: Opportunities and challenges. *Current Nanoscience*, *1*(1), 47–64. doi:10.2174/1573413052953110

Vauthier, C., Labarre, D., & Ponchel, G. (2007). Design aspects of poly(alkylcyanoacrylate) nanoparticles for drug delivery. *J. Drug Target.*, *15*, 641.

Vecchio, G., Galeone, A., Brunetti, V., Maiorano, G., Rizzello, L., Sabella, S., Cingolani, R., & Pompa, P. P. (2012). Mutagenic effects of gold nanoparticles induce aberrant phenotypes in Drosophila melanogaster. *Nanomedicine; Nanotechnology, Biology, and Medicine*, *8*(1), 1–7. doi:10.1016/j.nano.2011.11.001 PMID:22094122

Vecchio, G., Galeone, A., Brunetti, V., Maiorano, G., Sabella, S., Cingolani, R., & Pompa, P. P. (2012). Concentration-dependent, size-independent toxicity of citrate capped AuNPs in Drosophila melanogaster. *PLoS One*, *7*(1), e29980. doi:10.1371/journal.pone.0029980 PMID:22238688

Velappan, S., Nivedhita, P., Vimala, R., & Raja, S. (2020). Role of nano titania on the thermomechanical properties of silicon carbide refractories. *Ceramics International*, *46*(16), 25921–25926. doi:10.1016/j.ceramint.2020.07.077

Venkataraju, J. L., Sharath, R., Chandraprabha, M. N., Neelufar, E., Hazra, A., & Patra, M. (2014). Synthesis, characterization and evaluation of antimicrobial activity of zinc oxide nanoparticles. *Journal of Biochemical Technology*, *3*, 151–154.

Vercauteren, J., Deforche, K., Theys, K., Debruyne, M., Duque, L. M., Peres, S., Carvalho, A. P., Mansinho, K., Vandamme, A.-M., & Camacho, R. (2008). Mansinho K, Vandamme AM, Camacho R: The incidence of multidrug and full class resistance in HIV-1 infected patients is decreasing over time (2001-2006) in Portugal. *Retrovirology*, *5*(1), 12. doi:10.1186/1742-4690-5-12 PMID:18241328

Verheyen, E., Schillemans, J. P., Van Wijk, M., Demeniex, M. A., Hennink, W. E., & Van Nostrum, C. F. (2011). Challenges for the effective molecular imprinting of proteins. *Biomaterials*, *32*(11), 3008–3020. https://doi.org/10.1016/j.biomaterials.2011.01.007

Verma, A., & Mehata, M. S. (2016). Controllable synthesis of silver nanoparticles using Neem leaves and their antimicrobial activity. *J. Radiat. Res. Appl. Sci.*, *9*(1), 109–115. doi:10.1016/j.jrras.2015.11.001

Verma, M. L., Kumar, P., Sharma, D., Verma, A. D., & Jana, A. K. (2019). Advances in Nanobiotechnology with Special Reference to Plant Systems. In *Plant Nanobionics* (pp. 371–387). Springer. doi:10.1007/978-3-030-12496-0_13

Vilalta-Clemente, A., & Gloystein, K. (2008). Principles of Atomic Force Microscopy (AFM). *Proceedings of Physics of Advanced Materials Winter School.*

Villa, L. L., Costa, R. L. R., Petta, C. A., Andrade, R. P., Ault, K. A., Giuliano, A. R., Wheeler, C. M., Koutsky, L. A., Malm, C., Lehtinen, M., Skjeldestad, F. E., Olsson, S.-E., Steinwall, M., Brown, D. R., Kurman, R. J., Ronnett, B. M., Stoler, M. H., Ferenczy, A., Harper, D. M., ... Barr, E. (2005). Prophylactic quadrivalent human papilloma virus (types6,11,16, and 18) L1virus-like particle vaccine in young women: A randomised double blind placebo controlled multicenter phase II efficacy trial. *The Lancet. Oncology*, *6*(5), 271–278. doi:10.1016/S1470-2045(05)70101-7 PMID:15863374

Vimala, R., Charumathi, D., & Das, N. (2011). Packed bed column studies on Cd (II) removal from industrial wastewater by macrofungus Pleurotus platypus. *Desalination*, *275*(1-3), 291–296. doi:10.1016/j.desal.2011.03.014

Vimbela, G. V., Ngo, S. M., Fraze, C., Yang, L., & Stout, D. A. (2017). Antibacterial properties and toxicity from metallic nanomaterials. *International Journal of Nanomedicine*, *12*, 3941–3965. doi:10.2147/IJN.S134526 PMID:28579779

Virlan Maria, J. R., Daniela, M., Radu, R., Cristina, M. S., Alexandra, T., Bogdan, C., & Maria, G. (2016). Organic Nanomaterials and Their Applications in the Treatment of Oral Diseases. *Molecules (Basel, Switzerland)*, *21*(2), 207. doi:10.3390/molecules21020207 PMID:26867191

Voicu, G., Oprea, O., Vasile, B. S., & Andronescu, E. (2013). Antibacterial activity of zinc oxide-gentamicin hybrid material. *Digest Journal of Nanomaterials and Biostructures*, *8*, 1191–1203.

Vollath, D. (2013). *Nanoparticles-Nanocomposites–Nanomaterials: An Introduction for Beginners*. John Wiley & Sons.

Vunain, E., Mishra, A. K., & Mamba, B. B. (2016). Dendrimers, mesoporous silicas and chitosan-based nanosorbents for the removal of heavy-metal ions: A review. *International Journal of Macromolecules*, *86*, 570–586. doi:10.1016/j.ijbiomac.2016.02.005 PMID:26851359

Wagemaker, M., Borghols, W. J. H., & Mulder, F. M. (2007). Large Impact of Particle Size on Insertion Reactions. A Case for Anatase Li_xTiO_2. *Journal of the American Chemical Society*, *129*(14), 4323–4327. doi:10.1021/ja067733p PMID:17362005

Wagner, S., Gondikas, A., Neubauer, E., Hofmann, T., & von der Kammer, F. (2014). Spot the Difference: Engineered and Natural Nanoparticles in the Environment—Release, Behavior, and Fate. *Angewandte Chemie International Edition*, *53*, 12398–12419. doi:10.1002/anie.201405050

Walia, S., Shah, C. M., Gutruf, P., Nili, H., Chowdhury, D. R., Withayachumnankul, W., Bhaskaran, M., & Sriram, S. (2015). Flexible metasurfaces and metamaterials: A review of materials and fabrication processes at micro- and nano-scales. *Applied Physics Reviews*, *2*(1), 011303. doi:10.1063/1.4913751

Walling, M. A., Novak, J., & Shepard, J. R. E. (2009). Quantum Dots for live cell & in vivo imaging. *International Journal of Molecular Sciences*, *10*(2), 441–491. doi:10.3390/ijms10020441 PMID:19333416

Walther, A., Timonen, J. V., Díez, I., Laukkanen, A., & Ikkala, O. (2011). Multifunctional high-performance biofibers based on wet-extrusion of renewable native cellulose nanofibrils. *Advanced Materials*, *23*(26), 2924–2928.

Wang, S., Kang, L., & Werner, D. H. (2017). Hybrid resonators and highly tunable terahertz metamaterials enabled by Vanadium Dioxide (VO_2). *Scientific Reports*, *7*(1), 4326-1-4326–4328. doi:10.103841598-017-04692-8

Wan, G., Ruan, L., Yin, Y., Yang, T., Ge, M., & Cheng, X. (2016). Effects of silver nanoparticles in combination with antibiotics on the resistant bacteria Acinetobacter baumannii. *International Journal of Nanomedicine*, *11*, 3789–3800.

Wang, D. W., Li, F., Zhao, J., Ren, W., Chen, Z. G., Tan, J., Wu, Z. S., Gentle, I., Lu, G. Q., & Cheng, H. M. (2010). Fabrication of Graphene/Polyaniline Composite Paper via In Situ Anodic Electropolymerization for High-Performance Flexible Electrode. *ACS Nano*, *3*(7), 1745–1752. doi:10.1021/nn900297m PMID:19489559

Wang, D., Jiang, J., Tao, L., Kou, Z., & Yao, L. (2017). Experimental investigation on a novel cold storage defrosting device based on electric heater and reverse cycle. *Applied Thermal Engineering*, *127*, 1267–1273. doi:10.1016/j.applthermaleng.2017.08.122

Wang, G., Zhang, L., & Zhang, J. (2012). A review of electrode materials for electrochemical supercapacitors. *Chemical Society Reviews*, *41*(2), 797–828. doi:10.1039/C1CS15060J PMID:21779609

Wang, H. E., Cheng, H., Liu, C., Chen, X., Jiang, Q., Lu, Z., ... Martinu, L. (2011). Facile synthesis and electrochemical characterization of porous and dense TiO_2 nanospheres for lithium-ion battery applications. *Journal of Power Sources*, *196*(15), 6394–6399. doi:10.1016/j.jpowsour.2011.03.085

Wang, H., Tan, T. A., Yang, P., Lai, M. O., & Lu, L. (2011). High-rate performances of the Ru-doped spinel $LiNi_{0.5}Mn_{1.5}O_4$: Effects of doping and particle size. *The Journal of Physical Chemistry C*, *115*(13), 6102–6110. doi:10.1021/jp110746w

Wang, J. L., Li, Z. H., Yang, J., Tang, J. J., Yu, J. J., Nie, W. B., Lei, G. T., & Xiao, Q. Z. (2012). Effect of Al-doping on the electrochemical properties of a three-dimensionally porous lithium manganese oxide for lithium-ion batteries. *Electrochimica Acta*, *75*, 115–122. doi:10.1016/j.electacta.2012.04.136

Wang, J., Zhang, S. Q., Guo, Y. Z., Shen, J., Attia, S. M., Zhou, B., Zheng, G. Z., & Gui, Y. S. (2001). Morphological effects on the electrical and electrochemical properties of carbon aerogels. *Journal of the Electrochemical Society*, *148*(6), D75–D77. doi:10.1149/1.1368104

Wang, L., Ma, A., Tan, Y., Cui, X., & Cui, H. (2012). Study on Solar-Assisted Cascade Refrigeration System. *Energy Procedia*, *16*, 1503–1509. doi:10.1016/j.egypro.2012.01.236

Wang, L., Zhao, J., Guo, S., He, X., Jiang, C., & Wan, C. (2010). Investigation of SnO_2-modified $LiMn_2O_4$ composite as cathode material for lithium-ion batteries. *International Journal of Electrochemical Science*, *5*, 1113–1126.

Wang, L., Zhao, W., & Tan, W. (2008). Bioconjugated silica nanoparticles: development and applications, Bioconjugated silica nanoparticles: development and applications. *Nano Research*, *1*(2), 99–115. doi:10.100712274-008-8018-3

Wang, M., Liu, Y., Ren, G., Wang, W., Wu, S., & Shen, J. (2018). Bioinspired carbon quantum dots for sensitive fluorescent detection of vitamin B12 in cell system. *Analytica Chimica Acta*, *1032*, 154–162. doi:10.1016/j.aca.2018.05.057 PMID:30143213

Wang, P., Nasir, M. E., Krasavin, A. V., Dickson, W., Jiang, Y., & Zayats, A. V. (2019). Plasmonic metamaterials for nanochemistry and sensing. *Accounts of Chemical Research*, *52*(11), 3018–3028. doi:10.1021/acs.accounts.9b00325 PMID:31680511

Wang, Q., Wen, X., & Kong, J. (2019). Recent progress on uric acid detection: A review. *Critical Reviews in Analytical Chemistry*, *50*(4), 359–375. https://doi.org/10.1080/10408347.2019.1637711

Wang, R., & Xue, X. (2018). Theranostical application of nanomedicine for treating central nervous system disorders. *Science China. Life Sciences*, *61*(4), 392–399. doi:10.100711427-017-9292-7 PMID:29675554

Wang, S., Mamedova, N., Kotov, N. A., Chen, W., & Studer, J. (2002). Antigen/antibody immunocomplex from CdTe nanoparticle bioconjugates. *Nano Letters*, *2*, 817–822.

Wang, S., Sun, H., Ang, H. M., & Tadé, M. O. (2013). Adsorptive remediation of environmental pollutants using novel graphene-based nanomaterials. *Chemical Engineering Journal*, *226*, 336–347. doi:10.1016/j.cej.2013.04.070

Wang, T., Jin, X., Chen, Z., Megharaj, M., & Naidu, R. (2014). Green synthesis of Fe nanoparticles using eucalyptus leaf extracts for treatment of eutrophic wastewater. *The Science of the Total Environment*, *466–467*, 210–213. doi:10.1016/j.scitotenv.2013.07.022 PMID:23895784

Wang, T., Zou, M., Jiang, H., Ji, Z., Gao, P., & Cheng, G. (2011). Synthesis of a novel kind of carbon nanoparticle with large mesopores and macropores and its application as an oral vaccine adjuvant. *European Journal of Pharmaceutical Sciences*, *44*(5), 653–659. doi:10.1016/j.ejps.2011.10.012 PMID:22064451

Wang, X., Dennis, M., Jiang, J., Zhou, L., Zhai, X., & Lipiński, W. (2019). Performance of a novel cold thermal storage material in an emulated air conditioning system using different storage strategies. *International Journal of Refrigeration*, *104*, 259–269. doi:10.1016/j.ijrefrig.2019.05.038

Wang, X., Ishida, T., & Kiwada, H. (2007). Anti-PEG IgM elicited by injection of liposomes is involved in the enhanced blood clearance of a subsequent dose of PEGylated liposomes. *Journal of Controlled Release*, *119*, 236–244. doi:10.1016/j.jconrel.2007.02.010

Wang, Y., Pan, C., Chu, W., Vipin, A., & Sun, L. (2019). Environmental remediation applications of carbon nanotubes and graphene oxide: Adsorption and catalysis. *Nanomaterials (Basel, Switzerland)*, *9*(3), 439. doi:10.3390/nano9030439 PMID:30875970

Wang, Z. L., & Song, J. H. (2006). Piezoelectric Nanogenerators Based on Zinc Oxide Nanowire Arrays. *Science*, *312*(5771), 242–246. doi:10.1126cience.1124005 PMID:16614215

Wani, A. H., & Shah, M. A. (2012). Article. *Journal of Applied Pharmaceutical Science*, *2*, 40–44.

Ward, M. B., Brydson, R., & Cochrane, R. F. (2006). Mn nanoparticles produced by inert gas condensation. *Journal of Physics: Conference Series*, *26*(1), 296–299. doi:10.1088/1742-6596/26/1/071

Warheit, D. B., Laurence, B. R., Reed, K. L., Roach, D. H., Reynolds, G. A. M., & Webb, T. R. (2004). Comparative pulmonary toxicity assessment of single-wall carbon nanotubes in rats. *Toxicological Sciences*, *77*, 117–125.

Waterhouse, D. N., Madden, T. D., Cullis, P. R., Bally, M. B., Mayer, L. D., & Webb, M. S. (2005). Preparation, characterization, and biological analysis of liposomal for mulations of vincristine. *Methods in Enzymology*, *391*, 40–57. doi:10.1016/S0076-6879(05)91002-1 PMID:15721373

Weerapreeyakul, N., Hollenbeck, R. G., & Chikhale, P. J. (2000). Stability of bioreductive drug delivery systems containing melphalan is influenced by conformational constraint and electronic properties of substituents. *Bioorganic & Medicinal Chemistry Letters*, *10*(21), 2391–2395. doi:10.1016/S0960-894X(00)00496-0 PMID:11078186

Wegner, G. J., Lee, H. J., Marriott, G., & Corn, R. M. (2003). Fabrication of histidine-tagged fusion protein arrays for surface plasmon resonance imaging studies of protein - protein and protein - DNA interactions. *Analytical Chemistry, 75*(18), 4740–4746. https://doi.org/10.1021/ac0344438

Wei-Chiang, S., Xiantang, D., Feener, E. P., & Ryser, H. J. P. (1989). The intracellular release of methotrexate from a synthetic drug carrier system targeted to Fc receptor-bearing cells. *Journal of Controlled Release, 10*(1), 89–96. doi:10.1016/0168-3659(89)90020-5

Wei, Q., Wang, X., Sun, D.-W., & Pu, H. (2019). Rapid detection and control of psychrotrophic microorganisms in cold storage foods: A review. *Trends in Food Science & Technology, 86*, 453–464. doi:10.1016/j.tifs.2019.02.009

Weishaupt, K. R., Gomer, C. J., & Dougherty, T. J. (1976). Identification of singlet oxygen as the cytotoxic agent in photo-inactivation of a murine tumor. *Cancer Research, 36*(7 Part 1), 2326–2329. PMID:1277137

Weissleder, R., Elizondo, G., Wittenburg, J., Rabito, C. A., Bengele, H. H., & Josephson, L. (1990). Ultrasmall superparamagnetic iron oxide: Characterization of a new class of contrast agents for MR imaging. *Radiology, 175*, 489–493.

Welford, K. (1991). Surface plasmon-polaritons and their uses. *Optical and Quantum Electronics, 23*, 1–27. https://doi.org/10.1007/BF00619516

West, J. L., & Halas, N. J. (2000). Applications of nanotechnology to biotechnology commentary. *Current Opinion in Biotechnology, 11*(2), 215–217. doi:10.1016/S0958-1669(00)00082-3 PMID:10753774

White, B., Stackhouse, T., & Holcombe, J. (2009). Magnetic γ-Fe2O3 NPs coated with poly-L-cysteine for chelation of As (III), Cu (II), Cd (II), Ni (II), Pb (II) and Zn(II). *Journal of Hazardous Materials, 161*(2-3), 848–853. doi:10.1016/j.jhazmat.2008.04.105 PMID:18571848

WHO. (2016). *Global Tuberculosis Report*. World Health Organization.

WHO. (2019). *Number of people (all ages) living with HIV Estimates by WHO region*. https://apps.who.int/gho/data/view.main.22100WHO?lang=en

Wickline, S. A., Neubauer, A. M., Winter, P., Caruthers, S., & Lanza, G. (2006). Applications ofnanotechnology to atherosclerosis, thrombosis, and vascular biology. *Arteriosclerosis, Thrombosis, and Vascular Biology, 26*(3), 435–441. doi:10.1161/01.ATV.0000201069.47550.8b PMID:16373609

Wilkinson, J. M. (2003). Nanotechnology applications in medicine. *Med Device Technol., 14*, 29-31.

Winter, M., & Besenhard, J. O. (1999). Electrochemical lithiation of tin and tin-based intermetallics and composites. *J. Electrochim. Acta, 45*(1-2), 31–50. doi:10.1016/S0013-4686(99)00191-7

Wolf, A. M. D., Wender, R. C., Etzioni, R. B., Thompson, I. M., D'Amico, A. V., & Volk, R. J. … Smith, R. A. (2010). American cancer society guideline for the early detection of prostate cancer: Update 2010. *CA: A Cancer Journal for Clinicians, 60*(2), 70-98. doi:10.3322/caac.20066

Wolf, M. J., Amrein, H., Izatt, J. A., Choma, M. A., Reedy, M. C., & Rockman, H. A. (2006). Drosophila as a model for the identification of genes causing adult human heart disease. *Proceedings of the National Academy of Sciences of the United States of America, 103*(5), 1394–1399. doi:10.1073/pnas.0507359103 PMID:16432241

Wong, Z. J., Wang, Y., O'Brien, K., Rho, J., Yin, X., Zhang, S., Fang, N., Yen, T. J., & Zhang, X. (2017). Optical and acoustic metamaterials: superlens, negative refractive index and invisibility cloak. *Journal of Optics, 19*(8), 084007-1-084007–084013. doi:10.1088/2040-8986/aa7a1f

Wood, R. W. (1902). XLII. On a remarkable case of uneven distribution of light in a diffraction grating spectrum. *The London, Edinburgh and Dublin Philosophical Magazine and Journal of Science*, *4*(21), 396–402. https://doi.org/10.1080/14786440209462857

Wu, C., Mosher, B. P., & Zeng, T. (2006). One-step green route to narrowly dispersed copper nanocrystals. *Journal of Nanoparticle Research*, *8*(6), 965–969. doi:10.100711051-005-9065-2

Wu, D., Liu, Y., Yu, Z., Chen, L., Ma, R., Li, Y., Li, R., & Ye, H. (2016). Wide-angle, polarization-insensitive and broadband absorber based on eight-fold symmetric SRRs metamaterial. *Optics Communications*, *380*, 221–226. doi:10.1016/j.optcom.2016.06.023

Wu, H. M., Belharouak, I., Abouimrane, A., Sun, Y. K., & Amine, K. (2010). Surface modification of $LiNi_{0.5}Mn_{1.5}O_4$ by ZrP_2O_7 and ZrO_2 for lithium-ion batteries. *Journal of Power Sources*, *195*(9), 2909–2913. doi:10.1016/j.jpowsour.2009.11.029

Wu, H. M., Tu, J. P., Chen, X. T., Li, Y., Zhao, X. B., & Cao, G. S. (2007). Effects of Ni-ion doping on electrochemical characteristics of spinel $LiMn_2O_4$ powders prepared by a spray-drying method. *Journal of Solid State Electrochemistry*, *11*(2), 173–176. doi:10.100710008-005-0082-y

Wu, H. M., Tu, J. P., Yuan, Y. F., Li, Y., Zhao, X. B., & Cao, G. S. (2005). Structural, morphological and electrochemical characteristics of spinel $LiMn_2O_4$ prepared by spray-drying method. *Scripta Materialia*, *52*(6), 513–517. doi:10.1016/j.scriptamat.2004.10.037

Wu, L., & Ritchie, S. (2006). Removal of trichloroethylene from water by cellulose acetate supported bimetallic Ni/Fe nanoparticles. *Chemosphere*, *63*(2), 285–292. doi:10.1016/j.chemosphere.2005.07.021 PMID:16226292

Wulff, G. (1995). Molecular imprinting in cross-linked materials with the aid of molecular templates - A way towards artificial antibodies. *Angewandte Chemie International Edition in English*, *34*(17), 1812–1832. https://doi.org/10.1002/anie.199518121

Wu, V. M., & Uskoković, V. (2017). Population Effects of Calcium Phosphate Nanoparticles in *Drosophila melanogaster*: The Effects of Phase Composition, Crystallinity, and the Pathway of Formation. *ACS Biomaterials Science & Engineering*, *3*(10), 2348–2357. doi:10.1021/acsbiomaterials.7b00540 PMID:29862315

Wu, W. Y., & Ting, J. M. (2002). Growth and characteristics of carbon films with nano-sized metal particles. *Thin Solid Films*, *420*, 166–171. doi:10.1016/S0040-6090(02)00804-0

Xia, H., Luo, Z., & Xie, J. (2012). Nanostructured $LiMn_2O_4$ and their composites as high-performance cathodes for lithium-ion batteries. *Progress in Natural Science*, *22*(6), 572–584. doi:10.1016/j.pnsc.2012.11.014

Xiao, L., Zhao, Y., Yang, Y., Cao, Y., Ai, X., & Yang, H. (2008). Enhanced electrochemical stability of Al-doped $LiMn_2O_4$ synthesized by a polymer-pyrolysis method. *Electrochimica Acta*, *54*(2), 545–550. doi:10.1016/j.electacta.2008.07.037

Xiao, X., Lu, J., & Li, Y. (2010). $LiMn_2O_4$ microspheres: Synthesis, characterization and use as a cathode in lithium ion batteries. *Nano Research*, *3*(10), 733–737. doi:10.100712274-010-0037-1

Xia, Y., Zhang, W. K., Huang, H., Gan, Y. P., Tian, J., & Tao, X. Y. (2011). Self-assembled mesoporous LiFePO4 with hierarchical spindle-like architectures for high-performance lithium-ion batteries. *Journal of Power Sources*, *196*(13), 5651–5658. doi:10.1016/j.jpowsour.2011.02.044

Xie, L., Gao, W., Shu, J., Ying, Y., & Kono, J. (2015). Extraordinary sensitivity enhancement by metasurfaces in terahertz detection of antibiotics. *Scientific Reports*, *5*(1), 1–4. doi:10.1038rep08671 PMID:25728144

Xie, T., Chen, Z., Ma, R., & Zhong, M. (2017). A wide-angle and polarization insensitive infrared broad band metamaterial absorber. *Optics Communications*, *383*, 81–86. doi:10.1016/j.optcom.2016.08.058

Xie, Y., He, Y., Irwin, P. L., Jin, T., & Shi, X. (2011). Antibacterial activity and mechanism of action of zinc oxide nanoparticles against Campylobacter jejuni. *Applied and Environmental Microbiology*, *77*(7), 2325–2331. doi:10.1128/AEM.02149-10 PMID:21296935

Xi, L. J., Wang, H. E., Lu, Z. G., Yang, S. L., Ma, R. G., Deng, J. Q., & Chung, C. Y. (2012). Facile synthesis of porous $LiMn_2O_4$ spheres as positive electrode for high-power lithium ion batteries. *Journal of Power Sources*, *198*, 251–257. doi:10.1016/j.jpowsour.2011.09.100

Xing, T., Sunarso, J., Yang, W., Yin, Y., Glushenkov, A. M., Li, L. H., Howlett, P. C., & Chen, Y. (2013). Ball milling: A green mechanochemical approach for synthesis of nitrogen doped carbon nanoparticles. *Nanoscale*, *5*(17), 7970–7976. doi:10.1039/c3nr02328a PMID:23864038

Xiu, Z., Zhang, Q., Puppala, H. L., Colvin, V. L., & Alvarez, P. J. J. (2012). Negligible particle specific antibacterial activity of silver nanoparticles. *Nano Letters*, *12*(8), 4271–4275.

Xu, H., Wang, H., Zhang, Y., He, W., Zhu, M., Wang, B., & Yan, H. (2004). Hydrothermal synthesis of zinc oxide powders with controllable morphology. *Ceramics International*, *30*(1), 93–97. doi:10.1016/S0272-8842(03)00069-5

Xu, W., Xie, L., Zhu, J., Wang, W., Ye, Z., Ma, Y., Tsai, C., Chen, S., & Ying, Y. (2017). Terahertz sensing of chlorpyrifos-methyl using metamaterials. *Food Chemistry*, *218*, 330–334. doi:10.1016/j.foodchem.2016.09.032 PMID:27719917

Xu, W., Yuan, A., Tian, L., & Wang, Y. (2011). Improved high-rate cyclability of sol–gel derived Cr-doped spinel $LiCr_yMn_{2-y}O_4$ in an aqueous electrolyte. *Journal of Applied Electrochemistry*, *41*(4), 453–460. doi:10.100710800-011-0255-6

Xu, X., Peng, B., Li, D., Zhang, J., Wong, L. M., Zhang, Q., Wang, S., & Xiong, Q. (2011). Flexible visible-infrared metamaterials and their applications in highly sensitive chemical and biological sensing. *Nano Letters*, *11*(8), 3232–3238. doi:10.1021/nl2014982 PMID:21696183

Yadav, S. K. (2017). Realizing the Potential of Nanotechnology for Agriculture and Food Technology. *Journal of Tissue Science & Engineering*, *8*(01), 195. doi:10.4172/2157-7552.1000195

Yallappa, S., Manjanna, J., & Dhananjaya, B. L. (2015). Phytosynthesis of stable Au, Ag and Au–Ag alloy nanoparticles using J. sambac leaves extract, and their enhanced antimicrobial activity in presence of organic antimicrobials. *Spectrochimica Acta. Part A: Molecular and Biomolecular Spectroscopy*, *137*, 236–243. doi:10.1016/j.saa.2014.08.030 PMID:25222319

Yamaki, J., Takatsuji, H., Kawamura, T., & Egashira, M. (2002). Thermal stability of graphite anode with electrolyte in lithium-ion cells. *Solid State Ionics*, *148*(3-4), 241–245. doi:10.1016/S0167-2738(02)00060-7

Yamamoto, O., Ohira, T., Alvarez, K., & Fukuda, M. (2010). Antibacterial characteristics of $CaCO_3$–MgO composites. *Materials Science and Engineering B*, *173*(1-3), 208–212. doi:10.1016/j.mseb.2009.12.007

Yam, K. L., Takhistov, P. T., & Miltz, J. (2005). Intelligent packaging: Concepts and applications. *Journal of Food Science*, *70*, R1–R10.

Yang, B., Lv, S., Chen, F., Liu, C., Cai, C., Chen, C., & Chen, X. (2016). A resonance light scattering sensor based on bioinspired molecularly imprinted polymers for selective detection of papain at trace levels. *Analytica Chimica Acta*, *912*, 125–132. doi:10.1016/j.aca.2016.01.030 PMID:26920781

Yang, J., Guo, F., Hua, J., Li, X., Wu, W., Qu, Y., & Tian, H. (2012). Efficient and stable organic DSSC sensitizers bearing quinacridone and furan moieties as a planar π-spacer. *Journal of Materials Chemistry*, *2012*(22), 24356–24365. doi:10.1039/c2jm31929b

Yang, J., Hou, B., Wang, J., Tian, B., Bi, J., Wang, N., Li, X., & Huang, X. (2019). Nanomaterials for the removal of heavy metals from wastewater. *Nanomaterials (Basel, Switzerland)*, *9*(3), 424. doi:10.3390/nano9030424 PMID:30871096

Yang, J., Wang, B. F., Wang, K., Liu, Y., Xie, J. Y., & Wen, Z. S. (2003). Si/c composites for high capacity lithium storage materials. *Electrochemical and Solid-State Letters*, *6*(8), A154–A156. doi:10.1149/1.1585251

Yang, J., Winter, M., & Besenhard, J. (1996). Small particle size multiphase Li-alloy anodes for lithium-ion-batteries. *Solid State Ionics*, *90*(1-4), 281–287. doi:10.1016/S0167-2738(96)00389-X

Yang, K., Han, Q., Chen, B., Zheng, Y., Zhang, K., Li, Q., & Wang, J. (2018). Antimicrobial hydrogels: Promising materials for medical application. *International Journal of Nanomedicine*, *13*, 2217–2263. doi:10.2147/IJN.S154748 PMID:29695904

Yang, K., Yu, W., Huang, G., Zhou, J., Yang, X., & Fu, W. (2020). Highly sensitive detection of Staphylococcus aureus by a THz metamaterial biosensor based on gold nanoparticles and rolling circle amplification. *RSC Advances*, *10*(45), 26824–26833. doi:10.1039/D0RA03116J

Yang, K., Zhang, L., Liang, Z., & Zhang, Y. (2012). Protein-imprinted materials: Rational design, application and challenges. *Analytical and Bioanalytical Chemistry*, *403*(8), 2173–2183. https://doi.org/10.1007/s00216-012-5840-y

Yang, L., & Li, Y. (2006). Simultaneous detection of *Escherichia coli* O157:H7 and *Salmonella Typhimurium* using quantum dots as fluorescence labels. *Analyst (London)*, *131*, 394–401.

Yang, N., Zhai, J., Wang, D., Chen, Y., & Jiang, L. (2010). Two-dimensional graphene bridges enhanced photoinduced charge transport in dye-sensitized solar cells. *ACS Nano*, *4*(2), 887–894. doi:10.1021/nn901660v PMID:20088539

Yang, Q., Agouri, S., Tyrrell, J., & Walsh, T. (2018). Heavy metal resistance genes are associated with blaNDM-1 and blaCTX-M15 carrying *enterobecteriaceae*. *Antimicrobial Agents and Chemotherapy*, *62*(5), e02614–e02642. doi:10.1128/AAC.02642-17 PMID:29507071

Yang, Q., Wang, S., Fan, P., Wang, L., Di, Y., Lin, K., & Xiao, F. S. (2005). pH-responsive carrier system based on carboxylic acid modified mesoporous silica and polyelectrolyte for drug delivery. *Chemistry of Materials*, *17*(24), 5999–6003. doi:10.1021/cm051198v

Yang, R., Qin, Y., Dai, L., & Wang, Z. L. (2009). Power generation with laterally packaged piezoelectric fine wires. *Nature Nanotechnology*, *4*(1), 34–39. doi:10.1038/nnano.2008.314 PMID:19119280

Yang, W., Ni, M., Ren, X., Tian, Y., Li, N., Su, Y., & Zhang, X. (2015). (. Graphene in supercapacitor applications. *Current Opinion in Colloid & Interface Science*, *20*(5-6), 416–428. doi:10.1016/j.cocis.2015.10.009

Yang, W., Wan, F., Wang, Y., & Jiang, C. (2009). Achievement of 6.03% conversion efficiency of dye-sensitized solar cells with single-crystalline rutile TiO2 nanorod photoanode. *Applied Physics Letters*, *95*(13), 133121. doi:10.1063/1.3240870

Yang, X., Wang, Q., Wang, K., Tan, W., Yao, J., & Li, H. (2006). Electrical switching of DNA monolayers investigated by surface plasmon resonance. *Langmuir*, *22*(13), 5654–5659. doi:10.1021/la052907m PMID:16768490

Yang, Y., Qu, L., Dai, L., Kang, T. S., & Durstock, M. (2007). Electrophoresis Coating of Titanium Dioxide on Aligned Carbon Nanotubes for Controlled Syntheses of Photoelectronic Nanomaterials. *Advanced Materials*, *19*(9), 1239–1243. doi:10.1002/adma.200602181

Yang, Y., Xie, C., Ruffo, R., Peng, H., Kim, D. K., & Cui, Y. (2009). Single nanorod devices for battery diagnostics: A case study on LiMn2O4. *Nano Letters*, *9*(12), 4109–4114. doi:10.1021/nl902315u PMID:19807129

Yang, Z., Cao, G. S., Xie, J., & Zhao, X. B. (2012). Oleic acid-assisted preparation of LiMnPO4 and its improved electrochemical performance by Co doping. *Journal of Solid State Electrochemistry*, *16*(3), 1271–1277. doi:10.100710008-011-1523-4

Yang, Z., Choi, D., Kerisit, S., Rosso, K. M., Wang, D., Zhang, J., Graff, G., & Liu, J. (2009). Nanostructures and lithium electrochemical reactivity of lithium titanites and titanium oxides: A review. *Journal of Power Sources*, *192*(2), 588–598. doi:10.1016/j.jpowsour.2009.02.038

Yan, H., & Row, K. H. (2006). Characteristic and synthetic approach of molecularly imprinted polymer. *International Journal of Molecular Sciences*, *7*(5), 155–178. https://doi.org/10.3390/i7050155

Yan, J., Wei, T., Shao, B., Ma, F., Fan, Z., Zhang, M., Zheng, C., Shang, Y., Quian, W., & Wei, F. (2010). Electrochemical properties of graphene nanosheet/carbon black composites as electrodes for supercapacitors. *Carbon*, *48*(6), 1731–1737. doi:10.1016/j.carbon.2010.01.014

Yao, T., Gu, X., Li, T., Li, J., Li, J., & Zhao, Z. … She, Y. (2016). Enhancement of surface plasmon resonance signals using a MIP/GNPs/rGO nano-hybrid film for the rapid detection of ractopamine. *Biosensors and Bioelectronics, 75,* 96-100. doi:10.1016/j.bios.2015.08.027

Yao, K., Salvador, M., Chueh, C. C., Xin, X. K., Xu, Y. X., de Quilettes, D. W., Hu, T., Chen, Y. W., Ginger, D. S., & Jen, A. K. Y. (2014). General Route to Enhance Polymer Solar Cell Performance using Plasmonic Nanoprisms. *Advanced Energy Materials*, *4*(9), 1289–1295. doi:10.1002/aenm.201400206

Yella, A., Lee, H. W., Tsao, H. N., Yi, C., Chandiran, A. K., Nazeeruddin, M., Diau, E. W.-G., Yeh, C.-Y., Zakeeruddin, S. M., & Gratzel, M. (2011). Porphyrin-sensitized solar cells with cobalt (II/III)-based redox electrolyte exceed 12 percent efficiency. *Science*, *334*(6056), 629–634. doi:10.1126cience.1209688 PMID:22053043

Yhee, J. Y., Son, S., Kim, S. H., Park, K., Choi, K., & Kwon, I. C. (2014). Self-assembled glycol chitosan nanoparticles for disease-specifc theranostics. *Journal of Controlled Release*, *193*, 202–213. doi:10.1016/j.jconrel.2014.05.009 PMID:24845129

Yianoulis, P., & Giannouli, M. (2008). Thin Solid Films and Nanomaterials for Solar Energy Conversion and Energy Saving Applications. *Journal of Nano Research*, *2*, 49–60. doi:10.4028/www.scientific.net/JNanoR.2.49

Yilma, A.N., Singh, S.R., Dixit, S., & Dennis, V.A. (2013). Anti-inflammatory effects of

Yılmaz, F., Saylan, Y., Akgönüllü, S., Çimen, D., Derazshamshir, A., Bereli, N., & Denizli, A. (2017). Surface plasmon resonance based nanosensors for detection of triazinic pesticides in agricultural foods. In A. M. Grumezescu (Ed.), New pesticides and soil sensors (pp. 679–718)., https://doi.org/10.1016/b978-0-12-804299-1.00019-9.

Yilmaz, E., Majidi, D., Ozgur, E., & Denizli, A. (2015). Whole cell imprinting based Escherichia coli sensors: A study for SPR and QCM. *Sensors and Actuators. B, Chemical*, *209*, 714–721. https://doi.org/10.1016/j.snb.2014.12.032

Ying, J., Jiang, C., & Wan, C. (2004). Preparation and characterization of high-density spherical $LiCoO_2$ cathode material for lithium ion batteries. *Journal of Power Sources*, *129*(2), 264–269. doi:10.1016/j.jpowsour.2003.10.007

Ying-Yu, M., Ke-Tao, J., Shi-Bing, W., Hui-Ju, W., Xiang-Min, T., & Dong-Sheng, H. (2017). *Molecular Imaging of Cancer with Nanoparticle-Based Theranostic Probes*. Hindawi Contrast Media & Molecular Imaging Volume.

Yi, T. F., Zhu, Y. R., Zhu, X. D., Shu, J., Yue, C. B., & Zhou, A. N. (2009). A review of recent developments in the surface modification of $LiMn_2O_4$ as cathode material of power lithium-ion battery. *Ionics*, *15*(6), 779–784. doi:10.100711581-009-0373-x

Yi, T., Hu, X., Wang, D., & Huo, H. (2008). Effects of Al, F dual substitutions on the structure and electrochemical properties of lithium manganese oxide. Journal of University of Science and Technology Beijing, Mineral, Metallurgy. *Material*, *15*(2), 182–186.

Yiwei, T. (2011). Health impact and safety of engineered nanomaterials. *Chemical Communications*, *47*(25), 7025–7038. doi:10.1039/c0cc05271j PMID:21479319

Yokoyama, M., Miyauchi, M., Yamada, N., Okano, T., Sakurai, Y., Kataoka, K., & Inoue, S. (1990). Polymer micelles as novel drug carrier: Adriamycin-conjugated poly(ethylene glycol)-poly(aspartic acid) block copolymer. *Journal of Controlled Release*, *11*(1-3), 269–278. doi:10.1016/0168-3659(90)90139-K

Yokoyama, M., Okano, T., Sakurai, Y., Ekimoto, H., Shibazaki, C., & Kataoka, K. (1991). Toxicity and antitumor activity against solid tumors of micelle-forming polymeric anticancer drug and its extremely long circulation in blood. *Cancer Research*, *51*, 3229–3236. PMID:2039998

Yola, M. L., Atar, N., & Eren, T. (2014). Determination of amikacin in human plasma by molecular imprinted SPR nanosensor. *Sensors and Actuators. B, Chemical*, *198*, 70–76. https://doi.org/10.1016/j.snb.2014.02.107

Yola, M. L., Eren, T., & Atar, N. (2014). Molecular imprinted nanosensor based on surface plasmon resonance: Application to the sensitive determination of amoxicillin. *Sensors and Actuators. B, Chemical*, *195*, 28–35. https://doi.org/10.1016/j.snb.2014.01.011

Yoo, E., Okata, T., Akita, T., Kohyama, M., Nakamura, J., & Honma, I. (2009). Enhanced electrocatalytic activity of Pt subnanoclusters on graphene nanosheet surface. *Nano Letters*, *9*(6), 2255–2259. doi:10.1021/nl900397t PMID:19405511

Yoon, G., Kim, I., & Rho, J. (2016). Challenges in fabrication towards realization of practical metamaterials. *Microelectronic Engineering*, *163*, 7–20. doi:10.1016/j.mee.2016.05.005

Yoshino, M., Kubota, Y., Nakagawa, Y., & Terano, M. (2019). Efficient fabrication process of ordered metal nanodot arrays for infrared plasmonic sensor. *Micromachines*, *10*(6), 27–30. doi:10.3390/mi10060385 PMID:31181766

Yotsuyanagi, T., & Hazemoto, N. (1998). Cationic liposomes in gene delivery. *Japanese Journal of Clinical Medicine*, *56*, 705–712. PMID:9549361

Young, L. S., Searle, P. F., Onion, D., & Mautner, V. (2006). Viral gene therapy strategies:from basic science to clinical application. *The Journal of Pathology*, *208*(2), 299–318. doi:10.1002/path.1896 PMID:16362990

Yousaf, S. A., & Salamat, A. (2008). *Effect of heating environment on fluorine doped tin oxide (f: SnO/sub 2/) thin films for solar cell applications*. Faculty of Engineering & Technology.

Yuan, X. C., Ong, B. H., Tan, Y. G., Zhang, D. W., Irawan, R., & Tjin, S. C. (2006). Sensitivity-stability-optimized surface plasmon resonance sensing with double metal layers. *Journal of Optics. A, Pure and Applied Optics*, *8*(11), 959–963. https://doi.org/10.1088/1464-4258/8/11/005

Yu, C., Fan, S., Sun, Y., & Pickwell-Macpherson, E. (2012). The potential of terahertz imaging for cancer diagnosis: A review of investigations to date. *Quantitative Imaging in Medicine and Surgery*, *2*(1), 33–45. doi:10.3978/j.issn.2223-4292.2012.01.04 PMID:23256057

Yu, D., & Dai, L. (2010). Self-Assembled Graphene/Carbon Nanotube Hybrid Films for Supercapacitors. *The Journal of Physical Chemistry Letters*, *1*(2), 467–470. doi:10.1021/jz9003137

Yue, J., Feliciano, T. J., Li, W., Lee, A., & Odom, T. W. (2017). Gold nanoparticle size and shape effects on cellular uptake and intracellular distribution of siRNA nanoconstructs. *Bioconjugate Chemistry, 28*(6), 1791–1800. doi:10.1021/acs.bioconjchem.7b00252 PMID:28574255

Yue, X., & Dai, Z. (2018). Liposomal nanotechnology for cancer theranostics. *Current Medicinal Chemistry, 25*(12), 1397–1408.

Yu, J. Y., Jiao, S. Q., Nawaz, T., Wang, S. Q., & Wei, T. X. (2019). Surface plasmone resonance sensor for biomimetic detection of progesterone with macroporous molecularly imprinted polymers prepared by visible light. *IOP Conference Series. Materials Science and Engineering, 688*(3). https://doi.org/10.1088/1757-899X/688/3/033032

Yu, L., Qiu, J. J., Cheng, H., & Luo, Z. H. (2013). Facile preparation of gold nanoparticles using the self-assembled ABC non-amphiphilic fluorosilicone triblock copolymer template. *Materials Chemistry and Physics, 138*(2-3), 780–786. doi:10.1016/j.matchemphys.2012.12.060

Yusof, Y. (2016). Enhanced Structural, Thermal, and Electrical Properties of Multiwalled Carbon Nanotubes Hybridized with Silver Nanoparticles. Journal of Nanomaterials. *Article ID, 6141496*, 1–9.

Yu, Z. M., & Zhao, L. C. (2007). Structure and electrochemical properties of $LiMn_2O_4$. *Transactions of Nonferrous Metals Society of China, 17*(3), 659–664. doi:10.1016/S1003-6326(07)60152-6

Zahid, N., Ali, A., Manickam, S., Siddiqui, Y., & Maqbool, M. (2012). Potential of chitosan-loaded nano-emulsions to control different Colletotrichum spp. And maintain quality of tropical fruits during cold storage. *Journal of Applied Microbiology, 113*(4), 225–239. doi:10.1111/j.1365-2672.2012.05398.x PMID:22805053

Zain, N. M., Stapley, A. G., & Shama, G. (2014). Green synthesis of silver and copper nanoparticles using ascorbic acid and chitosan for antimicrobial applications. *Carbohydrate Polymers, 112*, 195–202.

Zalba, B., Marin, J. M., Cabeza, L. F., & Mehling, H. (2003). Review on thermal energy storage with phase change: Materials, heat transfer analysis and applications. *Applied Thermal Engineering, 23*(3), 251–283. doi:10.1016/S1359-4311(02)00192-8

Zambrano-Zaragoza, M. L., Mercado-Silva, E., Gutiérrez-Cortez, E., Cornejo Villegas, M. A., & Quintanar-Guerrero, D. (2014). The effect of nano-coatings with α-tocopherol and xanthan gum on shelf-life and browning index of fresh-cut "Red Delicious" apples. *Innovative Food Science & Emerging Technologies, 22*, 188–196. doi:10.1016/j.ifset.2013.09.008

Zandi, K., Weisany, W., Ahmadi, H., Bazargan, I., & Naseri, L. (2013). Effect of Nanocomposite-Based Packaging on Postharvest Quality of Strawberry during Storage. *Bulletin of Environment. Pharmacology and Life Sciences, 2*(5), 28–36.

Zayats, A. V., & Smolyaninov, I. I. (2003). Near-field photonics: Surface plasmon polaritons and localized surface plasmons. *Journal of Optics. A, Pure and Applied Optics, 5*(4), S16–S50. doi:10.1088/1464-4258/5/4/353

Zeiny, A., Haruna, M. A., & Wen, D. (2019). Aqueous lithium bromide nano-solution for solar absorption refrigeration systems. *AIP Conference Proceedings, 2123*, 020083. doi:10.1063/1.5117010

Zeltins, A. (2012). Construction and characterization of viruslike particles: A review. *Molecular Biotechnology, 53*(1), 92–107. doi:10.100712033-012-9598-4 PMID:23001867

Zeng, J. L., Sun, L. X., Xu, F., Tan, Z. C., Zhang, Z. H., Zhang, J., & Zhang, T. (2007). Study of a PCM based energy storage system containing Ag nanoparticles. *Journal of Thermal Analysis and Calorimetry, 87*(2), 369–373. doi:10.100710973-006-7783-z

Zeng, J., Roberts, S., & Xia, Y. (2010). Nanocrystal-based time-temperature indicators. *Chemistry (Weinheim an der Bergstrasse, Germany), 16*, 12559–12563.

Zeng, S., Hu, S., Xia, J., Anderson, T., Dinh, X., Meng, X., Coquet, P., & Yong, K. (2014). Graphene-MoS_2 hybrid nanostructures enhanced surface plasmon resonance biosensors. *Sensors and Actuators. B, Chemical, 207*, 801–810. doi:10.1016/j.snb.2014.10.124

Zhang, Q., Jing, L., Wang, Y., Zhang, J., Ren, Y., & Wang, Y. … Liedberg, B. (2014). Surface plasmon resonance sensor for femtomolar detection of testosterone with water-compatible macroporous molecularly imprinted film. *Analytical Biochemistry, 463,* 7-14. doi:10.1016/j.ab.2014.06.014

Zhang, B., Li, Y., & Fang, C. Y. (2009a). Receptor- mediated cellular uptake of folate conjugated fluorescent nanodiamonds: A combined ensemble and single- particle study. *Small, 5*, 2716–2721.

Zhang, C. H., Liu, L. W., Liang, P., Tang, L. J., Yu, R. Q., & Jiang, J. H. (2016). Article. *Analytical Chemistry, 88*, 447–452.

Zhang, L. L., & Zhao, X. S. (2009). Carbon-based materials as supercapacitor electrodes. *Chemical Society Reviews, 38*(9), 2520–2531. doi:10.1039/b813846j PMID:19690733

Zhang, L., Zhu, C., Chen, C., Zhu, S., Zhou, J., Wang, M., & Shang, P. (2018). Determination of kanamycin using a molecularly imprinted SPR sensor. *Food Chemistry, 266*, 170–174. https://doi.org/10.1016/j.foodchem.2018.05.128

Zhang, M., Lv, J., Li, F.-F., Bao, N., Wang, A.-J., Feng, J.-J., & Zhou, D.-L. (2014). Urea assisted electro_chemical synthesis of flower_like platinum arrays with high electrocatalytic activity. *Electrochimica Acta, 123*, 227–232. doi:10.1016/j.electacta.2014.01.054

Zhang, Q. F., & Cao, G. Z. (2011). Nanostructured photoelectrodes for dye-sensitized solar cells. *Nano Today, 6*(1), 91–109. doi:10.1016/j.nantod.2010.12.007

Zhang, Q. F., Yodyingyong, S., Xi, J. T., Myers, D., & Cao, G. Z. (2012). Oxidenanowires for solar cell applications. *Nanoscale, 4*(5), 1436–1445. doi:10.1039/C2NR11595F PMID:22200055

Zhang, Q., Rao, Y., Jiao, Y., Li, L., Li, Y., & Jin, L. (2017). preparation and performance of composite building materials with phase change material for thermal storage. *Energy Procedia, 143*, 125–130. doi:10.1016/j.egypro.2017.12.659

Zhang, S. S. (2006). A review on electrolyte additives for lithium-ion batteries. *Journal of Power Sources, 162*(2), 1379–1394. doi:10.1016/j.jpowsour.2006.07.074

Zhang, S., Sun, D., Fu, Y., & Du, H. (2003). Recent Advances of Superhard Nanocomposite Coatings: A Review. *Surface and Coatings Technology, 167*(2–3), 113–119.

Zhang, W., Han, Y., Chen, X., Luo, X., Wang, J., Yue, T., & Li, Z. (2017). Surface molecularly imprinted polymer capped Mn-doped ZnS quantum dots as a phosphorescent nanosensor for detecting patulin in apple juice. *Food Chemistry, 232*, 145–154. doi:10.1016/j.foodchem.2017.03.156 PMID:28490057

Zhang, X., Fan, Y., Qi, L., & Li, H. (2016). Broadband plasmonic metamaterial absorber with fish-scale structure at visible frequencies. *Optical Materials Express, 6*(7), 2448–2457. doi:10.1364/OME.6.002448

Zhang, Y., Li, R., Jiang, Y., Zhao, B., Duan, H., Li, J., & Feng, Z. (2011). Morphology evolution of ZrB2 nanoparticles synthesized by sol–gel method. *Journal of Solid State Chemistry, 184*(8), 2047–2052. doi:10.1016/j.jssc.2011.05.040

Zhang, Y., Schlachetzki, F., Li, J. Y., Boado, R. J., & Pardridge, W. M. (2003). Organ specific gene expression in the rhesus monkey eye following intravenous nonviral gene transfer. *Molecular Vision, 9*, 465–472. PMID:14551536

Zhang, Y., Tang, Z. R., Fu, X., & Xu, Y. J. (2010). TiO_2 Graphene Nanocomposites for Gas-Phase Photocatalytic Degradation of Volatile Aromatic Pollutant: Is TiO_2 Graphene Truly Different from Other TiO2 Carbon Composite Materials? *ACS Nanotechnology, 4*(12), 7303–7314. doi:10.1021/nn1024219 PMID:21117654

Zhang, Y., Tapas, R. N., Hao, H., & Weibo, C. (2013). Biomedical Applications of Zinc Oxide Nanomaterials. *Current Molecular Medicine, 13*(10), 1633–1645.

Zhang, Y., Wei, J., Yuan, Y., & Yue, T. (2019). Diversity and characterization of spoilage-associated psychrotrophs in food in cold chain. *International Journal of Food Microbiology, 290*, 86–95. doi:10.1016/j.ijfoodmicro.2018.09.026 PMID:30317110

Zhang, Z., Ding, H., Yan, X., Liang, L., Wei, D., Wang, M., Yang, Q., & Yao, J. (2018). Sensitive detection of cancer cell apoptosis based on the non-bianisotropic metamaterials biosensors in terahertz frequency. *Optical Materials Express, 8*(3), 6951–6957. doi:10.1364/OME.8.000659

Zhang, Z., Huang, J., Dong, B., Yuan, Q., He, Y., & Wolfbeis, O. S. (2015). Rational tailoring of $ZnSnO_3$ /TiO_2 heterojunctions with bioinspired surface wettability for high-performance humidity nanosensors. *Nanoscale, 7*(9), 4149–4155. doi:10.1039/C4NR07559E PMID:25665734

Zhao, W., Wu, W., & Xu, X. (2007). Oral vaccination with liposome- encapsulated recombinant fusion peptide of urease B epitope and cholera toxin B subunit affords prophylactic and therapeutic effects against H.pylori infection in BALB/cm ice. *Vaccine, 25*(44), 7664–7673. doi:10.1016/j.vaccine.2007.08.034 PMID:17913305

Zhao, Y., Chu, J., Li, S. H., Chen, Y., Sheng, G. P., Chen, Y. P., Li, W. W., Liu, G., Tian, Y. C., Xiong, Y., & Yu, H. Q. (2011). Preparation of Pt-Fe2O3 nano-electrode array on gold nano-wires and its application to the catalytic degradation of methyl orange. *Chemical Engineering Journal, 170*(2–3), 440–444. doi:10.1016/j.cej.2010.11.104

Zhao, Y., Sultan, D., Detering, L., Cho, S., Sun, G., Pierce, R., Wooley, K. L., & Liu, Y. (2014). Copper-64-alloyed gold nanoparticles for cancer imaging: Improved radiolabel stability and diagnostic accuracy. *Angewandte Chemie, 126*(1), 160–163. doi:10.1002/ange.201308494 PMID:24272951

Zheludev, N. I. (2011). A roadmap for metamaterials. *Optics and Photonics News, 22*(3), 30–35. doi:10.1364/OPN.22.3.000030

Zheludev, N. I., & Kivshar, Y. S. (2012). From metamaterials to metadevices. *Nature Materials, 11*(11), 917–924. doi:10.1038/nmat3431 PMID:23089997

Zheng, J. P., Cygan, P. J., & Jow, T. R. (1995). Hydrous Ruthenium Oxide as an Electrode Material for Electrochemical Capacitors. *Journal of the Electrochemical Society, 142*(8), 2699–2703. doi:10.1149/1.2050077

Zheng, J., Li, S., Xu, Y., & Zheng, X. (2019). Effect of oxalic acid on edible quality of bamboo shoots (Phyllostachys prominens) without sheaths during cold storage. *Lebensmittel-Wissenschaft + Technologie, 109*, 194–200. doi:10.1016/j.lwt.2019.04.014

Zheng, L., Zhang, W., & Liang, F. (2017). Experiment Study on Thermal Conductivity of Microcapsule Phase Change Suspension Applied to Solar Powered Air Conditioning Cold Storage System. *Procedia Engineering, 205*, 1237–1244. doi:10.1016/j.proeng.2017.10.364

Zhou, C. (2013). Theoretical analysis of double-microfluidic-channels photonic crystal fiber sensor based on silver nanowires. *Optics Communications, 288*, 42–46.

Zhou, H., Li, D., Hibino, M., & Honma, I. (2005). A self-ordered, crystalline-glass, mesoporous nanocomposite for use as a lithium-based storage device with both high power and high energy densities. *Angewandte Chemie International Edition, 44*(5), 797–802. doi:10.1002/anie.200460937 PMID:15612076

Zhou, W. J., He, B. L., & Li, H. L. (2008). Synthesis, structure and electrochemistry of Ag-modified $LiMn_2O_4$ cathode materials for lithium-ion batteries. *Materials Research Bulletin, 43*(8), 2285–2294. doi:10.1016/j.materresbull.2007.08.013

Zhou, X., Zhou, D.-Y., Liu, Z.-Y., Yin, F.-W., Liu, Z.-Q., Li, D.-Y., & Shahidi, F. (2019). Hydrolysis and oxidation of lipids in mussel Mytilus edulis during cold storage. *Food Chemistry*, *272*, 109–116. doi:10.1016/j.foodchem.2018.08.019 PMID:30309519

Zhou, Y. K., Shen, C. M., Huang, J., & Li, H. L. (2002). Synthesis of high-ordered $LiMn_2O_4$ nanowire arrays by AAO template and its structural properties. *Materials Science and Engineering B*, *95*(1), 77–82. doi:10.1016/S0921-5107(02)00197-6

Zhu, G., Yang, R., Wang, S., & Wang, Z. L. (2010). Flexible High-Output Nanogenerator Based on Lateral ZnO Nanowire Array. *Nano Letters*, *10*(8), 3151–3155. doi:10.1021/nl101973h PMID:20698630

Zhu, H. T., Lin, Y. S., & Yin, Y. S. (2004). A novel one-step chemical method for preparation of copper nanofluids. *Journal of Colloid and Interface Science*, *277*(1), 100–103. doi:10.1016/j.jcis.2004.04.026 PMID:15276044

Zhu, H., Guo, Z., & Liu, W. (2016). Biomimetic water-collecting materials inspired by nature. *Chemical Communications (Cambridge)*, *52*(20), 3863–3879. doi:10.1039/C5CC09867J

Zhu, J., Yan, F., Guo, Z., & Marchant, R. E. (2005). Surface modification of liposomes by saccharides: Vesicles and stability of lactosyl liposomes studied by photon correlation spectroscopy. *Journal of Colloid and Interface Science*, *289*(2), 542–550. doi:10.1016/j.jcis.2005.03.088 PMID:15922349

Zhukovskii, Y. F., Balaya, P., Kotomin, E. A., & Maier, J. (2006). Evidence for Interfacial-Storage Anomaly in Nanocomposites for Lithium Batteries from First-Principles Simulations. *Physical Review Letters*, *96*(5), 058302. doi:10.1103/PhysRevLett.96.058302 PMID:16487002

Zhu, N., Luan, H., Yuan, S., Chen, J., Wu, X., & Wang, L. (2010). Effective dechlorination of HCB by nanoscale Cu/Fe particles. *Journal of Hazardous Materials*, *176*(1-3), 1101–1105. doi:10.1016/j.jhazmat.2009.11.092 PMID:19969417

Zhu, X., Wu, D., Wang, W., Tan, F., Wong, P. K., Wang, X., & Qiao, X. (2016). Highly effective antibacterial activity and synergistic effect of Ag-MgO nanocomposite against Escherichia coli. *Journal of Alloys and Compounds*, *684*, 282–290. doi:10.1016/j.jallcom.2016.05.179

Zilli, D., Bonelli, P. R., & Cukierman, A. L. (2006). Effect of alignment on adsorption of multi-walled carbon nanotube arrays. *Nanotechnology*, *17*, 5126. doi:10.1088/0957-4484/17/20/016

Zong, L., Li, M., & Li, C. (2017). Bioinspired Coupling of Inorganic Layered Nanomaterials with Marine Polysaccharides for Efficient Aqueous Exfoliation and Smart Actuating Hybrids. *Advanced Materials*, *29*(10), 1604691. doi:10.1002/adma.201604691

Zook, J., Halter, M., Cleveland, D., & Long, S. (2012). Disentangling the effects of polymer coatings on silver nanoparticle agglomeration, dissolution, and toxicity to determine mechanisms of nanotoxicity. *Journal of Nanoparticle Research*, *14*(10), 1–9.

Zuhong, L., Yangjun, C., Ya, Y., Yan, Y., & Yanhong, Z. (2019). Recent Advances in Nanomaterials-Based Chemo-Photothermal Combination Therapy for Improving Cancer Treatment. Review article. *Frontiers in Bioengineering and Biotechnology*.

Zulfiqar, F., Navarro, M., Ashraf, M., Akram, N. A., & Munné-Bosch, S. (2019). Nanofertilizer use for sustainable agriculture: Advantages and limitations. *Plant Science*, *289*, 110270. doi:10.1016/j.plantsci.2019.110270 PMID:31623775

About the Contributors

Mohd Amin Bhat is a Teaching and Research Assistant at Sathyabama University, India.

* * *

Jahangir Ahmad is currently working in the Department of Chemistry, Govt. Degree College, Udhampur, Jammu. Dr. Jahangi did his masters in Chemistry from University of Kashmirand doctorate from National Institute of Technology Srinagar.

Shabir Ahmad Akhoon did his MSc in Physics from the Department of Physics., University of Kashmir. He did his PhD from National Institute of Technology, Srinagar. Currently, he is working as an assistant professor in the Department of Applied Sciences, University of kashmir. His core research interests are Nanotechnology and Energy.

Basharat Ahmad Bhat is working as Research Scholar in the Department of Bioresources, University of Kasmir. He has obtained his Bachelors in Science(B.Sc) from S.P College Srinagar Kashmir in 2010 and M.Sc Bio-Resources from Kashmir University in the year of 2012-2014. He obtained his M.Phil in Plant Molecular Biology from BGSB University in 2016-2018, Rajouri, India. Currently he is pursuing his Ph.D in Bio-Resources from Department of Bio-Resources in collaboration with BGSB University, Department of Biotechnology. He is working on DNA Fingerprinting of Medicinal Plants, DNA Barcoding, Plant Metagenomics, Plant Transcriptomics, Free Radical Biochemistry and Green synthesis of Nanoparticles.

Brij Bhushan is a researcher involved in recovery of resources by integration of membrane technology from wastewater, activated carbon development and its use in wastewater treatment. Actively involved in research since the last 8 years. PhD from IIT Roorkee and postdoc from UPC, Barcelona, Spain. Currently working as Associate Professor at Graphic Era University, Dehradun.

Arghya Chakravorty is a Ph.D. scholar at Centre for Nanotechnology Research, VIT - Vellore. He is a 25 years old young, passionate & enthusiastic researcher holding three Indian patents; contributed in a total of nine book chapters of different renowned international publishers like Elsevier, Springer, CRC Press, and IGI Global - USA. Recently he has worked with pioneer nanotechnologist Prof. Seeram Ramakrishna & the manuscript has been accepted by a renowned journal of Elsevier. On his Ph.D. project, he is concentrating on "Theranostics and bio-sensing application of MXene". As a research scholar, he has been very accommodating, efficient, and self-driven. His ability to grasp quickly has made him a valuable member of our team within a short span. He was never reluctant to experiment on what he understood and kept working patiently on it after giving careful thought. Despite his own work being pretty exhaustive, he would always be very polite in helping other team members with their work. This has resulted in him developing a fine rapport with all his team members and colleagues alike. He possesses an immensely strong analytical sense and research-oriented bent of mind. Even, as PI he has completed two interdisciplinary minor non-profit projects in collaboration with North University of China & HUST Wuhan and successfully presented at RECYCLE 2020, hosted by IIT- Guwahati. Furthermore, his ability to express and share views with other scientists and peers indicates that he has good communication and interpersonal skills.

Yi Lin Chan was born in Perak, Malaysia, in 1992. He received his Bachelor of Science (Applied Physics) with Honour in 2016 and Master of Science in 2019 from Universiti Tun Hussein Onn Malaysia (UTHM), Batu Pahat, Johor, Malaysia. He is currently pursuing his Doctor of Philosophy in Science at Faculty of Applied Sciences and Technology, UTHM. His research interests include material science, composite material and microwave characterization.

Moharana Choudhury is an activate environmentalist and researcher has written/edited 2 Nos of Books and more than 25 Nos of research articles in national, international journals, proceedings as international repute. He has written many articles and scientific reports in popular magazines. He is the fellow, founder and life member of several academic societies among them "Voice of Environment" (A Youth Environmental Organization) is well known for its promising Environmental initiatives and works so far.

Mintu Maan Dutta obtained his Ph.D. degree in 2020 from Department of Chemistry, Gauhati University, Assam. He has carried out his research work under the supervision of Professor Prodeep Phukan. His PhD. thesis entitled "Surface functionalized magnetic nanoparticles as catalyst for organic transformations". He has co-authored number of publications in reputed journals that includes Dalton Transactions, Catalysis Communications, ChemistrySelect etc. He has also co-authored couple of book chapters in IGI global, Lambert Academic publishing respectively. He obtained his M.Sc degree from Gauhati University, Assam with specialization in Physical Chemistry in 2014 and B.Sc. degree from Cotton College in 2012. His current research interest includes heterogeneous catalysis, organic synthesis.

Manish K Dwivedi, Ph.D. scholar in the Department of Biotechnology, Indira Gandhi National Tribal University, Amarkantak, Madhya Pradesh, has completed his M.Phil. and M.Sc. in Biochemistry from Awadesh Pratap Singh University, Rewa, MP. He has been awarded gold medals during M.Sc. and M. Phil. His areas of interest are infectious disease biology and drug development. He has published several national and international papers.

Fahmiruddin Esa was born in 1984. He graduated from Universiti Putra Malaysia (UPM) with a Bachelor's degree in Physics in 2006. Two years later, he furthered his studies at Universiti Teknologi Malaysia (UTM) and obtained Master of Science (Physics) by coursework in 2010. He began his Ph.D. study a year later in Microwave at the Faculty of Science, UPM, and completed it in 2015. He is currently a lecturer at Department of Physics and Chemistry, Faculty of Applied Sciences and Technology,

Universiti Tun Hussein Onn Malaysia (UTHM), Pagoh campus, Malaysia. His research interest is in experimental and simulation for the characterisation techniques of microwave-absorbing material.

Manzoor Ahmad Mir holds Master's Degree in Zoology from HNBG Central University after qualifying prestigious National level CSIR-JRF-NET examination and worked jointly for his Ph. D at Jawaharlal Nehru University New Delhi and CSIR-Institute of Microbial Technology Chandigarh in the field of Immunology and Cell Biology. He currently teaches Endocrinology, Animal Physiology, Immunology and Developmental Biology at the Department of Bioresources, University of Kashmir, and has been a Research Scientist at SATCAS Stroke Research Chair Majmaah University KSA. Dr Manzoor has research and has attended many courses and conferences on immunology, cancer Biology, stroke biology and endocrinology at USA, UK, Kuwait, China, UAE and Saudi Arabia. His basic research interests include molecular immunology, Tuberculosis immunology, Cancer and Stroke Biology. He has published more than 50 high-impact research papers and book chapters, in recognition of which he has received several awards and Royalties from international publishing houses. Dr. Manzoor has authored several books with international publishers like Elsevier USA and Nova Science Publisher USA. He is currently receiving Royalty from Academic Press USA for his book in the field of Immunology entitled "Developing costimulatory molecules for immunotherapy of diseases". Dr. Manzoor is on the editorial board of some prestigious journals from DOVE medical press New Zealand and Springer Plus UK and has been an invited speaker at various scientific meetings/conferences within India and abroad. He is member of many scientific organizations and societies like International Immunology Association, Indian Association of Immunology, Indian National Science Association, IMMUNOCON etc. Dr Manzoor was awarded Teachers Associate Research Exellence Fellowship (TARE) by DST Govt of India. He has been awarded Summer Research Fellowship Programme (SRFP-2019) by Indian Academy of Sciences and National Science Academy. Dr Manzoor has developed Massive Open Online Course (MOOCs) in Immunology for UG students by sanctioned by UGC- Consortium for Educational Communication (CEC) SWAYAM Ministry of HRD Govt of India. He has been awarded another MOOC Course on Endocrinology by Academic advisory committee of CEC-UGC.

Rizwana Mobin is working as Assistant Professor in the Department of Industrial Chemistry, Govt. College for Women, Cluster University, Srinagar, India. She received her B.Sc. Hons., Masters and Ph.D (Applied Chemistry) from Aligarh Muslim University, Aligarh, India on the topic "Studies on Thin-Layer Chromatographic Analysis of Surfactants". She has been the recipient of the Gold medal at Masters level. She has published several research articles in international journals of repute and six book chapters in knowledge-based book editions published by renowned international publishers. She has edited books with Materials Research Forum U.S.A. Her research expertise includes thin-layer chromatography, development of new methodologies involving green solvent system for the analysis of surfactants and food dyes.

Kapilan N. is working as Professor and Head of Mechanical Engineering Department, Nagarjuna College of Engineering and Technology. Having more than 22 years of teaching and research experience. Published more than 52 papers in journals and 18 papers in conference. Authored one text book and four book chapters. Received research funding work US$ 75,000 from various funding agencies. Filed a patent and received best paper presentation awards in conferences.

Anima Nanda holding the post of Director – IQAC at Sathyabama Institute of Science and Technology (Deemed to be University), Chennai, India. She was also the Dean for the School of Bio & Chemical Engineering has credited with Ph. D. degrees in Microbiology from Berhampur University, Odisha. Dr. Nanda is a renowned professor heading four departments like, Department of Biomedical Engineering, Department of Biotechnology, Department of Bioinformatics and Department of Chemical Engineering with specialized in Microbial Nanotechnology. Her laboratory studies on the role of bacteria and fungi in human health by using nanotechnology to have a better control over broad spectrum antibiotics. Her publications proved the novel bio-nanomaterials synthesized in her lab by using various fungi and bacteria isolated from various sources have a targeted therapy against human pathogenic and broad spectrum antibiotic resistant bacteria in Septicemia (MRSA and MRSE), Multi Drug Resistant Tuberculosis (MDR Tb) and Extra Drug Resistant Tuberculosis (XDR Tb). In addition to this Dr. Nanda has been heavily involved in promoting microbial nanotechnology as the cornerstone in the field of biology in India. Currently she has two ongoing Govt. of India sponsored projects worth of 1.85 crore and two are in process. She has research tie up with reputed institutions in National and international level. She has worked with several eminent personalities of the world at various places. Apart from this she has more than 168 publications in high impacted national and international journals. To her credit she has produced 11 Ph. D. students and 7 are continuing. She has delivered more than 73 lecturers as an invited speaker in national and international level. To her credit, Dr. Nanda has one patents on staircase climbing wheel chair for physically challenged person. She has honored with Fellow of Natural Resources and Conservation and Fellow of Indian Aerobiological Society and also received twice best teacher award, gold medalist, and best project award, chaired number of technical sessions and life member of varied societies including American Nano Society and Indian Nanomedicine and a reviewer of nature scientific journal.

Joan Nyika is an Environmental Science PhD student at the University of South Africa and a Tutorial Fellow at the Technical University of Kenya, Geoscience and the Environment Department. She obtained a Bsc. degree in Biochemistry and Molecular Biology from the Jomo Kenyatta University of Agriculture and Technology in 2011. She also obtained an Msc degree in Land and Water Management from the University of Nairobi and, Kenya in 2017. Her PhD work revolves around solid waste management and the effects of landfill leachate on soil and groundwater. She has also done research on the use of microbes for pollutant bioremediation and phytoremediation. She has interests in sustainable environmental management, water management, ecological and ecosystem management. Joan has published more than 15 articles and 6 book chapters in peer reviewed journals and books, respectively. She has and is mentoring both undergraduate and diploma students and has more than 5 years experience teaching and training in environmental science.

Vidhya P. is working as Assistant Professor in SRSMN Government First Grade College and having more than 15 years of teaching and research experience. Published research papers in Journals and conferences. Authored a textbook.

Tauseef Ahmad Rangreez has worked as PI/postdoctoral fellow at National Institute of Technology, Srinagar, India. He completed his Ph.D in Applied Chemistry, from Aligarh Muslim University, Aligarh, India on the topic "Development of Nanostructure Organic-Inorganic Composite Materials based Sensors for Inorganic Pollutants". He worked as Project Fellow under the UGC Funded Research Project entitled "Synthesis, characterization and application of biocompatible surfactant based hydrogels". He completed his Masters in Chemistry from Jamia Hamdard, New Delhi. He has published his work in number of peer reviewed journals, wrote book chapters and edited books with Springer and Materials Research Forum, U.S.A. His research interests includes ion exchange materials, development of nano-composite sensors for heavy metals and biosensors.

Gulzar Ahmed Rather works in the department of biomedical engineering Sathyabama University Rajiv Gandhi Salai, Chennai, Tamil Nadu, 600119 India as a full-time Ph.D. Scholar. He has registered the department in the year 2017. He is working on nanobiotechnology under the guidance of Prof. Anima Nanda, Dean, and Prof. in the Department of Biomedical Engineering. He has completed his M.Sc in Biochemistry in 2014, from the Department of Biochemistry, Kashmir University. He has done the projecton the level of evaluation of knowledge, attitude, and behavior of people about Alternative Medicine. He has got more than two-years of teaching experience as a biology lecturer, from 2014-2016. He has attended the 8th JK Science Congress at the University of Kashmir. International seminar on Accu-Pressure at the University of Kashmir. Expert Lecture on Stem Cell Therapy for Brain Tumors by Dr.KhalidShah, Faculty at Harvard MedicalSchool, Boston. Attend FivedaysFirstNationalworkshopontechniques in biotechnology (NWTBT-17) Which was organized by the Department of Biotechnology, School of Bio and chemical engineering Sathyabama University (18th to 22nd, 2017). Attended three days National workshop on Animal cell line techniques (NACL-2017) 22nd to 24th August 2017. He has received the best paper award in a'International conference on Bioengineering on health and environment-2018. He has attended and published papers in the 6thInternational Conference on Nanotechnology for the better living 7-11April 2019 jointly organized by the National Institute of Technology (NIT) Srinagar and the Indian Institute of Technology (IIT) Kharagpur. Besides doing a Ph.D. he is also teaching students' biochemistry at B.Tech. level in the Department of Biomedical Engineering, from time to time he also attended ISRO exam duties as an invigilator.

Vipin Saini is an Assistant Professor in the School of Environment and Natural Resources, at Doon University, Dehradun. He has obtained his Ph.D. degree in Chemistry (Environmental Chemistry) from IIT Roorkee, 2007, and from 2007-2013 he has worked in different postdoctoral fellowships in Europe. He works on multidisciplinary Material & Environmental Chemistry. So far he has worked with several distinguished research groups from reputed universities of Germany, Belgium, Portugal, and Spain. His expertise involved the development of nano-scale properties in bulk material using innovative techniques, like Nanocasting, Self-assembly, Sol-gel, Hydrothermal, and Impregnation and so on. His key areas of research are Natural materials based Nanoporous materials, Innovative nanoporous adsorbent materials for selective adsorption of gaseous and aqueous pollutants, Valorisation of wastes and by-products, Light-harvesting for environmental applications.

Siva Sankar Sana is working as a postdoctoral fellow. He is working on polymer nanocomposites and green synthesis of metal nanoparticles and their biological applications.

Man Seng Sim was born in Johor, Malaysia, in 1993. In 2017, he received the Bachelor of Science in Applied Physics from Universiti Tun Hussein Onn Malaysia (UTHM). In 2019, he received the Master of Philosophy in Electrical Engineering from Universiti Teknologi Malaysia (UTM). He is currently a Ph.D. candidate at School of Electrical Engineering in UTM. His research interests are in electromagnetic metamaterials, microwave sensors, and material characterization techniques.

Ashaq Hussain Sofi did his MSc in Physics from the Department of Physics., University of Kashmir. He did his PhD from National Institute of Technology, Srinagar. Currently, he is working a Lecturer in the Department of Physics, GDC-Ganderbal, University of kashmir. His core research interests are Nanotechnology and Energy.

R. Vimala is currently an Associate Professor at Vellore Institute of Technology, Vellore, Tamil Nadu, India. She completed her Ph. D in Environmental biotechnology in 2010 from VIT, Vellore. Her research focus is on the synthesis and characterization of nanoparticles for various applications viz.drug delivery, environmental remediation, agriculture etc. She has published more than 40 research papers in peer-reviewed national and international journals. She has guided 3 Ph. D scholars and more than 30 master student projects. She has more than 13 years of teaching experience and was associated with UG and PG students.

Kok Yeow You was born in 1977. He obtained his B.Sc. Physics (Honours) degree in Universiti Kebangsaan Malaysia (UKM), in 2001. He pursued his M.Sc. in Microwave at the Faculty of Science in 2003, and his Ph.D. in Wave Propagation at the Institute for Mathematical Research in 2006 in Universiti Putra Malaysia (UPM), Serdang, Selangor, Malaysia. He has recently worked as a senior lecturer at the School of Electrical Engineering, Faculty of Engineering, Universiti Teknologi Malaysia (UTM), Skudai, Johor, Malaysia. His main personal research interest is in the theory, simulation, and instrumentation of electromagnetic wave propagation at microwave frequencies focusing on the development of microwave passive devices and sensors for medical and agricultural application.

Index

A

B

C

D

E

F

G

O

P

Q

R

S

T

W

Z

www.ingramcontent.com/pod-product-compliance
Lightning Source LLC
LaVergne TN
LVHW060356300926
849162LV00006B/1276